Caring
and Curing

Coordinating Editors

Martin E. Marty   James P. Wind

An ornamental rose opens each chapter of the book, celebrating the rose's long medicinal history.

*The ancients used roses in salves, decoctions, bathwater, puddings, and preserves; Romans wore rose wreaths to counteract the intoxicating effects of wine; Greek philosopher Theophrastus (ca. 372–287 BC) and Greek physician Dioscorides (1st cent. AD) assigned rose hips particular medicinal value; and Roman naturalist Pliny the Elder (ca. 23–79 AD), in his monumental **Historia Naturalis,** lists 32 remedies made from rose petals and leaves.*

Rose hips have long been in official pharmacological use for their refrigerant and astringent properties and are still used today in certain medications.

Caring
and Curing

Health and Medicine
in the Western
Religious Traditions

EDITED BY

Ronald L. Numbers
Darrel W. Amundsen

MACMILLAN PUBLISHING COMPANY
A Division of Macmillan, Inc.
NEW YORK

Collier Macmillan Publishers
LONDON

Macmillan Publishing Company
A Division of Macmillan, Inc.
866 Third Avenue, New York, N. Y. 10022

Collier Macmillan Canada, Inc.

Library of Congress Catalog Card Number: 86-3030

Printed in the United States of America

printing number
    4   5   6   7   8   9   10

Library of Congress Cataloging in Publication Data

Caring and curing.

    Bibliography: p.
    1. Health—Religious aspects.   2. Medicine—
Religious aspects.   1. Numbers, Ronald L.   II. Amundsen,
Darrel W. [DNLM: 1. Religion and medicine.
BL 65.M4 C277]
BL65.M4C37 1986   261.5'6   86-3030
ISBN 0-919270-6

Contents

29.39

v

89793

Foreword

To describe this as a collection of historical essays is to risk losing all readers except historians. To lose them would be unfortunate, for the essays are designed to be of use and of help to professionals in medicine and religion as well as to people who are or would like to be involved with the "caring and curing" of themselves and others.

Historians by profession look backward, and essays by and for them will necessarily dwell on the past. Yet they do not live in the past. They share the present with people who want to know about what it means to care and to cure now, today, and what it might take to be well tomorrow. The authors of these chapters were assigned the task of being faithful to what has gone before and to be mindful of the need to make available data and concepts from the past that would be helpful for the future.

If on first appearance it would seem that historians alone care about health traditions, a second glance shows that not to be the case. Each individual has a "medical history." For some it is informal, unwritten. The body carries this history in the form of wounds, scars, limps, postures, tumors, and atrophied muscles—just as it may bear the marks of well-being in the form of strong muscles, healthy lungs, and bright countenance. Those who wish to minister to individuals must learn to read these evidences of what has occurred to them. Many individuals also have formal, written medical histories, filed in the offices of physicians or recorded on applications for insurance policies. The data of these records help their readers understand the person's past for the sake of present and future.

As with individuals, so with social groups. They, too, have medical histories. In order to interpret the life of a culture, it is extremely important to know whether it has hospitals, honors medical science, cherishes folk wisdom, is marked by belief in the supernatural. Whoever needs convincing that history, the past, has a shaping role in group well-being need only observe what happens when a modern techno-logical health facility is "dropped down" on an unprepared and suspicious culture by professionals who are not mindful of the attitudes of the people who make up that culture. Similarly, to see what happens when people are deprived, by economic circumstance or "Acts of God," of the kind of medical care they have known and come to expect is to relearn the power of history and tradition.

Traditions of medical history often follow secular patterns. They run across divisions between developed and developing or rich and poor nations, between social classes, between nations with their separate heritages, and the like. Yet the more a secular or pluralist society has come to think of itself as distanced from its religious roots, the more it has become evident that these roots are long, deep, entangling, possibly nurturing, and possibly strangling. While each health-seeking individual is likely to improvise in order to meet current needs, he or she will tend to draw on a repertory of options made available in a spiritual heritage.

For that reason, this book and those like it are becoming practical necessities. In a diverse society it is impossible for healing professionals to have all of the options in the front of their minds. They need reference books. How does one deal medically with a member of the Jehovah's Witnesses, a Hispanic or Southeast Asian refugee, or an Orthodox Jew when it comes to medical matters? Do Mormons and Seventh-day Adventists have peculiar views of the body and health? What do Christian Scientists believe? What is a permissible range of options for a Catholic when it comes to decisions about "euthanasia"? Do evangelical and fundamentalist Protestants make special demands and have special resources? What has exposure to the secular order done to the "mainline" groups?

If this book is what one of our advisers called a "data bank" of the sort physicians have been seeking, it is also designed for lay people— lay in medicine as well as religion—to understand not only their own traditions but also those of others. This is a time in which people not only seek their own roots and set out to firm up their own identities. They find good reason to try to understand those of others, both in order to live with them and to draw upon what might be borrowed from them. That is why an interreligious collection such as this has special value in a dynamic culture.

The modern biomedical enterprise—with its threefold work of knowledge acquisition, technology development, and care delivery—urgently needs the guiding visions and values embodied in the faith traditions. When technological momentum or economic necessity alone guides the health care enterprise, the sustaining impulses of respect, meaning, and purpose often fall aside. These essays present in historical perspective the substance of this perennial wisdom.

This volume deals with religions that are often broadly described as "Western" because, whatever their origins may be, they are now associated with the world called the West; its forthcoming companion treats a variety of "World Religions" which, while they may be at home in the West, have their chief influence elsewhere. The books are issued from The Park Ridge Center, an Institute for the Study of Health, Faith, and Ethics. A denominational adjective characterizes the host institution, the Lutheran General Health Care System, but it is clear from the structure and content of the book that the initiators at all points have an ecumenical, indeed interfaith, outlook and intention.

To that end, The Park Ridge Center entrusted the first volume to two accomplished historians, inviting them to select the most highly regarded professionals in various traditions. All contributors are critical scholars, not apologists or public relations experts. No one can be representative of all aspects of these traditions, internally divided as most of them are. All of them can be representative of the scholarly conscience and the impulse to be fair. They can then contribute to the acts of "caring and curing" by faithful fulfillment of their assignments. While the coeditors will do their own acknowledging, we will join the company of readers in thanking Professors Numbers and Amundsen for their vision and scrupulous attention to detail in producing this work.

Martin E. Marty, President
The Park Ridge Center
Park Ridge, Illinois

Acknowledgments

The production of this volume has involved a cast of dozens, whose contributions made this book possible and to whom we owe an immense debt. This historical investigation originated as an undertaking of Project Ten, created in 1980 by Lutheran General Hospital in Park Ridge, Illinois, in an attempt to examine the ethics and theology of medicine. When The Park Ridge Center superseded Project Ten in 1985, it inherited this volume-in-the-making and fostered its completion.

Above all, this volume is the result of both the initial vision and continuing sustenance of George B. Caldwell, President of Lutheran General Health Care System, who provided the institutional base that allowed our effort to reach fruition. Crucial financial aid came from Naurice Nesset, Ph.D., founder of Lutheran General Hospital as well as the first chairman of its board of directors and its first president and chief executive officer, whose generous contribution underwrote much of the scholarly research that went into producing this work; and Martin Staunt, a Chicago-area designer and manufacturer of dental equipment and long-time benefactor of Lutheran General Hospital, whose assistance allowed the completion of this project. Lawrence E. Holst, chairman of the Division of Pastoral Care at Lutheran General Hospital and chairman of Project Ten's management team, linked Mr. Staunt's interest to Project Ten's needs and cogently argued for the clinical relevance of this undertaking.

Other Project Ten and Park Ridge Center staff members played equally important roles. The editors of the series in which this volume appears, historians Martin E. Marty and James P. Wind, offered advice and encouragement at every stage of the project and oversaw the evolution of the book from outline to bound volume. Mary-Carroll Sullivan critically and perceptively evaluated each chapter proposal. Bioethicist Kenneth L. Vaux served as theological consultant to the project. Last, but certainly not least, David T. Stein, Project Ten administrator, provided the kind of behind-the-scenes support, from negotiating contracts to distributing manuscripts, that most editors only dream of.

In November, 1983, Dr. Stein orchestrated a three-day conference in Chicago that brought together the various contributors to this volume. Particularly valuable were the criticisms and suggestions offered by six invited historical consultants: Catherine Albanese, Theodore Dwight Bozeman, Lawrence T. Geraty, Nathan O. Hatch, Thomas A. Kselman, Mark A. Noll, and Jan Shipps. Later, after the contributors had completed their essays, we drew on the good will and expert advice of forty scholars (two per chapter), whose identities must unfortunately remain anonymous. Their expertise saved us from many a slip and contributed greatly to the overall quality of this book.

During the process of preparation and production, we were fortunate to have the assistance of a number of highly skilled and agreeable secretaries: Jane Frey, Lois Frey, and Lorraine Bunch at Park Ridge; Carolyn Hackler at the University of Wisconsin–Madison; and Kathy Robinson and Kim Koenig in Bellingham, Washington. Kathleen A. Cahalan at The Park Ridge Center adroitly followed the manuscript through the final stages of publication. At Macmillan Publishing Co., we had the pleasure of working with Charles E. Smith, vice president and publisher, and Elyse Dubin, editorial supervisor.

Finally, each of us has some personal debts to acknowledge. During the period from 1983–1985, the Menninger Foundation in Topeka, Kansas, provided Ronald L. Numbers with office space and a supportive environment in which to work away from home. He is particularly grateful to Paul W. Pruyser, then director of the Foundation's Department of Education, who arranged for his appointment as a Postdoctoral Fellow in Interdisciplinary Studies. He also wishes to thank his wife, Janet, for her support and understanding and Judith Walzer Leavitt, chair of the Department of the History of Medicine, University of Wisconsin–Madison, for arranging time for him to work on this volume. Darrel W. Amundsen is grateful to his wife, Jean, for her patience with him in his taking on responsibilities connected with this volume when time was precious owing to considerable overcommitment. He is also indebted to the Bureau for Faculty Research, Western Washington University, for the assistance that they have rendered in various ways.

Contributors

DARREL W. AMUNDSEN (Ph.D., University of British Columbia, 1980) is Professor of Classics at Western Washington University, where he has taught since 1969. He is the author of numerous essays on the history of ancient and medieval medicine, particularly medical ethics. A frequent participant at conferences on medicine and values, he currently serves on the editorial boards of the *Journal of Medicine and Philosophy* and the *Bulletin of the History of Medicine*.

JOHN E. BOOTY (Ph.D., Princeton University, 1960) teaches Anglican Studies at the University of the South, where, from 1982 to 1985, he served as dean of the School of Theology. An ordained Episcopal priest, he has written extensively on English church history, including books on *John Jewel as Apologist of the Church of England* (1963), *The Church in History* (1979), and *The Godly Kingdom of Tudor England* (1981). He is a former fellow of the National Endowment for the Humanities and, in 1985–1986, was a visiting professor and research fellow at the Divinity School of Yale University.

LESTER E. BUSH, JR. (M.D., University of Virginia, 1968) is a consultant in preventive medicine with the United States government and lives in Gaithersburg, Maryland. In addition to his strictly medical activities, he has written a number of articles on Mormon history that have appeared in the *Bulletin of the History of Medicine*, the *Journal of Mormon History*, and *Dialogue: A Journal of Mormon Thought*, of which he was associate editor from 1976 to 1982. He is the coeditor of *Neither White nor Black: Mormon Scholars Confront the Race Issue in a Universal Church* (1984) and the author of a forthcoming book on *Health and Medicine in the Mormon Tradition*. He has twice won the Best Article prize awarded annually by the Mormon History Association.

WILLIAM H. CUMBERLAND (Ph.D., University of Iowa, 1958) is Professor of History and Chairperson of the Division of Social Sciences, Philosophy and Religion at Buena Vista College in Storm Lake, Iowa, where he has taught since 1958. He is the author of a *History of Buena Vista College* (1966), a biography of *Wallace M. Short: Iowa Rebel* (1983), and various articles on socialism and radicalism in Iowa. His interest in the history of Jehovah's Witnesses dates from the writing of "A History of the Jehovah's Witnesses" for his doctoral dissertation.

ELLIOT N. DORFF (Ph.D., Columbia University, 1971) is Provost and Professor of Philosophy at the University of Judaism in Los Angeles. He also serves as a lecturer at the UCLA School of Law and as chairman of the Los Angeles Jewish Hospice Commission. A Conservative rabbi, he is the author of *Jewish Law and Modern Ideology* (1970), *Conservative Judaism: Our Ancestors to Our Descendants* (1977), and, with Arthur Rosett, *A Living Tree: Materials on the Jewish Legal Tradition with Comparative Notes* (forthcoming).

GARY B. FERNGREN (Ph.D., University of British Columbia, 1973) is Professor of History at Oregon State University, where he has taught since 1970. He has published extensively on the social history of medicine and the history of medical ethics, including chapters (co-authored with Darrel W. Amundsen) in *Health/Medicine and the Faith Traditions,* ed. Martin Marty and Kenneth L. Vaux (1982). A practicing evangelical, he has had a longstanding interest in the history of the evangelical-fundamentalist movement.

STANLEY SAMUEL HARAKAS (Th.D., Boston University, 1965) is Professor of Christian Ethics at Holy Cross Greek Orthodox School of Theology in Brookline, Massachusetts, where he has also served as dean. A priest of the Greek Orthodox Archdiocese of North and South America, under the Ecumenical Patriarchate of Constantinople, he is a past president of the Orthodox Theological Society in America. His several books include *Contemporary Moral Issues Facing the Orthodox Christian* (rev. ed., 1982), *Let Mercy Abound: Social Concern in the Greek Orthodox Church* (1983), and *Toward Transfigured Life: The* Theoria *of Eastern Orthodox Ethics* (1983).

DAVID EDWIN HARRELL, JR. (Ph.D., Vanderbilt University, 1962) is University Scholar and Chairman of the Department of History at the University of Alabama in Birmingham, having previously served as Distinguished Professor of History at the University of Arkansas and as Senior Fulbright Lecturer at the University of Allahabad in India. His many publications include a two-volume social history of the

Disciples of Christ (1966, 1973), *All Things Are Possible: The Healing and Charismatic Revivals in Modern America* (1975), and *Oral Roberts: An American Life* (1985). He co-edits the series "Minorities in Modern America" for Indiana University Press.

WALTER KLAASSEN (D. Phil., Oxford University, 1960) is Professor of History at Conrad Grebel College, University of Waterloo, Ontario, Canada. A specialist in the history of Anabaptism, he is the author of *Michael Gaismair: Revolutionary and Reformer* (1978), *Anabaptism: Neither Catholic nor Protestant* (rev. ed., 1982), and a forthcoming study of "Eschatology and Millennium in the Radical Reformation." He formerly edited the *Mennonite Quarterly Review* and currently edits *The Conrad Grebel Review: A Journal of Christian Inquiry.* From 1970 to 1983 he served as director of the Institute of Mennonite Studies in Elkhart, Indiana.

DAVID R. LARSON (D. Min., School of Theology at Claremont, 1973; Ph.D., Claremont Graduate School, 1982) is Associate Professor of Christian Ethics and Associate Director of the Center for Christian Bioethics at Loma Linda University, where he teaches ethics to medical, dental, nursing, and public-health students. An ordained Seventh-day Adventist minister, he has contributed numerous articles on medical and sexual ethics to Adventist journals.

SPENCER LAVAN (Ph.D., McGill University, 1970) is Associate Professor and Chairman, Department of Medical Humanities, University of New England College of Osteopathic Medicine. He is the author of *The Ahmadiyah Movement: A History and Perspective* (1974) and *Unitarians and India: A Study in Encounter and Response* (2nd ed., 1984) and co-author of *Alone/Together: Essays in the History of Liberal Religion* (1979). From 1978 to 1982 he was president of the Unitarian Universalist Historical Society; since 1984 he has edited the *Journal of Medical Humanities and Bioethics.*

CARTER LINDBERG (Ph.D., University of Iowa, 1965) is an associate professor in the School of Theology of Boston University. He is a past president of the Society for Sixteenth Century Studies (1978–1979) and a former research professor at the Centre d'Etudes Oecumeniques in Strasbourg, France (1979–1982). Among his numerous publications are *The Third Reformation? Charismatic Renewal and Lutheran Tradition* (1983), *Piety, Politics and Ethics: Studies in Honor of George W. Forell* (edited, 1983), and *Poverty and Church Care of the Poor from the First to the Sixteenth Centuries* (forthcoming).

RONALD L. NUMBERS (Ph.D., University of California, Berkeley, 1969) is Professor of the History of Medicine and the History of Science at the University of Wisconsin-Madison. His publications include *Ellen G. White: Prophetess of Health* (1976), *Almost Persuaded: American Physicians and Compulsory Health Insurance, 1912–1920* (1978), and *God and Nature: Historical Essays on the Encounter between Christianity and Science* (co-edited, 1986). The recipient of fellowships from the Josiah Macy, Jr. Foundation and the John Simon Guggenheim Foundation, he spent 1983–1985 as a Fellow in Interdisciplinary Studies at the Menninger Foundation in Topeka, Kansas.

MARVIN R. O'CONNELL (Ph.D., University of Notre Dame, 1959) is Professor of History at the University of Notre Dame, where, from 1974 to 1980, he served as chairman of the Department of History. He is the author of a number of books including *Thomas Stapleton and the Counter Reformation* (1964), *The Oxford Conspirators: A History of the Oxford Movement, 1833–1845* (1969), and *The Counter Reformation, 1559–1610* (1974), which appeared in the Rise of Modern Europe series edited by William L. Langer. During 1985–1986 he held a Senior Research Fellowship from the National Endowment for the Humanities.

ALBERT J. RABOTEAU (Ph.D., Yale University, 1974) teaches American religious history in the Department of Religion at Princeton University. His book *Slave Religion: The "Invisible Institution" in the Antebellum South* (1978) won the National Religious Book Award in 1979. He has served on the council of the American Society of Church History and on the editorial boards of *Church History, Journal of the American Academy of Religion,* and *Historical Magazine of the Protestant Episcopal Church.* He has received awards from the American Council of Learned Societies and the National Endowment for the Humanities.

RENNIE B. SCHOEPFLIN (Ph.D. candidate, University of Wisconsin-Madison) is Assistant Professor of History at Loma Linda University. A specialist in the history of science and medicine, he is co-author of "Ministries of Healing: Mary Baker Eddy, Ellen G. White, and the Religion of Health," in *Women and Health in America: Historical Essays,* ed. Judith Walzer Leavitt (1984) and author of "Christian Science" in *Unorthodox Medicine in American Society,* ed. Norman Gevitz (forthcoming). His dissertation title is "Christian Science Healing in American Society: Theory and Practice from 1865 to 1910."

JAMES H. SMYLIE (Ph.D., Princeton Theological Seminary, 1958) is Professor of American Church History at Union Theological Seminary in Virginia. His publications include *Presbyterians and the American*

Revolution: A Documentary Account (edited, 1974), *Presbyterians and Biblical Authority* (edited, 1981), and *American Presbyterians: A Pictorial History* (1985). An ordained Presbyterian minister, he is editor of the *Journal of Presbyterian History.* He has served as secretary (1963–1974) and as a member of the council of the American Society of Church History and as a member of the editorial council of *Theology Today.*

HAROLD Y. VANDERPOOL (Ph.D., Harvard University, 1971) is Associate Professor of the History of Medicine in the Institute for the Medical Humanities, University of Texas Medical Branch in Galveston. He is the editor of *Darwin and Darwinism: Revolutionary Insights Concerning Man, Nature, Religion and Society* (1973), co-editor of *Ethics and Cancer: An Annotated Bibliography* (1984), and author of numerous articles in journals and encyclopedias. In 1975–1976 he held a Kennedy Foundation Fellowship in Medical Ethics. His current research includes a study of the medical theory and practice of John Wesley and his eighteenth-century contemporaries.

GRANT WACKER (Ph.D., Harvard University, 1979) is Associate Professor of Religious Studies, University of North Carolina at Chapel Hill, where he teaches the history of religion in America. He is the author of *Augustus H. Strong and the Dilemma of Historical Consciousness* (1985) and *Primitive Pentecostalism: Social and Cultural Origins in America, 1870–1930* (forthcoming). He has been the recipient of awards from the Lilly Foundation and the National Endowment for the Humanities.

TIMOTHY P. WEBER (Ph.D., University of Chicago, 1976) is Associate Professor of Church History at Denver Conservative Baptist Seminary and pastor of Heritage Baptist Church in Aurora, Colorado. His publications include *Living in the Shadow of the Second Coming: American Premillennialism, 1875–1925* (1979), an enlarged edition of which, covering the years up to 1982, appeared in 1983, and *The Almost Chosen People: A Documentary History of American Evangelicalism* (forthcoming).

GEORGE HUNTSTON WILLIAMS (Th.D., Union Theological Seminary, 1946) is Hollis Professor of Divinity Emeritus at Harvard University. Among his many books are *The Radical Reformation* (1962), *Wilderness and Paradise in Christian Thought* (1962), and, most recently, an English translation and annotated edition of Stanislaus Lubieniecki's *History of the Polish Reformation* (1985). He has served as president of the American Society for Reformation Research and of the American Society of Church History and on the editorial boards of numerous journals. He has received several honorary degrees as well as awards from the John Simon Guggenheim Foundation and the National Endowment for the Humanities.

List of Abbreviations

Books of the bible are abbreviated throughout this work in the following shortened forms.

Old Testament

Genesis	Gn	Proverbs	Prv
Exodus	Ex	Ecclesiastes	Eccl
Leviticus	Lv	Song of Songs	Sg (Song)
Numbers	Nm	Wisdom	Wis
Deuteronomy	Dt	Sirach	Sir
Joshua	Jos	Isaiah	Is
Judges	Jgs	Jeremiah	Jer
Ruth	Ru	Lamentations	Lam
1 Samuel	1 Sm	Baruch	Bar
2 Samuel	2 Sm	Ezekiel	Ez
1 Kings	1 Kgs	Daniel	Dn
2 Kings	2 Kgs	Hosea	Hos
1 Chronicles	1 Chr	Joel	Jl
2 Chronicles	2 Chr	Amos	Am
Ezra	Ezr	Obadiah	Ob
Nehemiah	Neh	Jonah	Jon
Tobit	Tb	Micah	Mi
Judith	Jdt	Nahum	Na
Esther	Est	Habakkuk	Hb
1 Maccabees	1 Mc	Zephaniah	Zep
2 Maccabees	2 Mc	Haggai	Hg
Job	Jb	Zechariah	Zec
Psalms	Ps(s)	Malachi	Mal

New Testament

Matthew	Mt	1 Timothy	1 Tm
Mark	Mk	2 Timothy	2 Tm
Luke	Lk	Titus	Ti
John	Jn	Philemon	Phlm
Acts of the Apostles	Acts	Hebrews	Heb
Romans	Rom	James	Jas
1 Corinthians	1 Cor	1 Peter	1 Pt
2 Corinthians	2 Cor	2 Peter	2 Pt
Galatians	Gal	1 John	1 Jn
Ephesians	Eph	2 John	2 Jn
Philippians	Phil	3 John	3 Jn
Colossians	Col	Jude	Jude
1 Thessalonians	1 Thes	Revelation	Rv
2 Thessalonians	2 Thes		

Introduction

To the casual observer, medicine and religion may appear to have little connection except in the names of some hospitals and in the claims of some TV evangelists. Appearances, however, can be deceiving. Many religious traditions possess a rich, though largely forgotten, heritage of involvement in medical matters, and even today religious values continue to influence the attitudes and behavior of many people throughout the world toward sickness, sexuality, and lifestyle—to say nothing of such controversial issues as abortion and euthanasia. The essays in this volume seek to illuminate the history of health and medicine within the various Judeo-Christian traditions. In so doing, they promise not only to clarify our understanding of the past but to serve as a practical guide for the present, sensitizing physicians, chaplains, nurses, and other health-care professionals to the possible importance of religion in their patients' lives.

Both Jews and Christians have long stressed the importance of caring for the human body. Chapter 1 recounts that the Talmud went so far as to prohibit Jews from living in a city in which there was no physician, and Chapter 2 recalls that healing miracles marked the birth of Christianity. In fact, according to the medical historian Henry Sigerist, Christianity entered the world as a "religion of healing." During the early Middle Ages (Chapter 3), Christian priests and monks often ministered to bodies as well as souls, and the "angelical conjunction" of spiritual and physical healing, as the Puritan divine Cotton Mather called it, continued with varying emphasis well into the nineteenth century. The ranks of cleric-physicians (mentioned in several chapters) included some of the most prominent pioneers in the annals of early American church history: John Clarke, one of the Baptist founders of Rhode Island; Francis Makemie, who helped bring Presbyterianism to America; Henry Melchior Muhlenberg, the patriarch of American Lutheranism; and Samuel Seabury, the first bishop of the Protestant Episcopal Church of the United States of America.

1

At least three denominational founders devoted part of their time to healing the sick. John Wesley, the father of Methodism, not only studied medicine in preparation for his mission to North America, but established several medical dispensaries and wrote one of the most popular medical manuals of his time (Chapter 11). Mary Baker Eddy practiced both homeopathy and a form of mesmerism before creating a church of her own, Christian Science, which emphasized spiritual and physical healing (Chapter 15). Ellen G. White, the Seventh-day Adventist prophetess, at times administered hydropathic treatments to family and friends and personally supervised the founding of a chain of sanitariums (Chapter 16).

Since late antiquity, when Eastern Orthodox Christians established the first hospitals (Chapter 5), religious organizations have frequently led the way in providing for the institutional care of the sick. During the late nineteenth and early twentieth centuries, all the major religious bodies in America—Catholic, Protestant, and Jewish—established hospitals, and by the mid-twentieth century, church-related hospitals were caring for over a quarter of all hospitalized patients in the United States. As illustrated in many chapters, these institutions came into existence for a number of reasons: to convert unbelievers, to care for communicants in a supportive setting, to provide professional opportunities for members of the faith, and to create good will in the community. Foreign medical missions served similar purposes. Although medical missionaries dated back to early modern times, the age of the trained medical missionary did not dawn until the 1830s and 1840s, when the exploits of two Christian doctors, Peter Parker and David Livingstone, touched off a medical-missionary movement that eventually involved most major denominations and that remained vigorous for over a century.

Until recently, Catholic and Protestant nursing orders often cared for the sick, both at home and abroad. Since the founding of the Sisters of Charity of St. Vincent de Paul in the seventeenth century, thousands of Catholic nuns have served as nurses in both religious and secular hospitals (Chapter 4). Protestants had nothing comparable until the 1830s, when a Lutheran pastor in Germany, Theodore Fliedner, founded a nursing school in Kaiserswerth to train "deaconesses" for a life of service (Chapter 6). Other denominations soon followed the Lutheran example, and Florence Nightingale, who visited Kaiserswerth in 1851, created a secular version of the deaconesses.

Many chapters in this book shed light on the increasingly divergent paths taken by medicine and religion in modern times, especially at the institutional level. For millennia, medicine and religion had been so tightly intertwined in the lives of most Christians and Jews that people tended to view sickness and health in supernatural terms. But by the nineteenth century, divinity and medicine had coalesced into distinct professional entities, each set off by well-marked boundaries. And by the mid-twentieth century, most denominationally affiliated hospitals were distinguished more by their names than by their medical practices, admissions policies, or the religious beliefs of their staffs. The nature of medical missions also changed radically. As early as the 1930s, a Baptist commission investigating mission activities called for less evangelism and more humanitarianism. "The use of medical or other professional service as a direct means of making converts, or public [religious] services in wards and dispensaries from which patients cannot escape, is subtly coercive, and improper," concluded the commission (Chapter 10).

As scientific medicine, symbolized by the germ theory of disease, gathered momentum in the nineteenth century, supernatural explanations of disease increasingly gave way to naturalistic ones, and the commonly shared values of medicine rather than distinctive religious beliefs more and more determined attitudes toward sickness and health. Although the religious sects succumbed less quickly than the mainline denominations to the homogenizing influence of modern medicine, even they did not escape its pervasive influence. The practices of Mormon and Adventist physicians, for example, have become virtually indistinguishable from those of other doctors; in the early 1980s surgeons from these two traditions captured headlines for their technological accomplishments—experiments with artificial and baboon hearts—rather than for theological reasons (Chapters 14 and 16). Even Pentecostals, long suspicious of modern medicine, began seeking its benefits—a shift marked by the opening in 1978 of Oral Roberts' City of Faith Medical and Research Center in Tulsa, where patients could benefit from both medical and spiritual therapy (Chapter 19).

But the desacralization of healing at the institutional level tells only one side of the history of medicine and religion in the modern world. Paradoxically, at the very time that the germ theory of disease was revolutionizing etiological theory in the late nineteenth century, faith healing was experiencing a major revival, especially among Protestants, who had traditionally associated miraculous healings with such "popish" practices as pilgrimages to shrines and appeals to relics. By the 1980s perhaps as many as 100,000,000 charismatic Christians in the world professed a belief in divine healing (Chapter 19), and millions of pilgrims each year traveled to Lourdes in search of a healing miracle (Chapter 4). In the face of the ethical dilemmas created by the ability of medical technology to determine matters of life and death, many religious organizations and individuals turned to their religious traditions for moral guidance.

To explore the multifaceted relationship between health and medicine, on the one hand, and the western religious traditions, on the other, contributors were recruited who displayed both a sensitivity to the values of the tradition they were to investigate and an ability to look critically at that tradition. We gave each author a virtually impossible assignment: to address a list of topics ranging from sickness and health to death, sexuality, medical ethics, and efforts to care for and cure the ill; to construct a historical narrative that emphasized the issues most central to the tradition being discussed; to cover not only what was taught from the pulpit but what was practiced by the person in the pew; and to write in nontechnical language that could be readily understood by nonspecialists. Although the social history of medicine and religion sometimes got slighted, the resulting essays form a comprehensive yet readable survey of health and healing in the western religious traditions—the first of its kind.

CHAPTER 1

The Jewish

Tradition

Elliot N. Dorff

The Jewish tradition traces its roots to Abraham. The patriarchal stories of the Bible reflect the migration of the ancient Hebrews from Mesopotamia to Canaan and from there to Egypt. Jewish history continues with the Exodus from Egypt; the Sinai event; the gradual conquest of Canaan during the period of Joshua, the Judges, and the Kings; the building of the First Temple and, with it, the first Jewish commonwealth under Solomon; the splitting of the Jewish commonwealth into northern and southern kingdoms around the year 930 B.C.E.; the conquest and dispersion of the northern kingdom by Assyria in 722 B.C.E.; and the conquest and exile of the southern kingdom by the Babylonians in 586 B.C.E., and with that the destruction of the First Temple and the first Jewish commonwealth. All of these events are familiar from their biblical accounts.

Jews established a strong community in Babylonia that continued to exist for another fifteen hundred years under the Persians and then the Muslims. A number of Jews returned to rebuild the temple in 516 B.C.E., and with that the second Jewish commonwealth was born. It continued to exist in Israel through Greek and Roman conquest until 70 C.E., when the Romans destroyed the Second Temple and, with it, the second Jewish commonwealth.

Jews continued to exist in Israel in fairly large numbers for the next three hundred years, but their situation became increasingly dire, and the focus of Jewish history shifted to the community in Persia. The Persian Jewish community was at the forefront of world Jewry through the Muslim period, extending to approximately 1050 C.E., but there were sizeable Jewish communities in Israel, North Africa, and southern Europe during that time.

Beginning around the year of 1000 C.E. and extending to the fifteenth century, the Jewish communities of North Africa and western Europe became the major centers of Jewish culture. Jews, expelled from the western Mediterranean region and western Europe in the fourteenth and fifteenth centuries, moved to eastern Europe and the eastern Mediterranean basin, where they were concentrated until the late nineteenth and early twentieth centuries. At that time, because of persecution in Russia and the development of Zionism, a movement to reconstitute Jewish national life in the ancient homeland, many Jews moved to America and Israel, although the majority of them remained in eastern Europe until they were slaughtered in the Nazi Holocaust.

The largest Jewish community in the mid-1980s lives in the United States (approximately 5.7 million Jews), the second largest lives in Israel (approximately 3.3 million Jews), and the next largest lives in Russia (approximately 1.7 million Jews), although the Russian Jewish community is assimilating quickly under immense political pressure. There are also large Jewish communities numbering in the hundred thousands in France, Great Britain, Canada, and Argentina, and there are sizeable but somewhat smaller Jewish communities in Australia, South Africa, and Mexico. It can be said truthfully that Jews live in almost every country of the world, including those that are currently hostile to Judaism and Israel. That is the result of the remarkable fact that Jews lived without a homeland for close to nineteen hundred years, the only people to survive under those conditions. Although it is difficult to determine exactly how many Jews there are in the world today, demographers estimate that there are about thirteen million.[1]

Jewish belief centers on the revelation of God at Sinai contained in the Torah (the Five Books of Moses) and on the historical relationship of God to the Jewish people from the time of Abraham through the Exodus and on to the present day. Traditional Jews consider themselves bound by the commandments of God as articulated in Jewish law. Because Jewish law gives Judaism a distinctly activist cast, even those Jews who do not observe the law often are actively involved in many projects for the improvement of life on earth. Jewish values concentrate on the life of the family and the community, education throughout life, historical rootedness, and hope for a Messianic future in which all peoples will come to know God and follow Jewish law. In that way, Jews understand themselves as having a mission of demonstrating morality to the world and being, in Isaiah's terminology, "a light unto the nations."[2] For Jews, the land of Israel is the Jewish homeland not only because many of the critical events in the birth and development of Judaism took place there, but also because God gave the land to the Jews according to Scripture. Although Jews understand themselves as having a divine mission, that mission is to be carried out by example rather than by actively pursuring converts; in fact, Judaism has historically been reluctant to accept converts. While Jewish law specifies many particulars about the actions of Jews, Jewish belief is much less determined. Consequently, Judaism has a long history of lively intellectual debate on philosophical issues, and rabbis have taken theological positions ranging from supernaturalism to naturalism, from rationalism to mysticism, and from a community-based revelational understanding of Jewish law to an individualistic, existential understanding of it.

Traditional and liberal manifestations of Judaism exist in most countries. In the United States there are four movements: the Reform Movement, the Reconstructionist Movement, the Conservative Movement, and the Orthodox Movement. Orthodox Jews believe that the Torah is the literal word of God and that Jewish law is to be determined by reference to the codes and responsa of the past. Conservative Jews believe that all Jewish sources must be understood in their historical context and that Jewish law developed historically as well. Therefore, while Conservative Jews consider Jewish law binding, they are more willing than Orthodox Jews to make changes in its content in response to modern needs. Reconstructionist and Reform Jews do not consider Jewish law to be binding, although many voluntarily choose to observe sections of it. The Reconstructionist Movement possesses a greater sense of community than the Reform Movement and hence offers more encouragement to adopt the folkways of the People of Israel. Autonomy is a central value for the Reform Movement. Thus for Reform Jews the law is at most a resource that the individual may choose to consult in making a decision; it is certainly not the authoritative command of God. These represent the positions of the rabbis of the various movements, but for the lay people, family history, convenience, and friendships are at least as important in choosing an affiliation as ideology and practice. Therefore, Jews might be members of synagogues that are affiliated with one movement or another even though their own personal philosophies and practices do not coincide with those of the institutions that they join.

While the Torah serves as the constitution of the Jewish people, Judaism is based upon the interpretation of that constitution by the rabbis in each generation. Consequently, biblical verses give some direction to Jewish medical ethics, but most of its content comes from rabbinic literature.

The primary sources of rabbinic discussions and decisions on medical matters in the ancient world were the Mishnah, edited by Rabbi Judah, the president of the Sanhedrin, in the year 220 C.E.; and the Palestinian (or Jerusalem) and Babylonian Talmuds, edited in approximately 400 and 500 C.E., respectively. Other ideational material that forms the philosophical background for rabbinic decisions appears in the various collections of Midrash. These homilies and stories were edited during the Middle Ages, but consist of sources from the periods of the Mishnah and the Talmud.

The Mishnah and the two Talmuds were produced at a time in which there was a fairly clear line of authority within the Jewish community. That was not the case from the Middle Ages on. Consequently, two genres of legal literature—responsa and codes—appeared.

When a question was raised on any issue, the rabbi of a community might answer it. If he had a question, he would address it to some other rabbi whom he respected, and that rabbi would write a response. This literature is called the *responsa literature*. The Hebrew term is more explicit: Its translation is "questions and answers." There are responsa on all sorts of subjects from the eighth century on, during which responsa have served as the major source of ongoing Jewish law. Any rabbi can issue a responsum, and there is no mechanism within the Jewish community to determine which of several conflicting answers is the authoritative Jewish position.

Codes answered the need for a practical, summary statement of Jewish law. Aside from the Mishnah, the two codes that are most often cited are the *Mishneh Torah,* written by Moses Maimonides (Moses ben Maimon, 1135–1204) in the twelfth century, and the *Shulhan 'arukh,* written by Joseph Caro (1488–1575) in the sixteenth century with notes by Moses Isserles. The task of writing a code is a long and comprehensive one, and consequently most of Jewish attitudes on contemporary medical issues are based on modern responsa rather than on codes.

Although the Jewish tradition placed great emphasis on its holy texts and their exegesis, the customs of the people and the general wisdom that they heard in the streets played a crucial role in shaping Jewish practice. As one might expect, folk wisdom and practice were not always consistent with the thought and instructions of the Rabbis; consequently, we must be careful to take both elements of the tradition into account in order to understand it properly.

The point should not be exaggerated, however. Because there was no central body dispensing law during most of Jewish history, the Rabbis, who created the texts, generally lived among the people in small communities and were therefore cognizant of folk practices. More often than not they considered custom as a source of binding law. All Israel stood at Sinai, they noted, and therefore in addition to the holy texts the practices of the people could serve as an indication of revelation. As Hillel the Elder (first century) put it, "Leave it to the people of Israel: if they are not prophets, they are the children of prophets!"[3] Moreover, in many cases there simply was no law, and then custom was explicitly invoked to fill the void. Thus the discrepancy between Jewish folk practices and Jewish law is often not great.

Jewish Views of the Body

God created bodies as well as minds, emotions, and wills. Therefore, for the Rabbis—the sages of the Mishnah, Talmud, and Midrash—the body was a good thing. It was, in fact, God's masterpiece, proving his infinite goodness and boundless wisdom, and the Rabbis waxed eloquent in admiring its intricate construction. The body could be abused in the process of sinning, but so could the soul. Neither was solely responsible for sin. Thus the body was not a "prison house" for the soul, as it was in many of the traditions influenced by Gnosticism and other Greek schools of thought. It was the vehicle by which God's purposes could be carried out if one used it correctly.[4]

Because the body was God's creation, it was right to enjoy its legitimate pleasures and wrong to deny them to oneself. In sharp contrast to elements of the Christian tradition, the Jewish tradition strongly denounced asceticism and monasticism. The Rabbis assumed that God wanted his creatures to be happy and therefore that it was sinful deliberately to shun physical happiness and material well-being. "In the Hereafter" they declared, "a man will have to stand judgment and give reckoning for all that his eyes saw but he did not eat."[5] Similarly they noted that the Nazirite, who had taken a vow to abstain for a time from drinking wine, had to bring a sin offering after the period had elapsed according to *Numbers* 6:11, "because he has sinned against the soul." The Rabbis then asked: "Against which soul has he sinned?" The answer:

> He withheld himself from wine. And we may apply the argument *a fortiori:*
> If a person who withholds himself from wine is called a sinner, how much
> more so is he a sinner who withholds himself from all enjoyments.[6]

Judaism recognized limitations on the pursuit of bodily pleasures, but because God had determined the limits of that pursuit within the law, any assumption of further limits on the part of human beings was an act of both pride and ingratitude.

The Rabbis assumed that human bodies were God's property, which he leased for the duration of one's life. If a person were to rent an apartment, he or she would not have the right to destroy it, but would have the responsibility to take reasonable care of it. In the same way, because a person's body was on loan, one did not have the right to destroy it by suicide, but rather had the responsibility to take care of it. This was taken very seriously: One was even required to violate any commandment except those prohibiting murder, idolatry, and incest in order to save one's life. Consequently, according to the Talmudic rabbis, "it is forbidden to live in a city in which there is no physician," for doing so would expose a person's body to an unacceptable degree of risk and would prevent the person from fulfilling his or her responsibility to care for it.[7] Moreover, matters of hygiene, diet, exercise, and sleep were subjects for legal obligations within Judaism, not just matters of sensible living. So, for example, the following story was told about Hillel, one of the most important Jewish leaders of the early first century:

> When he had finished the lesson with his students, he accompanied them part of the way. They said to him, "Master, where are you going?" "To perform a religious duty." "Which religious duty?" "To bathe in the bathhouse." "Is that a religious duty?" He answered them, "If somebody appointed to scrape and clean the statues of the king which are set up in the theatres and circuses is paid to do the work and furthermore associates with nobility, how much more so should I, who am created in the divine image and likeness, take care of my body!"[8]

Similarly, Maimonides, both a rabbi and a physician, devoted several chapters of his code to the obligations of diet, exercise, hygiene, and sleep, thereby indicating that these were legal obligations, not just practical advice.[9] He indicated the theological motivation for these rules explicitly:

> He who regulates his life in accordance with the laws of hygiene with the sole motive of maintaining a sound and vigorous physique and begetting children to do his work and labor for his benefit is not following the right course. A man should aim to maintain physical health and vigor in order that his soul may be upright, in a condition to know God. . . . Whoever throughout his life follows this course will be continually serving God, even while engaged in business and even during cohabitation, because his purpose in all that he does will be to satisfy his needs so as to have a sound body with which to serve God.[10]

This theological context also governed the corollaries of the Jewish view of the body in matters of diet, hygiene, and exercise. In each case it was the religious, not the pragmatic, motivation that was primary.

Judaism imposed a number of restrictions on the foods that Jews could eat. Any animals, fowl, or fish that Jews ate were to come from the limited list that the Bible allows (*Lv.* 11; *Dt.* 14); animals and fowl were to be slaughtered in a specific way designed to minimize the animal's pain; blood was to be drained from meat (*Lv.* 17:10–12; *Dt.* 12:23); and meat and dairy foods were to be separated in preparing, serving, and eating meals.

Many Jews and non-Jews have assumed that Jewish dietary laws were designed to maintain health. Some modern Jews even use that

explanation in order to justify their abandonment of those rules, reasoning that the work of the United States Food and Drug Administration makes the health measures involved in Jewish dietary laws unnecessary. The truth of the matter is that health was never given as the principal rationale for the dietary rules. Maimonides came closest. He thought that observing the dietary rules would benefit one's health by prohibiting dangerous and dirty foods and, more importantly, by curbing one's lust for food so that one did not take the desire for food as an ultimate end.[11] Even for him, however, the maintenance of health was not a necessary nor even a sufficient reason to observe the dietary rules; it was rather that God commanded them.

The Bible specifically indicated several times that the rationale for restricting the number of animals that could be eaten was to make the people of Israel holy (*Lv.* 11:43–45; *Dt.* 14:1–3, 21). The Rabbis carried this further:

> What does God care whether a man kills an animal in the proper way and eats it, or whether he strangles the animal and eats it? Will the one benefit Him, or the other injure Him? Or what does God care whether a man eats impure animals or pure animals? "If you are wise, for yourself are you wise, but if you scorn, you alone shall bear it" (*Prv.* 9:12). So you learn that the commandments were given only to purify God's creatures, as it says, "God's word is purified, it is a protection to those who trust in Him" (2 *Sm.* 22:31).[12]

Part of the confusion may well have resulted from the Bible's terminology in describing the dietary rules, for its Hebrew words *tahor* and *tameh* are often rendered "clean" and "unclean." They have nothing to do with sanitation, however, and are more properly rendered "pure" and "impure." The dietary restrictions probably began as a method to mark off the priests as special people. The rules were later extended to all Israelites to make them "a kingdom of priests and a holy nation" (*Ex.* 19:6), "a people consecrated to the Lord" (*Dt.* 14:21).

Similar remarks apply to hygiene. Thus the Talmud, commenting on the biblical verse "Sanctify yourselves and be holy" (*Lv.* 11:44) says, " 'Sanctify yourselves'—i.e. wash your hands before the meal, 'and be holy'—i.e. wash after the meal."[13] This was an application of priestly practice to the masses, for the meal was considered to be like a sacrifice on the altar; and consequently priestly rituals appropriate to handling sacrifices were also appropriate to eating an ordinary meal.[14] Similarly, it was forbidden to live in a town that had no public bathing facilities, because "physical cleanliness is conducive to spiritual purity," and the required morning ablution was seen as a reenactment of the priestly practice of washing hands before performing the Temple service.[15]

In addition to diet and hygiene, a third area that the Rabbis treated in distinctly religious terms was athletics. While they did not object to sports for purposes of physical exercise or as part of military training, until the modern period they largely frowned upon competitive sports "for the sake of the game." Their opposition was based upon two considerations. First, participation in athletics would rob time from what was really important, that is, study. Thus Salo W. Baron in his book on Jewish communities of the Middle Ages says:

> Sporadic voices in favor of recreational pauses [in the daily and yearly schedule of classes] were as ineffective as those which advocated physical exercises. Northern [European] Jewry, especially, had little use for physical education or sports, and paid little heed even to the demand of a talmudic sage that a father give his son instruction in swimming as a life-saving precaution.[16]

Even for Maimonides, the rabbi–physician, maintaining a healthy body was a religious obligation because it was a prerequisite for the well-being of the soul, which "alone is the source of eternal life."[17]

Moreover, athletics carried extremely negative connotations for Jews for historical reasons. Athletics were a central feature of the process of hellenization against which the Maccabees revolted in 168 B.C.E. (the Hanukkah story),[18] and ever since athletics have symbolized the essence of Gentile values that Jews should shun.

When cruelty to either humans or animals was involved in a sport, it was opposed for that reason as well as for the two general considerations just mentioned. Thus Josephus, a first-century Jewish historian, noted that to the Jews the Roman contests to the death between men and beasts were "a palpable breaking up of those customs for which they had so great a veneration."[19]

Despite these objections, there is some evidence of the participation of Jews in competitive sporting events in Wiesenfeld, Germany, in 1386 and in German and Italian games in the fifteenth century. These tourneys included running, jumping, throwing, and bowling. Ball games were popular in the sixteenth century—so much so that Moses Isserles specifically permitted them on the Sabbath and festivals "even for pure sport."[20]

It was not until the nineteenth and twentieth centuries, however, that Jews actively engaged in competitive sports. In western Europe this change resulted from their participation in the full culture of modern societies. In eastern Europe, it was the product of the new mood of self-assertion fostered by the Zionist movement. Even so, in many Jewish minds athletic prowess continued to carry the taint of being a Gentile value.[21]

A corollary of the requirement to take care of one's body was the obligation not to endanger it unduly. There are varying twentieth-century responsa on whether smoking is such an undue risk, with several Orthodox rabbis claiming that smoking is permissible in Jewish law and some Orthodox, Conservative, and Reform rabbis claiming that it is not.[22] Similar remarks apply to drugs. One may instruct the physician to use whatever experimental drugs have any chance of saving a life, however risky they may be, but one may not use addictive drugs simply for the purposes of achieving some kind of psychological or emotional high.[23] No Jewish source saw coffee, tea, or alcohol as a prohibited drug, but a number of contemporary respondents have prohibited the use of marijuana and, all the more so, harder drugs.[24] Alcohol, used in many Jewish rituals, has always been regarded as one of the legitimate pleasures of life. Intoxication, however, has been frowned upon, and alcoholism among Jews was rare until the last decade.[25]

Thus Jewish views on diet, hygiene, exercise, and protection of the body have distinctively religious roots apart from any pragmatic results they may foster. God gave life to be enjoyed, but pleasure must yield to health as a value because health is necessary for one to function as the servant of God.

The Etiology of Illness

Because God is the creator of everything, according to the Bible, he is ultimately the author of health and disease: "I deal death and give life; I wounded, and I will heal; none can deliver from My hand" (*Dt.* 32:39). The biblical authors depicted God as visiting illness on people as punishment for sins and as a means of expiation (for example, *Dt.* 28), and the Talmud followed suit: "There is no suffering without iniquity."[26] A tenth-century commentary put it graphically: "If a subject sins against his ruler, a blacksmith is commanded to fashion chains in which the ruler imprisons the sinner. When a man sins against the Lord, his limbs become his fetters."[27]

While this linkage between sickness and sin has been sustained in Jewish sources to this century, it has also been challenged throughout the ages. The *Book of Job* forcefully challenged this tenet, as does a popular, contemporary book by Rabbi Harold Kushner, *When Bad Things Happen to Good People.*[28] As difficult as it was to understand the suffering of individuals according to the calculus of sin and sickness, it was even more difficult to explain the suffering of the People of Israel on that basis. Consequently, Judaism developed a broad range of theodicies, but generally they addressed the degradation, death, destruction, and exile that Jews suffered rather than physical illness.

Wounds and dismemberment suffered in the course of persecutions were all seen as part of the broader question of how God could allow human beings to inflict suffering of all sorts on his covenanted people in the apparent absence of sin.

The causative properties of sin did not prevent the Rabbis of the Talmud from identifying physical causes of illnesses or from seeking to cure them. The most widely held view was that "blood is the chief cause of disease." Therefore they advised bloodletting once every thirty days for those under forty and less frequently for older people so that the bad blood could flow away.[29] Other carriers of disease mentioned in the Talmud include bile, the air, contaminated foods or beverages, bodily discharges, clothing, bath water, animals, and insects (especially flies and worms).[30] Lack of fluids was believed to lead to digestive disturbances; neglecting one's health, to fevers and colds. Injury to the spinal cord caused paralysis.[31] Excessive eating, fasting, drinking of liquor, and sexual activity were also thought to cause disease. Psychological causes were recognized too: "Three things weaken the strength of man: fear, trouble, and sin." Fear, by accelerating the pulse, had reportedly "slain many a person." The Rabbis also recognized the physiological implications of the psychological upset attendant upon changes in routine: "A change in habit is the beginning of illness."[32]

But sometimes sickness was not connected to sin or physical or psychological causes, but was rather attributed to the work of demons. Because of the difficulties in identifying divine or natural causes for disease, demons were the most commonly designated agents in Talmudic and medieval times, and belief in them continued until the twentieth century among the majority of Jews untouched by the Enlightenment.

The willingness of even the Rabbis to accept demonic etiologies despite the obvious conflict that they posed to the omnipotent rule of God indicates the perplexity and fear that people had in the face of disease. If pushed, Jewish leaders might claim that the demons were not as independent as they seemed and actually operated under God's overarching authority. It is notable, though, that Jewish sources seldom linked the work of demons to the previous sins of their victims, and thus Jews apparently acquiesced to the inconsistency of believing in both an omnipotent God and independent demons. The power of pain and fear was clearly greater than the quest for consistency.

The Agents of Cure

As mentioned earlier, the Talmud prohibited living in a city in which there was no physician.[33] This rule, eminently plausible on pragmatic grounds, represented a major historical and philosophical development.

Prior to the Hellenistic period, there is no evidence of a medical *profession* among the Hebrews. The Bible never uses the word "physician" *(rofeh)* to refer to human beings, except in describing foreign doctors whose treatments were being mocked.[34] The biblical objection to these practitioners was a theological one: Their treatments used magic and religious tenets and practices that were inconsistent with belief in God. Involvement in such practices, even as a patient, was therefore tantamount to idolatry. The Greeks, however, introduced a form of secular, "scientific" medicine that was not based upon such beliefs and acts. Thus Ben Sira, writing in the third century B.C.E., not only condoned the new medical art and its practitioners, but praised them as the fulfillment of God's will: "Honor a physician with the honor due to him for the uses which you may have of him, for the Lord created him. . . . The Lord created medicines out of the earth, and he who is wise will not abhor them."[35]

Scientific methods removed Jewish objections to medicine based on its former pagan associations, but there still remained a major theological problem in accepting the work of physicians to cure illness. God, after all, announced himself as healer in many places in the Bible, suggesting perhaps that medicine was an improper human intervention in God's decision to inflict illness.[36]

The Rabbis were aware of this line of reasoning, but they counteracted it by pointing out that God himself had authorized healing, in fact required it. They found that authorization and that imperative in two biblical verses: *Exodus* 21:19–20, according to which an assailant must insure that his victim is "thoroughly healed," and *Deuteronomy* 22:2, which instructed "And you shall restore the lost property to him." The Talmud understood the *Exodus* verse as giving "permission for the physician to cure." On the basis of an extra letter in the Hebrew text of the *Deuteronomy* passage, the Talmud declared that that verse included the obligation to restore a fellow man's body as well as his property; hence there was an obligation to come to the aid of another person in a life-threatening situation. On the basis of *Leviticus* 19:16 ("Nor shall you stand idly by the blood of your fellow"), the Talmud expanded the obligation of providing medical aid to encompass expenditure of financial resources for that purpose.[37] The commandment "And you shall love your neighbor as yourself" (*Lv.* 19:18) was used to exempt physicians from any liability for injuries they caused in the process of healing, for presumably the patient, like the physician himself, would be willing to take some risk to be healed.[38] In sum, Joseph Caro, author of the *Shulhan 'arukh,* said:

The Torah gave permission to the physician to heal; moreover, this is a religious precept and is included in the category of saving life; and if the physician withholds his services, it is considered as shedding blood.[39]

The following story from a tenth-century collection of Midrash indicates that the famous second-century Rabbis of whom it speaks recognized the theological issue involved, but it also indicates the clear assertion of the Jewish tradition that the physician's work was legitimate and, in fact, obligatory:

It once happened that Rabbi Ishmael and Rabbi Akiva were strolling in the streets of Jerusalem accompanied by another person. They were met by a sick person. He said to them, "My masters, tell me by what means I may be cured." They told him, "Do thus and so until you are cured." The sick man asked them, "And who afflicted me?" They replied, "The Holy One, blessed be He." The sick man responded, "You have entered into a matter which does not pertain to you. God has afflicted, and you seek to cure! Are you not transgressing His will?"

Rabbi Akiva and Rabbi Ishmael asked him, "What is your occupation?" The sick man answered, "I am a tiller of the soil, and here is the sickle in my hand." They asked him, "Who created the vineyard?" He answered, "The Holy One, blessed be He." Rabbi Akiva and Rabbi Ishmael said to him, "And you enter into a matter which does not pertain to you! God created the vineyard, and you cut His fruits from it." He said to them, "Do you not see the sickle in my hand? If I did not plow, sow, fertilize, and weed, nothing would sprout." Rabbi Akiva and Rabbi Ishmael said to him, "Foolish man! Have you never in your life heard that it is written, 'As for man, his days are as grass; as a flower of the field, so he flourishes' (Ps. 103:15)? Just as if one does not weed, fertilize, and plow, the trees will not produce fruit, and if fruit is produced but is not watered or fertilized, it will not live but die, so with regard to the body. Drugs and medicants are the fertilizer, and the physician is the tiller of the soil."[40]

Jews were obligated to heal non-Jews as well. This duty was based partly on a homiletic interpretation of Leviticus 25:35 and partly on the consideration that failing to do so would jeopardize friendly relations and bring about profanation of the Divine Name.[41] Some sources limited this obligation to Gentiles who accepted the seven Noahic laws, which were considered the minimal standards of humanity,[42] while others extended the obligation even to those who have not accepted those laws.[43] In practice, Jewish physicians during the Middle Ages commonly served Jews and Gentiles alike, even if it required desecration of the Sabbath.[44] This practice has been even more common in modern societies.

The result of these historical and philosophical developments was that Jews embraced medicine and ministered to both Jews and non-

Jews. Medieval Jews in southern Europe benefitted from, and contributed toward, the scientific advances of the Arabs. Jews in northern Europe, closed off from that enlightened spirit, contributed little to developments in medicine. Moreover, Jewish medical practitioners in the North mixed their medicine with a healthy dose of magic and folk remedies. Even so, Jewish physicians throughout Europe gained great popularity because of their medical expertise. Arabic and Greek medical works were available in Hebrew translations, but not in most European languages, and the Jews' propensity for travel and study made them aware of discoveries in other lands.

Paradoxically, because of the popular view that demons and magic were responsible for disease, the Jews' medical reputation enhanced the Christian perception of Jews as sorcerers, a development that later had both positive and negative consequences. On the one hand, Jewish doctors were very popular in northern Europe throughout the Middle Ages, despite stringent church prohibitions against consulting them and despite the constant warning of Christian clerics that Jews would turn their magic against their patients. On the other hand, every time a Jewish physician tried to help a Christian, he risked his life. If the Jew was successful, his reputation as a magician was enhanced along with the fear, respect, and animosity attendant thereto; if he failed, he often lost his own life. This was true of the very first Jewish physician on record in the West. Tzedkeiah, court physician to Emperor Charles the Bald, was accused of poisoning the emperor in 877 and undoubtedly was executed.

Beyond the Jews' medical knowledge, their involvement in international commerce further added to their reputation for sorcery, because most of the exotic elements of the medieval pharmacopoeia were imported from the East, and drugs and poisons were synonymous in the medieval mind. Thus in 1267 church councils in Breslau and Vienna forbade Christians to purchase foodstuffs from Jews lest they be poisoned, and during the fourteenth century thousands of Jews were massacred, accused of causing the Black Plague by poisoning the wells. One important element of Martin Luther's anti-Semitism was his belief about the superior medical knowledge and practices of the Jews:

> If they could kill us all, they would gladly do so, aye, and often do it, especially those who profess to be physicians. They know all that is known about medicine in Germany; they can give poison to a man of which he will die in an hour, or in ten or twenty years; they thoroughly understand this art.[45]

Luther aptly summarized the late medieval Christian view of both the positive and the negative implications of Jewish medical knowledge and practice.

Normally Jewish law permitted a physician to charge a fee for his services.[46] At the same time, there was great concern that medical services be available to the poor. The Talmud approvingly held up the example of Abba, the bleeder, who

> placed a box outside his office where his fees were to be deposited. Whoever had money put it in, but those who had none could come in without feeling embarrassed. When he saw a person who was in no position to pay, he would offer him some money, saying to him, "Go, strengthen yourself [after the bleeding operation]."[47]

The Middle Ages provided similar examples of the charity of Jewish physicians. The ethic must have been quite powerful, because it was not until the nineteenth century that a rabbi ruled that the communal court should force physicians to give free services to the poor if they did not do so voluntarily.[48]

The obligation to heal the poor devolved upon the community as well as the physician. Therefore the sick enjoyed priority over other indigent persons in their claim to private or public assistance. Joseph Caro recorded the view that while contributions to erect a synagogue were to take precedence over ordinary forms of charity, even the synagogue's needs must give way to the requirements of the indigent sick. And the sick could not refuse such aid if they required it to get well.[49]

Reliance on the generosity and ethical sensitivity of physicians for the care of the poor was the norm, but there were cases where Jewish communities organized medical care in a form of socialized medicine. In medieval Spain, for example, Jews played a prominent role in the state's program of socialized medicine, and in other places Jewish communities on their own hired surgeons, physicians, nurses, and midwives as salaried servants.[50] Whatever the arrangement, the community as well as the individual doctor was under the obligation to heal, and that was taken very seriously.

There is no evidence of hospitals in biblical or talmudic times, but there were "houses set apart" for lepers and, during the talmudic period, there were also marble operating rooms where surgeons did their work.[51] During the Middle Ages, Jewish communities had inns that served primarily to house poor or sick travelers and secondarily to nurse the ailing poor of the community itself—although the poverty and political insecurity of medieval Jewish communities made both types of service primitive.

The first Jewish hospitals designed exclusively for the sick were built in the last half of the eighteenth century in the enlightened countries of western and central Europe, where Jews could look forward to permanent settlement and better economic prospects. By 1933, Jewish hospitals existed in most countries in Europe; Poland alone had 48— nine percent of all of the hospitals in the country—with over 3,500 beds. This pattern of establishing hospitals continued in North America, although the rationale changed over time. The original motivation was to provide hospital care for Jewish patients in a Jewish atmosphere. After about 1920, when an increasing percentage of American Jews had become Americanized and consequently less interested in a specifically Jewish hospital environment, the justification for building and maintaining hospitals was increasingly to afford professional oppportunities to Jewish physicians, who suffered severe discrimination in gaining appointments to the staffs of other hospitals. After 1950, when such discrimination subsided and when less than a quarter of the patients in Jewish hospitals were Jewish, the rationale shifted once again: Jewish hospitals simply served the general community.[52]

The obligation to heal in Judaism extended beyond medical professionals to laypersons, who were required to visit the sick. That duty was seen specifically as a means of helping to cure the patient; therefore it was not only encouraged, but prescribed. In fact, one who refused to perform this duty was likened to a shedder of blood, because he thereby withheld a source of cure from the patient.[53] In their prayers every morning Jews recited a passage from the Talmud that depicted visiting the sick as one of ten ethical duties that had no specific limits and that gave "fruits which a person enjoys in this world while the stock remains for him in the World to Come."[54] In addition to being a legal and moral duty, it was "a religious precept" in the sense that it enabled one to imitate God.[55] The obligation devolved equally upon every Jew, even the old and the great, who were to visit their juniors and subordinates.[56]

Especially during the Middle Ages, Jews formed local societies to visit the sick, a practice modern congregations are beginning to revitalize.[57] It is the lay people who participate in these groups; rabbis simply do an equal share with the other members of the society. For the promotion of good neighborly relations, Jews are also obligated to visit non-Jewish patients.[58] Jewish law even provides some guidance as to what one is to do during the visit in order to maximize its good effects.[59]

Thus physicians, hospitals, and visitors all became important human agents of cure, but ultimately God was recognized as the Healer. Physicians were to be consulted only because they functioned as God's partners in treatment, not as his substitutes. Because of God's crucial role in curing, Jews were supposed to pray to God as part of the treatment; indeed, in the traditional liturgy even a healthy Jew was supposed to recite a prayer three times each weekday asking God to heal the sick. Similarly, before the prescribed monthly bloodletting, the Jew of Talmudic times was supposed to say:

> May it be your will, O Lord my God, that this operation be a cure for me, and may you heal me; for you are a faithful healer, and your cure is certain, since it is not the way of human beings to cure, but so they are accustomed.

After the bloodletting, the patient was to say: "Blessed be He Who heals without fee."[60] Moreover, because the ultimate cause of illness was presumed to be sin, the Talmud advised the sick to ask a sage to pray for them on the assumption that the sage's relatively unblemished record would aid them in pleading their case before God.[61] Thus Jews sought cure from both divine and human agents, assuming that the latter would succeed only if God willed them to do so.

Methods of Cure and Prevention

Using materials similar to a disease in order to cure it was widespread in both Talmudic and medieval times. As the English treated dog bites by applying "the hair of the dog that bit them," so the Mishnah prescribed using the lobe of the dog's liver.[62] The only Talmudic cure that Rabbi Jacob Mollin (1365–1427) endorsed was this:

> "When a bone sticks in one's throat, he should place a similar bone on his head and say, 'One, one, gone down, swallowed, swallowed, gone down, one, one.' " This cure is tested and proven, and so we may use it.[63]

To stop bleeding, Talmudic sources recommended parching some of the shed blood over a fire and then applying the dry, powdery product to the wound. They also suggested using contrary treatments: cold to cure fevers, and heat to cure chills.[64]

Among the treatments mentioned in the Talmud are diets, warm and cold compresses, sweating, rest, sunbaths, change of climate, hydrotherapy, psychotherapy, massages, and exercises.[65] Medicinal powders, liquids, and herbs were used, including even opium, but the Rabbis were wary of using drugs and cautioned against their overuse.[66] Meat, eggs, vegetables, and water were considered nourishing, but wine was placed at "the head of all medicine": "Only where there is no wine are drugs required."[67] Clean air and sunlight were considered the best cures.[68]

Medieval Jewish physicians rarely used Talmudic remedies. Some rabbis justified this by claiming that Talmudic cures were outdated. Rabbi Jacob Mollin, for example, suggested these reasons for abandoning them:

> One should not try any of the medicines, prescriptions or exorcisms recommended in the Talmud because no one today knows how they should be applied. If they should be tried nevertheless and found ineffective, the words of our sages would be exposed to ridicule.

Joseph Caro also advised against using Talmudic remedies because the medicines and personal habits recommended in the Talmud differed from those of medieval European communities. In seventeenth-century Poland, Rabbi Abraham Gombiner went even further, saying that many things mentioned in the Talmud were dangerous and ineffective "today because conditions and ways of living have changed."[69]

In place of Talmudic therapies, Jewish physicians used whatever was accepted medical procedure in their times, reasoning that the religious imperative was to cure and that the Talmudic prescriptions were simply suggestions based upon the medicine of that time. The one non-Jewish medical practice Jews consistently rejected for religious reasons was the use of human and animal blood. According to one scholar, "there is not a single instance in all of Jewish literature of the prescription of blood for internal medicine, and the very rarity of the suggestions that horse's blood, or the menses, may be applied externally serves only to bring out in bold relief the sharp prejudice against these usages."[70] In view of the medieval blood-libels against Jews, this is indeed ironic.

Biblical and Talmudic medicine proved more effective in preventing illness than in curing it. As the third-century Rabbi Samuel said, "Washing one's hands and feet in the morning is more effective than all the lotions in the world." Some of the preventive measures that the Bible and Talmud prescribed were remarkably advanced for their time. In cases of communicable diseases, Jews of biblical times disinfected clothing and objects by washing, fumigation, or fire. They also knew about the preventive significance of isolation (see *Lv.* 13–15). The rabbis similarly advised the public to avoid crowds and narrow streets during epidemics. Flies were to be avoided as carriers of disease. It was forbidden to dig wells near dumps and cemeteries. Water that had been left standing uncovered was considered unfit for human consumption, and water suspected of being contaminated had to be boiled before use. Food had to be served fresh and in clean dishes, and meat had to be cooked sufficiently to destroy any parasites it might harbor.[71]

Sages of the biblical and rabbinic periods roundly criticized faith healing. Anyone who consulted exorcists was cut off from the community (*Lv.* 19:31, 20:6), and the exorcists themselves were stoned to death (*Lv.* 20:27), because any form of magic was viewed as an "abomination to the Lord" (*Dt.* 18:10–12). Even the suggestion of sorcery was abhorred. Thus Moses' use of a copper serpent to heal the people from snakebites (*Nm.* 21:9), was easily misconstrued as cure through sorcery, and so—much to the delight of the later sages—it was destroyed by King Hezekiah (2 *Kgs.* 14:4). The Rabbis strongly condemned the use of incantation as part of treatment, especially when it involved biblical verses.[72]

As time went on, however, the Rabbis increasingly bowed to the fear and pain involved in being sick or wounded and ignored injunctions against magical cures. The fourth-century disputants Rava and Abayae agreed that "nothing done for the purposes of healing is to be forbidden as superstitious," and indeed the Talmud contains scores of references to the use of charms for healing.[73] During the Middle Ages, Rabbi Israel Isserlein (d.1460) faced the issue squarely. In answering a questioner, he wrote, "regarding your questions as to whether an invalid may consult a magician, know that we have found no explicit prohibition of such a course, for the biblical strictures against sorcerers do not apply in this case." Influenced by that advice, Rabbi Solomon Luria (1510–1573) ruled even more permissively that "if a serious illness is caused by magic or evil spirits, one may resort to a non-Jewish magician for a cure."[74]

But it was not necessary to consult a magician because Jewish physicians employed the entire range of magical remedies as a matter of ordinary practice, often with rabbinic sanction. Medieval remedies might have had therapeutic value, but it was the incantations that invariably accompanied them that the masses and, for that matter, many of the physicians regarded as the effective agent in the cure. Biblical verses and forms of God's name were used extensively,[75] and medieval Jews often borrowed both the form and content of incantations from neighboring Christian sources. Thus the ethical manual *Sefer Hasidim* (thirteenth century) specifically employed the German usage: "To cure a person who has been harmed by a demon, the charm must be repeated nine times, as they do in Germany."[76] Normally, Jews substituted a Jewish form for the Christian incantations they borrowed, but sometimes they acquiesced to the use of unaltered Christian incantations by non-Jewish doctors ministering to them. Rabbi Menahem of Speyer (fifteenth century) offered a justification for this: "The sounds effect the cure, and not the words of the incantation; therefore a Christian may be permitted to heal a Jew even if he invokes the aid of Jesus and the saints in his spell."[77]

Aside from incantations, physicians regularly employed other forms of magic for both cure and prevention. Medieval Jews who fell ill often changed their names and sometimes even adopted new parents so that their parents' names might be different as well. Eastern European Jews of the last several centuries improved on this scheme: They regularly chose some form of the Hebrew word for life *(hayyim)* for their new names in order to both hide the identity of the sick from the demons of the disease and also to force God, as it were, to sustain them through the power of the meaning of the new name.[78] To counteract the demons that inflict illness at night, before retiring one was to recite the "anti-demonic psalm" (generally identified as Psalm 91, but sometimes as Psalm 3), *Numbers* 6:24–27, and *Deuteronomy* 32:10–12.[79] Amulets were permitted with rabbinic approval; those written by a recognized physician were approved automatically. Jews commonly tied red ribbons to the beds of women who had just given birth to ward off the evil eye from both mother and child. When the plague devastated a community, its leaders inspected the *mezuzot,* the traditional signs on the doorposts containing two sections of the Torah, to determine if one was improperly written and therefore responsible for the infestation. Astrology also played a major role in medieval Jewish medicine. The planet Saturn governed illness and death; thus its movements and the waning and waxing of the moon were especially scrutinized in medical matters.[80]

Jewish curative and preventive medicine in Talmudic and medieval times was thus a combination of the empirical, the religious, and the magical. While some of the specific forms were distinctly Jewish (for example, the use of *mezuzot* to ward off disease), the substance of these measures was undoubtedly the product of the interaction between Jews and the non-Jews among whom they lived, who used similar empirical, religious, and magical measures.

Mental Health

If it was difficult to discover effective medications for the body, it was all the more difficult to treat illnesses of the mind. The Bible describes in detail the paranoid psychopathia and perhaps the epilepsy of King Saul, and others in the Bible and Talmud suffer from visual and auditory hallucinations, insanity, and "possession by demons or spirits."[81] Biblical prophets experienced trances and ecstasies. The ancient Jews interpreted such phenomena positively, as proof of divine contact, but the later tradition treated them negatively, as illness, and sought to exorcise the ghosts *(shedim)* or furies *(dybbuk)* that caused them. Music was used often in an attempt to seduce demons to leave the minds of the insane and thereby to calm and cure them.

Because insanity had legal implications, the Rabbis tried to define it as specifically as possible:

> Our Rabbis taught: Who is deemed an imbecile? He who goes out alone at night, and he who spends the night in a cemetery, and he who tears his garments. It was taught: Rabbi Huna said: he must do all of them [to be considered an imbecile]. Rabbi Johanan said: Even if [he does only] one of them. It was taught: Who is deemed an imbecile? One who destroys everything which is given to him.[82]

Maimonides notes, however, that these are to be construed as examples, not as an exhaustive definition of insanity.[83] Moshe Halevi Spero, a contemporary Orthodox psychologist, suggests specific criteria for determining mental disorders in the cases of a person who commits suicide or a woman who seeks an abortion or permission to use contraceptive devices for reasons of mental health. "Generally speaking," he says, "*shtus* (insanity) might denote one who has lost the ability to reason or make reality-based judgments. *Shtus* may also signify the loss of emotional control."[84]

The legal implications of insanity in Jewish law were many. The Rabbis of the Mishnah and Talmud exempted the insane from responsibility in both ritual and civil law, and they made the insane ineligible for certain legal roles (for example, being empowered as another person's legal agent).[85] The Talmud permitted lighting a candle in violation of the Sabbath rules for a woman in labor in order to spare her psychic anguish.[86] Citing that precedent, Nahmanides (thirteenth century) specifically included mental illness in the category of "saving one's life" (pikuah nefesh) so that almost all obligations and prohibitions could be laid aside in order to save a person's mental health as well as his or her physical health.[87] Other issues concerning the mentally ill that arose in Jewish law included defining the exact legal responsibility of someone who did not have free will (psychological determinism), who was under the influence of alcohol or drugs, who was a homosexual, or who wanted to abort a fetus.[88] Contemporary rabbinic authorities are increasingly interested in the progress of psychology as a science because of its legal as well as its therapeutic ramifications.

Especially because mental illness was often not curable, the Jewish tradition sought to prevent it by offering advice for maintaining mental health, often suggesting the cultivation of specific personal characteristics and values. The biblical *Book of Proverbs* provides an early instance of such advice. Perhaps the most famous example in Rabbinic literature is *Ethics of the Fathers (Avot),* a tractate of the Mishnah (edited 220

C.E.) which is read every Sabbath afternoon during the weeks between Passover and Shavu'ot (Pentecost). A thousand years later Maimonides wrote a book on personality traits in which he embraced the Aristotelian golden mean as the proper guideline. He suggested that one who was very calm, for example, should try to go to the other extreme in order to maintain a balance of spirit.[89] Jews in Medieval Spain also produced important psychological–ethical handbooks, including *Hovot ha-Levavot (Duties of the Heart)* by Bahya ibn Paquda (eleventh century); *Sefer ha-Hinukh (Book of Education)* by Aaron He-Levi of Barcelona (thirteenth century); and *Kad ha-Cemah (Measure of Flour)* by Bahya ben Asher (thirteenth century).[90] In the nineteenth and twentieth centuries the Musar movement spread through some Orthodox communities of eastern Europe, seeking to balance the heavy emphasis on study of texts and intellectual analysis that was common in traditional seminaries with materials and sessions devoted to moral and spiritual development.

In such ways, Jews sought to prevent and cure mental illness. After the bands of prophets during biblical times (see 1 *Sm.* 10:5–12; 19:8–24), we do not hear of Jewish communities isolating the mentally ill. The Rabbis limited the legal incapacities of the insane as much as possible, distinguishing between those times when a man was apparently sane and therefore legally capable and those times in which he was not.[91] However primitive their understanding of mental illness, Jews saw it as an illness and not as a moral fault. They therefore did not treat it as something for which one should repent or be punished, but rather sought to prevent or cure it as part of their general obligation to heal. This prepared the way for Sigmund Freud and many other Jews to develop and practice the modern medical forms of psychological care.

Sexuality

For Judaism, sexual relations are a good thing within marriage; in fact, they were prescribed in two separate commandments of God. One was the command to "be fruitful and multiply" (*Gn.* 1:28). The other asserts that a man must not withhold from his wife "her food, her clothing, or her conjugal rights" (*Ex.* 21:10). The fact that these were two separate commandments meant that a man's duty to have sexual relations with his wife was independent from his duty to propagate, and consequently the duty to fulfill the woman's sexual needs continued even after the man had fulfilled the duty to propagate; that is, after he had begotten two children, one male and one female, in accordance with the verse in *Genesis* 1:27, "male and female He created them."

The Rabbis of the Mishnah had no qualms about spelling out specifically how often a man should offer to have sexual relations with his wife in order to fulfill the commandment in *Exodus:*

> If a man forbade himself by vow to have intercourse with his wife, the House of Shammai ruled: she may consent to the deprivation for two weeks; the House of Hillel ruled: only for one week.
>
> Students may leave home to study the Torah without the permission of their wives for a period of thirty days; laborers for only one week.
>
> The times for conjugal duty prescribed in the Torah are: for men of independent means, every day; for laborers, only twice a week; for ass-drivers, once a week; for camel-drivers, once in thirty days; for sailors, once in six months. These are the rulings of Rabbi Eliezer.[92]

These rules clearly recognized a woman's need for sexual relations and granted legal status to that need by imposing an obligation on her husband.

The man also has sexual rights in marriage according to Jewish law, as the Mishnah specified:

> If a wife rebels against her husband, her marriage contract may be reduced by seven *denarii* per week. . . . For how long may the reduction continue to be made? Until a sum corresponding to her marriage contract has accumulated [at which time he may divorce her without giving her any monetary marriage settlement whatsoever]. . . . Similarly, if a husband rebels against his wife, an addition of three *denarii* a week is made to her marriage contract. . . .[93]

Underlying this obligation was the basic principle that sexual relations were a special form of communication and bonding between husband and wife. Sexual energies were thus to be channeled toward good purpose, that is, the strengthening of the marital bond. Consequently, all sexual relations outside marriage were prohibited, although premarital sex was punished much less harshly than adultery or incest.

Celibacy was frowned upon. Thus, despite Rabbi Hamnuna's scholarly reputation among his third-century colleagues, Rabbi Huna turned away from him in disgust, refusing to see him until he was married, for "He who is twenty years of age and is not married spends all of his days in . . . sinful thoughts." According to another rabbinic passage, "A man without a wife lives without blessing, without life, without joy, without health, and without peace. . . ." A medieval, mystical source carried this one step further: "The divine presence can rest only upon a married man because an unmarried man is but half a man and the divine presence does not rest upon that which is imperfect." So important was it to take a wife that Jews could "sell a scroll of the

Torah for the purpose of [having enough money to] marry." Such practices contrasted sharply with the ideal of monasticism held by a number of elements within Christianity.[94] This emphasis on marriage is in part an appreciation for the fullness of life it affords and its role in transferring Jewish culture to the next generation, but it is also a reaction to the fear of the power of sex. Marriage was a way to satisfy a man's sexual drive so that he could devote his life to the raising of a family, work, and study.

Jews shared the abhorrence of masturbation that characterized other societies. Interestingly, although legal writers did not debate the prohibition of this act, they had difficulty locating a biblical base for it, and no less an authority than Maimonides claimed that it could not be punishable by the court because there was not an explicit negative commandment to forbid it. In part, the prohibition undoubtedly stemmed from assumptions about the medical consequences of ejaculation, as Maimonides explained:

> Semen constitutes the strength of the body, its life, and the light of the eyes. Its emission to excess causes physical decay, debility, and diminished vitality. Thus Solomon, in his wisdom, says: "Do not give your strength to women" [*Proverbs* 31:3]. Whoever indulges in sexual dissipation becomes prematurely aged; his strength fails; his eyes become dim, a foul odor proceeds from his mouth and armpits; the hair of his head, eyebrows, and eyelashes drops out; the hair of his beard, armpits, and legs grows abnormally; his teeth fall out; and besides these, he becomes subject to numerous other diseases. Medical authorities have stated that for each one who dies of other maladies, a thousand are the victims of sexual excess.[95]

Although Jews feared the medical consequences of masturbation, Jewish sources did not prohibit it for those reasons, but rather because of the self-pollution involved and the murder of unborn generations. Of these two concerns, the former was far more pronounced, but the mystical tradition in Judaism gave particular emphasis to the latter theme. It pointed out that a man who masturbated was guilty not only of murder but of killing his own children; therefore, he was a criminal more reprehensible than any other. Moreover, the mystics claimed that even involuntary emissions of semen created demons, a notion common in folk literature. Thus the narrator in I. B. Singer's book, *Gimpel the Fool,* said: "I was not born. My father sinned as did Onan, and from his seed I was created—half spirit, half-demon." These notions gave graphic and harsh expression to the belief that exposed semen somehow contaminated the environment and tainted its holiness. Nevertheless, ejaculation was prized in heterosexual relations, even when it did not lead to procreation, for no "murder" took place, nor were the forces of evil enhanced.[96] Apparently, for the Talmud and the medievals even the medical hazards of ejaculation were inoperative during intercourse.

From biblical times, Jews had a similar abhorrence of menstruation. Great pains were taken to avoid the slightest contact, even between husband and wife, for the whole traditional lore threatened the direst of consequences for those who touched the menses (let alone had intercourse during its flow)—extending to the children of the offenders and to their lives in the hereafter. The Talmud even claimed that a snake threatening to bite a woman would glide hastily away if she simply announced, "I am menstruating!"[97] There is no doubt that the fear of menstruation must have made women feel contaminated. At the same time, both Maimonides and Caro permitted a menstruating woman to hold a Torah scroll and to study from it.[98] Based on these mixed signals, contemporary Jews speculate widely on the extent to which menstruation provided a biological rationale in Talmudic and medieval times for excluding women from certain ritual, legal, and social roles.

Children were always considered a blessing among Jews, who took many measures to cure barrenness and to prevent miscarriages. These included wearing a stone amulet; reciting designated biblical passages; imbibing one of the many fertility potions made from fecund animals like the hare or fish; eating spicy or heavy foods like strong wines, dairy products, eggs, garlic, and meat; and avoiding light or unseasoned foods like melons and fish. In thirteenth-century Germany, Judah the Pious used the fairly common therapeutic device of a symbolic burial in order to give a barren woman a new identity, thereby freeing her from the barrenness of her previous existence.[99]

It was important not only to have children, but right and proper children, and it was believed that the time of coition, its form, and the thoughts of the parents during it had a bearing upon the offspring's character. Friday night, the eve of the Sabbath, was considered to be the most propitious time, and if at all possible one was to take advantage of the beneficial effects of the waxing moon by having intercourse during the first half of the lunar month. The Talmud permitted non-vaginal sex, but medieval texts depicted fearful consequences for the children of parents who engaged in such practices. Parents were sternly warned not to have relations when they were on bad terms and not to think of other individuals or of unpleasant and unworthy things during coitus. "The embryo is formed in consonance with the thoughts and emotions of the parents," claimed the Talmud, "and the greatest part of infant mortality is due to neglect of this principle." Having the courage to take this theory to its logical conclusion, the rabbis noted that "most bastards are bright because the union of their parents is consummated in love and joy!" Because the mother's thoughts were decisive, medieval Jews were especially cautious about the influences on her—to the point of blindfolding her on the way home from the ritual bath that permitted intercourse after menses, so that she would not be distracted from thinking of pious men and thus would have a good chance of conceiving one.[100]

Despite the command to have two children and the ideal of having more, and despite the general prohibition against "wasting the seed," contraception was permitted under certain circumstances. In general, the tradition, both for exegetical and economic reasons, understood the command to propagate to obligate the male but not the female. That, plus the prohibition against masturbation, meant that female forms of contraception were permitted while male forms were not. Talmudic sources indicate that mechanical and oral forms of contraception were in practice then, but the specific circumstances under which female contraception was permitted are not clear. There was an ambiguous Talmudic ruling on the subject, and medieval commentators took varying positions. Those who followed the lead of Rashi (eleventh century), the most famous commentator on the Talmud (for example, Rabbi Meir Posner of eighteenth-century Danzig, Rabbi Akiva Eger of nineteenth-century Posen in Prussia, and Rabbi Moses Sofer of nineteenth-century Pressburg), allowed contraception when medical reasons required it, but not otherwise. The majority of authorities, however, followed the reading of Rabbenu Tam, one of Rashi's grandsons, who permitted women to use contraceptive devices even in situations where the mother's life was not directly threatened. Rabbi Solomon Luria, in sixteenth-century Poland, permitted women to use contraceptive devices even for non-therapeutic purposes.[101] Because propagation was commanded, it can be assumed that even liberal Jews would have limited the use of contraceptives to those couples who had already fulfilled the commandment by having a boy and a girl—unless, of course, the medical condition of the woman or fetus required it.[102]

In contemporary times, when couples frequently postpone marriage until after extended education and the initiation of a career, the modern Jewish movements have varied widely in their response to family planning. Some allow contraception even before having children, and that has been the practice of the vast majority of Jews. Because of the loss of one-third of the Jewish population during the Holocaust, and because of the high rate of intermarriage and the extremely low birth rate among Jews, Jewish religious leaders have increasingly stressed the need for Jews to propagate, thus tempering an otherwise liberal approach to contraception on the part of many non-Orthodox rabbis and most Jews.

Sterilization was traditionally prohibited by Jews because it mutilated God's property. However, a few recent responsa have addressed the new methods of sterilization through vasectomies and tubal ligations. Both traditional and liberal respondents have forbidden vasectomies on the basis of the rabbinic interpretation and extension of *Deuteronomy* 23:2: "No one whose testes are crushed . . . shall be admitted into the congregation of the Lord." Jewish responses to tubal ligations have been more permissive both because a woman does not come under that Deuteronomic prohibition and also because she is not obligated to procreate. All have agreed, however, that even male sterilization is permitted and perhaps even required if the man's life or health makes it necessary.[103]

The Bible proscribed homosexuality in the strongest of terms: "Do not lie with a male as one lies with a woman; it is an abomination" (*Lv.* 18:22). In light of that, Jewish homosexuals of times past hid their orientation as much as possible. In the last decade, however, as homosexuals of all religious persuasions have become more open about their sexual behavior, Jews have begun a rather painful reexamination of the traditional stance on this issue. The Reform movement has even accepted several avowedly homosexual congregations as full members of the Union of American Hebrew Congregations, although this was not accomplished without controversy. There have been several positions articulated within the Conservative movement, but none has been as liberal as the Reform policy, and Orthodox spokesmen have maintained the traditional abhorrence of homosexuality.[104]

Issues at the Beginning of Life

Traditional sources could not have contemplated modern reproductive technology, and so little was said that is directly relevant to many issues that it raises. Contemporary rabbis extend the law to cover these issues as lawyers and judges do in other legal systems—by analogy and by reference to the values behind the law.

According to Jewish law, adultery or incest does not take place until and unless the penis of the man enters the vaginal cavity of the woman. Consequently, the laws against adultery and incest do not apply to artificial insemination. Even the most stringent rabbinic authorities would permit a husband to have his semen implanted in the uterus of his wife. However, rabbis are much less sanguine about having some other man serve as the donor or using a surrogate mother, practices often prohibited on the basis of concern about unintentional incest in the next generation (that is, if the child of the artificial insemination happens to marry his or her natural half-brother or half-sister). Similiar remarks apply to in-vitro fertilization: There is no objection if the husband and wife are the donors and the zygote is implanted in the uterus of the wife. All of this, of course, is condoned only when conception cannot take place through sexual intercourse.

When a couple cannot have children, Jewish law permits adoption. Several passages in the Bible seem to indicate that there was a formal ceremony of adoption during biblical times, although that is not specified in any legal source of the Bible. Talmudic literature prescribed no formal ceremony, but rabbinic law stipulated that a child who lived with a man for six months or more legally became the child of that man—a provision recently used in a New York State civil case.[105]

Rabbinic sources understood the process of gestation in a developmental way. Specifically, within the first forty days after conception (within the first three months, according to some sources), they regarded the zygote as "simply water." That meant that abortion during that time was permitted for more reasons than it was during the second period of pregnancy, which lasted until the moment of birth (when the head emerged, or, if a breech birth, when the shoulders emerged). During that second period of gestation, Jewish law did not regard the fetus as a full-fledged human being with all the rights pertaining thereto, while the mother clearly was. Consequently, if the fetus threatened the life or health of the mother, then it had to be aborted, as the following Mishnah graphically stipulated:

> If a woman has [life-threatening] difficulty in childbirth, one dismembers the embryo in her, limb by limb, because her life takes precedence over its life. Once its head [or its "greater part"] has emerged, it may not be touched, for we do not set aside one life for another.[106]

While all Jewish sources have required abortion in order to preserve the life or organs of the mother, opinion has differed on how much of a threat to a woman's health the fetus must pose in justifying an abortion or requiring it. Citing a responsum by Rabbi Israel Mizrahi (eighteenth century), some authorities have permitted an abortion to preserve the mother's mental health. Some traditional rabbis have used the consideration of the mother's mental health as a roundabout way for justifying abortion in cases where amniocentesis has revealed that the child will be malformed or will have a genetic, degenerative disease like Tay-Sachs. They have engaged in that form of legal legerdemain because there is no justification in the traditional sources for abortion for reasons having to do with the health of the fetus; only the mother's health is a consideration. That, of course, is probably because until recently it was impossible to know very much about the fetus before birth. Noting that fact, some Conservative and Reform rabbis claim that we now can and should establish the fetus' health as an independent consideration when judging whether an abortion is justified.[107]

In practice, Jews who wish an abortion rarely worry about a justification—to the extent that among Jews in Israel, who number approximately 3.5 million, there were at least 600,000 abortions between
the state's founding in 1948 and 1975. That is a particularly problematic
phenomenon for the contemporary Jewish community because Jews are
barely reproducing themselves in Israel and are falling far short of that
in the United States, where the Jewish reproductive rate is approximately
1.6 or 1.7 children per couple. Consequently, even those rabbis who
are liberal in their interpretation of Jewish abortion law also are calling
for Jews to marry and to have children so that the Jewish people and
Judaism can continue for more than another generation or two.[108]

Issues at the End of Life

The criterion of death in Jewish law was based upon the passage in
Genesis 7:22, "All creatures in whose nostrils was the breath of life."
Because the Bible identified life with breathing, and because testing the
breath of a person was easy (one simply put a feather to the nostrils
of a patient), Jews used the breath test to determine death. One position
in the Talmud required that there also be cessation of heartbeat, a
condition some medieval sources considered to be the primary factor
in ascertaining death, with cessation of breath simply indicating loss
of cardiac function. Because of a comment of Isserles on the *Shulhan
'arukh* (1567) that we are no longer competent to determine the exact
moment of death, during the last several hundred years people normally
have waited for periods extending between twenty minutes and an
hour after cessation of both breath and heartbeat before beginning
preparations for burial.[109]

Traditional Judaism has not allowed cremation, because that constitutes destruction and desecration of God's property. However, many
authorities have permitted the use of organs for the life or health of
other living human beings, because that does not desecrate the dead
person, but rather, honors him or her. The one complicating factor is
that the person must legally be dead before the bodily part may be
transplanted. Consequently, there is no problem, for example, in willing
the corneas of one's eyes to another because they are usable for as
long as twenty-four hours after death. Because of doubts about the
moment of death, transplanting vital organs such as the heart or kidneys
is much more complicated for Jews. Some Conservative and Reform
authorities permit organ transplants after a flat electroencephalogram
reading.[110]

Similiar considerations apply to autopsies. Although rabbis differ as
to how specific the reason must be in order to justify an autopsy, if

there is some medical or legal reason for doing an autopsy, Judaism allows it. In the landmark decision on this, Ezekiel Landau (eighteenth century) permitted autopsies only when life depends upon this particular autopsy. Modern means of communication have ironically led Orthodox rabbis to be more restrictive in permitting autopsies on the grounds that autopsies done elsewhere may yield the desired information, while the same improved communications have prompted Reform Rabbi Solomon Freehof to claim that the "at hand" requirement is no longer necessary because people everywhere will benefit from the new medical knowledge revealed by an autopsy.[111]

Jewish sources have classified active means of euthanasia as murder, even when the motivation of the perpetrator was benign. They have, however, allowed passive euthanasia when a cure is no longer possible. Although the sources have not put it in quite this way, the general principle is that Jews are commanded to cure, but not to perpetuate life beyond its natural bounds. Two Talmudic passages and one thirteenth-century responsum described situations in which it was permissible to let nature take its course.[112] The principle embodied in these sources was later incorporated into the glosses of Rabbi Moses Isserles on the *Shulhan 'arukh* (sixteenth century) as follows:

> One in a dying condition is considered a living being in all respects. . . . Whoever closes the eyes [of the dying person] is regarded as one who sheds blood. . . . *Gloss:* . . . It is likewise forbidden to do anything to hasten the death of one who is in a dying condition. For example, if one has been in a dying condition for a long time and could not depart, we may not remove the pillow or the mattress from under him just because some say that there are feathers from some fowl which cause this prolongation of death. Similarly, we may not move him from his place. . . . However if there is anything which causes a hindrance to the departure of the soul, e.g. if near the house there is a knocking sound of a wood cutter, or there is salt on his tongue, and these hinder the departure of the soul, it is permitted to remove it, for there is no direct action involved since he merely removes the hindrance.[113]

The thirteenth-century source actually *prohibited* any action that might lengthen the patient's agony by preventing his quick death, and it forbade those attending at the moment of death to cry lest the noise restore the soul to the deceased. Some later authorities even prohibited the use of medicines to "delay the departure of the soul."[114] Modern technology has obviously made these questions considerably more complicated by enhancing the ability to maintain many bodily functions artificially, thereby blurring the distinction between life and death. Contemporary rabbis therefore differ markedly on many of the particular questions that have arisen in this regard.[115] Whatever their differences, they all attempt to balance the tradition's underlying principles of respect for life against the permission, and perhaps the obligation, to let nature take its course at some point.

Judaism thus has had a long history of dealing with medical questions. Its answers have been informed by its fundamental theory of the body as the creation and property of God on loan for the duration of life. Although the following Mishnah is written as a warning to witnesses in capital cases and not in a medical context, it offers a fitting expression of the sacredness of life within Judaism that makes concern for the well-being of the body a matter of divine import:

> Only one man was originally created in order to teach the lesson that if one destroys a single person, Scripture imputes it to him as if he had destroyed the whole population of the world. And if he saves the life of a single person, Scripture imputes it to him as though he had saved the whole world.[116]

Notes

Citations in the Mishnah are noted with tractate, chapter, and section, e.g., *Bava Kamma* 8:1. References to the *Babylonian Talmud* are either preceded by "B.T." or carry no prefix before the name of the tractate and the page number in the standard, Bomberg edition (e.g., B.T. *Bava Kamma* 86a, or, simply *Bava Kamma* 86a). References to the *Palestinian Talmud* are preceded by "P.T.," to the *Mishneh Torah* of Maimonides by "M.T.;" and to the *Shulhan 'arukh* by Caro (with glosses by Isserles) by "S.A."

The Mishnah has been translated in one volume by Herbert Danby (London, 1933) and in six volumes by Philip Blackman (London, 1955). The Babylonian Talmud has been translated in thirty-five volumes under the general editorship of I. Epstein (London, 1935–1959). Most of Maimonides' *Mishneh Torah* has been translated in twenty-one volumes under the general editorship of Leon Nemoy (New Haven, 1949–1979). The major collection of Midrash, Midrash Rabbah, consisting of rabbinic commentaries on the Torah (Pentateuch) and the five scrolls read in the synagogue *(Song of Songs, Ruth, Lamentations, Ecclesiastes,* and *Esther)* has been translated in ten volumes under the editorship of H. Freedman and Maurice Simon (London, 1939–1951). Jacob Neusner is in the process of translating the Palestinian Talmud under the title of *The Talmud of the Land of Israel* (Chicago, 1983–1984), ten volumes of which have appeared as of this writing. The *Shulkhan 'arukh* has not been translated.

1. Milton Himmelfarb and David Singer, eds., *American Jewish Yearbook, 1983* (New York, 1982), 83:275–279.
2. Isaiah 49:6; see also Isaiah 51:4.
3. *Tosefta, Pisha* 4:14; B.T. *Pesahim* 66a.
4. See *Berakhot* 61a, b; *Sanhedrin* 38a; *Genesis Rabbah* 1:3; *Exodus Rabbah* 24:1; and *Numbers Rabbah* 18:22 for examples of the Rabbis' praise of the body. See *Sanhedrin* 91a, b; *Shabbat* 152b; and *Genesis Rabbah* 67:3 for examples of the interaction of body and soul in

determining the virtuous or sinful nature of a person. See also A. Cohen, *Everyman's Talmud* (New York, 1949), pp. 67–78, 88–95, on these topics.

5. P.T. *Kiddushin* 66d.
6. *Ta'anit* 11a; See also M.T. *Laws of Ethics* 3:1.
7. On the primacy of preserving life over other commandments, see *Yoma* 83–84; M.T. *Shabbat,* ch. 2. On the requirements to live where there is a physician, see P.T. *Kiddushin* 66d; see also B.T. *Sanhedrin* 17b.
8. *Leviticus Rabbah* 34:3.
9. M.T. *Laws of Ethics,* chs. 3–5.
10. Ibid. 3:3; see also 4:1.
11. Maimonides, *Guide for the Perplexed,* M. Friedlander, trans. (London, 1904) Part III, chs. 33, 35, 48.
12. *Tanhuma Buber,* Shemini, 15b; see also *Genesis Rabbah* 44:1 and *Leviticus Rabbah* 13:3.
13. *Berakhot* 53b.
14. See ibid. 55a, *Sotah* 4b.
15. *Sanhedrin* 17b; *Avodah Zarah* 20b; P.T. *Shabbat* 1:3; Solomon Ganzfried, *Kitzur Shulhan Arukh* (translated by Hyman E. Goldin as "Code of Jewish Law," New York: 1927), Part 1, ch. 2:1.
16. Salo Wittmayer Baron, *The Jewish Community,* 3 vols. (Philadelphia, 1948), 2:197–198.
17. Maimonides, *Guide,* Part 3, ch. 27.
18. *1 Maccabees* 1:15.
19. *Antiquities* XV 8:1.
20. S.A. *Orah Hayyim* 308:45 and 518:2.
21. See, for example, Simon Greenberg, *A Jewish Philosophy and Pattern of Life* (New York, 1981), pp. 416–417.
22. See J. Bleich, "Smoking," *Tradition* 16:4 (Summer 1977), 130–133 for a review of Orthodox opinions. The Rabbinical Assembly, the association of Conservative rabbis, has passed a resolution forbidding smoking; see *Proceedings of the Rabbinical Assembly* 44 (1983), p. 182. For a Reform position, see Solomon Freehof, *Reform Response for Our Time* (Cincinnati, 1977), ch. 11.
23. See Sidney B. Hoenig, "The Use of Drugs: An Historic Excursion," in Leo Landman, ed., *Judaism and Drugs* (New York, 1973), pp. 39–50; Walter S. Wurzburger, "The Jewish Attitude Toward Psychedelic Religion," ibid., pp. 135–143; David Novak, "Alcohol and Drug Abuse in the Perspective of Jewish Tradition, *Judaism* 33 (1984): 221–232. On the use of experimental drugs to cure or to relieve pain, see J. David Bleich, *Judaism and Healing: Halakhic Perspectives* (New York, 1981), pp. 116–122, 137–139.
24. See Landman, L., ed., *Judaism and Drugs;* Menachem M. Brayer, "Drugs: A Jewish View," in Fred Rosner and J. David Bleich, eds., *Jewish Bioethics* (New York, 1979), pp. 242–250; Alex J. Goldman, *Judaism Confronts Contemporary Issues* (New York, 1978), ch. 10; Novak, "Alcohol."
25. See "Drunkenness," *Encyclopedia Judaica* 6:237–241; Goldman, *Judaism;* Novak, "Alcohol."
26. *Shabbat* 55a; see also *Sanhedrin* 101a.
27. *Midrash Tadshe* 16.
28. See *Menahot* 29b for a powerful Talmudic example.

29. *Bava Batra* 55b; *Shabbat* 129b.
30. *Berakhot* 25a; *Shabbat* 109b; *Ta'anit* 21b; *Ketubbot* 20a, 77a; *Gittin* 70a; *Avodah Zarah* 30a; *Hullin* 48a; etc.
31. *Shabbat* 41a; *Bavia Metzia* 107b; *Hullin* 51a.
32. *Gittin* 70b; *Sanhedrin* 100b; *Ketubbot* 100a.
33. See Note 7.
34. See *Jeremiah* 8:22; *Hosea* 5:13; *Job* 13:4; 2 *Chronicles* 16:12.
35. *Ecclesiasticus* 38:1–12.
36. E.g. *Exodus* 15:26; *Deuteronomy* 32:39; *Isaiah* 19:22, 57:18–19; *Jeremiah* 30:17, 33:6; *Hosea* 6:1; *Psalms* 103:2–3, 107:20; *Job* 5:18.
37. *Bava Kamma* 85a; *Sanhedrin* 73a.
38. *Sanhedrin* 84b and Rashi's commentary there. See also Nahmanides (1194–1270), *Kitvei Haramban*, Bernard Chavel, ed., (Jerusalem, 1963), vol. 2, p. 43.
39. S.A. *Yoreh De'ah* 336:1.
40. *Midrash Temurrah*, as cited in *Otzar Midrashim*, J. D. Eisenstein, ed., 2 volumes (New York: 1915), 2:580–581.
41. See Rashi's commentary on *Pesahim* 21b for the *Leviticus* homily. See *Gittin* 5:8–9; *Avodah Zarah* 26a; *Bava Kamma* 113b; and *Gittin* 61a for the concern for good relations and honoring God.
42. *Avodah Zarah* 26a; M.T. *Laws of Idolatry* 10:2. The Noahic laws, which, according to Talmudic traditions, had been given to all descendants of Noah, prohibit murder, theft, incest, idolatry, blasphemy, and tearing a limb from a living animal, and they require the establishment of civil laws and courts (*Sanhedrin* 56a).
43. *Gittin* 70a and the commentary of *Tosafot* there; *Tur, Yoreh De'ah* 158 and the commentary of *Bet Yosef* there.
44. See Harry Friedenwald, *The Jews and Medicine* (Baltimore, 1944), pp. 47, 560, 564 ff., 570, 591, 622. On violating the Sabbath to treat a non-Jew, see *Yoma* 84b; S.A. *Orah Hayyim* 329:2; 330:2; *Even Haezer* 4:34; Me'iri, *Bet Habehirah* (Bnei Brak, Israel: 1966) on *Yoma* 84b and 85a, pp. 249–253.
45. Luther is quoted in Joshua Trachtenberg, *Jewish Magic and Superstition* (New York, 1939), p. 6. On the relationship between the Jews and the Black Plague, see Seraphine Guerchberg, "The Controversy Over the Alleged Sowers of the Black Death in the Contemporary Treatises on Plague," in *Change in Medieval Society*, ed. Sylvia L. Thrupp (New York, 1964), pp. 208–224.
46. *Bava Kamma* 8:1; B.T. *Bava Kamma* 85a.
47. *Ta'anit* 21b.
48. Rabbi Eleazar Fleckeles, *Teshuvah Meahavah* (Prague, 1808) III, on *Yoreh De'ah* 336.
49. S.A. *Yoreh De'ah* 249:16; 255:2.
50. See Baron, *The Jewish Community*, 2:115, 329.
51. 2 *Kings* 15:5; 2 *Chronicles* 26:21; *Bava Metzia* 83b.
52. See "Hospitals," *Encyclopedia Judaica* 8:1033–1040; David Rosner, *A Once Charitable Enterprise: Hospitals and Health Care in Brooklyn and New York, 1885–1915* (New York: 1982).
53. *Nedarim* 40a; see also M.T. *Laws of Mourning* 14:4.
54. *Shabbat* 127a.
55. *Sotah* 14a. Visiting the sick is called "a religious precept" in S.A. *Yoreh De'ah* 335:1.

56. S.A. *Yoreh De'ah* 335:2.
57. Baron, *Jewish Community*, 1:362 ff, 2:327 ff.
58. S.A. *Yoreh De'ah* 151:12 and 335:9.
59. Ibid. 335.
60. *Berakhot* 60a.
61. *Bava Batra* 116.
62. *Yoma* 8:5.
63. *Ta'ame Ha Minhagim* II, 41a, cited in Trachtenberg, *Jewish Magic*, p. 196. See also *Shabbat* 67a; Sherira Gaon, *Takhkemoni* (Bern:1910), vol. 1, p. 71.
64. See also Trachtenberg, *Jewish Magic*, pp. 196–197 and n. 7 on p. 304.
65. *Shabbat* 40a; *Gittin* 70b.
66. *Avodah Zarah* 11a; P.T. *Abodah Zarah* 2:2, 40d; *Pesahim* 113a.
67. *Berakhot* 40a, 44b, 57b; *Bava Batra* 58b.
68. *Ketubbot* 110b. A compendium of rabbinic cures can be found in *Gittin* 68b–70b and in Cohen, *Everyman's Talmud*, pp. 250–259.
69. Tosafot, *Mo'ed Katan* 11a; Jacob ben Moses Mollin, *Yalkutai Maharil* (Segal), cited in Fred Rosner, *Medicine in the Bible and the Talmud* (New York, 1977), p. 21. See also Solomon Luria, *Yam Shel Shlomo*, "Kol Basar," Section 12; Caro, *Kesef Mishneh* commentary to M.T. *Laws of Ethics* 4:18; Gombiner, *Magen Avraham* commentary to S.A. *Orah Hayyim* 173.
70. Trachtenberg, *Jewish Magic*, p. 203.
71. *Shabbat* 108b, which quotes Samuel; *Bava Kamma* 60b; *Ketubbot* 77a; *Tosefta Bava Batra* 1; *Avodah Zarah* 27b; *Sanhedrin* 9a.
72. *Berakhot* 10b; *Shevuot* 15b; *Sanhedrin* 10:1; B.T. *Sanhedrin* 101a.
73. *Shabbat* 67a; *Gittin* 69a.
74. Israel Isserlein, *Pesakim Uketavim* (Furth, 1778) 96; Solomon Luria, *Responsa* (Furth, 1768), no. 3.
75. *Sefer Gematriot*, a fourteenth-century German–Jewish work that lists such cures, is translated in Trachtenberg, *Jewish Magic*, pp. 109–111. *Sefer Raziel*, compiled in the thirteenth century but containing much Geonic material, has directions for the use of the names of God; see *ibid.*, p. 97.
76. Judah he-Hasid, *Sefer Hasidim* (Bologna, 1538), par. 1153.
77. See Trachtenberg, *Jewish Magic*, pp. 200–201, and the references there.
78. Ibid., pp. 137, 204–206, and *passim*.
79. *Shevuot* 15b; see also Trachtenberg, *Jewish Magic*, pp. 107–113, 198.
80. Trachtenberg, *Jewish Magic*, pp. 46–47, 110–113, 133, 144, 146–147, 194, 252, 259.
81. Julius Preuss, *Biblical and Talmudic Medicine*, Fred Rosner, trans. (New York, 1978), ch. 11. Fred Rosner, *Medicine in the Bible and the Talmud*, (New York, 1977), p. 32, classifies King Saul as suffering from "a paranoid psychopathia." See M. Gorlin, "Mental Illness in Biblical Literature," *Proceedings of the Association of Orthodox Jewish Scientists*, 1 (1970): 43–62.
82. *Hagigah* 3b–4a; see also Tosefta, *Terumot* 1:3; B.T. *Shabbat* 105b; *Sanhedrin* 65b; *Niddah* 17a.
83. M.T. *Laws of Testimony* 9:9–11, and see the commentary of the *Kesef Mishneh* there.
84. Moshe Halevi Spero, *Judaism and Psychology: Halakhic Perspectives* (New York, 1980), p. 175; see pp. 174–178 generally.

85. *Hagigah* 1:1; *Bava Kamma* 8:4; *Gittin* 23a; S.A. *Hoshen Mishpat* 188:2.
86. *Shabbat* 128b.
87. *The Writings of Nahmanides*, trans. C. Chavel, 2 volumes, (New York, 1968), 2:43.
88. On all of these, cf, Spero, *Judaism and Psychology*, chs. 3, 9, 11, and 12.
89. M.T. *Laws of Ethics*, chs. 1–3.
90. Translated into English by C. Chavel under the title *Encyclopedia of Torah Thoughts* (New York, 1980).
91. Tosefta, *Terumot* 1:3; see also B.T. *Rosh Hashanah* 28a; *Yevamot* 31a, 113b; *Ketubbot* 20a.
92. *Ketubbot* 5:6.
93. Ibid. 5:7.
94. *Kiddushin* 29b–30a; *Midrash Psalms* on *Psalm* 59:2; *Zohar Hadash* 4.50b; *Megillah* 27a. See 1 *Corinthians* 7:25–40.
95. Maimonides, *Mishnah Commentary, Sanhedrin* 7:4; M.T. *Laws of Ethics* 4:19.
96. *Zohar*, "Vay'hi," 219b; "Bereshit," 19b, 54b; "Emor," 90a. See David Feldman, *Marital Relations, Birth Control, and Abortion in Jewish Law* (New York, 1968), p. 120 and Part 3 generally on this topic.
97. *Shabbat* 110a.
98. M.T. *Laws of the Torah Scroll* 10:8; S.A. *Yoreh De'ah* 282:9.
99. Trachtenberg, *Jewish Magic*, pp. 33–34, 137, 184–190, and 295, note 3.
100. *Ibid.*, pp. 184–190. For the Talmudic passages cited, see *Ketubbot* 48a; *Nedarim* 20a; *Shevuot* 18b. See also Feldman, *Marital Relations*, pp. 155–163.
101. The chief Talmudic sources on contraception are *Yevamot* 12b and 65b. For a thorough discussion of this, see Feldman, *Marital Relations*, Chs. 9–13.
102. Ibid., pp. 224–225.
103. M.T. *Laws of Forbidden Intercourse* 16:2,6; S.A. *Even Haezer* 5:2; Bleich, *Judaism and Healing*, p. 65; David M. Feldman and Fred Rosner, eds., *Compendium on Medical Ethics* (New York, 1984), pp. 46–47; Solomon B. Freeehof, "Sterilizing Husband," in *Reform Responsa* (Cincinnati, 1960), pp. 206–208.
104. See Goldman, *Judaism Confronts*, ch. 12, for a good summary of the positions. See also Reform Rabbi Solomon B. Freehof, "Judaism and Homosexuality: A Responsum," *C.C.A.R. Journal* 20:3 (Summer 1973): 31–33; Sanford Ragins, "An Echo of the Pleas of Our Fathers," ibid., pp. 41–47; and Conservative Rabbi Herschel J. Matt, "A Jewish Approach to Homosexuality," *Judaism* 27 (1978): 13–24.
105. Wener v. Wener 59 Misc. 2d 959, 301 N.Y. Supp. 2d 237 (Sup.Ct. 1969); and see appeal, 35 App. Div. 2d 50, 312 N.Y. Supp. 2d 815 (2d Dept. 1970).
106. *Ohalot* 7:6.
107. Mizrahi, *Responsa Pri Ha-aretz* (Jerusalem, 1899), vol. 3, *Yoreh De'ah*, no. 2. See Feldman, *Marital Relations*, pp. 284–294 and chs. 14–15 generally for an analysis of the historical sources on abortion. See also Alex J. Goldman, *Judaism Confronts*, ch. 3, for an overview of contemporary opinions within the Jewish community.

108. This is the figure cited by Dr. Haim Sadan, Advisor to Health Minister, Eliezer Shostak, in 1982; see *Jerusalem Post Magazine,* November 12, 1982, p. 8. Rabbi Jakobovits puts the number at one million; see Jakobovits, *Jewish Medical Ethics* (1975 edition), pp. 278–279.
109. *Yoma* 85a; S.A. *Orah Hayyim* 330:5. See Bleich, *Judaism and Healing,* pp. 148–153, for the various opinions on the relative weight given to the two criteria and on how long after death one must wait.
110. See Goldman, *Judaism Confronts,* ch. 13.
111. Ibid., ch. 6; Jakobovits, *Jewish Medical Ethics,* pp. 132–152, 278–283.
112. *Ketubbot* 104a; *Avodah Zarah* 18a; Rabbi Judah the Pious, *Sefer Hasidim,* nos. 723, 234.
113. S.A. *Yoreh De'ah* 339:1.
114. *Bet Ya'akov* no. 59; *Gilyon MaHaRSHa* on *Yoreh De'ah* 339:1; *Iggrot Moshe, Yoreh De'ah,* 2, no. 174.
115. See Goldman, *Judaism Confronts,* ch.11; Symposium on the California Natural Act (statements by Elliot Horowitz, Max A. Forse, Seymour Siegel, Moshe D. Tendler, and Hillel Cohn), *Sh'ma* 7 (1977): 93–102.
116. *Sanhedrin* 4:5.

CHAPTER 2

The Early

Christian

Tradition

DARREL W. AMUNDSEN
GARY B. FERNGREN

Christianity originated within the framework of Palestinian Judaism. Its founder was Jesus of Nazareth (ca. 4 B.C.E.–ca. C.E. 30), who, in a public ministry that lasted about three years, announced the coming of God's kingdom, which had long been awaited by the Jews. His ministry of preaching, teaching, and healing attracted widespread popular attention as well as growing opposition from Jewish religious leaders and ended with his death by crucifixion. Shortly after his death, a group of his followers in Jerusalem (led by the disciples that he had gathered around him) proclaimed that he had risen from the dead and ascended into heaven. They viewed his resurrection as the authentication of his claim to be the Jewish Messiah, the Son of God, who had by his death on the cross atoned for the sins of his people.

Jesus' followers carried the new faith throughout Palestine, where they initially sought converts among fellow Jews. The earliest significant attempt to win gentile (non-Jewish) converts to Christianity was made by the Apostle Paul. Born Saul of Tarsus (d. ca. C.E. 67), Paul was an early Jewish opponent of Christianity before his remarkable conversion to the new religion. Following his conversion, he made several missionary journeys throughout the Roman Empire and established churches in a number of important cities. By about C.E. 60, the new faith had been carried by Paul and others to most parts of the eastern Mediterranean and as far west as Rome. By the middle of the second century there were thriving Christian communities in all major and most minor cities of the Roman Empire. With the success of Paul's missionary activity among gentiles, tension developed over the question of whether gentile converts should be made to observe Jewish rites such as circumcision and traditional dietary practices. Paul's recommendation that they should not be required to do so was accepted by a council of Jesus' disciples (the apostles). As Jewish opposition to Christianity hardened and gentiles adopted the new faith in increasing numbers, Christianity's connection with Judaism gradually lessened.

Because the earliest Christians were Jews, who viewed Jesus' life and ministry as the fulfillment of Judaism, they regarded the Old Testament Scriptures as authoritative. In the first generation, the teachings of Jesus and the apostles were transmitted orally. As the apostolic writers committed their teaching to writing, their works began to circulate among the churches. These works included the four Gospels, *Acts,* and various letters (epistles) written by Paul and other apostles either to specific churches or to the churches in general. Some writings attributed to the apostles were accepted as unquestionably genuine and therefore authoritative, while the genuineness of others was disputed. In the third and fourth centuries, attempts were made to establish a canon of apostolic writings. The present New Testament canon of twenty-seven books finally received formal sanction in the churches by the Councils of Hippo (393) and Carthage (397).

In the first centuries of Christianity there were many attempts to define and systematize belief. In the controversies over doctrine that divided the early church, theologians sought to determine orthodoxy ("right belief"). Any belief that deviated from orthodoxy was called "heresy." One of the earliest (it appeared already in the first century) was Gnosticism, which regarded the material world as evil and sought salvation in esoteric knowledge. Probably the most important doctrinal dispute in the early church was over Arianism, a belief named after an Alexandrian priest, Arius (ca. 260–336), who taught that Jesus was a created being and therefore not coeternal with God the Father. The controversy split the church in the fourth century. Given the diversity of belief that likely existed at the local level in the early church, orthodoxy developed gradually over several centuries and came to be defined through the establishment of the New Testament canon, by councils, and in creeds that the majority of the Christian community accepted as authoritative statements of doctrine.

At first, Christianity was regarded by the Roman government as a Jewish sect and it benefited from special privileges enjoyed by the Jews. In C.E. 64, however, Nero accused the Christians of having set fire to Rome and began actively to persecute them. Thereafter, Christians faced persecution that was sometimes widespread and sometimes sporadic for the next 250 years. The Romans regarded them as traitors, for their refusal to offer sacrifice to the Roman emperor as a god; and atheists, for their failure to participate in public pagan worship. Rumor and mistrust led to charges against them of cannibalism, incest, and hatred of humankind. Full-scale systematic persecution throughout the Roman Empire broke out in the third century, culminating in violent persecution under the emperor Diocletian that began in 303. In 313, the emperor Constantine, who in the previous year had been converted to Christianity, issued (with his co-emperor Licinius) the Edict of Milan, which ended persecution and made Christianity for the first time a legal religion.

The reign of Constantine (312–337) marked a significant turning point in the history of Christianity. With the exception of Julian the Apostate (361–363), all subsequent Roman emperors professed Christianity and favored it in both policy and legislation. An alliance between church and state began that remained a constant, although frequently tense and conflictive, feature of western Christianity through the Middle Ages. Constantine provided public support for the church, granted various immunities and privileges to the clergy, strengthened church law by imposing the force of civil sanctions, attempted to suppress heresy, and sought, by summoning a church council in 325 at Nicaea, to settle the dispute between orthodox and Arian Christians. Although paganism remained the official Roman religion for most of the fourth century, it declined rapidly. In 391 the emperor Theodosius closed pagan temples, forbade public pagan worship, and made Christianity the official Roman religion.

Another significant event of Constantine's reign was his removing (in 330) the capital of the Roman Empire to the Greek city of Byzantium, which he renamed Constantinople. In 395 the Roman Empire was permanently divided, and this political separation ultimately led to the division of the church. In spite of heresies and schisms, the church had hitherto remained unified, although the western and eastern branches had begun to assume their own distinct theological and cultural identities in late antiquity. After 395 they increasingly diverged, although the division between eastern and western Christianity was not made official until the Great Schism of 1054.

One of the most notable developments in Christianity in late antiquity was the growth and spread of monasticism. Monasticism originated in Egypt with St. Anthony (251–356), the first well-known monk. It was an outgrowth of asceticism, a movement that encouraged Christians to lead holy lives by practicing mortification of the flesh. The earliest monks were hermits, or anchorites, who renounced the world and led solitary lives that were marked by self-denial and spiritual contemplation. In the fourth and fifth centuries, anchoritic monasticism began to give way to cenobitic monasticism, in which monks lived together in an ordered community. Monasticism was introduced into the West in the fourth century, where it gradually gained acceptance, particularly in the form developed by St. Benedict (480–543), who established several monasteries in Italy and composed a monastic rule that emphasized practicality and charity. Thereafter monasticism grew quickly in both the East and West. Monasteries came to be venerated as models of Christian society and exercised enormous influence.

Important for his influence on later western Christianity was Augustine (354–430), a transitional figure who represents a blending of Christianity and the classical tradition. The end of Augustine's long life marked a symbolic watershed in western Christianity. When he died in 430, Rome had already been sacked (twenty years earlier) by the barbarian Goths and North Africa was in the process of being conquered by the Vandals. The Roman world was rapidly disintegrating, as its western half was undergoing conquest by Germanic peoples from the North, some already Christianized, and was being drawn into the emerging European world of the Middle Ages.

––––––––––•⟨∞⟩••––––––––

The New Testament has much to say (both directly and indirectly) about health and healing. The writings that came to form the New Testament grew out of the faith of the earliest Christian communities and contain a great deal of diversity of theme and emphasis that reflects the diversities of that faith. While it is possible to see different theologies and motifs in these writings, the divergent traditions clearly formed a larger conceptual whole, which suggests that for all their differences, early Christians had much in common. It would be misleading to ignore the different perspectives of the writers of the New Testament, but it would be equally misleading to overlook their basic underlying faith, which gave a sense of unity and corporate belonging to the early Christians.

Health and Healing in the New Testament

The core of New Testament belief was the proclamation that God had provided salvation for the human race through his son Jesus Christ, who had made possible the restoration of a fellowship with God that had been broken by sin. For the writers of the New Testament, salvation resulted in the incorporation of believers into the body of Christ (the church) and their participation in the fellowship of Christ and fellow Christians. Reconciliation with God brought salvation from sin and from the consequences of sin and promised eternal life with Christ. In this life Christians could expect to be sustained by the grace of their heavenly

Father, who loved them and caused everything to work together for their good, including suffering, which the New Testament taught them to expect. God's grace was manifested in a fellowship based upon faith and trust in Christ in the midst of both those afflictions that were common to humanity and those that were peculiar to Christians. The writers of the New Testament never suggested that Christians should expect a life free from suffering. Whatever afflictions they experienced they should regard as only temporary and of little consequence when compared to the joys of heaven (eternal life; the absence of death; perfect health; and, above all, God's presence). "We do not lose heart," wrote the Apostle Paul. "Though our outer nature is wasting away, our inner nature is being renewed every day. For this slight momentary affliction is preparing us for an eternal weight of glory beyond all comparison" (2 Cor. 4:16–17).[1]

Suffering itself was seen by several New Testament writers as part of God's training, by which Christians would grow toward spiritual maturity (Heb. 12:7–11; 1 Pet. 4:12). They viewed affliction as being designed by God to weaken the ties of the Christian to the ephemeral lures of this world (see Jn. 17:14–16; Col. 3:2; 1 Pet. 1:24–25). New Testament writers saw suffering as purposive: It corrected specific sins or weaknesses, increased self-knowledge, stimulated Christian graces (such as humility, patience, and faith), and increased dependence upon Christ (Rom. 5:2–5; Jms. 5:10–11; 1 Pet. 1:6–7). These beneficial effects were possible only if faith and trust in Christ transformed suffering into a positive element. An illustration of this attitude was provided by Paul's response to his "thorn in the flesh," which appears to have been a chronic illness or disability.[2]

> And to keep me from being too elated by the abundance of revelations, a thorn was given me in the flesh, a messenger of Satan, to harass me. . . . Three times I besought the Lord about this, that it should leave me, but he said to me, "My grace is sufficient for you, for my power is made perfect in weakness." I will all the more gladly boast of my weakness that the power of Christ may rest upon me. For the sake of Christ, then, I am content with weaknesses, insults, hardships, persecutions, and calamities; for when I am weak, then I am strong. (2 Cor. 12:7–10)[3]

For Paul, strength came through weakness, while strength to endure affliction was given by Christ and resulted from dependence on him.

The emphasis of the New Testament on suffering and affliction as an expected part of the Christian's lot in life seems at variance with the numerous accounts of miraculous healing in the Gospels and Acts. The Gospels record some thirty-five instances of Jesus' healing (among others) the blind, the deaf, the dumb, the lame, lepers, those with disabled limbs, and those suffering from paralysis. Jesus is even said on several occasions to have raised the dead. There was no single pattern to his healings. He is reported to have healed both individuals and groups, in some cases with and in some cases without physical contact. The healings were occasionally attributed to Jesus' compassion, but more often were described as mighty works or signs of the presence of God's kingdom (see *Mt.* 11:2–5, which echoes the language of *Is.* 35 and 61; and *Lk.* 11:17–22). In *Acts,* several accounts of healing miracles by the apostles are recorded. They include healing the lame (3:1–11, 14:8–10), a paralytic (9:33–34), and a man suffering dysentery (28:8), as well as raising two people from the dead (9:36–41; 20:9–12). The Apostle Paul indicated that healing was practiced in the early church as one of several "gifts of the Spirit" (1 *Cor.* 12:9). The Epistle of James describes a rite of healing in which the elders of the local congregation anointed the sick with oil and prayed for their recovery (*Jas.* 5:14–15). How extensively it was employed we do not know.

In spite of the frequent reference to miraculous healing, the New Testament indicates that early Christians continued to suffer from illness. Paul recorded his sorrow over the serious illness of his friend Epaphroditus, whose gradual recovery caused him great joy (*Phil.* 2:25–27). On one occasion he was constrained to leave his companion Trophimus sick in Miletus even though he deeply missed him (2 *Tm.* 4:20). Thus one finds in the New Testament cases of ordinary sickness, some of which were healed by ordinary means and some of which remained unhealed, that existed side by side with instances of sickness that were healed miraculously. The presence of miraculous healing was regarded by early Christians as evidence that the messianic age had come, but they do not appear to have expected that God intended to heal all disease miraculously. In fact, the New Testament epistles, which were intended to provide normative apostolic instruction to the churches, have little to say about physical healing. There is, however, in the epistles an underlying emphasis on the importance of the corporate body of Christians in aiding the individual in all aspects of life (both spiritual and physical) by providing spiritual direction, comfort, and physical sustenance.

It is an underlying assumption of the New Testament, which was taken over from the Old Testament, that all affliction has sin (generically in the human race) as its ultimate cause. Early Christians hesitated, however, to ascribe the immediate cause of affliction in every case to the sufferer's personal sin. Jesus' response to questions raised about the sinfulness of some Jews who had been violently or accidentally killed was that they were not greater sinners than others (*Lk.* 13:1–5). Popular opinion often viewed sickness as punishment for sin. But when Jesus' disciples encountered a man who had been born blind, they asked,

"Who sinned, this man or his parents, that he was born blind?" Jesus replied, "It was not that this man sinned or his parents, but that the works of God might be manifested in him" (*Jn.* 9:2–3; see also 11:4). Yet in the same account Jesus told a man whom he had healed, "Sin no more, that nothing worse befall you" (*Jn.* 5:14), suggesting that Jesus himself in some cases viewed personal sin as the cause of sickness. This view was echoed by Paul, who maintained that some sickness and even death were the result of abuse of the Eucharist or Lord's Supper (1 *Cor.* 11:27–32).

The Gospels indicate that Jesus distinguished between ordinary sickness and sickness that he attributed to demon possession. On one occasion he referred to a woman who had "a spirit of infirmity" as one "whom Satan bound" (*Lk.* 13:11 and 16). Elsewhere he is described as having healed "all that were oppressed by the devil" (*Acts* 10:38). In these instances, however, New Testament writers seem to have understood disease as resulting from the effects of sin on the human race. While they did not attribute most disease to demon possession, they attributed some. Jesus is recorded as having cured a man who was dumb and possessed of a demon by expelling the demon (*Mt.* 9:32–33; see also 12:22). In every case in which disease was directly ascribed to possession, Jesus is said to have accomplished the healing by exorcism. Whether New Testament writers ascribed illness to natural or demonic causes, they viewed all suffering, including sickness, in reference to its ultimate spiritual significance in the life of the individual afflicted.

In contrast to various strains of Greek thought, which disparaged the body, regarding it as the prison of the soul, the New Testament viewed the human body as God's creation, which would one day experience redemption and resurrection. If Christ became flesh and dwelt among humankind, then flesh could not be evil in itself. The body was the dwelling place of God's Holy Spirit (*Rom.* 8:11). The care of the body was stressed with a view to guarding it from sin (1 *Cor.* 3:16–17), especially from such sexual sins as adultery, fornication, and homosexuality (1 *Cor.* 6:18–20). But there was more than a hint that the body itself was thought to deserve care. Paul said that no one ever hated his own flesh, but that one nourished it and cherished it, as Christ cared for the church (*Eph.* 5:29). In a passage that was probably written against Gnostic teaching, Paul also condemned the abusing of one's body as false wisdom (*Col.* 2:23). One can draw the inference that it was regarded by most first-century Christians as proper to care for one's body, to pray for good health, and to seek to maintain or restore it. On the other hand, undue solicitation for the body or a desperate clinging to life was regarded as a contradiction of the role that New Testament writers assigned to the body. The Christian was expected to have mastery over the body, because it served the will, but not contempt for it. However, the goal of the Christian life was spiritual (not physical) well-being, and the New Testament indicates that ill health and suffering could be used by God to contribute to that goal.

Although the writers of the New Testament saw sickness, like suffering generally, as potentially profitable in the life of the Christian, they did not view it as good in itself. There is considerably more emphasis in the New Testament on hope and joy than on affliction and sorrow. Christians were urged to rejoice always, even when suffering, because their hope was anchored in a spiritual dimension that sought the joys of heaven rather than of earth (*Phil.* 4:4; 2 *Cor.* 6:10; *Ti.* 2:12–13). The Christian's hope was grounded in God's love for all persons, which was the source of the love that Christians were to manifest first to fellow Christians and then to all humanity (1 *Jn.* 4:7–21). Love indeed was to predominate in the Christian's life to the point that one ought to be willing to lay down one's life for another (1 *Jn.* 3:16). The suffering of others should elicit sympathy and concern from Christians (see *Rom.* 12:15). According to the practical Epistle of James, while concern for another's spiritual needs was vitally important, it was not to take the place of providing obvious physical or material necessities (*Jas.* 1:27). One finds a much stronger imperative to alleviate the ills of others than to seek to lessen one's own sufferings. Christians viewed Jesus himself as the supreme example of this disposition, and he had commanded that his followers love their neighbors as themselves. The illustrations of charity that Jesus had given to his disciples in the Sermon on the Mount were very practical: "I was hungry and you gave me food, I was thirsty and you gave me drink, I was a stranger and you welcomed me, I was naked and you clothed me, I was sick and you visited me, I was in prison and you came to me. . . . As you did it to one of the least of these my brethren, you did it to me" (*Mt.* 25:35–40). Jesus' words, as reported by Matthew, warned his followers that God would ultimately judge the authenticity of their faith by their active benevolence toward others.

The Developing Church, Circa 100–400 C.E.

The Christian faith, as it was proclaimed by the early church, sought primarily the eternal salvation of souls, but it had implications as well for life in this world. It introduced, in the words of Henry Sigerist,

> the most revolutionary and decisive change in the attitude of society toward the sick. Christianity came into the world as the religion of healing, as the

joyful Gospel of the Redeemer and of Redemption. It addressed itself to the disinherited, to the sick and the afflicted, and promised them healing, a restoration both spiritual and physical. . . . It became the duty of the Christian to attend to the sick and poor of the community. . . . The social position of the sick man thus became fundamentally different from what it had been before. He assumed a preferential positon which has been his ever since.[4]

Early Christian literature is full of admonitions to care for the sick.[5] Although concern for the ill was urged upon all Christians in the early church, it increasingly became the specific duty of deacons and deaconesses to report cases of sickness or poverty to the local bishop.[6] After the legalization of Christianity, bishops acquired a civic status similar to that of important government officials and assumed the responsibility of managing large-scale charitable efforts.[7]

On several occasions, Christians demonstrated great courage in their care of the sick during outbreaks of the plague. In the mid–third century, during a plague that ravaged the Mediterranean area and northern Africa in particular, Christians brought aid to fellow Christians and pagans alike who were suffering from the pestilence. Contemporary accounts describe their zeal as nearly suicidal.[8] Somewhat later there appeared a group of Christians called the *Parabolani* ("the reckless ones"), who were so named because of their devotion to caring for the sick during times of pestilence.[9] So well known were the Christians for their acts of charity that the pagan emperor Julian the Apostate complained that the "impious Galileans support not only their own poor but ours as well."[10] In general there was no religious or ethical motivation for charity in the pagan classical world. Among the Greeks and Romans, benevolence manifested itself in civic philanthropy on behalf of the entire community rather than in private charity undertaken for individuals in need, such as the sick, widows, or orphans.[11] In spite of the emphasis of the Hellenistic and Roman philosophical sects (such as the Stoics) on the brotherhood of all persons, pagan philosophers discouraged private charity that was based on pity or emotion rather than on reason. In contrast to the pagan attitude, later Judaism (in the Apocrypha and the Talmud) placed great importance on the duty of almsgiving and this emphasis was taken over by Christianity. Like Judaism, Christianity taught that the human race had been created in the image of God *(imago Dei)*, but that this image had been defaced by sin.[12] According to the doctrine of the Incarnation, God had assumed human flesh in Jesus Christ, who gave himself as a ransom for the sins of the world *(Jn.* 1:14). The Incarnation was rooted in God's self-giving love for the human race *(agape).*

The Christian belief that human beings were created in God's image, particularly viewed in the light of the Incarnation, had two important consequences for the development of Christian ethics. The first was the impetus that it gave to Christian benevolence. The New Testament was clear in teaching that one could not claim to love God without also loving one's fellow human beings (see 1 *Jn.* 4:20–21). It was Christian concern for all persons, who bore God's image, particularly for those who were in need, that led to the establishment of the first hospitals in the fourth century. Christian hospitals *(xenodochia)* began to be erected within a generation or two after Christianity became a legal religion. One of the earliest, and probably the best known, was the Basileias, which was founded in about 372 by Basil the Great, who was bishop of Caesarea in Cappadocia. Basil provided as well accommodations for travellers and apparently a section for the treatment of lepers. The hospital had both nurses and medical attendants. Gregory of Nazianzus (330–389), who had seen the Basileias, described it in enthusiastic terms:

> Go forth a little from the city, and behold the new city, the treasure-house of godliness . . . in which disease is investigated and sympathy proved. . . . We have no longer to look on the fearful and pitiable sight of men like corpses before death, with the greater part of their limbs dead [from leprosy], driven from cities, from dwellings, from public places, from watercourses . . . Basil it was more than anyone who persuaded those who are men not to scorn men, nor to dishonour Christ the head of all by their inhumanity towards human beings.[13]

Basil's hospital provided a model for many others that spread throughout the eastern Roman Empire and from there into the West in the fifth century. Pagans recognized hospitals as distinctly Christian organizations, but their existence spurred Julian the Apostate to establish some pagan hospitals in order to emulate the Christians. Christian hospitals often had separate houses set apart for travellers, orphans and foundlings, the aged, and the poor.

A second consequence of the Christian doctrine that the human race was created in God's image was the concept that every human being, as God's creation and as a soul that Christ died to redeem, had inherent value and therefore ought to be protected and nourished. In the Graeco-Roman world, claims to human worth or dignity depended on citizenship, status, or virtue, but not on inherent right.[14] If an outgrowth of the Christian belief in the inherent worth of all human beings was the impetus that it gave to caring and compassion, another consequence was a resounding condemnation of abortion, infanticide, the exposure of children, euthanasia (either as homicide or suicide), and the gladiatorial games. To the Christians, the fact that pagan society permitted unwanted human life (particularly helpless life) to be eliminated, while it showed great cruelty to those who had been condemned, revealed its basic wickedness. Christians sought in particular to protect unborn and newborn life.[15] Abortion was widely practiced in antiquity, but Christian authors from at least the second century without exception condemned the practice. Thus Tertullian (ca. 160/70–ca. 215/20) wrote:

> For us, indeed, as homicide is forbidden, it is not lawful to destroy what is conceived in the womb while the blood is still being formed into a man. To prevent being born is to accelerate homicide, nor does it make a difference whether you snatch away a soul which is born or destroy one being born. He who is a man-to-be is man, as all fruit is now in the seed.[16]

By the fifth century many Christians came to consider abortion worse than murder, because the fetus could not be baptized and was thus thought to be condemned to hell.[17] Allowing children to die by exposure to the elements was very widely practiced in the ancient world and had for centuries represented the commonest form of population control.[18] Christians strongly attacked the practice, which they regarded as no less objectionable than infanticide. They also condemned contraception because it prevented the existence of life that God had intended. Conception, gestation, birth, and nurture were regarded by Christians as a continuous process, with which one should not interfere at any point. In a well-known passage, Augustine equally denounced as "lustful cruelty or cruel lust" contraception, abortion, and infanticide.[19] But condemnation of contraception in the early church appears not to have been as uniform as the Christian attitude toward abortion and infanticide.[20] After Christianity was legalized in the fourth century, it gradually introduced major changes in the moral climate of the Roman world. Under successive Christian emperors (beginning with Constantine), legislation was issued that aimed at protecting newborn infants from exposure. Even more influential than imperial legislation, however, were the decisions of church councils that condemned abortion, infanticide, and exposure, and imposed severe penance, and in some cases even excommunication from the church (with its corollary of eternal damnation). By its strong denunciation of these practices, the church portrayed them as the most heinous of sins and it undergirded its moral stand by imposing strong sanctions against those Christians who violated its teaching.[21]

While homicide was viewed as a reprehensible sin, suicide was not specified as worthy of particular condemnation in Christian teaching until the second century (although there is no reason to suppose that Christians before then viewed it as anything less than homicide). In the classical world, suicide was not condemned and, in fact, it was often idealized as a noble form of death. The Christian apologist Justin Martyr (ca. 100–165), anticipating the suggestion by a pagan that Christians should simply kill themselves and go immediately to heaven, responded that "we shall, if we so act, be ourselves acting in opposition to the will of God."[22] Clement of Alexandria, also writing in the second century, flatly stated that it was not permitted to Christians to kill themselves, while the author of the roughly contemporaneous *Shepherd of Hermas* wrote that whoever did not save someone who was driven to suicide by calamities "commits a great sin, and becomes guilty of his blood."[23] Augustine was the first Christian author to discuss suicide extensively.[24] "We are," he writes, "among evils which we ought patiently to endure until we arrive among those goods where nothing will be lacking to provide us ineffable delight, nor will there then be anything that we are obliged to endure."[25] Elsewhere he condemned suicide to escape illness or physical disability.

The contrast of the inexpressible bliss of heaven with the evils that must be endured on earth is a theme frequently encountered in early Christian literature. The Christian's attitude toward death was often contrasted in the early church with that of the pagan. While Christians believed that pagans trembled with fear in the face of death, they exhorted one another to rejoice at the prospect of the future life that awaited them.[26] According to Peter Brown, "the early church tended to leapfrog the grave. The long process of mourning and slow adjustment to the great sadness of mortality tended to be repressed by a heady belief in the afterlife."[27] But death remained for Christians the "last enemy" that must be confronted in order to arrive at the perfect happiness of heaven.[28] Many Christians anticipated heaven for the absence of suffering, both physical and mental, that they hoped to attain. They expected to receive that "perfect health of the body," which was immortality.[29]

It has been argued that early Christians rejected secular medicine for several centuries, depending instead on miraculous healing or healing by spiritual means.[30] Christians certainly continued to seek divine healing in the early centuries of Christianity, particularly through prayer and anointing with oil, the latter being employed both by the clergy and by lay men and women. In the *Canones Ecclesiastici* and *Bishop Serapion's Prayer Book*, which date from the mid–fourth century, there are prayers for the consecration of oil to be used against fever, sickness, and demons. Other means of sacramental healing and exorcism are mentioned in Christian writings as early as the mid–second century. Most prominent were healing by the laying on of hands and by the sacraments of baptism and the Eucharist or Lord's Supper. The use of the Eucharist for healing grew in the church, with the result that much later Caesarius of Arles (470–543) advised: "Let him who is sick receive the body and blood of Christ, and then let him anoint his body."[31] Early Christians do not, however, seem for the most part to have rejected the use of physicians.[32] With the exception of Luke, whom Paul calls "the beloved physician" (*Col.* 4:14), we find no specific mention of Christian physicians before the mid–second century, when reference is made to a physician who was put to death as a martyr at Lugdunum (Lyons). Yet when Christians began to establish hospitals in the fourth century, they often employed physicians, while at the same time continuing to seek and to claim miraculous healing. If we examine the writings of the Fathers of the church in the first four centuries of Christianity we find, in fact, numerous indications that many early Christians were not hostile to secular medicine and the restoration of health by physicians. Origen (ca. 185–ca. 254) referred to medicine as "beneficial and essential to mankind."[33] Clement of Alexandria (ca. 155–ca. 220) spoke of it as God's gift to the human race that was discovered by reason.[34] John Chrysostom (ca. 344/354–407) acknowledged physicians and medicine as gifts of God.[35] Not atypical of the early Fathers in his attitude to medicine was Basil the Great (ca. 329–379), who wrote to his fellow monks:

> We must take great care to employ this medical art, if it should be necessary, not as making it wholly accountable for our state of health or illness, but as redounding to the glory of God . . . In the event that medicine should fail to help, we should not place all hope for the relief of our distress in this art. . . . Yet, to reject entirely the benefits to be derived from this art is the sign of a pettish nature. . . . We should neither repudiate this art altogether nor does it behoove us to repose all our confidence in it. . . . When reason allows, we call in the doctor, but we do not leave off hoping in God.[36]

He goes on to say that the Christian should receive medical healing with thanksgiving. The Fathers generally agreed. A few (like Tatian, Marcion, and Arnobius) rejected secular medicine, but most believed that God could and did heal both through means and apart from means.[37] It is reasonable to conclude that Christians in the earliest centuries of the church generally sought healing through traditional medicine as well as by means of sacramental or spiritual healing.

The Influence of Asceticism, Magic, and the Cult of Saints

A number of new developments occurred in late antiquity that came to have a marked influence on Christian attitudes to health and healing.

Prominent among them were the rise of asceticism, the increasing resort to magic and superstition, the veneration of relics, and the growing importance of holy men. Asceticism (the practice of strict self-denial as a spiritual discipline) began to exercise a strong influence on Christianity in the third and fourth centuries. New Testament writers had urged self-denial in the form of moral purity, detachment from the world, and rejection of its pleasures.[38] The asceticism that was introduced into Christianity in the third century, however, went considerably beyond the New Testament pattern. It idealized virginity and preached contempt of the material world in general and of the body in particular. In its mildest form (among the Encratites) it involved continence and abstinence from wine and meat. In its more extreme forms it held that only the spiritual world was good, while the material world was evil and must be rejected. This dualism, which lay behind much of the new asceticism, characterized some late Greek philosophies and religious groups (particularly the mystery religions) and can even be found in Jewish writings of the first century B.C. It was adopted in the second century after Christ by Christian heretical groups such as the Gnostics, Manicheans, and Marcionites. Some church Fathers (such as Clement of Alexandria and Origen) disparaged the body but developed a theological basis for asceticism that was not rooted in the dualistic rejection of the material world. Most Fathers, however, regarded the body as morally neutral, potentially either a temple or a tomb, which must be subservient to the soul in its warfare against sin.[39]

The dualistic outlook, with its disparagement of the body, was widely held by pagans in late antiquity and it had a strong appeal to Christians.[40] According to E.R. Dodds, "pagans and Christians (though not all pagans or all Christians) vied with each other in heaping abuse on the body; it was 'clay and gore,' 'a filthy bag of excrement and urine'; man is plunged in it as in a bath of dirty water."[41] Whereas earlier Christians had regarded suffering as a necessary part of life in this world, which God sometimes used for spiritual edification, they did not for the most part actively seek it. Many ascetics, however, sought suffering for expiatory, propitiatory, or purificatory ends by abusing their bodies, which they thought to be the prison of their souls. The ascetics' mortification of the flesh not infrequently manifested itself in extreme ways. An early monk, Macarius, as penance for having angrily killed a fly, for six months permitted poisonous flies to sting his naked flesh. With the spread of monasticism in the fourth and fifth centuries, the influence of asceticism grew, but not all forms of monasticism placed the same emphasis on the mortification of the body. In general, eastern monasticism (especially in its earlier anchoritic form) emphasized the mortification of the flesh, while western monasticism discouraged it in extreme forms in favor of a disciplined life that was characterized by practicality and charity. When Christianity became a legal religion in 313 and Christians no longer suffered persecution, ascetics replaced martyrs in the popular mind as the new spiritual heroes.[42] Because ascetics had overcome the material world, they enjoyed an exalted position in the society of the eastern Roman Empire. They became the new spiritual elite and their life of rigid self-denial came to be viewed by ordinary Christians as a daily martyrdom. From the mid–fourth century, most of the leaders of the church in both the East and West regarded asceticism as the path to spiritual perfection.

With the new asceticism came an increasing belief in demonic activity as a cause of disease. Early Christian literature identified three sources of disease or illness: God, demons, and nature. They did not regard them, however, as mutually exclusive. While Christians hesitated to attribute specific cases of illness directly to God, the more they stressed his sovereignty, the more they saw him as the ultimate cause, regardless of whether the immediate cause was demonic or natural. Demonology occupies a large place in the writings of the church Fathers, all of whom believed in the existence of demons and in their widespread activity. Late antiquity was, in the words of one scholar, "an age which was hag-ridden with the fear of demonic forces dominating every aspect of life and death."[43] The belief was widespread among Christians that demons caused disease that manifested itself in ordinary symptoms, which could be distinguished from demonic possession. Possession also manifested itself in disease or madness, which could be treated by exorcism. Christians did not view all madness as possession. Jerome believed that some who were "melancholy mad" needed the help of a physician more than his advice.[44] The evidence suggests that early Christians generally distinguished between demonic possession and illness. It appears that in the second and third centuries Christians attributed a relatively small proportion of physical (as distinct from mental) illnesses to demonic possession. In the late fourth century, however, there was a marked increase in Christian belief in demonic activity, the result perhaps of the burgeoning cult of saints and relics. Even then cases that were specified as demonic possession usually exhibited a diverse range of bizarre aberrations rather than symptoms that were viewed as physical illness.[45]

In late antiquity, magic came increasingly to be used for healing by Christians and pagans alike. By the late third century the old Roman religious institutions had lost their appeal to all social classes. There existed a spiritual void that was filled by a variety of new religious manifestations, including the growing influence of magic, which was felt even in the highest intellectual circles.[46] Roman law had from the earliest times strictly prohibited malicious magic (magic used to harm) and harshly punished its practitioners.[47] But benevolent magic, such as that which the elder Roman Cato (234–149 B.C.E.) had employed for the cure of sprains, was not condemned by law. The Theodosian Code states regarding magic (in a law promulgated by Constantine) that "remedies sought for human bodies shall not be involved in criminal accusation."[48] Augustine, however, and other church Fathers considered dependence on magical powers and devices reprehensible, because they attributed those powers to demonic forces.[49] For more than three centuries Christians had condemned the use of all magic, including charms and amulets. Thus John Chrysostom commended in a sermon a mother who preferred to allow her sick child to die rather than to use amulets, even though she believed that such means would be effective and was urged by Christian friends to use them.[50] In the fourth century, however, as increasing numbers of nominal Christians entered the church following its legalization and growing respectability, they brought pagan attitudes and practices (such as magic) with them. Augustine complained of Christians who consulted astrologers after having unsuccessfully sought healing through prayer and natural remedies.[51] He wrote of Christian mothers who, in seeking healing for their children, used amulets and incantations and sometimes even offered sacrifices to the pagan gods in the hope of obtaining a cure.[52]

It was not always clear to Christians, however, what constituted magic. Augustine maintained that it was one thing to consume an herb for stomach pain and quite another to wear the herb around one's neck for the same purpose. He approved of the former practice, which he called a wholesome mixture; he condemned the latter as a superstitious charm. He conceded, however, that wearing an herb around one's neck might be effective because of its natural virtue and thought it acceptable as long as incantations and magical symbols were not used in conjunction with it.[53] The confusion regarding what constituted magic is evident also in Augustine's indignation at Christians who mingled the name of Jesus with their incantations and in his ambivalence concerning mothers who saw baptism as a possible remedy for the healing of their sick children.[54] Augustine himself had, as a boy, begged his mother Monica to allow him to be baptized when he was sick, not only for the sake of his soul but for physical healing as well.[55]

There were always some Christians in the early church who believed that miracles were a continuing phenomenon that were not limited to the apostolic age. Mention of healing miracles like those performed by Jesus and his disciples is, however, infrequent and guarded in Christian literature of the second and third centuries. A significant change in this regard occurred about the middle of the fourth century, when there was a pronounced increase in the number of miracles reported and in their sensational and magical character.[56] The source of this phenomenon was probably the ascetics or holy men of the East (like St. Anthony and his disciple Pachomius), who came to exercise widespread influence in the fourth century, and whom popular legend credited with many miracles. Miracle-workers had appeared from time to time in the early centuries of Christianity, but they were usually the founders of new and often heretical Christian sects, whose miracles were attributed by the orthodox to demonic powers. The desert fathers, however, were for the most part orthodox and as their reputation grew, they were eagerly sought out by ordinary Christians for spiritual counsel.

Athanasius wrote a life of St. Anthony shortly after the latter's death in 356 and it was soon translated into Latin and created a new genre of literature, hagiography. Lives of saints proliferated, inspired by the enormous popularity of Athanasius' work, and they came to constitute the most popular form of Christian literature in the fourth and fifth centuries. These lives described the miraculous exploits that had come to be attributed to the ascetics: their casting out of demons, miraculous healing of diseases, and raising from the dead. The holy men were said to effect cures by prayer, making the sign of the cross, laying their hands on the afflicted, or applying bread, oil, water, or garments that they had blessed. Typical of these lives was Jerome's life of Hilarion (ca. 291–371), a disciple of St. Anthony, whom Jerome credited with having performed many miracles of healing. They included restoring sight to a woman who had been blind for ten years, curing paralysis and dropsy, and casting out demons from those who had been possessed (including a possessed camel who had been responsible for many deaths).[57] Stories abounded of every kind of physical disability being healed by holy men: leprosy, madness, paralysis, the loss of fingers, and severe wounds. Miracles of healing were also attributed to bishops like Ambrose (ca. 339–397), the influential bishop of Milan. Many of the healings involved the use of what can only be called "Christian magic." For many Christians the name of Jesus became an irresistible spell and the sign of the cross an all-powerful charm.

Associated with the cult of holy men was the growing importance of relics (the material remains of saints or objects that had some contact with them). The remains of the earliest Christian martyrs had been venerated because the martyrs were thought to have been especially blessed of God, since they had proven their faith by offering their lives in death. Hence their tombs were honored and attracted pilgrims, who began to attribute miracles and cures to them. Before long, miracle-working power was believed to reside not only in the bones of the martyrs and holy persons, but in their garments and objects with which they had been associated. The relics of saints or martyrs extended to posterity the benefits that the saints had conferred on those in need during their own lifetime. The large number of converts from paganism after the legalization of Christianity brought into the church from pagan cults a reverence for relics. Their veneration had begun in the second century, but from the mid–fourth century there was a rapid increase in the quest for relics and the building of shrines, which were accompanied by numerous healings and manifestations of demonic activity. "Like the old gods," writes A. H. M. Jones,

> they cured the sick, gave children to barren women, protected travellers from perils of sea and land, detected perjurors and foretold the future. Some acquired widespread fame for special power. SS. Cyrus and John, the physicians who charged no fee, were celebrated for their cures, and their shrine at Canopus, near Alexandria, was thronged by sufferers from all the provinces, as in the old days had been the temple of Asclepius at Aegae. But the main function of the saints and martyrs in the popular religion of the day was to replace the old gods as local patrons and protectors.[58]

The cult of the saints was not, however, simply a manifestation of popular religion that was limited to ignorant or ordinary Christians. Such was the spirit of the age that Christian leaders, including many of the Fathers of the church, like Ambrose and Augustine, believed in the miracle-working power of saints and supported the founding of shrines in which to house their relics.[59] Ambrose discovered the remains of two martyrs (Gervasius and Protasius), which he believed that God revealed to him. He attributed many miracles (particularly cures of demoniacs and healings) to their remains, which he deposited beneath the altar of a new basilica in a place in which he had intended his own remains to rest.[60] Interestingly the Arians in this case were skeptical about the purported healings, while the orthodox accepted them. Augustine had, in his earlier writings, essentially denied the continuation of miracles into his own age and seemed little interested, and indeed somewhat impatient with, the question of whether miracles of the kind performed by Jesus and the apostles were still performed. His emphasis was on "healing the eyes of the heart" rather than on the miraculous cure of bodily ills. He had witnessed a few healing miracles but he spoke little about them until his later years, when he gradually acquired an interest in the contemporary miracles that were being widely reported by Christians in northern Africa. He began to keep records, hoping to give the miracles greater publicity as an aid to converting pagans. In less than two years he recorded seventy. Most are healings, but there are some accounts of those who had been raised from the dead. Many of them are said to have resulted from the healing power of relics, such as contact with a piece of cloth that someone had laid on the tomb of a martyr. Augustine recorded several of these stories in the last book of his *City of God*.[61] They represent a strange assortment of wonders and in general suggest a credulity that was widespread among all classes in Augustine's own day.[62]

With the widespread appeal of magical charms and relics in the fourth century, and the expectation of miraculous healing that could be gained from them, it is surprising to find that many (and perhaps most) Christians continued to seek healing from physicians. While there are only scattered references to Christian physicians before the fourth century (perhaps owing to the paucity of our sources), thereafter they appear with regularity. Because Christians regarded medicine as a superlative vehicle for compassion, Christian physicians were sometimes exhorted to combine spiritual and medical care. Basil of Caesarea wrote to the physician Eustathius: "And your profession is the supply vein of health. But, in your case especially, the science is ambidextrous, and you set for yourself higher standards of humanity, not limiting the benefit of your profession to bodily ills, but also contriving the correction of spiritual ills."[63] There is no evidence of the extent to which ordinary Christian physicians set for themselves "higher standards of humanity" in treating their patients. But there is ample evidence to indicate that a number of priests and monks in late antiquity were physicians, who sought to blend their spiritual and medical interests into a concern for the spiritual and physical condition of those whom they treated. With the growth of Christian hospitals in the fourth and fifth centuries, maintained either by monastic communities (of which they were sometimes a part) or by bishops, it appears that a number of priests and monks took up the practice of medicine.[64] Such a monk was Hypatius, who lived in the fifth century and who became the abbot of a monastery in Halmyrissos in Thrace that was celebrated for its humanitarian work among the poor. Hypatius became familiar with the art of Hippocrates and treated those who had been denied treatment by other physicians. He later moved to Bithynia, where he organized a monastery and continued his humanitarian work.[65]

Although the literature of early Christianity reveals an appreciation of medicine as a means of healing the ill, it also exhibits a concern for the proper use of medicine to promote spirituality. Little was said in condemnation of physicians for wrongly using their art, except against those who performed abortions or (occasionally) against those who excessively warned their patients of the rigors of self-denial. Rather, Christian writers repeatedly exhorted the sick not to disregard the fact that the physician was merely a servant of God who worked within the created order. Medicine, they said, could only be used properly as long as both patients and physicians acknowledged that all healing ultimately came from God, who sometimes worked through physicians, and that the health of the soul must have priority over the care of the body.[66] They regarded the right use of medicine as a compelling test of Christians' priorities and of their dependence upon God. John Chrysostom cautioned against making one's body the mistress of one's life in respect to its legitimate needs of food, shelter, clothing, and medical care.[67] Ambrose criticized those who, when ill, called physicians but prayed for healing only if their efforts failed. Their faith, he maintained, was in medicine, not in God. The Christian's priorities should be directed to eternal rather than temporal values.[68] Augustine said that some Christians, when desperate, would throw themselves at the feet of a physician and beg to be restored to health. "Do whatever you want, only cure me," was their plea.[69] He observed that many, when faced with troubles, would cry out, "O God, send me death; hasten my days!" But when sickness came, they would rush to the physician and promise him money and rewards for healing.[70] He condemned as incompatible with dependence on God the attitude of Christians who would do anything to live for a few more days.[71] Warnings against an undue solicitation for the body and a too ardent desire to cling to life are common in the works of Christian writers of the fourth and fifth centuries.

Conclusion

Christians from the New Testament period through the fifth century relied on a number of different means of healing. The New Testament suggests that while Jesus and the apostles healed miraculously on occasion, Christians for the most part neither expected miraculous healing for all their illnesses nor failed to seek medical assistance by ordinary means (see 1 *Tim.* 5:23). A rite of sacramental healing (by prayer and anointing) existed in the New Testament period and it appears to have continued in use throughout the early centuries of Christianity. It probably, in fact, was the commonest form of spiritual or divine healing employed in the early church. In the New Testament, Christians were warned to expect suffering, because God sometimes worked through suffering (physical or otherwise) to produce spiritual edification. This theme is found frequently in the church Fathers as well. In general they regarded physical health as a relative good, but not an end in itself and by no means essential to spiritual health, which they considered more important. Yet most maintained that the body was to be reasonably cared for because God had provided the means for its care.[72] Health was a blessing from God, but God sometimes used poor health as a spiritual discipline.[73] Sickness could serve to correct one's sins, refine, admonish, produce patience, lessen pride, make the afflicted an example of fortitude and virtue to others, increase one's dependence on God, and make one mindful of eternity and mortality.[74] Thus Christians should rejoice in sickness as well as in health.

In the fourth century, new influences began to make their mark on Christian belief and practice. The rise of asceticism produced among some Christians a disdain for the body and an encouragement to its mortification. While the influence of asceticism was powerful, it did not entirely overwhelm or displace earlier Christian emphases. The fourth century saw as well a tendency among Christians to regard magic as efficacious in healing and to seek miraculous healing from relics. Yet Christians also continued to seek out physicians and to depend on traditional spiritual means of healing, such as prayer and sacramental anointing. Moreover, the strong element of compassion and charity, which had remained a constant feature of Christianity since its beginning, manifested itself in the fourth century in the establishment of hospitals, which provided medical treatment in the context of philanthropy and humanitarian concern. It appears that, for the period under survey, several approaches to health and healing, involving both secular and spiritual means, although sometimes antithetical to each other, existed side by side among Christians. Some tension was inevitable, but there was a surprising degree of complementarity.

NOTES

1. Quotations from the New Testament are taken from the Revised Standard Version of the Bible.
2. For a discussion of the nature of Paul's illness, see Klaus Seybold and Ulrich B. Mueller, *Sickness and Healing,* trans. Douglas W. Stott (Nashville, 1981), pp. 171–182.
3. See also *Galatians* 4:13–14, where Paul speaks of the same or another illness with which he was afflicted.
4. Henry Sigerist, *Civilization and Disease* (Ithaca, NY, 1943), pp. 69–70.
5. See, e.g., Hippolytus, *Apostolic Tradition,* canon 20; Polycarp, *Epistle* 6; Pseudo-Clement, *De Virginitate;* Tertullian, *Ad Uxorem* 2.4; Justin, *Apology* 1.67; Jerome, *Epistle* 52.15–16.
6. *Apostolic Constitutions* 3.19.
7. See Bernard Cooke, *Ministry to Word and Sacraments: History and Theology* (Philadelphia, 1976), pp. 353–355.
8. Eusebius, *Ecclesiastical History* 7.22.7–8; see also Pontius, *The Life and Passion of Cyprian* 9–10.
9. See "Parabolani" in *The Oxford Dictionary of the Christian Church,* ed. F.L. Cross (London, 1958), pp. 1012–1013.
10. Julian, *Epistle* 22.
11. See Darrel W. Amundsen and Gary B. Ferngren, "Philanthropy in Medicine: Some Historical Perspectives," in *Beneficence and Health Care,* ed. Earl E. Shelp (Dordrecht, 1982), pp. 1–31, especially pp. 1–12.
12. See Gary B. Ferngren, "The *Imago Dei* and the Sanctity of Life: The Origins of an Idea," in *Euthanasia and the Newborn: Criteria for In-*

fanticide in the Twentieth Century, eds. R. M. McMillan, H. T. Engelhardt, and S. F. Spicker (Dordrecht/Boston, 1986).

13. *Oration* 20. Quoted in W. Smith and S. Cheetham, *A Dictionary of Christian Antiquities,* vol. 1 (London, 1875), s.v. "Hospitals," p. 786.

14. See John M. Rist, *Human Value: A Study in Ancient Philosophical Ethics* (Leiden, 1982).

15. See, e.g., Justin Martyr, *Apology* 1.27; Minucius Felix, *Octavius* 30; *Didache* 2; *The Epistle of Barnabas* 19.5; *The Epistle to Diognetus* 5.6; *Apostolic Constitutions* 8.3; Tertullian, *Apology* 9 and *Ad Nationes* 1.15; Clement of Alexandria, *Christ the Educator* 21; Lactantius, *The Divine Institutes* 5.9 and 6.20. For discussions of abortion and infanticide (including exposure) see John T. Noonan, Jr., "An Almost Absolute Value in History," in *The Morality of Abortion: Legal and Historical Perspectives,* ed. John T. Noonan, Jr. (Cambridge, MA, 1970), pp. 7–18; John Connery, *Abortion: The Development of the Roman Catholic Perspective* (Chicago, 1977), pp. 33–64; Igino Giordani, *The Social Message of the Early Fathers,* trans. A. Zizzamia (Boston, 1977), pp. 243–252.

16. *Apologeticum ad nationes* 1.15. Quoted in John T. Noonan, Jr., "An Almost Absolute Value in History," p. 12.

17. See Gary B. Ferngren, "The Status of Defective Newborns from Late Antiquity to the Reformation," in McMillan, Engelhardt, and Spicker, *Euthanasia and the Newborn.*

18. See Darrel W. Amundsen, "Medicine and the Birth of Defective Children: Approaches of the Ancient World," in McMillan, Engelhardt, and Spicker, *Euthanasia and the Newborn.*

19. *De nuptiis et concupiscentia* 1.15.17.

20. See John T. Noonan, Jr., *Contraception: A History of Its Treatment by the Catholic Theologians and Canonists* (Cambridge, MA, 1966), pp. 56–139.

21. See Ferngren, "The Status of Defective Newborns."

22. Justin Martyr, *Apology* 2.2.

23. Clement of Alexandria, *Stromateis* 6.9; *Shepherd of Hermas* 10.4 (compare Polycarp, *Epistle to the Philippians* 10.3; Lactantius, *On the Workmanship of God* 4 and *The Divine Institutes* 3.18).

24. *City of God* 1.20–27.

25. *City of God* 19.4.

26. See, for example, Cyprian, *De Mortalitate* 2, 5, 7, 14, 18–19, and 26 (which was written while Carthage was suffering from the plague).

27. Peter Brown, *The Cult of the Saints: Its Rise and Function in Latin Christianity* (Chicago, 1981), pp. 69–70.

28. Augustine, *Epistle* 243.11; *City of God* 13.6.

29. Augustine, *Epistle* 123.3; see also *Sermon* 240.3 and compare Irenaeus, *Against the Heretics* 5.12.6.

30. See V. G. Dawe, *The Attitude of the Ancient Church Toward Sickness and Healing* (unpublished doctoral dissertation, Boston University School of Theology, Boston, 1955); E. Frost, *Christian Healing,* 2nd ed. (London, 1954); and M. T. Kelsey, *Healing and Christianity in Ancient Thought and Modern Times* (New York, 1973).

31. *Sermon* 66.3. Quoted in W. Smith and S. Cheetham, *A Dictionary of Christian Antiquities,* vol. 2 (London, 1880), s.v. "Unction," p. 2004.

32. See Darrel W. Amundsen, "Medicine and Faith in Early Christianity," *Bulletin of the History of Medicine* 56 (1982): 326–350. There is a fairly extensive literature on medicine in the early church, particularly in studies of the extent and literary use of medical knowledge by individual church Fathers. See A. Harnack, "Medicinische aus der ältesten Kirchengeschichte," *Texte Untersuchungen Gesch. altchristlichen Literatur* 8 (4) (1892): 37–152; Stephen d'Irsay, "Patristic Medicine," *Annals of Medical History* 9 (1927): 364–378; "Christian Medicine and Science in the Third Century," *Journal of Religion* 10 (1930): 515–544; H. J. Frings, *Medizin und Arzt bei den griechischen Kirchenvätern bis Chrysostomos* (Bonn, 1959); H. Schedewaldt, "Die Apologie der Heilkunst bei den Kirchenvätern," *Veröffentlichungen Internat. Gesellschaft Gesch. Pharmazie* 26 (1965): 115–130.

33. *Contra Celsum* 3.12.

34. *Stromateis* 6.17; *Christ the Educator* 1.2.6.

35. *Homily 8 on Colossians.*

36. *The Long Rule* 55. Quoted in Amundsen, "Medicine and Faith," pp. 338–339.

37. See Amundsen, "Medicine and Faith," pp. 343–348.

38. See *Romans* 8:13; 1 *Corinthians* 9:25–27; *Colossians* 3:5.

39. See, e.g., Clement of Alexandria, *Stromateis* 3.7; Lactantius, *The Divine Institutes* 5.22; Ambrose, *Epistle* 63.91; Augustine, *De Vera Religione* 20.40. See also Frank Bottomley, *Attitudes to the Body in Western Christendom* (London, 1979); and Margaret Miles, *Fullness of Life: Historical Foundations for a New Asceticism* (Philadelphia, 1981).

40. See E. R. Dodds, *Pagan and Christian in an Age of Anxiety* (New York, 1970), pp. 7–36.

41. Ibid., p. 29.

42. See W. H. C. Frend, *Martyrdom and Persecution in the Early Church* (Oxford, 1965), pp. 356, 548.

43. Michael Green, *Evangelism in the Early Church* (Grand Rapids, MI, 1970), p. 190; see also F. van der Meer, *Augustine the Bishop: The Life and Work of a Father of the Church,* trans. B. Battershaw and G. R. Lamb (London, 1961), pp. 67–75; and Peter Brown, *Augustine of Hippo* (Berkeley, CA, 1969), p. 395.

44. Jerome, *Epistle* 125.16; see also Augustine, *De Cura pro Mortuis Gerenda* 12.14.

45. For a vivid description, see van der Meer, *Augustine the Bishop,* p. 539.

46. See A. A. Barb, "The Survival of Magic Arts," in *The Conflict Between Paganism and Christianity in the Fourth Century,* ed. Arnaldo Momigliano (Oxford, 1963), p. 115; Dodds, *Pagan and Christian,* pp. 125–126; A. H. M. Jones, *The Later Roman Empire, 284–602: A Social, Economic, and Administrative Survey* (Oxford, 1964), p. 962; Peter Brown, *The Making of Late Antiquity* (Cambridge, MA, 1978), pp. 60–66.

47. See Clyde Pharr, "The Interdiction of Magic in Roman Law," *Transactions of the American Philological Association* 63 (1932): 269–295.

48. *Codex Theodosianus* 9.16.3.

49. See Augustine, *City of God* 10.9; and Benedicta Ward, *Miracles and the Medieval Mind: Theory, Record, and Event, 1000–1215* (Philadelphia, 1982), p. 9.

50. John Chrysostom, *Homily 8 on Colossians.*

51. See Mary Emily Keenan, "Augustine and the Medical Profession," *Transactions of the American Philological Association* 67 (1936): 184.
52. Ibid., p. 184.
53. Augustine, *On Christian Doctrine* 2.45.
54. See Claude Jenkins, "Saint Augustine and Magic," in *Science, Medicine, and History: Essays on the Evolution of Scientific Thought and Medical Practice Written in Honour of Charles Singer,* ed. E. A. Underwood (London, 1953), p. 135; and Keenan, "Augustine and the Medical Profession," p. 184.
55. Augustine, *Confessions* 1.10.17.
56. See Cooke, *Ministry to Word,* p. 356; Jones, *Later Roman Empire,* pp. 912–913.
57. Smith and Cheetham, *Dictionary of Christian Antiquities,* vol. 2, s.v. "Wonders," p. 2042.
58. Jones, *The Later Roman Empire,* p. 961.
59. See Arnaldo Momigliano, "Popular Religious Beliefs and the Later Roman Historians," in *Popular Belief and Practice* (Studies in Church History 8), eds. G. J. Cuming and Derek Baker (Cambridge, 1972), pp. 17–18.
60. Ambrose, *Epistle* 22; see also Augustine, *Confessions* 40.7 and *City of God* 22.8.
61. *City of God* 22.8.
62. For discussions of Augustine's belief in miracles see van der Meer, *Augustine the Bishop,* pp. 539–557; and Brown, *Augustine of Hippo,* pp. 413–418.
63. Basil of Caesarea, *Epistle* 189.
64. For a recent discussion of the origin and growth of early Christian hospitals, see Timothy S. Miller, *The Birth of the Hospital in the Byzantine Empire* (Baltimore, 1985).
65. See Demetrios J. Constantelos, *Byzantine Philanthropy and Social Welfare* (New Brunswick, NJ, 1968), pp. 95–96.
66. See, e.g., Jerome, *On Isaiah* 8; Augustine, *Tractate 30 on John 3; On Christian Doctrine* 4.16.33.
67. John Chrysostom, *Homily 14 on Romans.*
68. Ambrose, *On Cain* 1.40.
69. Augustine, *Sermon* 80.3.
70. Augustine, *Sermon* 84.1.
71. Augustine, *Sermon* 344.5.
72. E.g., Tertullian, *De Corona* 8; Clement of Alexandria, *Stromateis* 6.17; *Christ the Educator* 1.2.6; Origen, *Homily 18 on Numbers* 3; *Annotations on III Kings* 15.13; *Homily 1 on Psalm 37*:1; *Contra Celsum* 3.12; Basil of Caesarea, *The Long Rule* 55; Gregory of Nyssa, *Life of St. Macrina;* John Chrysostom, *Homily 8 on Colossians;* Augustine, *On Christian Doctrine* 4.16.33.
73. E.g., Augustine, *Tractate 30 on John* 1; *Tractate 32 on John* 9; *On the Good of Marriage* 9; *City of God* 9.13 and 22.24; *Epistle* 130; Jerome, *Epistles* 10 and 39; Cassian, *Conference of Abbot Theodore* 3.
74. E.g., Tertullian, *On Purity* 13; Clement, *Stromateis* 7.14; Origen, *Contra Celsum* 8.56; *Shepherd of Hermas* 6.3; Cyprian, *De Mortalitate* 8; Ambrose, *Concerning Repentance* 1.13.61 and 63; *Epistle* 79; Eusebius, *Ecclesiastical History* 7.22.6; Cassian, *Conference of Abbot Theodore* 3; Jerome, *Epistles* 38.2 and 108.19; Basil, *The Long Rule* 55; Gregory

Nazianzen, *Epistle* 31; *Panegyric on Basil* 26; *On the Death of His Father* 28; John Chrysostom, *Homily 1 on the Statues; Homily 8 on Colossians; Homily 33 on Hebrews* 8; *Homily 38 on John* 2; Augustine, *Epistles* 130 and 38.1; *On Psalm* 39:18.

CHAPTER 3

The Medieval
Catholic Tradition

DARREL W. AMUNDSEN

The date that marks the beginning of Roman Catholicism is a matter of some debate. Surely its roots go back to the earliest decades of Christianity, but the distinct identity of that enormously complex structure that was Medieval Catholicism developed only gradually. In 380, in response to the teaching known as Arianism, which held that Christ was a created being neither co-equal nor co-eternal with God the Father, the Roman Emperor Theodosius I decreed that all people of the Empire must adhere to that religion "which the divine Peter the Apostle transmitted to the Romans . . . that is followed by the Pontiff Damasus and by Peter, bishop of Alexandria." That religion was the historical Christianity that had, during the preceding centuries, formulated among numerous other dogmas the doctrine of the Trinity as finally expressed in the Nicene Creed (325). Damasus is significant as the first bishop of Rome to articulate the conviction that the holder of that office was the direct successor to the apostle Peter, upon whom it was claimed that Christ had said that he would build his church (*Mt.* 16:18–19). This principle, which was the foundation of the papacy, was even more forcefully advanced by two subsequent bishops of Rome, Leo I (440–461) and Gelasius I (492–496), the latter of whom insisted that the bishop of Rome (later known as the pope) had the authority to judge secular rulers but was himself subject to no man.

The most fundamental feature of the Catholic Church in the Middle Ages was its nearly complete identification with organized society in western Europe, at least in theory if not always in practice. The church became possibly the most thoroughly integrated religious system in human history. It was not a voluntary association because, from the late fourth century, all members of organized society in the West, except for a small number of Jews who were tolerated and a few heretics who were excluded from society and intermittently persecuted, had to be part of it. Only obedient believers could enjoy full rights within it and, consequently, rights within the various secular states of western Europe, whose relationship with the church was often fraught with tensions and conflicting claims of authority and jurisdiction. As many scholars have observed, the church was "the ark of salvation in a sea of destruction." Being in this ark provided the only assurance of meaning and purpose in this life and confidence in respect to the next, which was the exclusive possession of the ark's occupants. All of life, indeed the entire cosmos and people's place within it, could be understood only with reference to the church, which had the obligation to direct and regulate the details of human life. The medieval Catholic Church had as its head a single spiritual and temporal power, the pope, who sometimes claimed ultimate and absolute power within western European society.

Pope Gregory I (590–604) gave to the medieval papacy its distinct character, claiming universal (catholic) jurisdiction over all Christendom and proclaiming a Christian commonwealth in which the pope and the clergy were to exercise authority and responsibility for ordering society. He was a significant figure also for being the first pope zealously to support monasticism and to stress the cult of saints and relics, ascetic virtues, and demonology, which were the most distinct features of early medieval Catholicism. Additionally he was active in sponsoring missionary activity to the pagans, sending Augustine (who was later consecrated as Archbishop of Canterbury) to convert the pagan English in 596.

The Middle Ages began as classical civilization was nearing collapse in western Europe and closed when the conversion of western Europe to Christianity was nearly complete. At the beginning of the fourth century, Christianity in the West was a religion of a small minority. By the end of that century, most of the aristocracy and the urban population had been converted. It took centuries more, however, before Christianity meaningfully penetrated the peasant population of western Europe who, even when ostensibly converted, still continued to practice some form of ancestral paganism, however modified by Christian influence. The barbarian invasions of western Europe in the fifth century complicated the life of the church. The barbarians were almost all pagan. Many were converted to the Arian form of Christianity; others were gradually converted to Catholicism through missionary activity. Arians were finally brought into the Catholic fold by the end of the sixth century.

The centuries from about 500 to 1050 were, for the most part, chaotic and unsettled in western Europe with the notable exception of the time of the so-called Carolingian Renaissance. Poverty, famine, plague, disorder, and commercial atrophy typified much of the early Middle Ages. Numerous monasteries provided a symbol of stability in the midst of instability, an image of eternal order in a world of change that, when supplemented by local parishes, represented the intrusion of the licit supernatural into the lives of a society riddled by the reality of the evil supernatural. It was an age in which the ostensibly miraculous was common and expected, but never any less awe-inspiring on that account. The locus of the licit supernatural was the cult of saints and relics.

The high Middle Ages (1050–1300) were marked by enormous economic and religious changes. The period opened with a rapidly accelerating growth of economic development: rise of urbanization, colonization on all frontiers, expanding commercial enterprise within western Europe, and trade with the East, stimulated in part by the Crusades. It was a time of significant population growth, an age in which numerous complex problems produced by rapid social change gave rise to the need for more sophisticated solutions than old secular and religious mechanisms were able to provide. Expert knowledge and competence were being demanded in every sphere of life. Education was still dominated by the clergy, but was increasing dramatically, especially due to the creation and growth of universities. Theological debate stimulated by renewed philosophical analysis captured the minds of intellectual giants, for example Thomas Aquinas (1225–1274). Canon law, which was virtually in a state of chaos at the beginning of this period, had developed into a vastly complex and intricate science before 1300.

Although the aspects of life controlled by direct appeal to the supernatural were decreasing in number, the authority of the church over the individual was broadening through its increasingly efficient mechanisms of moral coercion and social control. The catalyst of much of this development was the papacy. This period opened with popes who were zealous to put into practice the papal authority that had been usually present only in theory, and closed with a succession of lawyer–popes, who were the embodiment of a strong papal monarchy.

The late Middle Ages (1300–1545) began with a strong papal monarchy that may have seemed indestructible but was soon weakened significantly. Papal hegemony was decreased by the rise of strong national monarchies headed by kings who coveted absolute jurisdiction over their lands, which were inhabited by people whose sense of national and ethnic identity was increasing. In 1309 the papacy moved to Avignon, France, where it remained until 1377, appearing to many as simply a tool of the French monarch. The Avignonese Papacy led to the Great Schism, lasting from 1378 to 1417, a time that saw two, and then (from 1409) three, concurrent lines of popes. All claimed exclusive rights to the papal office and excommunicated each other. By the time that this division ended, the prestige and authority of the papacy had been enormously weakened. Shortly thereafter, the effects of the Italian Renaissance were evidenced in the beginning of a line of "Renaissance popes." Some were pious and distinguished humanists, others were of very questionable spiritual qualifications and moral integrity.

In 1348–1349 a plague called the Black Death ravaged Europe, killing at least a quarter of the population. The impact of this and subsequent epidemics of pestilential disease, combined with numerous social, economic, and political developments, contributed to a laicization of European society. The towns and cities became hotbeds of dissent, both political and religious. Varieties of subversive religious movements surfaced. Corruption in the medieval church, both real and alleged, became increasingly a matter of concern to a growing number of clergy and laymen. Attempts to remove certain abuses, periodically initiated by various popes and by some monastic movements, met usually with limited success. Other reform efforts within the church were unsuccessful because those seeking reform did not limit their efforts to dealing with the spiritual and moral laxity so prevalent within the church, but also sought to change some of the theology of the church that seemed to contradict Scripture. Such were John Wycliffe (ca. 1329–1384), Jan Hus (1373–1415), and Martin Luther (1483–1546), the last of whom in great part perpetrated the Protestant Reformation, which brought to an end the medieval Catholic Church, a structure that had exercised nearly exclusive authority in religion in western Europe for a millennium. The reaction of the Catholic Church to the Protestant Reformation was the Counter Reformation, through which the church removed many abuses that had been weakening it internally and created a structure of practice and belief embodied in the decrees of the Council of Trent, which convened in 1545.

The Early Middle Ages (500–1050)

Early in the fourth century (313), official persecution of Christians by the imperial government ceased. By the end of the century (391), Christianity became the official religion of the Empire, and all public forms of paganism were outlawed. That which had been the religion of a small minority in the western half of the Empire now became the religion of all, at least in form. Church and state joined hands, the latter in an effort to suppress, and the former in an attempt to replace with Christian ideas and practices, whatever expressions of paganism remained.

The nature of Christian practices and even some beliefs undergirding those practices seem to have changed in late antiquity. It is a commonplace to attribute this change to the entry into the church, after the legalization of Christianity, of a vast number of pagans who brought with them a rich diversity of pagan superstitions that were soon clothed in quasi-Christian garb. In this view a small theological elite, frustrated in their efforts to suppress the superstitious beliefs and practices of this horde of "converts," sought to accommodate, adapt, and gradually Christianize their religious expression. This interpretation, although correct to a limited extent, is inaccurate and simplistic. Before the Christianization of the Empire, indeed even by the late third century, discernible changes had begun to occur in the Mediterranean ethos, affecting Christians and pagans alike. These changes affected people's perception, understanding, and definition of the supernatural and their relationship and accessibility to it.[1] New relationships were evident both at a sociopolitical level, as the structure of late Roman society was undergoing enormous change, and at the religious level as contact with the supernatural assumed new forms. New religious expressions emerged as people sought to relate to bewilderingly varied manifestations of the supernatural that were an integral part of even their most mundane affairs. The church clearly distinguished between the licit and illicit supernatural. And any contact with the supernatural was illicit if the church did not dispense it.

While the battle against the residue of paganism in the Mediterranean ethos of late antiquity was being waged by state and church, the western half of the Empire was slowly falling to incursions of primarily Germanic barbarians, some of whom had already been converted to the Arian heresy and were, within two centuries, to be won over to Catholicism. The rest were pagans who were gradually converted by Catholic missionaries. In spite of enormous diversity among the converted barbarian peoples of Europe during the early Middle ages, two factors created a significant degree of homogeneity. First, all had their distinct ancestral religions that, although greatly varied, possessed commonalities of thought and expression typical of folk paganism generally. This folk paganism, essentially pantheism, was so much a part of the very rhythm of their lives that it remained, for most of them, a vitally real, if officially suppressed and experientially submerged, current of their subconscious being and identity. Secondly, all had in common the same alternative to their folk paganism. That was Roman Catholicism, which consistently declared their folk paganism to be both real and evil, and could tolerate no alternative to itself. Accordingly, the church sought to channel their individual and communal impulses and wants into sources of actualization and fulfillment that were within the ordered structure of Catholic liturgy, sacraments, and the cult of saints and relics.

There were of course some, who usually became clergy, who embraced Christianity with such fervency and commitment that they utterly repudiated all association with their ancestral paganism, seeing all folk religious practice as magical and demonic. In a sense it is proper to speak of the clergy as an elite. But without significant qualifications, so to speak would be grossly misleading, for, when reading the literature written during the early Middle Ages, one is struck by "the common credulity and lack of critical sense which underlay the observances of literate and illiterate alike."[2] We may call the clergy a theological elite, an intellectual elite, especially because nearly the only literate people were clergy, and, to an extent, a social elite. But their eliteness was not manifest in their belief in a practice of religion that was, at a functional level, theological while that of the masses was superstitious, that the former was sophisticated while the latter was vulgar. Granted, the former had a theologically reasoned structure that could not be articulated in the latter; but at a functional level there was often very little significant difference except that the former was licit while the latter was not, and the licit declared the illicit to be evil and fought against it vigorously. While the early medieval church never denied the reality of the supernatural power that undergirded folk paganism, it did seek to meet the needs of pagan converts by substituting beliefs and practices that had already become part of the Christian experience in the West. It also permitted certain strictly pagan practices to continue as long as they were conducted in the vicinity of churches and not in traditional sites like sacred groves.

The conversion of western Europe during the early Middle Ages hinged on combatting one form of the supernatural with another. Gaining the religious loyalty of pagans depended upon missionaries convincing them that Christianity's power to aid them was greater than that of their pantheistic folk paganism. And the greatest display of Christianity's power was in the miracles worked by the cult of saints and relics. One of the most spectacular manifestations of this cult was the shrine of Saint Martin at Tours. Between 563 and 565, Nicetus, bishop of Trier, wrote to Clotsinda, Catholic queen of the Arian Lombards, urging her to help win her Arian husband, King Alboin, to the Catholic religion. Among other things, he suggested:

> If the King chooses let him send his men to [Gaul], to the Lord Martin [at Tours], at his feast . . . where every day we see the blind receive their sight, the deaf their hearing, and the dumb their speech. What shall I say of lepers or of many others, who, no matter with what sickness they are afflicted, are healed there year after year? . . . What shall I say of the [shrines of the] Lord Bishops Germanus [of Auxerre], Hilary [of Poitiers], or Lupus [of Troyes], where so many wonders occur every day, so great that I cannot express them in words: where the afflicted (those having demons) are suspended and whirled round in the air and confess the [power of the] Lords I have named? You have heard how your grandmother . . . led the Lord Clovis to the Catholic Law, and how, since he was a most astute man, he was unwilling to agree to it until he knew it was true. When he saw that the things I have spoken of were proved he humbly prostrated

himself at the threshold of the Lord Martin [at Tours] and promised to be baptized without delay.[3]

The cult of saints and relics was the single most important force in the conversion of Western Europe. The literature of the early Middle Ages is rife with examples of miracles wrought through the relics of the saints. In 601 Pope Gregory I wrote to Augustine of Canterbury, a missionary whom he had sent to England, congratulating him on his successes in converting through his miracles the Anglo-Saxons, whose souls "are drawn by outward miracles to inward grace."[4] Gregory recognized that when pagans were converted to Christianity, the process of transformation was often both precarious and lengthy. He wrote to Mellitus, who was en route to England, that "it is doubtless impossible to cut out everything at once from their stubborn minds: just as the man who is attempting to climb to the highest place, rises by steps and degrees and not by leaps." Accordingly, Gregory ordered that their idols should be destroyed but their temples should be allowed to stand, be purified with holy water, and furnished with altars and relics, so that

> they should be changed from the worship of devils to the service of the true God. When this people see that their shrines are not destroyed they will be able to banish error from their hearts and be more ready to come to the places they are familiar with, but now recognizing and worshipping the true God. And because they are in the habit of slaughtering much cattle as sacrifices to devils, some solemnity ought to be given them in exchange for this. So on the day of the dedication or the festivals of the holy martyrs, whose relics are deposited there, let them make themselves huts from the branches of trees around the churches which have been converted out of shrines, and let them celebrate the solemnity with religious feasts. Do not let them sacrifice animals to the devil, but let them slaughter animals for their own food to the praise of God, and let them give thanks to the Giver of all things for his bountiful provision.[5]

Gregory's letter advocated both condemnation and accommodation. While accommodation involved a degree of condescension, condemnation did not, and throughout the early Middle Ages, condemnation of pagan practices was incessant.[6]

During the frequent outbreaks of plague that afflicted Europe in sixteen waves from 541 to 767, and especially during early episodes, people fled to pagan alternatives.[7] In the British Isles, Cuthbert (ca. 634–687) sought to convert the people "from a life of foolish habits to a love of heavenly joys. For many of them also at the time of the plague, forgetting the sacred mystery of the faith into which they had been initiated, took to the delusive cures of idolatry"[8] In France, 150 years later, Jonas of Orleans complained that people hastened to sorcerers when sick.[9]

Attempts to deal with relapses into paganism or participation in pagan practices varied. Early medieval law was concerned with any unauthorized religious or superstitious practice. Like Roman law,[10] the secular codes of the early Middle Ages adamantly forbade the use of malicious magic. But they differed from Roman law in prohibiting a wide variety of pagan practices such as "nocturnal sacrifices to devils," "infamous rites," going to a soothsayer for divination, incantation, performing sacrilege generally, worshipping at "a tree which the rustics call holy and at springs."[11] One of Charlemagne's laws specified some thirty superstitious practices as illicit[12]; another directed that "every bishop carefully visit his diocese each year and that he take pains . . . to prohibit pagan celebrations and diviners or soothsayers or auguries, amulets, incantations, and all kinds of pagan filth."[13] A half century earlier Pope Gregory II had commended Bishop Boniface to the Christians of Germany. Boniface's mission was to deal with those who had been "led astray by the wiles of the devil and now serve idols under the guise of the Christian religion." Boniface was enjoined to enlighten them with his preaching.[14] Twenty years later (742) Boniface presided over a church council that decreed that "in accordance with the canons each bishop should take care . . . that the people of God should not do pagan things but should abandon and repudiate all the filthy practices of the gentiles, be it sacrifices to the dead or divination or immolation of sacrificial animals, things which ignorant people do in the pagan way next to churches in the name of the holy martyrs or confessors."[15]

Numerous church synods and councils had addressed the problem of continuing pagan practices. Walter Ullmann writes that the conciliar "decrees against superstition are so numerous that one is justified in the assumption that [the practices that they repeatedly prohibited] were general and widespread." Commenting on the motivation behind these conciliar actions, he asserts that the promulgators of such decrees "cared for what may be termed the public health of society, public health understood not in terms of physical well-being, but in terms of protecting and if necessary immunizing and inoculating the mind of the people against infectious diseases of a pandemic kind."[16]

Throughout the Middle Ages, the well-being of the corporate body of Christ was, above all else, the major concern of those who sought to protect the community from all incursions of contaminating influence, whether of paganism (including magic in its manifold varieties) or heresy. For salvation was only through the church; all else led to damnation. For the hierarchy of the church, and for those clergy about whom we have information, well-being found expression in personal piety, self-denial, ascetic practices, missionary zeal, and a deep pastoral concern for the well-being of the large numbers of people, mostly peasants, whose conception of well-being was significantly different from their own. Tension between these two groups arose from their markedly discordant conceptions of well-being. The well-being that was common probably to the majority of the laity during the early Middle Ages was essentially mundane. But this mundane sphere was intimately connected with the supernatural that permeated all aspects of their lives. Their well-being depended upon a sustained harmony with their whole environment, a harmony of well-being congruous with the very rhythm of their lives. When this harmony was marred by any cacophony, it could be restored only through rituals and magical manipulations that had proven efficacious in bringing their lives back into harmony with the properly integrated order for their world. Sometimes the church, through its liturgy, sacraments, and especially through the cult of saints and relics, was able to contribute to this process. But it was seldom able to satisfy the deepest cravings of the peasant population for sustained periods; life was too tumultuous and uncertain during these centuries. For them, well-being was the state of being in the right relationship with the totality of their environment. The well-being that Christianity offered was to be in a right relationship with God, which depended upon being in a right relationship with the church. Although the church provided mechanisms for sustaining and restoring equilibrium at a mundane level, the ultimate orientation and objective was always with a view to eternity, whereas the deepest yearnings of the peasants were predominantly temporal. Hence the tension illustrated by the efforts of the clergy, law, and councils to deal with the continued recurrence of illicit practices.

Although this tension endured throughout the Middle Ages at least in remote areas, it gradually diminished, particularly in the last century of the primitive age of medieval Catholicism. This process was aided by the organization of rural parishes (effective in few areas before the tenth century),[17] which made possible relatively close contact between the clergy and the majority of the people generally. The people needed to be protected from themselves, from Satan, from all evil influences, from sin itself. This was accomplished in part through pastoral teaching and exhortation. Even more intimate, however, was the personal encounter of clergy with laity in systematic efforts to identify and deal with specific sins. These efforts took the form of interrogation by the clergy and confession, repentance, and penance by the laity. The most useful tool for this process was the penitential literature that was produced in abundance during the early Middle Ages. These handbooks of penance essentially were guides for clergy that enumerated and discussed a wide and imaginative variety of sins for which specific acts of penance were prescribed. Probably more than any other, sexual sins aroused the attention of the authors of these handbooks. Adultery, fornication, sodomy, homosexuality, masturbation, and bestiality were treated with great thoroughness.[18]

Significantly less attention was paid to categories of sin other than sexual, but concern with superstitious practices was a strong contender for second place in these handbooks. Wilfrid Bonser writes of the penitentials that "the magical practices especially attacked may be divided into the following categories: (1) idolatry and worship of 'demons' in general; (2) the cult of the dead; (3) the worship of nature (trees, wells, stones, fire, etc.); (4) pagan calendar customs and festivals; (5) witchcraft and sorcery; (6) augury and divination; and (7) astrology."[19] Beginning with *The Penitential of Finnian* (ca. 525–550), the prescribing of penance for any kind of pagan practice became a constant feature.[20] With some regularity, pagan methods of healing or preserving health were mentioned. The placing of a child upon a roof or into (or on) an oven for the cure of a fever was frequently condemned.[21] The oven (or hearth) was the place where the guardian spirits of the house dwelt; spirits who might aid healing also resided on the roof.[22] One penitential condemns a woman's tasting her husband's blood as a remedy,[23] and another prescribes penance for drinking blood or urine, probably consumed for health-related reasons.[24] Two penitentials condemn the practice of the burning of grain at the place where a man has died, for preserving or restoring the health of the living.[25] One also assigns penance if on account of illness one bathes below a mill. The penance is much more severe if this act was accompanied by an incantation.[26] The same penitential also deals with the sin of uttering incantations while collecting medicinal herbs. Instead of incantations, one should recite the Creed or the Lord's Prayer while gathering the herbs.[27] Three centuries later, the same advice appears in *The Corrector and Physician* of Burchard of Worms.[28] In this work there are, among numerous interrogations regarding superstitious practices, the following concerning sickness and healing:

> Have you come to any place to pray other than a church or other religious place which your bishop or your priest showed you, that is, either to springs or to stones or to trees or to crossroads, and there in reverence for the place lighted a candle or a torch or carried there bread or any offering or eaten there or sought there any healing of body or mind? If you have done or consented to such things, you shall do penance for three years on the appointed fast days. Have you done what some do when they are visiting any sick person? When they approach the house where the sick person lies, if they find a stone lying nearby, they turn the stone over and look in the place where the stone was lying [to see] if there is anything living under it, and if they find there a worm or a fly or an ant or anything that moves, then they aver that the sick person will recover. But if they find

there nothing that moves, they say he will die. If you have done or believed in this you shall do penance for twenty days on bread and water.[29]

Only two penitentials referred to permitted means of healing. The prologue to *The Penitential of Cummean* (ca. 650) quotes *James 5:14–16*, suggesting anointing with oil for healing.[30] The so-called *Roman Penitential of Halitgar* (ca. 830) included a prayer to be said over the sick: "O God, Who gave to Your servant Hezekiah an extension of life of fifteen years, so also may your greatness raise up Your servant from the bed of sickness unto health. Through our Lord Jesus Christ."[31] Because the penitentials were concerned with sin, it is not remarkable that they had so little occasion to speak of licit means of healing. It would not be surprising, however, if they had much to say about sickness, especially given the assumed relationship of sin and sickness in medieval Christian thought. This, however, is not the case, for the penitentials mentioned sickness very little. One stipulated that any individual who became ill during penance should be permitted to receive the sacrament of communion.[32] There is no indication that the sickness was regarded as a punishment for sin, because the penitent was to resume penance if he or she recovered from his illness. Nothing here was even implied about causality.

The penitentials addressed the issue of causality only when insanity led to suicide.[33] *The Penitential of Theodore* (668–690) specified that "if a man is vexed by the devil . . . and slays himself, there may be some reason to pray for him if he was formerly religious."[34] Other reasons for insanity leading to suicide were then given: despair, fear, unknown reasons, or a sudden seizure.[35] *The Burgundian Penitential* (ca. 700–725) referred to wizards taking away the minds of men by the invocation of demons or by rendering them mad.[36] Here the emphasis was on the sin of practicing wizardry, whereas in the former the concern was with the sin of self-destruction, while insanity was only a mitigating factor. Because it is so common to assume that in the early Middle Ages demonic causality was accepted for most disease, and certainly for mental illness, such natural causes as despair, fear, sudden seizure, and "unknown reasons" may surprise us. Such explanations, however, occur with some frequency. For instance, when Richer of Rheims wrote his *Historia* between 991 and 998, he thus described the death of King Odo: "On account of his extreme nervousness he began to suffer from insomnia, the aggravation of which brought about the loss of reason . . . he died from what some call mania, others madness."[37] And in 1023, Fulbert of Chartres, when comparing the functions of priests and physicians, said that "it is a physician's duty to offer those who are suffering from depression, insanity, or any other illness what he has learned in the exercise of his art."[38] Jerome Kroll is undoubtedly right when he says of this period that "mental and spiritual illnesses were attributed as much to overwork, overeating, and overindulgence in sexual activity as to climatic conditions, magic spells, and demonic possession."[39] There is, however, considerable ambiguity in the literature. This ambiguity arises from two different sources. First, there was much imprecision in identifying the causes of mental illness. The second source of ambiguity is the failure of the modern reader to enter sufficiently into the early medieval structure of reality in which ultimate and proximate causality may be spoken of in the same breath without any distinction being made, and an intermediate (usually demonic) causality mingled in with the former two. Any one of the three may be mentioned as the cause of a particular condition, and taken by the modern reader as the author's perceived sole cause, whereas the choice of that cause was simply determined by the author's desire to emphasize one with no intention of making it appear exclusive. This applies not only to considerations of madness but also, indeed even more so, to sickness generally.

A degree of demonic causality was seen in many conditions, and some people may have attributed nearly every adverse condition to demons. But the sources adequately demonstrate that on the whole God was viewed as the ultimate dispenser of human suffering, including sickness. As a general rule, when early medieval sources mentioned direct demonic involvement, which they frequently did, the condition was clearly regarded as possession, whether accompanied by sickness or not. They delighted in relating stories of exorcisms, but they were equally eager to tell of healings through relics from which exorcism is absent. Furthermore, the most holy of the saints could not conceivably have been possessed by demons, but yet were frequently ill; some indeed seemed to gain a high degree of sanctity through their sicknesses.

Another commonplace encountered in modern assessments of the early Middle Ages is the assertion that early medieval people saw sin as the cause of most sickness. Here there is room for much confusion because the relationship of sin with sickness can appear at three different levels. First, sin was certainly regarded by early medieval authors as the cause of sickness in the sense that without sin there would have been no material evil. This, although not expressed, was an underlying assumption of the sources. Second, one's own general sinfulness was often given as the cause of one's own sicknesses. Third, sickness, it was thought, might result from specific sin. This last statement is very seldom encountered except in denunciations of and warnings to entire communities, and then the emphasis was often on general moral laxity, which makes it nearly indistinguishable from the second category. We should also note that it is one thing to maintain that a person is sick as a punishment for a specific sin to which one is obstinately and tenaciously clinging, but it is quite another matter to attribute one's own sickness to one's general sinfulness and see the sickness as part of God's punitive and refining process.

There is, in the literature, a definite appreciation of God's hand in a Christian's suffering and of the salutary effects of sickness in the Christian's life. Pope Gregory I, in his pastoral handbook, wrote that "the sick are to be admonished so that they will feel that they are the sons of God because the scourge of discipline chastizes them." They were also exhorted "to maintain the virtue of patience."[40] We must bear in mind that the concept of discipline here was by no means limited to punishment. Indeed, the predominant emphasis in the term was on training or edification. For example, Bede, a contemporary of the events he described, said of the Abbess Aethelburh: "Now in order that her strength, like the apostle's, might be made perfect in weakness, she was suddenly afflicted with a most serious bodily disease and for nine years was sorely tried, under the good providence of our Redeemer, so that any traces of sin remaining among her virtues through ignorance or carelessness might be burnt away by the fires of prolonged suffering."[41] Aethelburh died of her disease. Bede also saw benefit derived from acute conditions. For example, he wrote that the merits of the saintly Germanus were increased by the suffering caused by an injury. Germanus was miraculously healed after a short period.[42] Bede's account of the suffering of Bishop Benedict and one of his colleagues is typical of the attitudes expressed in the literature:

And not long after, Benedict also began to be wearied by the assault of illness. That the virtue of patience might be added, to give conclusive proof of such great zeal for religion, Divine Mercy laid them both up in bed by temporal illness that, after sickness had been conquered by death, God might restore them with the endless rest of heavenly peace and light. Sigfrid, punished . . . by long internal suffering, drew toward his last day, and Benedict, during three years, gradually became so paralyzed that all his lower limbs were quite dead . . . to exercise him in the virtue of patience. Both men sought in their suffering ways to give thanks to their Creator, and always to be occupied with the praises of God and with teaching the brethren.[43]

Such attitudes, of course, were not typical of all people during the early Middle Ages. Some might admire the spiritual fortitude manifested in the sanctified suffering of a select, holy few whose actions were much more admired than emulated. Although the well-being of these few might be enhanced by suffering, the perceived well-being of the semi-Christianized pagans of the early Middle Ages was destroyed or at least disrupted by sickness. Their eager, indeed frantic, quest for the healing that was itself a restoration of well-being indicates that their sense of wellness was tied to temporal and material considerations.

In their efforts to deal with the spiritual needs of the majority, the clerical minority sought to maintain a delicate balance between meeting the people's temporal and material wants on the one hand and their eternal and spiritual needs on the other. There was a long and evolving tradition of physical healing in Christianity. There was an equally long tradition in Christianity to provide for spiritual healing; indeed, the very essence of Christianity had that as its goal. This tradition also assumed new forms, or at least was manifested in new emphases, in late antiquity and even more so in the early Middle Ages, when the expectation of Christ's return, which had always been present to some degree in Christianity, assumed an air of impending destruction and doom precipitated by God's wrath. While the mechanisms for physical healing were exploited in missionary activities and in pastoral efforts to keep the flock from reverting to pagan healing methods, the message of impending doom was proclaimed in an attempt to wean the flock from the temporal to the eternal, and from the material to the spiritual, to realign their well-being from a present horizontal to a future vertical orientation. Plague proved to be most useful in this effort. We have noted earlier that Europe was afflicted by sixteen waves of plague from 541 to 767, during the early occurrences of which Christians often relapsed into pagan practices. But plague was a two-edged sword, and in the long run the effect was less to stimulate people to concern for the well-being of their bodies than to direct their concern to escaping the eternal consequences of the wrath of God. Plague "mainly had the effect of making them more amenable to certain Christian beliefs and practices. Seen as one element in a whole set of calamities and signs, the plague settled in people's minds a concrete expectation of the Last Judgement . . . . [It] explained calamities as retribution for collective sin, instilled notions of a wrathful God . . . and gave rise to an apocalyptic and millenarian mentality."[44] Pope Gregory I was obsessed by the plague. Gregory assumed the papacy during a time of plague (590) and "preached a sermon . . . declaring the plague to be a punishment from God and calling upon the people to do penance and repent of their sins. He ordered them to pray and sing psalms for three days, and at the end of that time arranged for a massive city-wide litany. . . . No less than eighty people dropped dead of the plague during the procession."[45]

About 150 years later, Bede, in his *Ecclesiastical History,* marveled that the Anglo-Saxons were not turned from their wicked ways by a devastating visitation of the plague[46] and in his *Life of St. Cuthbert* he referred to the plague as "a blow sent by God the Creator."[47] Bede was not only interested in the theological nature of plague, but also in its natural explanation. In his *De Natura Rerum* he asserted that plague was "produced from the air when it has become corrupted" and then hastened to add parenthetically "in accordance with the deserts of men."[48] Although Gregory, Bede, and churchmen generally saw the plague as punishment imposed by God, it does not follow that they also viewed those stricken by the plague as especially great sinners. When the pestilence hit Britain, Bede recorded the death of the "blessed Boisil," who had predicted three years earlier that he himself would die of the plague. Cuthbert also came down with the plague at the same time but did not die of it.[49]

Personal sanctity was no guarantee of avoiding plague. Being afflicted with it was no sign of personal sin. Plague and all other sicknesses were designed for the purpose of adjusting people's minds to eternal and spiritual verities. And repentance, regardless of the level of one's own personal sanctity, was always appropriate. But such views were not always consonant with the heart of the masses and even of some clergy. Around 829, part of southern France was hit by a very painful epidemic. Terror-stricken people bringing offerings flocked to the shrine of Fermin, hoping to be cured. No one was cured. Agobard, bishop of Lyons, "was particularly critical of the willingness of the clergy who accepted these offerings to keep them to their profit. He suggested that plagues visited on men by God required not simply payment but repentance. . . ."[50] Bishop Agobard's criticism of the lack of repentance on the part of those who hoped to be healed at the shrine of Fermin was consistent with the theology of the time. It was, however, discordant with the emphasis and orientation of the thriving cult of saints and relics during the early Middle Ages.

As Christianity expanded northward during the early Middle Ages, the cult of saints and relics was imported into the realm of the barbarians, and for many who were converted, the bones of holy men and their relics became the very core of Christianity, taking the place of theological subtleties that they could not hope to understand. For a millennium the beliefs and miraculous practices associated with the cult of saints and relics dominated western Christianity. Each shrine and its immediate vicinity were viewed as being inhabited by a powerful presence, and it was believed that the saints were especially responsive to prayers made near their relics. For the physically ill or maimed or demon-possessed, these shrines became a focal point for hope, comfort, healing, and a social and spiritual reintegration throughout the Middle Ages. But especially during the early Middle Ages, when the cult of saints and relics was a substitute for some of the pagan practices that had provided security by maintaining or restoring social cohesiveness, the importance of the cult is best understood in view of its identity with the welfare of the community rather than the welfare of the individual. The festival of a saint, celebrated at his shrine, as Peter Brown says,

> made plain God's acceptance of the community as a whole: his mercy embraced all its disparate members, and could reintegrate all who had stood outside in the previous year. . . . The terror of illness, of blindness, of possession . . . resided in the fear that, at that high moment of solidarity, the sinner would be seen to have been placed by his affliction outside the community. . . . Hence [these were] miracles of reintegration into the community.[51]

The cult of saints and relics provided stability and safety for a society in which individuals were of little importance, because individuals' meaning, security, indeed their well-being itself, derived from their oneness with their community.[52]

Although not the sole means of healing in the church's repertoire, the cult of saints and relics overshadowed all other sources of licit miraculous healing. Prayer was a mechanism for hope, but it lacked both the glamor and efficacy of the cult of saints and relics. Even prayer itself was so frequently made to or through saints and their relics that it seems to be nearly subsumed under the cult. Another healing medium was the practice of anointing with oil for healing, as directed in *James* 5:14–16. The practice prescribed there appears to have received little attention in the post-apostolic church. Perhaps the earliest direct application was in a letter by Pope Innocent I in the early fifth century.[53] This letter addressed the question of whether consecrated oil could be taken home and used privately for healing (as was the practice, apparently) or could only be administered by a priest. Innocent allowed this nonclerical practice to continue, which it did for much of the early Middle Ages.[54] It is difficult to tell how popular this procedure was with the common people. When Caesarius of Arles, in the early sixth century, complained about people reverting to pagan practices when sick, he said: "How much more right and salutary it would be if they made haste to the church . . . and piously anointed themselves and their family with holy oil; and in accordance with the words of the Apostle James received not only health of the body but also pardon of their sins."[55] The connection between physical healing and the forgiveness of sin, the latter being under the exclusive province of the clergy, caused the demise of anointing with oil for the healing of the sick in medieval Catholicism. Through a rather circuitous route, the anointing of the sick for physical healing became associated in practice with penitential anointing, which could be administered only by a priest. Because penitential anointing carried with it several stipulations as to conduct (including a permanent renouncing of marital relations and of the eating of meat), it was quite understandably put off until the last moment. It became known in the tenth or eleventh century as extreme unction and for the most part lost any of its effective connection with physical healing, usurping the significance of the *viaticum*, the administration of communion to those in danger of death.

We see in Caesarius' statement a desire for the cure of the body to be combined with the cure of the soul. This is by no means peculiar to him or to his time. It has been and remains at least a latent source of tension in Christianity. Spiritual models for physical healing controlled by the church were least productive of tension. Pagan or magical models obviously went beyond simple tension because they were declared illicit. The greatest tension was produced by natural or medical healing models. They were sometimes essentially neither strictly medical nor magical, quasi-medical healing models as it were. A good example is provided by the *De Medicamentis* of Marcellus of Bordeaux (fifth century) which was designed to show people how to treat their own ills by learning to employ the occult virtues of plants, gems, and other natural properties. This curious mixture of classical pharmacology, local herb lore, and Greco-Roman and Celtic spells offered, in the words of Peter Brown, "a model of direct and unmediated dependence of the individual on his environment."[56] And it was an environment regarded as alive with hidden but exploitable powers.[57] Basically this kind of healing effort could be something as innocent as simple folk-medicine, but when it employed any means that were, or appeared to be, magical or pagan, it assumed a dangerous ambiguity. Against such sometimes ambiguous practices the early medieval church waged considerable combat. It was particularly the use of spells or incantations in connection with herbs, gems, and the like, that frustrated the church. We have already seen mention of this in the penitential literature that recommended the substitution of the Creed and the Lord's Prayer for pagan utterances.[58]

The tension between the church and such folk medicine arose from the potential for even temporary dependence upon a source that either was not compatible with Christianity or could be employed without reference to it. Most obviously, the use of incantations and spells in conjunction with folk remedies had to be replaced with Christian formulae. But even if folk medicine were employed without the use of any illicit procedures, the attitude of the one using the remedies was important, because a dependence upon the power of the herbs and gems without reference to their creator was regarded as improper for a Christian. The latter of these two objections to folk medicine could also be applied to the secular medicine practiced by physicians.

It is not uncommon to see in modern discussions of the Middle Ages assertions or implications that the medieval church was hostile to science, especially to medicine, and disparaged its practice as a threat to the spiritual health of the physically ill. Such a picture is false. It may, however, appear on the surface to be at least partially true. For example, miraculous healings abound in much of the literature. The spectacular nature of these healings is highlighted when the failures of physicians were mentioned in particular cases. Several times in the two accounts of the life of Cuthbert, individuals were miraculously healed whom doctors could not help "with their compounds and drugs" or "with all their care."[59] One of the most enthusiastic recorders of miracles was Gregory of Tours (sixth century). He especially seemed to delight in describing the abysmal failures of physicians whose patients subsequently found healing at the shrine of St. Martin. But Gregory definitely used Greco-Roman medical handbooks and pharmacological guides himself.[60] Likewise, Pope Gregory I, who more than any other individual shaped the ethos of early medieval Catholicsm with its emphasis on miraculous healings, the cult of saints and relics, and demonology, had a fascination with medicine. Because of his almost constant illnesses, he kept an Alexandrian physician in permanent attendance. When a friend of his living in Ravenna was sick, Gregory solicited the opinions of all the physicians he knew and passed them on to his ill friend. Tradition also has it that he cured a Lombard king's stomach ailment by prescribing a milk diet.[61]

Medicine was a standard part of the medieval curriculum and it is not uncommon to encounter educated clerics requesting medical handbooks[62] and both seeking and giving medical advice. Bishop Fulbert of Chartres (early eleventh century) outdid Pope Gregory I by not only sending medical advice but also a variety of medicines to a sick friend.[63] On another occasion he wrote to a fellow bishop: "Believe me, father, I have not prepared any ointments since I was raised to the bishopric. But the little that is left of what a doctor gave to me I am sending as a gift . . . with the prayer that Christ, the author of good health, may make it help you."[64]

The closing comment in this letter is important: The cure comes from God. This theme was a constant undercurrent, and occasionally voices were raised to remind people that when they are ill their hope should not be placed in drugs and remedies but in God, who gave these substances their efficacy. Physicians likewise were urged to place their faith in God and to extend charity to the destitute ill. This latter advice appeared in some treatises on medical etiquette from the early Middle Ages. One of these, from the eighth century, urged the physician to serve rich and poor alike, and to look for eternal rather than material rewards.[65] The identity of the authors and the intended audience of these treatises is unknown. These writings are part of a fairly large body of medical manuscripts that reflect a sustained tradition of Greco-

Roman medicine. References to physicians are frequently encountered in all genres of literature. These physicians were of two basic categories: strictly secular practitioners and cleric–physicians, often monks. Occasionally, physicians schooled in Constantinople or Alexandria appear. Now and then we also encounter Jewish or Islamic physicians, who were trained in the much more medically sophisticated environment of the East. But the vast majority undoubtedly were Catholics born and trained in western Europe who were little more than craftsmen who had acquired their medical skills by apprenticeship. Even those who were trained at Salerno in Italy, of whom we hear a little by the tenth century, were essentially craftsmen. Our knowledge is very inadequate of the wide variety of secular physicians who tended the ills of the probably relatively small minority of the population who could pay for their services. The vast majority of people who sought nonmiraculous healing had to rely upon traditional folk remedies or seek help from such clergy as possessed medical knowledge or skill.

The duty to visit and care for the sick is clearly given in the Gospel and is repeatedly encountered in the literature of early Christianity.[66] Care of the poor and infirm was enjoined by various councils throughout these centuries.[67] It was the bishop's responsibility to administer the funds for the care of the poor and sick. Bishops were directed to provide accommodations for the destitute. These buildings were originally called *xenodochia,* a term that eventually gave way to *hospitia* or *hospitalia.* These were usually attached to a cathedral or other church.[68] It is a mistake to envision these facilities for the most part as hospitals in anything approaching the modern sense.[69] Some, particularly in the sixth and seventh centuries, were designed for the extension of medical care by a staff of trained physicians, but these were probably an exception.[70] The vast majority of *xenodochia* simply provided refuge in the form of shelter, food, and a few amenities.

The *xenodochia* that survived the chaos of the disintegration of the Carolingian Empire usually became the property of monasteries. In the early Middle Ages, monasteries were also places of refuge for the poor and the sick. The *Rule* of Benedict (sixth century), which governed the vast network of Benedictine monasteries that spread throughout western Europe during these centuries, addressed health needs. One passage specified that the cellarer give care to fellow monks who were ill.[71] In another passage he was admonished to "take the greatest care of the sick, of children, of guests, and of the poor, knowing without doubt that he will have to render account for all these on the Day of Judgement."[72] The availability of those qualified to give medical care certainly varied from monastery to monastery. Both accounts of the life of Cuthbert tell of a young paralytic monk who was sent by his abbot to Cuthbert's monastery, not to be healed by Cuthbert's relics, but because there were "very skilled" physicians there. All their medical skills availed nothing, however, and the youth finally cried out for aid from the "heavenly Physician" and was cured through the relics (in this case the shoes) of the deceased Cuthbert.[73] This incident tells us that there were physicians who were viewed as "very skilled" at the monastery at Lindisfarne in the seventh century. Their work on this youth was undoubtedly performed in the infirmary, which was reserved for clerics. It tells us nothing about the availability of health care for the needy laity provided by monks. We do know that in the sixth century the sick came to the monastery at Iona for medical attention.[74] It is unlikely that the destitute sick were refused help when they presented themselves at a monastery, and the monasteries to which the sick would most likely come were those known for their competent physicians. Such care as was extended was ideally motivated by Christian charity and not by a desire for financial gain.

The High and Late Middle Ages (1050–1545)

The Cistercian abbott, Bernard of Clairvaux (1090–1153), wrote to an abbot of another monastery in response to the latter's demand that a monk who had fled to Clairvaux be returned to his former monastery. This monk's complaint was that his abbot "used him not as a monk but as a doctor" and forced him "to serve not God but the world; that in order to curry favour with the princes of this world he was made to attend tyrants, robbers, and excommunicated persons." His work apparently had resulted in much financial gain for his monastery. The monk had fled for the health of his soul. His abbot accused him of having left, "drawn away by his cupidity and curiosity to run around here and there selling his art." Bernard refused to force him to return.[75] It should be noted that shortly after Bernard's death, the Cistercians adopted a rule that none of the order's doctors could practice outside their monasteries or treat laymen.[76] That there were indeed monks who practiced medicine for their monasteries' or their own profit is clear from a canon promulgated by the Second Lateran Council of 1139 having the rubric, "Monks and canons regular are not to study jurisprudence and medicine for the sake of temporal gain." This canon condemned the impulse of avarice that caused some monks to pursue such studies: "[T]he care of souls being neglected . . . they promise health in return for detestable money and thus make themselves physicians of human bodies."[77] Although mention was also made that when acting as physicians, monks would see shameful things that were not appropriate for them, the major concern was that the study and practice of medicine and secular law were not appropriate for those whose lives were to be devoted exclusively to a religious life, if their motivation were financial gain. Two matters should be noted. First, this canon applied only to monks and canons regular and not to most clergy. Second, this canon was never incorporated into any official collection of canon law.

In 1163, at the Council of Tours, Pope Alexander III enacted a canon considerably weaker than the one just mentioned, which simply forbade monks and other regular clergy to leave their religious institutions for the study of medicine or secular law.[78] This canon, which said nothing about the practice of medicine by clergy, was included in the first officially promulgated major collection of canon law, the *Decretales* of Gregory IX (1234).[79] Another piece of papal legislation, a rescript of Honorius III issued in 1219 and also included in the *Decretales*,[80] extended the prohibition of the study of medicine and secular law essentially to all clergy whose livelihood was provided by the performance of spiritual duties. A vast number of clergy, however, still would not have been affected by this legislation. Even its prohibitions were significantly lessened by subsequent legislation.[81] By the end of the Middle Ages there was yet no prohibition of the practice of medicine by clergy in canon law. Surgery, however, was a different matter, because it involved the shedding of blood and much greater risk of harm to a patient, thus heightening the danger that a clerical practitioner might be held responsible for a patient's death. In 1215, at the Fourth Lateran Council, the practice of surgery was forbidden to clergy in major (holy) orders (subdeacons, deacons, and priests) but still permitted by those in minor orders (porters, acolytes, exorcists, and lectors).[82]

While medieval canon law never prohibited the practice of medicine by the clergy, there was obvious uneasiness on the part of the church about their motivation for engaging in such pursuits and the effects such endeavors would have on their spiritual obligations. The issue eventually grew nearly moot as more and more secular physicians were trained in the universities, one of many examples of the increasing involvement of the educated laity in areas previously dominated by the clergy. Medical and surgical practice by the clergy, however, continued to an extent throughout the Middle Ages, but the major motivation appears to have been for charity. For instance, a medical treatise was written in the thirteenth century by a member of a religious order to instruct his fellow clerics in medicine so that they could treat the poor gratis. They could receive fees from the rich.[83] Such treatises were fairly common. Numerous medical handbooks were also written by the clergy in order to help the poor help themselves. For example, Peter Hispanus, who became pope in 1276 as John XXI, was the probable author of the *Treasury for the Poor* that listed simple but salubrious herbs that the poor could gather for themselves.

It was especially in response to the widespread suffering and disease in the growing towns and cities of the late eleventh and twelfth centuries that Augustinian canons (who were like monks in that they lived under a rule but unlike them in that they did not remove themselves from society) and various lay brotherhoods established houses of charity that included institutions or facilities for the succor of the destitute ill.[84] A variety of what may be called hospitals were founded by kings, bishops, feudal lords, wealthy merchants, guilds, and municipalities as endowed charitable institutions that were then staffed by members of various orders, some of which, like the Knights Hospitallers of St. John of Jerusalem, were, as their nomenclature indicates, given to the tasks of charity. Numerous nursing orders arose whose members devoted their lives to caring for the destitute ill in these institutions. By the beginning of the thirteenth century, many hospitals had one or more trained physicians. The hospitals themselves were owned by church orders. During the thirteenth and fourteenth centuries, especially in Italy and Germany, the control of many of these institutions passed into the hands of municipal governments also as part of the general laicization of European society.[85]

The rapidly changing character of society in the high Middle Ages stimulated churchmen to subject the vagaries of the contemporary scene to both abstract and practical moral analyses. The theologians who engaged in such efforts during the twelfth century were the founding fathers of moral theology. The Parisian theologian Peter the Chanter is a good example.[86] His major work[87] consists of three parts, the first dealing with sacraments, the second with penance and excommunication, and the third with ways of resolving cases of conscience. Peter wrote this work in part to aid priests in the increasingly difficult task of determining what constituted sin in a society enormously more complex and confusing than that which had prevailed during the preceding centuries, when the penitential handbooks had proved quite adequate. The genre of aids to confessors, of which Peter's work is an early example, was significantly stimulated by a canon promulgated in 1215 by the Fourth Lateran Council, which a leading historian of the last century called "perhaps the most important legislative act in the history of the Church."[88] This canon,[89] which was soon incorporated into the *Decretales*,[90] required, under pain of excommunication, annual confession to one's own priest. This thoroughly publicized decree reached every level of medieval society.[91] The literature that arose in response to this need consisted of lengthy, finely reasoned tomes and short, practical confessional manuals (or *Summae*) to be used by confessors in their systematic interrogations of penitents. One *Summa*, the *Astesana* (ca. 1317), instructs the confessor to "scrutinize the conscience of the sinner in confession as a physician scrutinizes wounds and a judge a case."[92] Confessional examination was to penetrate into every area of life: birth, marriage, sex, the rearing of children, and vocational obligations.

The writers of these *Summae* appear to have been concerned with sexual morality more than with any other area. The thoroughness and interrogatory ingenuity of the probing of confessors into the sexual activities of penitents are really quite remarkable. Sexual sins were thus graded in order of gravity: unchaste kiss; unchaste touch; fornication; simple adultery; double adultery; rape or abduction of a virgin, of another's wife, or of a nun; incest; masturbation; unnatural relations within marriage; homosexuality; and bestiality. The last five of these were regarded as sins against nature. Thomas Tentler, an authority on the confessional literature of the late Middle Ages, writes: "Taken as a whole, the practical literature on sin and confession gave considerable attention to sins against nature. Medieval churchmen were devoted to the idea of the moral goodness of procreation and mistrustful of doing anything for pleasure. They accordingly conceived a horror of unnatural practices, which they sometimes defined with a startling comprehensiveness."[93]

Other sins against nature, such as contraception and abortion, were regarded both as sexual sins and, under some circumstances, as homicide. Both were fraught with interpretive problems during the period under consideration and have been discussed extensively by modern scholars.[94] Contraception and abortion, although treated separately, were oftentimes confused owing to the primitive understanding of fertilization and fetal development. The statements of Jerome and Augustine, made several centuries earlier than the period under consideration, that abortion was not counted as homicide unless the fetus was "formed," were incorporated into the early medieval penitentials and taken by Gratian, in the twelfth century, as meaning vivified or ensouled,[95] along the lines of Aristotelian embryonic theory. In the *Decretales,* two canons deal with abortion. One follows Gratian[96]; the other applies the penalty for homicide to contraception and to the induced abortion of a fetus at any stage of development.[97] Theologians, canonists, and the authors of *Summae* were split between these two positions. The more liberal of the two did not regard induced abortion as a mortal sin if performed within the first forty days in the case of a male fetus, eighty (or, according to some, ninety) days in the case of a female, and permitted abortion during these periods under a variety of extenuating circumstances. The stricter position generally forbade abortion at all times and under all circumstances. The conflict of interpretations between these two camps was not resolved until long after the period under consideration. Both, however, clearly condemned contraception and abortion as reprehensible if performed simply to vitiate normal procreative functions.

The writers of the *Summae* often had to interpret and apply fine points of canon law. While the *Summae* were not always totally consistent with one another, they were usually as consistent with canon law and theological opinion as these were with themselves. Some scholars say the effect of canon law and confessional interrogation on private morality was probably negligible. There is, however, good reason to believe that the hortatory impact of the pulpit and the coercive force of the confessional proved to be significant factors in shaping the moral attitudes, if not always the behavior, of a large portion of the population. Thomas Tentler writes that "it would have been impractical and self-defeating" for the authors of the *Summae* "to appeal to ideas and expectations that were novel, irrelevant, or unintelligible." He sees in this literature "the practicality of men who understood the inherent power of the system placed at the disposal of every rank of ecclesiastical authority."[98] He considers the confessional system of the late Middle Ages to have been a "most effective means of social control" because of its "clear and explicit expectations, clear and direct accountability." He says of the *Summae* that "they are, if any books ever were, devoted to the clarification, definition, and publication of expectations, as well as to the assertion of the legitimacy of the authority of priest over penitents and the hierarchy over the church."[99] It was perhaps due to the educational efficacy of the confessional, supplemented by the pulpit, that such conditions of religious law and order prevailed in the western church that the Greek Orthodox monk Barlaam in the early fourteenth century was moved to remark: "The whole people is ruled by laws, even the smallest matters are subject to regulation and orderly administration." He was not only struck by the all-pervasive character of canon law, but also by the reverence that people seemed to have for it "as the ordinances of Christ himself."[100]

Sometimes this reverence was for religious principles whether or not they had been specifically embodied in canon law and inculcated through the church's mechanisms of moral instruction. A good example of this involves the attitudes of physicians toward an obligation made in 1215 by the Fourth Lateran Council that required physicians to ensure that their patients make confession to a priest before undertaking treatment.[101] This canon, which was included in the *Decretales*,[102] reads:

Since bodily infirmity is sometimes caused by sin, the Lord saying to the sick man whom he had healed: "Go and sin no more, lest some worse thing happen to thee" (John 5:14), we declare in the present decree and strictly command that when physicians of the body are called to the bedside of the sick, before all else they admonish them to call for the physician of souls, so that after spiritual health has been restored to them, the application of bodily medicine may be of greater benefit, for the cause being removed the effect will pass away. We publish this decree for the reason that some, when they are sick and are advised by the physician in the course of the sickness to attend to the salvation of their soul, give up all hope and yield more easily to the danger of death. If any physician shall transgress this decree after it has been published by the bishops, let him be cut off from the church till he has made suitable satisfaction for his transgression. And since the soul is far more precious than the body, we forbid under penalty of anathema that a physician advise a patient to have recourse to sinful means for the recovery of bodily health.[103]

Even before this obligation was imposed, we find the author of an anonymous twelfth-century treatise dealing with medical etiquette suggested the following to his fellow physicians: "When you reach [a patient's] house and before you see him, ask if he has seen his confessor. If he has not done so, have him either do it or promise to do it. For if he hears mention of this after you have examined him and have considered the signs of the disease, he will begin to despair of recovery, because he will think that you despair of it too."[104] The author, of course, was part of a society that believed in the absolute necessity of confession before death for the health of the soul. Although he may not have considered it his spiritual duty to look after his patients' spiritual welfare, he certainly considered it potentially dangerous to patients to advise them to confess only when in dire straits. He makes no mention, however, of the relationship of sickness and sin.

In the late thirteenth or early fourteenth century, a treatise was written, later attributed to the physician Arnald of Villanova, that contains the following advice:

When you come to a house, inquire before you go to the sick whether he has confessed, and if he has not, he should immediately or promise you that he will confess immediately, and this must not be neglected because many illnesses originate on account of sin and are cured by the Supreme Physician after having been purified from squalor by the tears of contrition, according to what is said in the Gospel: "Go, and sin no more, lest something worse happens to you."[105]

This so strikingly resembles the canon of Lateran IV that it demonstrates the direct influence of canon law on a strictly secular piece of medical literature, as does the following passage in an anonymous plague tractate composed in 1411:

If it is certain from the symptoms that it is actually pestilence that has afflicted the patient, the physician first must advise the patient to set himself right with God by making a will and by making a confession of his sins, as is set forth according to the Decretals: since a corporal illness comes not only from a fault of the body but also from a spiritual failing as the Lord declares in the gospel and the priests also tell us.[106]

The author of this passage includes a provision not in medieval canon law, that the physician advise the patient to make a will. About a century earlier, similar advice was given by the physician Henri de Mondeville: "Do not let the patient be concerned about any business except spiritual matters only, such as confession and his will and arranging similar affairs in accordance with the rules of the Catholic faith."[107] The injunction concerning the making of a will was not in canon law, but in the confessional literature.

The Summae, as already mentioned, probed into all aspects of life, including one's vocation. Several professions, including medicine, were regarded as worthy of scrutiny because of their potential for sin.[108] Two matters raised by the canon of Lateran IV were considered by the authors of the Summae. The first was the physician's obligation to advise a patient to call a priest to hear his confession. The second was to refrain from advising sinful means to bring about a cure. The Summae specify as sin a physician's advising fornication, masturbation, incantations, consumption of intoxicating beverages, breaking the church's fasts, and eating meat on forbidden days. More problematic, however, was the question of calling a confessor, as is evident from the involved discussions in the Summae. Two reasons are given in the canon for the requirement: Because confession had a curative effect, it would either make physicians' attendance superfluous or more efficacious. Second, the practice of calling a confessor as a matter of course before undertaking treatment would dispel the notion that physicians only call for a confessor when they have given up hope for the recovery of a patient. The variety of problems that would arise in practice are very obvious. The authors of the Summae raised and discussed several questions: Does this apply to each and every case undertaken? Is it the physician's responsibility to ensure compliance? Must the physician withdraw from the case if the patient refuses to call a confessor? The authorities seldom agreed on the answers to these and related questions.

They were much more in accord on a variety of other matters. They agreed, for example, that a physician sins by practicing without being competent according to the accepted standards of the art; by failing to keep abreast of medical developments or to consult colleagues when in doubt about a case; by harming patients due to ignorance or negligence; or by experimenting on patients. Rash treatment was condemned as was the giving of medicines about which the physician is in doubt. They felt that patients would be much better off, under such circumstances, to be left in God's hands. In the case of patients for whom there was little hope of recovery, if the physician was unsure about the state of the patients' temporal affairs, he was obliged to inform them of impending death and advise them to make a will. A physician sinned if he withheld effective treatment so that he could increase his fee by prolonging the illness. The physician was obligated not to desert his patients even if there were virtually no hope of recovery and to extend care even if the patient refused to pay, if without such care the patient would die. The authors of *Summae* dealt with the question of treating the poor by following Thomas Aquinas' principle that because "no man is sufficient to bestow a work of mercy on all those who need it," charity ought first to be given to those with whom one is united in any way. Otherwise, if one "stands in such a need that it is not easy to see how he can be succored otherwise then one is bound to bestow the work of mercy on him." Accordingly, a physician was not obligated always to treat the destitute, "or else he would have to put aside all other business and occupy himself entirely" with them.[109] Most *Summae* maintained that the physician must treat the poor gratis only if it were evident that otherwise they would die. The sometimes crass expectations of some members of society for free medical care were a source of much frustration for many secular physicians in the high and late Middle Ages.[110]

There was considerable popular sentiment against physicians during this period. While physicians' greed topped the list of complaints,[111] their lack of concern for spiritual affairs came in a close second. The ill will that was felt appears to have been generated in great part by concern for the potential spiritual damage a physician could cause if he put the health of the patient's body ahead of the health of his soul. Undergirding this concern was the suspicion that, as the Latin adage goes, *"Tres medici, duo athei"* ("Out of three physicians, two will be atheists"). In the thirteenth century, the preacher Jacque de Vitry told his auditors that the advice of physicians was deleterious to their souls: "God says keep vigils; the doctors say go to sleep. God says fast; the doctors say eat. God says mortify your flesh; the doctors say be comfortable."[112] Such sentiments occurred with regularity in the homiletical literature and represented an extreme antipathy to secular medicine. More consonant with late medieval theology and canon law was a thirteenth-century sermon of Humbert de Romans to the brethren and sisters of the hospitals, in which he briefly directed his attention to physicians, urging them never to perform an operation

> that is doubtful without grave consultation and deliberation. So let them deal faithfully with their patients as to cause them as little expense as possible; let them take a moderate fee that their consciences be not hurt.

Above all let them beware of doing aught in their art against God in themselves or in others, lest whilst they heal bodies they kill souls, others or their own. Finally, let them have not as much confidence in their medicines as in their prayers, and let them have most in God.[113]

Humbert's advice, although given before many of the *Summae* had been written, bears some clear resemblance to their categories. Much of the criticism of the medical profession in late medieval literature seems to have been nearly modeled on the concerns expressed in the confessional literature.[114]

Given the interests of the Church in the spiritual well-being of its people, as illustrated by the canon of Lateran IV dealing with the spiritual obligations of physicians, it is not surprising that church authorities sought to impose and enforce a policy of restricting medical practice on Christian patients to Christian physicians, especially because the conduct of non-Christian physicians could not be checked by the confessional. Particularly during the thirteenth century we find church councils strictly forbidding Christians to obtain medical or surgical services from Jewish or Islamic physicians under pain of excommunication.[115] Nevertheless, many people, including religious leaders, continued to employ the services of non-Christian physicians in spite of such prohibitions.

In the confessional literature there was a much greater emphasis on the responsibility of a physician not to advise sinful means for restoring health than on the responsibility of the patient to refuse to follow such advice. However, several *Summae* discussed the obligations of patients.[116] A composite includes the following matters: Patients do not sin if they disobey their physicians, because physicians have no real authority over them but can only advise and exhort. It is, however, good to trust one's physician to the extent to which he is an expert in the art. If patients knowingly or by gross (thus inexcusable) ignorance consume something deadly, they sin. They do not sin mortally, however, if they intentionally consume a substance that they believe is not deadly if by so doing they are attempting to aggravate their illness.

The small amount of attention in the confessional literature to the sins of patients should not lead one to believe that theologians were unconcerned about the moral responsibilities of the sick. A good example of late medieval attitudes toward the conduct of patients is found in the sermons preached in 1498 and 1499 by Johann Geiler von Kaiserberg, a German priest and professor of theology. In one sermon entitled "Sick Fools," Geiler discussed seven follies of the ill.[117] The first four involved their relations with the medical art and its practitioners. Ill fools scorned medicine; deceived or disobeyed their physician; followed the physician's advice belatedly or distorted it so that it did not help.

These four were simply foolish. The confessional literature did not classify them as sins. The remaining three involved sin, although the first of these was potentially neutral, being pivotal in this list. They sought medicine and advice from "old women and from others who have never learned medicine." They searched "for medicine and health from witches and exorcisoresses of the devil." The most serious folly "is to neglect one's duty to God—to make use of medicine and not desire the help of God."

The last of these seven follies of the sick was a frequently repeated concern of medieval authors. It showed an attitude of independence, of sufficiency to maintain or restore one's health without reference to one's creator. The church could exhort, threaten, and plead against that attitude but could not effectively regulate or control the attitudes of the sick or of physicians toward the medical art, which was regarded as both a gift of the creator and as a potential lure away from submission to him.

Geiler complained that people sought the help of old women and others "who have never learned medicine," and searched "for medicine and health from witches and exorcisoresses of the devil." During the twelfth and thirteenth centuries, the practice of medicine had changed from a right to a privilege with the introduction of medical licensure and the development of medical and surgical guilds that sought and obtained monopolies in medical and surgical care in exchange for guarantees of high ethical standards and requisite training for all practitioners, which was the basis for the assurance of competence. When guilds petitioned for monopolies, they always emphasized that this was for the public good. Those who granted such monopolies concurred. In some communities the church granted and enforced the monopoly (e.g., Montpellier). In others, even though it had not granted the guild's charter, it helped enforce the guild's rights. In Paris, for example, both the medical and surgical corporations maintained a constant struggle against unlicensed practitioners. They often appealed to the church. The accused would be tried by a church court which would either excommunicate the defendant or threaten excommunication for a second offense. Very often the alleged charlatans were women.[118]

The majority of unlicensed practitioners probably employed techniques and substances typical of folk medicine without any magical formulae and charms. But because so many of these unlicensed practitioners were women, they readily evoked suspicion of engaging in witchcraft or other illicit practices. In dealing with the subject of illicit healing in the high and late Middle Ages, we enter a maze of confusion.[119] Beginning with the revival of learning in the twelfth century, scholars were increasingly interested in those realms of inquiry that we probably would label superstition. Their definitions of the demonic, magic, miracle, natural properties, and occult virtues seem to blend in with the pertinacious endurance of various strata of folk and pagan practices. In a hazy middle ground between magic and miracle was the realm of "natural medicine" or the exploitation of occult virtues, to which Geiler's fifth and sixth points both have reference. "Natural medicine" was not simply the folk medicine that unlicensed people practiced without proper medical training, but possessed the additional ingredient of techniques for releasing the occult virtues contained within the natural objects. This could be done illicitly through incantations or licitly through formulae prescribed by the church.

Penitential handbooks continued condemning pagan practices through the twelfth century.[120] But beginning in that century we find magic denounced less as paganism than as heresy. From the quagmire of definitional confusion that prevailed arose a renewed interest in astrology. Astrology had usually been either condemned by the church Fathers as demonic or dismissed as banal, and these attitudes prevailed during the early Middle Ages. In the twelfth century, however, Hugh of St. Victor distinguished between "natural astrology" and "superstitious astrology." William McDonald explains: "The former, also called scientific astrology, concerned itself with the constitution of physical bodies like illness and health, which varied according to the mutual alignments of the astral bodies. In contrast, superstitious astrology, also designated judicial and divinatory astrology, was concerned with chance happenings or future contingent events and with matters of free will."[121] This distinction, which did not originate with Hugh, was the basis for much of the discussion that continued well beyond the period under consideration. Various questions arose. Were the stars agents of action or simply its harbingers? If the licit branch of astrology was concerned with such physical matters as illness, could prognostication be made without dabbling in the illicit branch, especially if one did not presume upon the spiritual realm, which included reason and free will? Different answers were given by different people and debate raged. The physician who did not use astrology was regarded by many as either incompetent or negligent. In the late thirteenth century, Roger Bacon, in his *On the Errors of Physicians,* says that "a physician who knows not how to take into account the positions and aspects of the planets can effect nothing in the healing arts except by chance and good fortune."[122] Although there were some voices raised against the validity of "natural astrology," it had become so much a part of medicine by the close of the Middle Ages that in 1509 the English Franciscan monk Alexander Barclay could criticize medical quacks for their failure to heed astrological signs.[123]

The supposed prognostic benefits of astrology came to the fore, especially in attempts to explain and cope with the Black Death of

1348–1349 and the subsequent waves of pestilential disease that periodically ravaged Europe well beyond the end of the Middle Ages. William McDonald thus paraphrases the conclusion of a treatise written in the fifteenth century by Conrad Bosner:

> [E]verything is subservient to the divine will. God [ordains] the celestial bodies to carry out their influence and does not hinder the natural forces on earth as a consequence of man's offenses against heaven. Following from this, the apparent decisive influence of the stars is but a further manifestation of divine control, in that God tolerates and uses that influence as an agent of his will to punish man for sin and error.[124]

Just as in the early Middle Ages, plague and all epidemic diseases were regarded as visitations of God's wrath. God was commonly depicted showering arrows of vengeance on sinful humanity.[125] We have seen that in the early Middle Ages the plague had proved to be a very effective illustration of God's wrath and of the importance of eternal priorities and thus was instrumental in turning the peasants' attention from their temporal concerns. Popular reactions to the plague in the late Middle Ages demonstrated that the desires of the theologians of earlier centuries had in great part been fulfilled.

The church's reaction to the Black Death of 1348–1349, the most horrible pestilence ever to afflict Europe, is well illustrated by the actions taken by Pope Clement VI as soon as the plague hit Avignon, then the seat of the papacy. In addition to taking various measures to hinder contagion, he hired physicians to care for the afflicted, gave special indulgences to encourage the clergy to minister to those stricken, and instituted a special mass to implore an end to the plague.[126] Medical care was viewed as an immediate need to be given in an attempt to counter this affliction, of which God was viewed as the ultimate cause. This was by no means regarded as inconsistent with the equally important effort to approach God through a special mass. This compatibility, however, was marred when, on numerous occasions during the next several centuries, physicians' concerns with contagion were overruled by the church's popularly welcomed organization of massive processionals to implore God's mercy.[127] There were, of course, some clergy and some laymen who argued against the use of physicans during time of plague, either on the spiritual grounds that such efforts were inconsistent or on the pragmatic grounds that physicians' efforts at prophylaxis and treatment were obviously of little or no value. Although physicians were able to accomplish little or nothing for their patients who were afflicted with the plague, their efforts to deal with this scourge were often supererogatory.[128] "The prestige of doctors was not weakened by heavy plague mortality," writes Sylvia Thrupp, "for they could take credit for cases of recovery and by personal concern and courage they eased the atmosphere of fear. Popular devotion to a favorite doctor was expressed in terms of love and of the honor due a father by a son."[129]

In addition to providing medical care and instituting a special mass, Clement gave indulgences to clergy ministering to the stricken. These indulgences were regarded as absolving the sins of those to whom they were granted so that their sins would not require expiation in purgatory. Apparently death by plague came to be regarded by some as potentially expiatory in itself. John of Saxony, who wrote a treatise on plague during the first half of the fifteenth century, complained that some people disregarded the prophylactic advice of physicians during times of plague. He gave several reasons for this attitude, one of which was a prevailing fatalism, for some held that "the time of one's death has been established for every individual." Another reason was "the desire and hope for death. For I recall that in a certain great pestilence in Montpellier, when many men wished to die, on that account the pope gave to the dying absolution from punishment and guilt and thus they hoped to be carried to heaven immediately, and therefore they did not want physicians to prolong their lives."[130]

It was commonly held by all levels of society that one must suffer for one's sins, either in this life or in purgatory, although usually in both. This led to various reactions to the plague, one of which was the flagellant movement. Flagellation had existed in Christianity for centuries. It had been prescribed as a means of public penance in late antiquity and the early Middle Ages. It was also a part of monastic discipline. Additionally, it was a form of voluntary penance that, during the eleventh century, became widespread among monks and the laity. In the thirteenth century, owing in great part to the emphasis of the mendicant orders on identification with Christ's sufferings, the order of Penitents arose. Members of this order identified themselves so closely with Christ's sufferings that they believed they could contribute to the expiation of the sins of mankind by self-flagellation. In central Italy in 1260 a popular outbreak of flagellation was stimulated in part by a famine (1258) followed by an epidemic (1259). John Henderson remarks,

> One can understand how flagellation came to be seen as the obvious method of expiation when translated into the context of a mass movement characterized by a widespread belief that God was intent on punishing mankind. It provided immediate and violent release from guilt and in the very process of beating their bodies participants could feel that they were washing away their sins. Moreover, in this exercise they saw themselves as sharing the sufferings of Christ.[131]

Various officially authorized flagellant confraternities arose over the next century. While the Black Death was devastating Europe, the flagellant movement took on a popular fervor. Motivated by the hope of appeasing God, groups of people formed who believed that by flagellating themselves for a period of 33½ days they could bring about the end of the plague and then be themselves cleansed entirely of sin. This popular movement spread rapidly, beginning in June 1349, apparently in Germany, which was soon overrun by flagellant bands. Violence and disorder accompanied some of these groups and, when they reached Avignon in October 1349, Clement condemned their activities and ordered them to desist.[132] Although their disorder and the attendant violence contributed to Clement's decision to condemn them, his action should not be taken as a denial of their basic theology. Rather, his negative reaction was primarily precipitated by their having adopted a specific habit. He "saw the wearing of a habit as a sign of the flagellants' rejection of the authority of the church, believing they saw their exercise as an end in itself which led them to their salvation unaided by the priesthood."[133]

Sin was commonly regarded as the immediate cause of plague, or at least the catalyst behind God's sending plague. This was collective sin. Individual sin was seldom seen as the cause of sickness, whether mental illness or physical ailments.[134] One notable exception was leprosy, which was associated with a variety of sins, but especially with lust and pride.[135] By a strange irony to which medieval Catholic theology was conducive, lepers were also regarded as chosen by God for the privilege of suffering in this life in lieu of purgatory.[136] Most people who suffered from sickness in the late Middle Ages were, of course, not afflicted with either leprosy or plague. Some people when ill may have been burdened with a sense of guilt. If medieval theology in some ways fostered such an attitude, it did not, however, encourage it as a morbidly obsessive response to illness.

The canon of the Fourth Lateran Council, which required physicians to have their patients make confession to a priest, began with the clause, "Since bodily infirmity is sometimes caused by sin. . . ." Confession was thought to restore spiritual health. If the physical problem was exacerbated by a spiritual problem, after confession, medicine for the body would be more effective. If the physical affliction was caused by spiritual sickness, physical healing would directly result from confession. Richard Palmer remarks, "In catholic theology confession was of fundamental importance in the treatment of disease. It was probably the church's nearest approximation in the medieval and early modern periods to a formal ritual of healing."[137] This observation, although essentially correct, is easily misleading. It was of "fundamental importance" to the formulators of canon law and to many theologians during the late Middle Ages. On the very eve of the Reformation, Dietrich Coelde, the author of a famous and highly influential manual of spiritual instruction, stressed that the ill should first seek such cures as confession and the mass because sickness "generally comes from sins."[138] It does not follow that confession was stressed, however, in even a significant minority of those varied procedures available for physical healing which were loosely under the auspices of the church. Mention was made earlier of a ninth-century French bishop's frustration at the lack of repentance evidenced by those who had flocked to the shrine of Fermin for healing. His reaction was atypical of that time. As Patrick Geary says of this period, "The miraculous rather than the penitential aspects of devotion to relics seem to have formed . . . the basis for popular devotion to local and regional pilgrimage sites."[139] But a significant change occurred in the eleventh and twelfth centuries as a motivation other than healing arose for visiting shrines. Expiatory pilgrimage to various shrines greatly contributed to the forgiveness of their sins. The age of the penitential pilgrimage had begun, a striking feature of the closing centuries of medieval Catholicism. The rapid social changes and population growth that marked the eleventh and twelfth centuries had led to a stark sense of alienation that is so evident in the literature of that time.[140] The deep sense of sin and the fear of purgatorial fires coupled with a feeling of alienation fostered penitential pilgrimages. The vast majority of pilgrims undoubtedly were not seeking physical healing during the late Middle Ages. But when the sick came as pilgrims to shrines for healing, there appears to have been as little concern on the part of the clergy at the shrines to deal with the ill persons' spiritual state as there had been during the early Middle Ages. We know of at least one shrine that required those who came for healing to have proof that they had confessed to their parish priest before leaving home,[141] but this was probably an exception to the practice that prevailed at most shrines, because the shrine in question was of Mary, a rather late extension of the cult of saints and relics. The majority of the healing shrines of the late Middle Ages were repositories of the bones or relics of saints.

Ronald Finucane, a leading authority on the English shrines of the late Middle Ages, has found that ninety percent of the miracles that were recorded at English and continental shrines from the twelfth through the fifteenth centuries involved healings and alleviations of physical ills. Many of those seeking healing had first tried other available means. The clergy at these shrines responded to the failures of physicians with the same enthusiasm and motivation as had Gregory of Tours earlier. Finucane concludes that "it is clear that in practice most sick people called on both the power of saints and of trained physicians.

This was as true at the very top of the social ladder as at the bottom; as true for laymen as for clerics."[142]

Trafficking in relics was an enormously lucrative business. So numerous were the healing shrines of this period that control was difficult. The church made gallant efforts to authenticate miracles and to limit canonization of individuals whose remains were potential relics.[143] At the same time a concerted effort was made to direct popular devotion away from often quite minor, nondescript, or simply unapproved saints to Christ and Mary. This was eminently practical: They did not require canonization and their shrines needed no relics, only a crucifix or a statue of Mary.[144] This seems to have resulted in some redirecting of attention from the shrines of saints to these new focal points of devotion and miracles. Also, the relic value of the elements in the sacrament of communion was exploited by the "exposition" of the Host in a container in which it could be viewed and venerated during the mass.[145] Stories of healing miracles that occurred during the mass were very common in the late Middle Ages.

Although some voices in late antiquity questioned the theological validity of the cult of saints and relics, opposition to the cult was extremely rare in the Middle Ages. Individual relics were often discredited, and abuses abounded. A good example of a critic of the abuses of the cult of saints and relics is Guibert of Nogent, who wrote *The Relics of the Saints* around 1120. He was a critic of the abuses, not of the theology underlying the cult itself. "Guibert did not object in principle to their veneration, but he was profoundly uneasy about some of the features of the developing cult," observes Colin Morris. "In the eyes of God, he believes, it is genuine faith which counts, and a prayer made through a false saint will still be of avail if the petitioner honestly believes in his sanctity."[146] Many Catholics, ranging from Guibert in the twelfth century to Erasmus in the sixteenth, expressed concern about particular relics, shrines, or supposed saints and indignation about widespread abuses while yearning for a reform of medieval Catholicism within the grounds of accepted orthodoxy. Others, however, voiced a more general skepticism about the whole range of supposedly miraculous occurrences. Such were, for example, John Wycliffe (ca. 1329–1384) and the Lollards in England and Jan Hus (1373–1415) and his followers on the continent. Their desire for radical reform struck so deeply at the core of late medieval Catholic theology and practice that they appeared heretical in their denunciations of what they regarded as gross abuses, including allegedly miraculous performances under the auspices of corrupt clergy. In short, the cult of saints and relics and the cults of Christ and Mary were undergirded by the same theology that approved and stimulated the sale of indulgences, an abuse that incensed both Luther and Erasmus.

The removal of the healing shrines from countries that became Protestant left a void filled in part by the rise of a wide variety of practices that were labeled as magic and witchcraft, and were associated with "cunning men and wise women."[147] Interestingly, Lionel Rothkrug has suggested that in the Reformation in Germany, "areas rich in pilgrimage places remained Catholic, and those showing a paucity of sites embraced the Protestant faith."[148] This phenomenon had its roots in the differing religious emphases and cultural variations within Germany that contributed to the popularity of the rather sensationalistic shrines as an expression of lay piety in some areas and the rather quiet piety of, for example, the Brethren of the Common Life, in others. This is but one example of the enormous diversity that existed within Catholicism during the late Middle Ages. After commenting on Finucane's study, Richard Palmer remarks that "far less is known about the shrines of continental Europe [than about those of England]. In Italy the bodies of the saints were venerated. . . . But shrines . . . do not seem to have been places of healing in any way comparable to those of medieval England. In Italy if a sick person travelled at all he was probably *en route* to one of the flourishing medicinal spas."[149] The reader should be aware that the present study stresses the commonalities and homogeneity of medieval Catholicism. Finucane, who was himself quite aware of the enormous diversity within late medieval Catholicism, rightly emphasizes that

"the Church" is really a convenient expression almost devoid of meaning. At its extremes it embraced the Church of the Lateran in Rome and the Church as known, say, to the medieval villagers of Oxenton in rural Gloucestershire. There was not only an Italian and an English medieval Church, as a modern historian has emphasized,[150] there was a French Church and a Spanish, an Icelandic and a German, each with its own history, traditions, liturgical uses and saints. Within these Churches were hundreds of divisions subdivided again into thousands of smaller units, ending at last with a semi-literate cleric in some rude chapel in the midst of inhospitable forests or fields, surrounded by peasants who muttered charms over their ploughs and whispered magic words at crossroads. It was a very long way from pope or prelate to peasant–priest, a long way in distance, education, and attitude.[151]

Notes

1. See the numerous works of Peter Brown, especially *The Making of Late Antiquity* (Cambridge, MA., 1978), and *The Cult of the Saints: Its Rise and Function in Latin Christianity* (Chicago, 1981).

2. Derek Baker, *"Vir Dei:* Secular Sanctity in the Early Tenth Century," in *Popular Belief and Practice* (Studies in Church History 8), eds. G. J. Cuming and Derek Baker (Cambridge, 1972), p. 43.

3. Quoted in J. N. Hillgarth, ed., *The Conversion of Western Europe, 350–75* (Englewood Cliffs, NJ, 1969), pp. 78–79.

4. Bede, *Ecclesiastical History* 1.31, trans. B. Colgrove and R. Mynors (Oxford, 1969).

5. Bede, *Ecclesiastical History* 1.30. For a fascinating discussion of the survival of paganism in Anglo-Saxon England, see Wilfrid Bonser, *The Medical Background of Anglo-Saxon England: A Study in History, Psychology, and Folklore* (London, 1963), pp. 117–157.

6. See, for example, the sermons of Maximus of Turin and Martin of Braga in Hillgarth, ed., *Conversion of Western Europe,* pp. 54–63.

7. For a discussion of the nature and effects of plague in the early Middle Ages, see J.-N. Biraben and Jacques LeGoff, "The Plague in the Early Middle Ages," in *Biology of Man in History: Selections from the Annales: Économics, Sociétés, Civilsations,* eds. R. Forster and O. Ranum, trans. E. Forster and P. M. Ranum (Baltimore, 1975), pp. 48–80.

8. Bede, *Life of St. Cuthbert* 9, in *Two Lives of Saint Cuthbert,* ed. and trans. B. Colgrave (1939, rpt. New York, 1969).

9. Jonas of Orleans, *Institutio Laicalis* 3.14.

10. See Clyde Pharr, "The Interdiction of Magic in Roman Law," *Transactions of the American Philological Association* 63 (1932): 269–295.

11. Thus the laws of the Visigoths and Lombards. See Hillgarth, ed., *Conversion of Western Europe,* pp. 103–104.

12. Walter Ullmann, "Public Welfare and Social Legislation in the Early Medieval Councils," in *Councils and Assemblies* (Studies in Church History 7), eds. G. J. Cuming and Derek Baker (Cambridge, 1971), p. 35.

13. Quoted by John T. McNeill and Helena M. Gamer, *Medieval Handbooks of Penance* (New York, 1938), p. 389.

14. Quoted in Hillgarth, ed., *Conversion of Western Europe,* p. 133.

15. Quoted in Patrick J. Geary, "The Ninth-Century Relic Trade: A Response to Popular Piety?" in *Religion and the People, 800–1700,* ed. James Obelkevich (Chapel Hill, NC, 1979), p. 11.

16. Ullmann, "Public Welfare," pp. 35–36.

17. Janet L. Nelson, "Society, Theodicy and the Origins of Heresy: Towards a Reassessment of the Medieval Evidence," in *Schism, Heresy and Religious Protest* (Studies in Church History 9), ed. Derek Baker (Cambridge, 1972), pp. 75–76.

18. See McNeill and Gamer, *Handbooks of Penance, passim.*

19. Bonser, *Medical Background,* pp. 128–129.

20. See, e.g., McNeill and Gamer, *Handbooks of Penance,* pp. 78, 90, 120, 198, 206–207, 228–229, 246, 255, 288–289, 292, 302, 311, 318, 330–335.

21. *The Penitential of Theodore* (ca. 668–690) 1.15.2; *The Penitential Ascribed to Bede* (possibly early eighth century) 10.2; the so-called *Confessional of Egbert* (ca. 950–1000); penitential canons from Regino's *Ecclesiastical Discipline* (ca. 906) section 304.

22. Bonser, *Medical Background,* p. 248.

23. *The Penitential of Theodore* (ca. 668–690) 1.14.16.

24. *The Irish Canons* (ca. 675) 12. See McNeill and Gamer, *Handbooks of Penance,* p. 120 (n. 22 and references there to secondary literature).

25. *The Penitential of Theodore* (ca. 668–690) 1.15.3; *The Penitential of Silos* (c. 800) 11 (107).
26. *The Penitential of Silos* 11 (107).
27. Ibid., 7 (104).
28. Buchard of Worms, *The Corrector and Physician* 65; cf. *The Penitential of Theodore* 2.10.5.
29. Burchard of Worms, *The Corrector and Physician* 66 and 102; adapted from the translation in McNeill and Gamer, *Handbooks of Penance,* pp. 331, 335.
30. McNeill and Gamer, *Handbooks of Penance,* p. 100.
31. Adapted from the translation in McNeill and Gamer, *Handbooks of Penance,* p. 302.
32. The so-called *Roman Penitential of Halitgar* canons 81 and 82. See the discussion, with other references, in John T. McNeill, *A History of the Cure of Souls* (New York, 1951), p. 129.
33. With the possible exception of a totally enigmatic statement in the *Old Irish Penitential* (c.800) 1.20, in McNeill and Gamer, *Handbooks of Penance,* p. 159.
34. *The Penitential of Theodore* 2.10.1, 2 and 4. A similar passage occurs in *The Judgement of Clement* (ca. 700–750) 15, in McNeill and Gamer, *Handbooks of Penance,* p. 272.
35. *The Penitential of Theodore* 2.10.2 and 3.
36. *The Burgundian Penitential* canon 36. A similar passage occurs in the so-called *Roman Penitential of Halitgar* (ca. 830) canon 39.
37. Loren C. MacKinney, "Tenth-Century Medicine as Seen in the *Historia* of Richer of Rheims," *Bulletin of the Institute of the History of Medicine* 2 (1934): 361–362.
38. *Letter* 71 in *The Letters and Poems of Fulbert of Chartres,* ed. and trans. Frederick Behrends (Oxford, 1976), p. 121.
39. Jerome Kroll, "A Reappraisal of Psychiatry in the Middle Ages," *Archives of General Psychiatry* 29 (1973): 281.
40. Gregory the Great, *Regula Pastoralis* 3.12.
41. Bede, *Ecclesiastical History* 4.9.
42. Bede, *Ecclesiastical History* 1.19.
43. From Bede, *Vita Beatorum Abbatum,* as quoted in Hillgarth, ed., *Conversion of Western Europe,* p. 121.
44. Biraben and LeGoff, "Plague," p. 61.
45. Jeffrey Richards, *Consul of God: The Life and Times of Gregory the Great* (London, 1980), pp. 41–42.
46. Bede, *Ecclesiastical History* 1.14.
47. Bede, *Life of St. Cuthbert* 9.
48. Bede, *De Natura Rerum* 37.
49. Bede, *Life of St. Cuthbert* 8.
50. Geary, "Relic Trade," p. 12.
51. Brown, *Cult of the Saints,* p. 100.
52. For a discussion of healing by means of relics in Anglo-Saxon England, see Bonser, *Medical Background,* pp. 178–210.
53. See Bernhard Poschmann, *Penance and the Anointing of the Sick,* trans. F. Courtney (London, 1964), pp. 239–240.
54. See H. B. Porter, "The Origin of the Medieval Rite for Anointing the Sick or Dying," *Journal of Theological Studies* new ser., 7 (1956): 211–225.

55. Caesarius of Arles, *Sermon* 279.5, quoted by Poschmann, *Penance,* pp. 241–242.
56. Brown, *Cult of the Saints,* p. 117.
57. See Benedicta Ward, *Miracles and the Medieval Mind: Theory, Record and Event, 1000–1215* (Philadelphia, 1982), p. 11.
58. See the statements of Aelfric (ca. 955–1020), quoted by Bonser, *Medical Background,* pp. 118–119, 138.
59. *Anonymous Life of St. Cuthbert* 1.4 and 4.4; Bede, *Life of St. Cuthbert* 4; 23; 32.
60. See Pierre Riché, *Education and Culture in the Barbarian West: Sixth through Eighth Centuries,* trans. J. J. Contreni (Columbia, SC, 1976), pp. 204–206.
61. See Richards, *Consul of God,* p. 47; and Riché, *Education and Culture,* pp. 142–143.
62. For a discussion, see Darrel W. Amundsen, "Medicine and Surgery as Art or Craft: The Role of Schematic Literature in the Separation of Medicine and Surgery in the Late Middle Ages," *Transactions and Studies of the College of Physicians of Philadelphia* new ser., 1 (1979): 49–52; and Riché, *Education and Culture,* p. 386.
63. Fulbert of Chartres, *Letters* 47 and 48. For a more reticent attitude, see *The Letters of Gerbert with His Papal Privileges as Sylvester II,* trans. H. P. Lattin (New York, 1961), p. 188.
64. Fulbert of Chartres, *Letter* 24, trans. Behrends, pp. 45–47.
65. Loren C. MacKinney, "Medical Ethics and Etiquette in the Early Middle Ages: The Persistence of Hippocratic Ideals," *Bulletin of the History of Medicine* 26 (1952): 1–31.
66. *Matthew* 25:35–46; see Adolf Harnack, *The Expansion of Christianity in the First Three Centuries,* trans. J. Moffatt (1904–1905, reprinted Freeport, NY, 1972), p. 199.
67. See Ullmann, "Public Welfare," p.8.
68. See ibid., pp. 9–10.
69. This caution is convincingly expressed by Timothy S. Miller, "The Knights of St. John and the Hospitals of the West," *Speculum* 53 (1978): 709–733, especially pp. 709–712.
70. See ibid., "Knights of St. John," pp. 710–711.
71. Benedict, *Rule* 36.
72. Benedict, *Rule* 31, trans. Justin McCann, *Saint Benedict* (New York, 1937). Cp. the very elaborate and atypical instructions by Cassiodorus, *Introduction to Divine and Human Readings* 1.31.
73. Bede, *Life of St. Cuthbert* 45; *Anonymous Life of St. Cuthbert* 4.17.
74. See *Vita Sancti Columbae Auctore Adamnano,* ed. W. Reeves (Dublin, 1857), pp. 55 ff.
75. Bernard of Clairvaux, *Letters* 70 and 71 in *The Letters of St. Bernard of Clairvaux,* trans. Bruno Scott James (London, 1953), pp. 95–99.
76. Miller, "Knights of St. John," p. 714.
77. Canon 9, translation in R. J. Schroeder, *Disciplinary Decrees of the General Councils* (St. Louis, 1957), pp. 201–202.
78. A translation, as well as a discussion of all pertinent legislation, may be found in Darrel W. Amundsen, "Medieval Canon Law on Medical and Surgical Practice by the Clergy," *Bulletin of the History of Medicine* 52 (1978): 22–44.
79. *Decretales* 3.5.3.

80. Ibid. 3.50.10.
81. See Amundsen, "Canon Law," pp. 36–38.
82. Lateran IV, canon 18 = Decretales 3.50.9. See Amundsen, "Canon Law," pp. 40–43.
83. C. H. Talbot, Medicine in Medieval England (London, 1967), p. 96.
84. Miller, "Knights of St. John," pp. 714–717.
85. On hospitals and hospital orders in the high and late Middle Ages, see the secondary literature cited by Miller, "Knights of St. John," and by Brian Tierney, Medieval Poor Law: A Sketch of Canonical Theory and Its Application in England (Berkeley, 1959), notes accompanying pp. 85–87.
86. See John W. Baldwin, Masters, Princes, and Merchants: The Social Views of Peter the Chanter and His Circle (Princeton, NJ, 1970).
87. Summa de Sacramentis et Animae Consiliis.
88. Henry Charles Lea, A History of Auricular Confession and Indulgences in the Latin Church, 2 vols. (Philadephia, 1896), vol. 1, p. 230.
89. Lateran IV, canon 21. For a translation, see Oscar Watkins, A History of Penance, 2 vols. (London, 1920), vol. 2, pp. 748–749.
90. Decretales 5.38.12.
91. Thomas N. Tentler, "Response and Retractatio," in The Pursuit of Holiness in Later Medieval and Renaissance Religion, ed. Charles Trinkaus (Leiden, 1974), p. 134.
92. As quoted by Thomas N. Tentler, "The Summa for Confessors as an Instrument of Social Control," in The Pursuit of Holiness, p. 115.
93. Thomas N. Tentler, Sin and Confession on the Eve of the Reformation (Princeton, NJ, 1977), p. 207.
94. See especially John T. Noonan, Jr., Contraception: A History of Its Treatment by the Catholic Theologians and Canonists (Cambridge, MA, 1966); Noonan, "An Almost Absolute Value in History," in The Morality of Abortion: Legal and Historical Perspectives, ed. John T. Noonan, Jr. (Cambridge, MA, 1970), pp. 1–59; and John Connery, Abortion: The Development of the Roman Catholic Perspective (Chicago, 1977).
95. Gratian, Decretum C. 32 q. 2. c. 7.
96. Decretales 5.12.20.
97. Ibid., 5.12.5.
98. Tentler, Sin and Confession, p. xv.
99. Tentler, "Response and Retractatio," p. 137.
100. Quoted by Bernard J. Verkamp, The Indifferent Mean: Adiaphorism in the English Reformation to 1554 (Athens, OH, and Detroit, 1977), pp. 6, 9.
101. Lateran IV, canon 22.
102. Decretales 5.38.13.
103. In Schroeder, Disciplinary Decrees, p. 236.
104. Latin text in S. DeRenzi, Collectio Salernitana, 5 vols., (Naples, 1852–1859), vol. 2, p. 74.
105. Translation in Henry E. Sigerist, "Bedside Manners in the Middle Ages: The Treatise De Cautelis Medicorum Attributed to Arnald of Villanova," Quarterly Bulletin of the Northwestern University Medical School 20 (1946): 141.
106. Translation in Darrel W. Amundsen, "Medical Deontology and Pestilential Disease in the Late Middle Ages," Journal of the History of Medicine and Allied Sciences 32 (1977): 416.

107. Latin text in Paul Diepgen, *Die Theologie und der ärztliche Stand* (Berlin, 1922), p. 51, n. 287.
108. For a discussion, see Darrel W. Amundsen, "Casuistry and Professional Obligations: The Regulation of Physicians by the Court of Conscience in the Late Middle Ages," *Transactions and Studies of the College of Physicians of Philadelphia* new ser., 3 (1981): 22–39 and 93–112.
109. Thomas Aquinas, *Summa Theologiae* 2–2.71.1.
110. See Darrel W. Amundsen and Gary B. Ferngren, "Philanthropy in Medicine: Some Historical Perspectives," in *Beneficence and Health Care,* ed. Earl E. Shelp (Dordrecht, 1982), pp. 22–23.
111. See the discussion in G. R. Owst, *Literature and Pulpit in Medieval England: A Neglected Chapter in the History of English Letters and of the English People,* 2nd ed. (Oxford, 1961), pp. 349–351.
112. Quoted by Jonathan Sumption, *Pilgrimage: An Image of Medieval Religion* (Totowa, NJ, 1975), p. 80.
113. Sermon 40, quoted by Bede Jarrett, *Social Theories of the Middle Ages, 1200–1500* (1926; reprinted Westminster, MD, 1942), p. 223.
114. E.g., in the early fifteenth century John Mirfield and late in the same century the various authors of different versions of *The Ship of Fools.*
115. See P. Delaunay, *La médecine et l'Église: Contribution a l'histoire de l'exercise médical par les clercs* (Paris, 1948), pp. 11–12; and Darrel W. Amundsen, "Medical Legislation of the Assizes of Jerusalem," in *Proceedings of the XXIIIrd International Congress of the History of Medicine* (London, 1974), p. 521, n. 16.
116. The following works have a section devoted to the subject: Bartholomaeus de Sancto Concordio, *Summa casuum* (ca. 1338; Venice, 1473), copy at University of Pennsylvania, generally cited as *Pisanella;* Antoninus of Florence, *Summa Theologica* (or *Summa Moralis*) (1477; reprint of 1740 edition, Graz, 1959); Baptista Trovamala de Salis, *Summa de Casibus Conscientiae* (ca. 1480; Venice, 1495), copy at College of Physicians of Philadelphia, generally cited as *Baptistina;* Angelus Carletus de Clavasio, *Summa Angelica de Casibus Conscientiae* (ca. 1486; Lyons, 1494), copy at Free Library of Philadelphia generally cited as *Angelica.*
117. See Thomas G. Benedeck, "The Image of Medicine in 1500: Theological Reactions to *The Ship of Fools,*" *Bulletin of the History of Medicine* 38 (1964): 332–333.
118. See Pearl Kibre, "The Faculty of Medicine at Paris, Charlatanism and Unlicensed Medical Practices in the Later Middle Ages," *Bulletin of the History of Medicine* 27 (1953): 1–20.
119. See the discussion in the first chapter of Ward, *Miracles,* especially pp. 10–13.
120. E.g., *The Penitential of Bartholomew Iscanus,* in McNeill and Gamer, *Handbooks of Penance,* p. 350.
121. William C. McDonald, "Death in the Stars: Heinrich von Mügeln on the Black Plague," *Mediaevalia* 5 (1979): 97.
122. Roger Bacon, *On the Errors of Physicians* 144–145, as quoted by John M. Riddle, "Theory and Practice in Medieval Medicine," *Viator* 5 (1974): 169–170, n. 51.
123. Benedek, "Image of Medicine," pp. 336–337.
124. McDonald, "Death in the Stars," pp. 101–102.

125. Richard Palmer, "The Church, Leprosy, and Plague in Medieval and Early Modern Europe," in *The Church and Healing* (Studies in Church History 19), ed. W. J. Sheils (Oxford, 1982), p. 83.

126. C. Mollat, *The Popes at Avignon, 1305–1378* (London, 1963), p. 40.

127. See Palmer, "The Church, Leprosy, and Plague," pp. 94–99; and Carlo M. Cipolla, *Faith, Reason and the Plague in Seventeenth-Century Tuscany* (Ithaca, NY, 1979) and *Public Health and the Medical Profession in the Renaissance* (Cambridge, 1976).

128. Amundsen, "Medical Deontology," pp. 403–421.

129. Sylvia L. Thrupp, "Plague Effects in Medieval Europe," *Comparative Studies in Society and History* 8 (1966): 480–481. For the effects of the Black Death on the medical profession and on medical knowledge, see Robert S. Gottfried, *The Black Death: Natural and Human Disaster in Medieval Europe* (New York, 1983), pp. 104–128.

130. Latin text in Karl Sudhoff, "Pestschriften aus den ersten 150 Jahren nach der Epidemie des 'schwarzen Todes' 1348," *Sudhoffs Archiv* 16 (1924–1925): 26.

131. John Henderson, "The Flagellant Movement and Flagellant Confraternities in Central Italy, 1260–1400," in *Religious Motivation: Biographical and Sociological Problems for the Church Historian* (Studies in Church History 15), ed. Derek Baker (Oxford, 1978), p. 151. See also Norman Cohn, *The Pursuit of the Millennium* (London, 1970) for a discussion of the flagellant movement and related phenomena.

132. Mollat, *Popes at Avignon*, p. 41.

133. Henderson, "Flagellant Movement" p. 160.

134. See Kroll, "A Reappraisal of Psychiatry," pp. 276–283; George Rosen, *Madness in Society* (Chicago, 1968), ch. 7; and Ronald C. Finucane, *Miracles and Pilgrims: Popular Beliefs in Medieval England* (Totowa, NJ, 1977), p. 72.

135. Palmer, "The Church, Leprosy, and Plague," pp. 82–83.

136. Saul Nathaniel Brody, *The Disease of the Soul: Leprosy in Medieval Literature* (Ithaca, NY, 1974), p. 103.

137. Palmer, "The Church, Leprosy, and Plague," p. 85.

138. See Steven E. Ozment, *The Reformation in the Cities: The Appeal of Protestantism to Sixteenth-Century Germany and Switzerland* (New Haven, CT, 1975), p. 29.

139. Geary, "Relic Trade," p. 19.

140. Colin Morris, *The Discovery of the Individual, 1050–1200* (New York, 1972), p. 122.

141. Sumption, *Pilgrimage*, p. 144. See also Emma Mason, "Rocamadour in Quercy Above All Other Churches: The Healing of Henry II," in *The Church and Healing*, p. 52.

142. Finucane, *Miracles and Pilgrims*, p. 67.

143. See ibid., pp. 52–53; and Eugene A. Dooley, *Church Law on Sacred Relics* (Canon Law Studies 70) (Washington, DC, 1931).

144. Finucane, *Miracles and Pilgrims*, pp. 196–197.

145. Ibid., p. 198. See also Lionel Rothkrug, "Popular Religion and Holy Shrines: Their Influence on the Origins of the German Reformation and Their Role in German Cultural Develoment," in *Religion and the People*, pp. 28–29, and 36.

146. Colin Morris, "A Critique of Popular Religion: Guibert of Nogent on *The Relics of the Saints*," in *Popular Beliefs and Practices*, pp. 56 and 58.
147. See Finucane, *Miracles and Pilgrims*, pp. 214–215. This is an important aspect of Keith Thomas' thesis in *Religion and the Decline of Magic*, (London, 1971).
148. Rothkrug, "Popular Religion and Holy Shrines," p. 56.
149. Palmer, "The Church, Leprosy, and Plague," p. 87.
150. Finucane is speaking of R. Brentano, *Two Churches: England and Italy in the Thirteenth Century* (Princeton, NJ, 1968).
151. Finucane, *Miracles and Pilgrims*, pp. 10–11.

CHAPTER 4

The Roman

Catholic Tradition

Since 1545

MARVIN R. O'CONNELL

The history of the Roman Catholic Church between the Council of Trent (1545–1563) and the second Council of the Vatican (1962–1965) reveals the thought and action of a denomination, one Christian sect competing among many, which nevertheless continued to maintain its traditional universalist claims as the one true church. The spirit that dominated Catholicism during these four centuries was the spirit of the Counter Reformation—a conservative theology combined with strict discipline, heightened centralization, a static liturgy, and a carefully monitored popular piety. The victories of the Counter Reformation were many and impressive, especially at the beginning, between, say, 1550 and 1700. Much of Europe that had been lost to Protestantism during the early stages of the Reformation was regained. More important, in the long run, was the missionary endeavor Catholics took on, an enormously daunting task of worldwide evangelization which resulted ultimately in thriving churches in Asia, Africa, and the Americas. The Counter Reformation, no mere reaction, also represented an intense interior revival within Catholicism, signalled by a lively intellectual life, a host of innovative religious orders and methods of spiritual direction, a blossoming of new art forms, and several generations of mystics and martyrs.

The invested capital of this revival had to sustain the church through the bleak eighteenth century and beyond, when Catholicism, like all Christian denominations, suffered a crisis of institutional confidence as it tried to deal with the inroads of rationalism and with the incessant belligerance of the secular state. The French Revolution (1789) heralded the age of democracy and capitalism, which posed new and difficult challenges to Catholics, who were accustomed to living in agrarian and hierarchical societies. But although controversy and struggle were long and bitter, the church learned to adapt to the different economic and political realities without sacrificing its identity, and in some places, notably the United States, the local Catholic community flourished to an unprecedented degree. Not until the mid–twentieth century did the spirit of the Counter Reformation begin to show signs of faltering; its testy exclusiveness and its intellectual timidity seemed to Pope John XXIII (1958–1963) less open to the age than a church called "Catholic" ought to have been. So the pope summoned the second Council of the Vatican in order, in his own homely image, to throw open the windows of the church to the air and light outside. The Counter Reformation was over.

The Roman Catholic Church today counts about 750,000,000 communicants living on all continents and in all corners of the world. Its polity is episcopal, its bishops basing their claim to authority as teachers and sanctifiers of the people upon the continuation in themselves of the apostolic office. At their head is the pope, the Bishop of Rome, whose position is analogous to that of Peter among the original apostles. The theoretical and practical power of the papacy has increased markedly since the Council of Trent and especially since the first Council of the Vatican (1869–1870). Centralization of initiative and of decision making within the pope's own administration—the Roman curia—has kept pace with similar developments in secular governments over the past century and a half. The popes exercise the fullness of jurisdiction over every local church, and, since Vatican I, the right to employ the charism of infallibility, that is, the guarantee that when they speak formally and solemnly to the whole church on a matter of faith or morals the Holy Spirit will preserve them from teaching error. This privilege has been invoked only once since its conciliar definition in 1870, but the mere admission of it has greatly enhanced the popes' prestige as the primary teachers of the universal church. The second Council of the Vatican endorsed the unique authority of the papacy, yet it also attempted to broaden the notion of the governing office by giving new emphasis to the ancient doctrine of collegiality, that is, to the idea that the day-to-day mission of the church to evangelize—the ordinary magisterium—lies within the competence of the whole college of bishops, the apostolic college over which the successor of Peter presides. This constitutional model, with its mixture of monarchical and aristocratic elements, is fleshed out by the position assigned to laity and lower clergy, whose functions within the church are defined not by the application of a democratic principle, but by the degree to which they share in the redemptive work carried out by the bishops. That degree, in turn, is determined by the sacraments received; the laity, by virture of baptism and confirmation, play one role; the clergy, by having also been ordained, play another. The rest of the seven sacraments—penance, anointing of the sick, matrimony, and the Eucharist—are conceived of as having social as well as personal implications. The venerable tradition of seven central ritual acts was confirmed at Trent.

Specialized personnel within the Catholic Church fall into two large groups. Secular or diocesan priests are primarily (although not exclusively) ordained to perform sacramental service in the parishes under the direct supervision of the bishop of a diocese (that is, of a certain geographical area); they take no vows, although they do promise obedience to their bishop and abstinence from sexual activity (celibacy). Since Vatican II, secular priests have been aided in their ministry by deacons, an order of the primitive church only recently revived. The other large group is designated collectively religious, whose spiritual lives are defined by the vows of poverty, chastity, and obedience which they take upon themselves. Some religious are also priests—most Jesuits, for example—but by no means all. Generally speaking religious, whether priests or sisters or brothers, devote themselves to special works like education or nursing, and are directed not by the local bishop but by the officers of the particular order to which they belong—Franciscan, Dominican, Augustinian—which usually has its headquarters in Rome.

Modern secularization has taken its toll upon the Catholic community, especially in its former heartland, western Europe, where practice of the faith, insofar as it is statistically measurable, has fallen steadily throughout the twentieth century. At the same time, the church has put down deep roots in many countries of the Third World, with the result that in future years the designation "Catholic" may come to have a fuller meaning than it has enjoyed since the Reformation.

—————···◁◈▷···—————

One of the landmark events in the long and tumultuous history of Roman Catholicism was the general council that met intermittently at the northern Italian town of Trent between 1545 and 1563. The crisis that prompted Pope Paul III to convoke the first session of this assembly (1545–1547) and his immediate successors to reconvene it twice (1551–1552 and 1562–1563) was so serious that it appeared to have brought the Latin church and western Christendom to the verge of dissolution. There was, first of all, the devastating success of the Protestant Reformation which had spread with remarkable speed across northern Europe so that in less than thirty years new and thriving ecclesiastical organizations had sprung up in Germany, Switzerland,

England, and the countries of Scandinavia. Everywhere the church, which had long claimed to define itself by its universality, seemed to be crumbling beneath the assault of a different gospel preached with unprecedented vigor and excitement. Noblemen in Poland and Hungary, academics in France, artisans and entrepreneurs in the Netherlands, even learned and distinguished friars in Italy—none of them was left untouched by the zeal and forceful personalities of the reformers and by the attractiveness of their ideas.[1]

The desperate problem that Protestantism posed for the Roman Church was greatly compounded by its own internal disarray. The cry for reform of abuses had been loud and persistent for a century before Martin Luther posted his *Ninety-five Theses* upon the door of the castle–church in Wittenberg (1517). Indeed, local initiatives in Italy, the Netherlands, and elsewhere had demonstrated that much correction could be achieved thanks to the efforts of a particular preacher or religious institute. Luther himself had begun his career as a representative of an older German reform tradition which, up to his time, had not found it necessary to separate itself from the larger ecclesiastical system. The state of the church, it could be argued, was far better in 1517 than it had been in 1417. But revolutions are often the product of rising expectations, and the very success of reform in certain localities served to underscore the continuing pervasive decay and to contribute to the impatience of Christian men and women with the apparent reluctance of the church as a whole to put right the abuses that disfigured it. A venal, slothful, and ignorant clergy; a laity shot-through with superstition; colossal financial chicanery from indulgence-hawkers to corrupt officials of the Roman curia who routinely sold benefices and dispensations; an administrative chaos which made it virtually impossible to fix responsibility for the abuses and hence to apply the practical means to root them out; popes who were hedonists and simoniacs like Alexander VI (d. 1503) or warriors like Julius II (d. 1513) or dilettantes like Leo X (d. 1521)—all these were commonplace in Christian Europe at the moment the Protestant Reformation began. "According to the testimony of those who were then alive," wrote the Jesuit theologian Robert Bellarmine (1542–1621) nearly a century later, "there was an almost entire abandonment of equity in ecclesiastical judgments; in morals no discipline, in sacred literature no erudition, in divine things no reverence. Religion was almost extinct."[2]

Inevitably the doctrinal challenge to the Roman church merged with the universal revulsion at the abuses, with the result that from the beginning the word *reformation* possessed a certain ambiguity. For many—certainly for the great Protestant leaders like Luther and John Calvin—it meant primarily a reform of doctrine and the pastoral consequences that would necessarily follow. They pointed to the undeniable decay of ecclesiastical institutions as evidence, if not proof, that the synthesis of Catholic teaching that had emerged out of the middle ages was, at least, a distortion of divine revelation. Because the popes, they argued, taught false doctrines—particularly with regard to justification, merit, free will, and the value of human works—the church over which the popes presided had predictably suffered a moral and disciplinary collapse. Teach the truth as revealed in the Bible, the argument ran in effect, and the church will become what God intended it to be, the unspotted bride of Christ.[3]

But this causal link did not recommend itself to everyone. Indeed, it might be said that the fathers—that is, the bishops and the generals of religious orders who enjoyed the conciliar franchise—assembled at the Council of Trent precisely in order to deny it. Not that they denied the abuses. A curial commission nine years earlier had urged upon Paul III the most sweeping internal reforms and had beseeched the pope "to restore the name of Christ, forgotten by the people and by us, the clergy, to our hearts and to our works; to heal our ailments; to bring back the flock of Christ into the one fold; to remove us from the wrath of God and punishment earned by our deserts, which now threatens our very lives."[4] Such lamentations and beatings of the collective breast were typical and worked themselves with startling candor into the council's early debates. "We ourselves," cried Reginald Cardinal Pole (1500–1558), one of the council's presiding officers, at the session of 7 January 1546, "we ourselves are largely responsible for the misfortunes which have befallen us, for the rise of heresy, and the collapse of Christian morality, because we have failed to cultivate the field which was entrusted to us. We are like salt which has lost its savor. Unless we do penance, God will not speak to us."[5]

But to admit the widespread existence of the abuses, to assume the blame for them, even to recognize that "heresy" was nurtured by them, was not the same as assigning false doctrines as their cause. For the fathers of Trent and their Catholic contemporaries the abuses had flourished despite the teaching of the Roman Church, not because of it. For them "reformation" meant purging a system that was fundamentally sound but that had fallen victim over the past several centuries to human frailty and vice. What the Protestants had proposed, controversialist Thomas Stapleton (1535–1598) argued a few years after the Council of Trent, was

> not a reformation but a transformation. If they had not snatched away the substance of the Catholic faith, abolished the Christian sacrifice, denied the sacraments and altogether confused and upset due order and polity; had they instead proposed to criticize and correct the abuses and superstitions which had sprung up in various places on account of the crass negligence

of certain pastors, then the church of God would neither have called into question their zeal nor repudiated their counsel.[6]

The Council of Trent set for itself, therefore, two tasks. It aimed first to reassert in clear and unequivocal fashion what it conceived to be the true, traditionally received understanding of divine revelation; or, to put the same thing negatively, to refute the doctrinal innovations of the Protestant reformers. "For they are preaching a gospel other than the one we have received," wrote Stapleton. "It is not really a gospel at all, because it perverts the only true gospel of Jesus Christ. And so with reason the whole church of God says to them, 'Anathema.' "[7] At the same time the council determined to eliminate the financial, administrative, and pedagogical abuses that had led to the corruption of the clergy and the paganization of the laity, without, however, radically altering the ecclesiastical system in place. This two-fold purpose was reflected even in the procedure the council followed, in which both sets of problems were treated simultaneously: Dogmatic issues raised by the Protestants were considered one day, so to speak, and the correction of internal abuses the next.[8]

It would be hard to overemphasize the importance of the Council of Trent. The mind-set of modern Roman Catholicism was framed by its decrees and by the theologies based upon those decrees. Indeed, the very phrase *Roman Catholicism,* with its intrinsic semantic contradiction, could come to have meaning as a sectarian term in distinction to, say, Lutheranism or Calvinism only after Trent managed to stop the hemorrhaging within the older Christian body and to provide it with the tools of survival. To be sure, a stern price had to be paid for the success achieved by the fathers at Trent, a success that was in any event bound to be limited. All hope for the reunion of western Christendom faded when the Protestants were confronted by the conciliar decisions on justification, revelation, and the sacraments. The imposition by the council of a sharply rigorous discipline, however necessary it may have been, underscored the Roman Church's new and unfamiliar role as one Christian denomination competing among many others. Competitiveness bred exclusivity. It led inevitably to the development of a kind of siege mentality and just as inevitably to an increasing centralization of decision making with the pope and his curia, not only because the fathers of the council made the popes the special guardians of its testament, but also because a militant and embattled organization demanded for its existence—so it seemed—a unified command.

Catholicism has continued to claim to be the church of the apostles, but since the sixteenth century it has also been the "tridentine" church, the church reconstructed at Trent. In every phase of modern Catholic life, including that of the treatment of the sick, the teaching and the ideals enunciated at Trent have provided, until very recently, the ultimate norm of belief and practice. This is not to say that all Catholics in all places at all times agreed as to the interpretation of that teaching or even fully understood it, or that they consistently lived up to those ideals. But the stubborn application of the same measure to the activities of the largest single community of Christian believers, spread to every corner of the world over a span of four centuries, was itself enormously significant.

Trent, the Sacramental Principle, and Extreme Unction: The Anointing of the Dying

What little the fathers of the Council of Trent had to say explicitly about illness and its relief was confined to its statement about the sacrament of extreme unction. The brief decree, dated 25 November 1551, took up only a couple of pages of print. It was assertive rather than argumentative. Significantly, it followed directly upon the much longer decree on the sacrament of penance, because extreme unction was regarded by ancient tradition "as the completion not only of penance but also of the whole Christian life, which ought to be a continual penance." The ambiguity in the use of the word *penance* was accompanied by an obscurity as to the precise situation in which the sacrament was to be received. "This anointing is to be applied to the sick, but especially to those who are in such danger as to appear to be at the end of life, which is why it is also called the sacrament of the dying."[9] *The Catechism of the Council of Trent,* a manual of instruction for the use of parish priests issued just after the council, observed that extreme unction had been called in antiquity "the sacrament of the anointing of the sick," but it predictably followed the conciliar decree in restricting administration "to those only whose malady is such as to excite apprehension of approaching death."[10] Thus it would seem that the sacrament was to be administered only when medical authorities, echoing the Epistle of James, should advise "bringing in the priests of the church."[11]

Both the decree of Trent and the *Catechism* insisted that the primary object of extreme unction was the spiritual, not the physical, well-being of the afflicted person. The council employed familiar scholastic terminology:

> The thing signified [in the sacrament] is the grace of the Holy Ghost whose anointing takes away the sins if there be any still to be expiated, and also the remains of sin, and strengthens the soul of the sick person by exciting in him great confidence in the divine mercy, supported by which the sick

person bears more easily the miseries and pains of his illness and resists more easily the temptations of the devil.

Yet, once having established this point, the council added with more solemnity than precision: "At times, when expedient for the welfare of the soul, [extreme unction] restores bodily health."[12] The *Catechism* elaborated only by pointing a cautionary finger: "If in our days the sick obtain [recovery of physical health] less frequently, this is to be attributed, not to any defect in the sacrament, but rather to the weaker faith of a great part of those who are anointed with the sacred oil or by whom it is administered."[13]

Extreme unction, therefore, as the council defined it, shared in the sacramental principle, in an incarnational theology that stressed divine immanence in the human situation and was thus in marked contrast to that keystone of all classical Protestant teaching, the notion of the transcendence of God.[14] This was a crucial difference that cut across all issues, including that of health care. It manifested itself, to be sure, in ways that could be expressed propositionally. Trent thus differed from the Protestant reformers in seeing original sin as debilitating rather than as radically destructive. It differed from them also in relating grace to human merit and striving. The council proclaimed the essential freedom of the human will. But these were hardly more than abstract corollaries of its central vision of God as somehow fleshly, of its conviction that the very reality of God had been so closely mingled with the human that that reality could be captured in ritual and symbol, particularly in the seven sacraments and most particularly in the Eucharist. And such ritual, by conciliar definition, combined as necessary constituents the grossly material—a bit of bread, wine, water, oil—and the purified intention of the believer.

The spiritual system that emerged out of Trent was thus relatively optimistic, sensual, and anthropomorphic. It quite explicitly contradicted the evangel of the Protestant reformers by enhancing the value of good works and of human endeavor by describing grace as a phenomenon that could wax or wane, that could be gained and lost and regained again.[15] At the center of the panoply of good works, the council placed the seven sacraments, which produced their graceful results not so much by the inner and unseen dispositions of minister and recipient as by the proper application of form—for example, Christ's words at the last supper—to matter—bread and wine. So the Council gave its blessing to an older formulary; the sacraments, it said, performed *ex opere operato* (by virtue of their own inner coherence).

Trent in one sense taught an apotheosis of the material, the palpable, and the limited. Thus it defined the church not as an invisible congregation of the elect, but as the corporate body of all the baptized, which necessarily included the morally halt and lame. And what of the physically halt and lame? It stood to reason that if Christ could be brought down upon an altar in the shape of bread by the mumbled Latin of an insignificant and no doubt sinful priest, there should be available to the faithful similar if less noble rituals for a body suffering from one or another of the multitude of afflictions to which flesh is heir.

This conviction took root in the Catholic consciousness not so much because of the short and rather laconic conciliar decree on extreme unction as because of the overall consistency of the tridentine testament. So long as an infant science did not seriously dispute that all of nature was an intimate coupling of the material and spiritual—a view as old as Aristotle and the stuff of poets no less than of philosophers—it did not seem at all unlikely to the tridentine Catholic that an interventionist God should choose to intervene in behalf of his sick children by way of ritual and physical symbol.[16]

The Protestant Reformation with its emphasis upon transcendence was a radical effort to spiritualize the Christian vocation. The Council of Trent rejected this view in the name of a revelation that it construed to mean that the physical *qua* physical possesses an instrumental sacredness. The sacramental principle was wider than the seven sacraments. That there was great risk here of keeping open the door to those superstitious practices that had so outraged the reformers, the conciliar fathers were fully aware. Their awareness expressed itself in the legislation of internal reform they passed, which to a great extent was designed to provide well-ordered ecclesial life at the grass-roots level—witness the enormous attention paid at Trent to the education and demeanor of the parochial clergy. Many of the highly legalistic decisions of the Roman congregations over the next four centuries might be interpreted as responding to the same concern.

But, even so, there existed within the tridentine synthesis an intrinsic tension between the carefully nuanced conciliar and (subsequent) papal teaching and the popular reception and understanding of that teaching. This was a scandal to John Henry Newman (1801–1890), who complained some years before he became a Catholic that Roman officials had routinely failed to place "a practical restraint upon the *natural* tendency of their system."[17] Here was a shrewd observation. There did indeed lie at the heart of post-Reformation Catholicism a "natural tendency" to blur the distinction between genuinely religious activity and superstition—so much so that authority was often reluctant to insist upon the distinction in individual cases. *Tolerari potest* (let the practice be allowed) was not infrequently the decision handed down by a bemused diocesan chancery or Roman congregation. Given Trent's principles, there appears to have been little chance of avoiding the problem; the physical cries out for quantification, ritual invites repetition, and the use of symbols degenerates all too easily into magic. Trent tried to walk a fine line between the spiritualism of its sectarian opponents and an age-old paganism which deified the powers of nature. The Roman Catholic attitude toward illness and its treatment reflected this bold attempt at balance.

The Sacerdotal Mission

There existed within the Roman Catholic community a remarkable consistency in thought and action during the four centuries between the Council of Trent and the second Council of the Vatican (1962–1965). It is permissible, therefore, to make certain generalizations about the tridentine church that might be hazardous if applied to Catholicism before 1545 or since 1965. Attitudes, for example, toward sickness and death, toward sexual morality, and toward the relationship between cultic practice and healing did not differ markedly between, say, the late sixteenth and early twentieth centuries. This is not to say that such attitudes did not have deep medieval or even ancient roots, nor that there were not significant differences in detail in the application of tridentine principles from locality to locality or from group to group. Even so, the fathers of Trent did manage to establish a system with massive staying-power, not least perhaps because, with the emphasis they placed upon divine immanence and sacramentality, they proposed a doctrine and a spirituality that readily recommended themselves to the bulk of the Catholic people. Thus, when the development of scientific medicine in the nineteenth century posed new ethical questions, the Catholic response was a sophistication and elaboration of tridentine teaching, not a repudiation of it.

One safe generalization is that Trent, by insisting upon interlocking sacramentality with all phases of the Christian life, sharply intensified the clericalization of the Roman church. The necessity of a duly ordained priest to perform the sacred rituals was central to the functioning of the tridentine system. Nothing the council did was to be of more importance to the future of Catholicism than its delineation of the ideal priest. He was to be well if narrowly educated, decently but not extravagantly supported, wedded to his parish, subject to his bishop, sober, unworldly, and sustained in his vocation by the regular prayer of the breviary. He was still viewed as a member of a distinct caste— a world away in this regard, at least theoretically, from the Protestant preacher—but he was to see the justification of his status in sacramental service to those less spiritually endowed than he. In order to attain so far as was possible the realization of this ideal, the fathers of Trent set

out in detail the regulations of clerical residence, the financial arrangements, the type of professional training—in new institutions called
seminaries—out of which was to emerge this dominant father-figure of
tridentine Catholicism.[18]

Despite Trent's explicit injunction, however, a system of seminaries
developed only slowly and unevenly. Pius IV (d. 1565) tried to set a
good example by establishing the Collegio Romano within months of
the closure of the council.[19] His nephew, Charles Borromeo (1538–1584),
Archbishop of Milan, set up three seminaries in his vast diocese, and
the Primate of Portugal opened one in 1565. The newly founded (1540)
Society of Jesus was active and effective in this task of clerical education,
especially in Italy and Poland. But there was no seminary in Ireland,
thanks to English conquest and penal laws, until the end of the eighteenth century. The seminary at Eichstadt (1564) stood in lonely em-
inence among the great sees of the Holy Roman Empire until Münster
(1610) and Prague (1630) finally followed suit. There is some irony in
the fact that the seminary model eventually adopted everywhere else
came from France, where the government, jealous as usual of its
prerogatives, never allowed the formal promulgation of the disciplinary
decrees of the Council of Trent. Despite this typically gallican prohibition, Jacques Olier (1608–1657) and his colleagues at St. Sulpice in
Paris worked out in detail the curriculum, spirituality, and life-style
that were almost to define the training of the parish clergy until the
eve of the second Vatican Council.[20]

It need hardly be said that Trent's priestly ideal, like all other ideals,
was never entirely realized and that indeed the breaching of it was
common enough testimony to human frailty and to the limits of the
best-laid plans. Nevertheless, the fact remains that under the tridentine
dispensation the sluggard and the reprobate could no longer expect
ecclesiastical preferment. Gradually, as the turmoil and violence of the
wars of religion (1559–1648) subsided, the seminary-educated priests
became the norm, with the result that every village in those parts of
Europe still in communion with Rome had its own representative of
the Council of Trent. In that rural, parochial, largely illiterate world—
in that "universe of Peasants"[21] that Europe and Europe's dependencies
continued to be until the mid–nineteenth century, when technology
finally began to break down the walls of separation which had from
time immemorial divided one little region from another—the parish
priest was uniquely important. He might have been a brilliant or a dull
man, personally effective or ineffective; he might have been liked or
disliked or, sometimes, hated. He was never ignored. He and his
confreres, imbued with a stern self-confidence which was another tridentine characteristic, believed that they played by right the essential
role in daily Catholic life and were, besides, the lynch-pins of society,

because without them the parishes—the elemental social units—would not exist. Their people did not dispute them on this point nor did their bitterest enemies. For instance, the persecution of English Catholics during the reign of Elizabeth I (1558–1603) concentrated on destroying the priests trained in the seminaries-in-exile on the continent, on the assumption that once the priesthood was eliminated, the Catholic church as a viable entity would wither away. The queen's policy in this regard was eminently successful.[22]

The attitude of the parish priest, therefore, toward wellness and illness, caring and curing, and the rites of passage, although by no means the only factor, was crucially important in framing tridentine Catholicism's response to matters related to health care. And special emphasis needs to be given to the fact that the parish priest was both a preacher and a confessor to a degree uncommon among his pre-Reformation counterparts, who had offered mass, baptized, and witnessed marriages but who had been most of the time too ill-trained to impart any kind of formal instruction to the faithful. Increasingly during the years after Trent the parish priest—a regular and sustained presence in the local community, unlike the medieval friar who had performed these functions before, if indeed they had been performed at all—made his influence felt from the pulpit and through the grill of the confessional.[23]

In some places he made his presence felt in the direct practice of medicine. It is difficult to be precise as to where or when this so-called *medicina clericalis* was carried on, because strictly speaking it was against the canon law and therefore its practitioners tended to remain discreetly quiet about it. Trent had explicitly, if obliquely, confirmed earlier legislation on the subject by forbidding clerics to engage in any "secular" profession. Clerical medicine lingered on nevertheless, particularly in remote locations where a physician was not available and where the parish priest was virtually the only educated person in the area. There was, to be sure, an older tradition which linked religion and medicine to the extent that in the early middle ages almost all European medical practitioners were monks. But the legists of the thirteenth century had condemned this link, and chiefly for two reasons: first, because increasingly clerics had taken to the study and practice of medicine as a way of making money instead of as a way of performing gratis a work of Christian mercy in the relief of human suffering; second, because the skills available to the practitioner were so limited that many a patient died as a direct result of his ministrations, especially if a surgical procedure were involved. The law clearly reflected a fear that *medicina clericalis* could arouse widespread hatred against the clerical estate.[24]

There is enough evidence to suggest, however, that even centuries later, in tridentine times, clerics were still practicing some forms of medicine. In 1626, for example, the Congregation for the Propagation of the Faith (the Vatican bureau in charge of the missions) forbade priests in Bulgaria to "dispense medicines—and in particular laxatives—to the sick, whether they be of the Faith or not." But seven years later the same congregation granted permission to an English Jesuit (who had been trained as a physician before entering the society) to practice medicine on the mission, so long as such activity was not his principal occupation and so long as he took no money for it. In 1641 an even broader mandate was given to the missionaries, who were allowed to practice medicine as a means of aiding in the conversion of unbelievers, provided that they were "truly learned in the profession," that they performed no surgery, that they worked without compensation, and that there were no other doctors available.[25]

This last proviso touched upon a condition as common in parts of Europe as in the mission lands, and it led to a practical softening of the law's rigor, so much so that by the eighteenth century *medicina clericalis* was experiencing a kind of revival. Much of what the parish priest did for his people in this regard might be categorized as simple procedures in first aid. But not infrequently medical practice was carried much farther. For instance, a manual appeared in Italy in 1745 (and went into numerous printings) that instructed the parish priest on how to treat illnesses associated with childbirth and even on how to perform a cesarean section when necessary.[26]

Despite the survival of clerical medicine—abetted to some extent by Enlightenment intellectuals who praised it as the one useful service performed by an otherwise parasitic profession—the pastor's chief role in the drama of health care had to do with his task as sanctifier and spiritual teacher of his people. He had little enough to say about wellness as such, except that it was a gift of God, as fleeting as one of Shakespeare's seven ages of man, and as tenuous as the next pestilence or accident could make it. Here, he said continually, we have no lasting city, here we have no abiding stay. "Remember, man," he intoned each year at the beginning of Lent as he rubbed ashes upon the foreheads of his parishioners, "remember that thou art dust, and to dust thou shalt return." Pain is our lot in this valley of tears, for we are the banished children of Eve, the victims of our own sins and of all sin, redeemed by the suffering of Calvary and promised the robust health of a resurrected body only after we have endured a crucifixion of our own. Tridentine Catholicism was not a religion of social amelioration or of humanitarian concerns; it was as relentlessly other-worldly as its Calvinist rival.

The parish priest, therefore, had a great deal more to say about the other side of the coin, illness and its concomitant suffering. On this subject there was basic consistency throughout the tridentine period, with the tone set more by spiritual writers than by academic theologians. So Robert Bellarmine, the most distinguished of the thinkers to emerge during the era immediately after the council, expressed his conviction that human pain was a sharing in Christ's redemptive pain more eloquently and with far wider influence in a popular tract than he did in his massive formal tomes.[27] Francis de Sales (1567–1622), an even more influential teacher than Bellarmine, stated (1609) in his typically succinct manner the conventional wisdom: "We must accept the sickness that God wishes, in the place he wishes, among the Persons he wishes, and with the inconveniences he wishes."[28] Such views as these the parish priest was invited to ponder and to transmit to his people. Suffering was a *sine qua non* condition of sanctity; this was a dictum that tridentine Catholicism took for granted. Suffering was always judged as edificatory and expiatory if it were accepted in the right spirit. The Council of Trent had stubbornly reasserted the notion of the *temporal* punishment due to sin, punishment to be inflicted in time, either in this world or in purgatory. Clearly, pain and illness were part of the purging process—a kind of good work—through which believers had to pass before they could experience the blessed vision of peace. To suffer, therefore, was to embark upon "the royal road of the holy cross," and those who suffered most were deemed to be the holiest of all.[29]

Prudential limits, however, were placed upon this principle. The church militant admitted of many levels of spiritual capacity. Not everyone could raise pain to the level of ecstasy. Francis of Assisi (1182–1226), who had borne upon his body the very wounds of Jesus, could be admired by all but imitated by only a small elite. The parish priest urged acts of self-denial upon his people, especially during the formal penitential seasons preceding Christmas and Easter, during the "ember days" which marked the beginning of the four seasons, on the vigils of great feasts, and on every Friday. But his ordinary message to the men and women in the pews in front of him was a plea to accept humbly the physical pain which was all too familiar a part of their lives, and of his. One might well argue that stigmatics like Francis of Assisi could have been more easily venerated, and understood, in an age when childbirth, stone, amputation, toothache, and all other conceivable ills had to be endured with only minimal medical aid and with anesthetic which at best could only dull the agony. Sunday after Sunday, in any event, the people were likely to hear their parish priest invoke some variation on the Pauline theme that it was their vocation "to make up what is lacking in the sufferings of Christ," but to do so according to the spiritual rank with which God had endowed them.[30]

The discipline of knotted thongs, the bed of boards, and the hairshirt were reserved for the privileged few, and for them only under the strict supervision of a director.[31]

Not many of these clerics who did most to fashion the Catholic consciousness after the Council of Trent entered into the theologians' arcane discussions of how God permitted rather than caused sickness and pain, nor could they explain precisely what responsibility the devil had for human suffering. Formal exorcism was an exotic art, understood by few,[32] but demons were very real persons, their chief "a raging lion, seeking some one to devour,"[33] and it was a boldly enlightened priest indeed who discouraged his people from sprinklings of holy water or wearing of amulets designed to ward off that Satan who, in far-off days, had covered Job's body with boils and had flung him upon a dung heap. Priests and people were likely moreover to ascribe a specific suffering to a specific moral lapse, their own or others', a habit they maintained in the face of official ecclesiastical and theological disapproval. A particularly baneful result of this mentality was the savage persecution of those "witches" popularly believed to be in league with the devil—although of course such persecution was by no means a uniquely Catholic phenomenon.[34]

On another level—one upon which he may have felt surer of himself—the parish priest after the Council of Trent had to deal with problems related to health care from the point of view of moral obligation, and he had to begin with himself. He knew from his seminary training that he was bound under the penalty of grave sin to minister to the seriously sick and particularly to the dying among his parishioners, no matter what the inconvenience or even danger to himself. Ordinarily such ministry included a triad of sacraments: confession, anointing, and Viaticum (the Eucharist, that is, defined as food providing strength for the journey from one stage of life to the next). If the patient were unconscious, then the first and third of these ritual acts were necessarily omitted. The anointing could proceed in any case, and the priest was instructed by his rubrical books that he must be properly vested (wearing a stole, the sign of sacerdotal office), that he take care to join the form of the sacrament (the words, said in Latin: "Through this holy anointing, and through his most loving mercy, may the Lord forgive whatever you have done wrong" by the misuse of the senses) with the matter (the physical application of the oil specially blessed for the purpose by a bishop), and that he anoint the eyes, ears, nostrils, mouth, hands, and feet, six separate rites, each symbolizing the purgation of one of the senses that may have led the dying person into sin during his or her lifetime.[35] The priest could not evade his duty of ministration even at the risk of being infected himself. He could, however, take what the theological manuals called "prudent" precautions; a patient with a very infectious disease might be anointed on one organ only, or, if he had just confessed, the administration of extreme unction might be omitted altogether.[36]

It is worth noting that through these elaborate rules the sacramental system manifested itself as a great chain of being, for the sake of which the rubrical and casuistical demands were made. The tridentine Catholic firmly, if obscurely, believed that this particular dying person, by the eternal decision in the mind of God, was to be saved by the grace conferred by this particular administration of the sacrament, which God also foresaw would be administered at the risk of the life of this particular priest.

Those in the parish who were sick or wounded or simply so aged as to be in the danger of death could receive the sacrament. If the patient recovered and then fell ill once more, he could be anointed again any number of times. Those who were judged incapable of committing sin—small children, the permanently insane—were incapable of receiving extreme unction; the rule of thumb was that those who had no need of the sacrament of penance had no need either of the last anointing which, the Council of Trent had taught, was at root an extension of the church's penitential mission.[37] The deaf, dumb, and blind, by contrast, could be anointed because they may have been guilty of interior sins of thought or desire. A soldier on the field of battle, a felon about to be executed, or a traveller soon to embark upon a dangerous journey could not receive the sacrament, because the proximity of death in none of these cases stemmed from a present bodily infirmity. Opinions differed as to whether women in labor could be anointed; some parish priests did so on the ground that such a woman was genuinely ill, while others refrained, arguing that childbirth was simply the performance of a natural function. Pregnancy was never considered sufficient cause for administration of the sacrament.[38]

The appearance at the cottage door of the priest with a stole around his neck and a vial of holy oil in his hand often occasioned wails of grief from the sick person's friends and relatives, who saw this visitation as a sign that death would inevitably follow. Some even maintained that the administration of the "last sacraments" did the patients serious harm by convincing them they had no hope of recovery. So the parish priest had to remind his people regularly that to refuse the church's final ministrations was itself a mortal sin. Resistance, although it may have been widespread, was mostly impulsive and fleeting. In an age when life was usually "nasty, brutish and short," and when, among Catholic peoples, the sacramental principle loomed so large, the last rites enjoyed a status that no transitory emotions could dislodge.[39] Peter Canisius (1521–1597), the Jesuit writer whose celebrated *Catechism* went into 200 editions and was translated into twelve languages during his lifetime, probably expressed the settled view of most tridentine Catholics:

> Whereupon albeit the health of the body be not restored to the sick (for often we see the patient to die after the unction received), still in this sacrament there is special grace given most constantly to suffer the violence and trouble of sickness to the end, and afterward more patiently to receive death itself; and this it is that God has promised by his apostle: the prayer of faith will save the sick, and our Lord will ease him, and if he be in sins they shall be forgiven him.[40]

In the pulpit and the confessional the parish priest explained wellness, considered as a good in itself, under the rubric of the commandment "Thou shalt not kill." This was an imperative that applied first of all to oneself; direct suicide as well as any form of euthanasia was dismissed out of hand. The doctrine, however, was not without nuance; exceptional circumstances or the promotion of a greater good might on occasion necessitate a person taking action that would bring about his or her death. It was not deemed suicide, for example, if a soldier remained at a dangerous post even though he would be killed as a result, nor if a virgin, to preserve her chastity, were "to embrace even certain danger of death," so great a good was her "integrity." The distinction between killing oneself and accepting the *certain* danger of death may not always have been clear in practice, but the moralists from whom the parish priests learned their lessons were perfectly straightforward and unequivocal that nobody was obliged to exercise extraordinary means merely to stay alive: "The ill can be excused who, a little before death, out of humility or to give good example, seek to be gathered into the earth, because they do not thereby intend to shorten life."[41]

The requirement to preserve one's life naturally extended to one's health. The parish priest was concerned, however, to point out that maintenance of health had primarily an instrumental function; one must keep oneself strong, not for the sheer animal joy of it, but in order to do one's duty in justice and charity and to take upon oneself the acts of physical self-denial recommended, indeed mandated, by the church. The body was the temple of the Holy Spirit and thus had to be cherished and cared for. Self-mutilation of any kind was sternly forbidden, unless amputation of a limb was called for in order to save one's life. In such an instance the good of the whole prevailed over the survival of the infected part. "Those Parents sin grievously who have their sons castrated in order to enhance their singing, even if the boys consent." (There was little dissent from this judgment except, significantly, in Italy where one seventeenth-century moralist argued that castrati contributed to the common good, because, thanks to them, "the divine praises [were] sung more sweetly in churches.")[42]

Over time the body would gradually decay, or in the twinkling of an eye it would be destroyed. How or when or even why was a decision locked in the mind of God, and it was a feckless enterprise to rail against that unalterable decision. One Catholic preacher, in 1618, chided his congregation for its lack of Christian patience: "Those that are sick afflict themselves that they cannot be well in health. And those that are well do run into disorders as though they hastened to be sick. If anything be amiss, instead of seeking a remedy by patience, they are more angry and make it worse."[43]

Tridentine Catholics were instructed to seek other, more mundane remedies as well. Indeed, they were told that they could be guilty of serious sin if they failed to follow the "informed opinions" of their physician, even to the point of taking prescribed medicines. The doctor, for his part, approached the confessional aware that his profession imposed upon him a long list of possible moral violations. Did he try to treat a serious illness without sufficient skill, or neglect to engage in "special study" when a certain case required it? Did he substitute eccentric forms of treatment, without the support of substantial medical opinion, when more conventional procedures were available? Did he carelessly absent himself when his patient was in danger, or, if justifiably absent, did he prevent other doctors from treating the patient? Did he persuade his patient to indulge in any act "contrary to God's honor or command, for example, pollution, incantation, superstition?" Did he without due cause excuse his patient from the church's law of fasting? Did he see to it that a patient gravely ill saw his confessor? Did he charge too much for his services? Did he fail to treat a poor person in danger of death because he would not be paid? If a surgeon, did he cause an abortion, or did he, more broadly, refuse to take advice in difficult operations?[44]

A physician was admonished to ask himself such questions when he examined his conscience, and indeed some of these queries might have been addressed to him in the confessional box. He would not, however, presuming he was a married man, be asked everything about his sexual life. Confessors were repeatedly warned to use "the maximum circumspection" (the words of Charles Borromeo) in interrogating penitents about sexual matters.[45] Alphonsus Liguori (1696–1787) summed up the mature tridentine consensus in this way: "Ordinarily speaking, the confessor is not bound nor is it fitting for him to inquire about sins of the married in respect to the marital debt, except that, as modestly as he can, he may ask wives if they have rendered it, for example by asking them if they have obeyed their husbands in everything. About other things let him be silent unless asked."[46] The prudence thus recommended to the confessor—and to the preacher as well—represented a considerable shift from pre-tridentine practice.[47] The severe Augustinian tradition, which had a sexual as well as a broader doctrinal context and which was so easily identified in the Catholic mind with Luther and Calvin, survived after Trent only among those latter-day Augustinians, the Jansenists. This was no doubt a significant and influential survival, one more testimony to Augustine's persuasive genius; but it was never more than a minority position among tridentine Catholics at large and its impact lessened drastically once the great school of seventeenth-century French Jansenists had passed away.

Augustine (354–430) had taught that sexual intercourse even within marriage was permissible only with explicit procreative intent (a far different proposition from the one that was to daunt Catholics in the twentieth century, that every act of sexual intercourse *had to be open* to procreative possibility). To be sure, the tridentine church continued to denounce abortion as murder, extramarital sex as lechery, and masturbation as self-indulgence which could cause serious bodily defects like blindness. (Nocturnal, and hence involuntary, emission was, by contrast, described as conducive to "physical health.")[48] But the *Catechism of the Council of Trent* explained the causes of marriage in a manner to dismay Augustinian rigorists of whatever denomination: "First of all, nature itself by an instinct implanted in both sexes impels them to such companionship, and this is further encouraged by the hope of mutual assistance in bearing more easily the discomforts of life and the infirmities of old age. A second reason for marriage is the desire of a family."[49]

Such a doctrine of the primacy of mutual solace was in accord with the radical optimism of tridentine Catholicism. This is not to say that the procreative element was eliminated or even denigrated in the church's official teaching. It did mean, however, that intercourse between married persons was morally licit for some reasons—the fostering of love, physical health, even venereal pleasure which otherwise might be sought in an adulterous union—other than procreation. It also opened the door a crack to the permissibility of birth control. The understanding, in any case, of the phrase *marital debt* underwent a change of some magnitude. The manuals of moral theology that the parish priest consulted spoke often of the economic burdens large numbers of children imposed upon families, especially among the poor. Little if anything was said about the effect upon the health of a woman subjected to frequent pregnancies, perhaps because women neither had nor thought they ought to have an organized voice to raise such an issue. The only permissible way to limit the number of conceptions was by abstinence, and here at least a woman might be able under certain economic circumstances to refrain on occasion from paying the marital debt. So, at any rate, some theologians argued. But although they wrestled manfully with the problem, they could not find a universally acceptable solution that was also consistent with traditional norms of sexual morality. The law of nature demanded that the act of intercourse be complete and integral. The sin of Onan, who spilled his seed on the ground, was fiercely condemned in the Bible.[50] Moralists wrote, moreover, in and for a society in which great ignorance of physiology, especially female physiology, prevailed. What sort of noncoital intimacy was licit for married couples? Withdrawal of the penis followed by ejaculation *(coitus interruptus)* was clearly wrong, the moralists said. They were not quite sure about a withdrawal not followed by ejaculation *(amplexus reservatus);* some of them hedged by suggesting that this practice might be venially, not mortally, sinful. Did touches and kisses that might— very likely would—result in orgasm provide a morally allowable alternative? Little wonder that in this jungle the confessor was urged to tread warily and not to ask too many questions.[51]

There were other reasons, besides the absence of a feminist lobby, that the issue of birth control, muddled as it was in its details, remained quiescent within the Roman Church until nearly the end of the tridentine era. Infant mortality was high and population pressure virtually non-existent. (An exception perhaps was Ireland, but the famine crisis there in the 1840s led to later marriage and vast emigration rather than to any coherent policy of restricting conceptions.) An overwhelmingly rural culture continued to put a premium on offspring who could take their places within the farm economy; children, to use the biblical image, were like arrows in the quiver, like olive plants around the table. Contraceptive methods were crude, often ineffective, often the "poisonous potions" that women sometimes took in order to abort and which therefore were identified officially and popularly as homicidal. The condom appeared in the middle of the seventeenth century, but it was expensive and from a moral point of view represented simply another version of *coitus interruptus.* Finally, it is surely safe to say that the issue was not faced squarely, because those who framed the official position—the bishops who taught it authoritatively, the theologians who interpreted it, and the parish priests who transmitted it to the married people under their direct charge—were all without exception celibate males and therefore did not encounter the problem in their day-to-day—or perhaps one should say their night-to-night—lives.

It would be easy to conclude that because the Catholic clergy were not allowed to enjoy sexual pleasure they made it their business to restrict as much as they could the enjoyment of their lay co-religionists. Such a conclusion, however, would leave out of account the fact that sexual teaching and practice among tridentine Catholics did not differ markedly from what prevailed in the Christian world at large. Contraception was frowned upon by most major denominations until well into the twentieth century. Before that no Catholic spokesman, not even the most dour Jansenist, could outdo the bleak attitude toward all things sexual routinely voiced by puritan preachers in New England—happily married and well-adjusted men, one might suppose, with squads of dutiful children around them. Lack of sensitivity toward the sexual wants and needs of women was certainly not a Catholic preserve. Queen Victoria (1819–1901) was not a Catholic, but her abhorrence of the marriage bed—even though she shared it with a man she deeply loved—represented a long tradition and provided a pattern for generations of respectable, white, Anglo-Saxon, Protestant women.[52] Not before the triumph of secularism in the twentieth century was sexuality as such discovered to be a major health concern. Sexual "compatibility," understood in its emotional implications, would have seemed an effete concept to earlier times. Passion was a matter of animal vigor, particularly of masculine vigor. It is said that the young Louis XIV (1638–1715), when the urge was upon him, would go to his queen's boudoir; if she were indisposed for some reason, he, perfect gentleman that he prided himself upon being, would not disturb her, but instead would satisfy himself with the nearest available lady-in-waiting. The anecdote may not be true, but it is not without its point even so; the double standard, so pervasive at all levels of society, took it for granted that the only health issue involved in sexuality was the assuaging of the physical needs of a king or, indeed, of any normal male.

In theory, both Protestant and Catholic catechesis would have condemned the king's conduct as adultery. But there was a difference. Louis as a Catholic would go to confession (although in fact he seldom did so before old age) and, if he were genuinely sorry and resolutely determined not to repeat the misdeed, have the sin forgiven. The availability of the sacrament of penance—and not just to repair sexual transgressions—could conceivably cut two ways, and it probably did. Protestant critics of the sacramental system pointed to it as a source of the loose morals they discerned in Catholic countries like Italy and Spain; easy "forgiveness," they said, was an invitation to habitual vice. Tridentine Catholics responded that theirs was not a religion of instant and complete conversion, that the necessity imposed upon them of confessing their sins was itself a kind of deterrence as well as an occasion for nurturing within themselves sound dispositions of contrition and amendment. Evidence could no doubt be brought forward to support either position, although it might be harder to demonstrate that one nation was less sinful than another; that the moral tone of Georgian England, for example, was loftier than that of Leopoldine Austria. In any event, when it came to dealing with sexual questions within the tridentine church the parish priest, as always, acted as the agent between the official teachers and the men and women in the pews. And more often than not he developed a salty wisdom. One veteran pastor, who in his village church had heard thousands of confessions and, *ipso facto,* almost that many stories of sexual misconduct, counselled his younger brethren to be surprised at nothing they heard and to take into account that most of the people they served lived close to the stock.

The Popular Response

They were people of the earth, earthy. The large majority of tridentine Catholics, until well past 1900, wrenched their sustenance directly from the reluctant soil. Whether they lived in Catholicism's European heartland, or had emigrated to other temperate areas like Argentina, Australia, or the United States, or were indigenous populations in tropical places like the Philippines or Uganda, converted by missionaries active since the sixteenth century, they dwelt in a world in which staying alive from day to day was a constant struggle, a world of uncertainty and pain. They stood in awe of a powerful nature which appeared to them, as it had to their ancestors back through countless centuries, to combine hostility with caprice. Some years, to be sure, were fatter than others; some land was more fertile, some climates more benign. Through the cycles of inflation and depression some did better than others. But overall, theirs was a life of chronic shortage; overall, they endured inadequate diet, poor housing, and bad sanitation.[53] They suffered more and died sooner than it is possible for their descendants, who stand beyond the door of modernization opened by science and technology, ever fully to appreciate.

They were not, of course, without their joys, not strangers to merriment, festivals, and fresh wine. They had their moments of triumph and serene satisfaction. The frugality which was their ordinary lot made their feasts all the dearer to them. They were neither stuffed nor hollow men, although their eyes often glittered with hunger. The very severity of their existence lent zest and excitement to their lives, in contrast, perhaps, to the blandness of a consumerist and hedonist society, built upon the predictability of central heating, the contraceptive pill, and the welfare state. Whether they were "happier" than their descendants or not is a question no mere historian dares ask.

The genius of the tridentine system, but its danger also, was its capacity to mesh its doctrine and practice, based upon the principle of divine immanence, with the acquired habits of country people. Even the dullest peasant could understand the soothing and curative property of oil, the nutritive value of bread, and the cleansing effect of water.

The church provided blessings and a sacramental context for all the important human moments from the womb to the deathbed. Formal rites marked the merging of one season into the next. Blessings were furnished for crops, catches of fish, domestic animals, and farm implements. Special saints' day observances focused upon promoting the physical well-being of a particular parish or region. In times of pestilence, the local church often organized processions, mobs of frightened penitents in effect, to implore God to forgive the sinfulness which was conceived to be the cause of the calamity; this common and popular practice, when it defied, as it often did, official rules of quarantine, brought with it a confrontation between church and state.[54]

Beneath this institutionalized framework, and to some degree mingling with it, there existed a vast underworld of cultic activities which had their beginning long before Trent—in many instances indeed long before the advent of Christianity—and which breathed the immemorial rhythms of the countryside as much as they did any religious sensibility. It was to be expected in an age of primitive and sometimes fraudulent medical care, if any care at all was available, that many such activities should be oriented toward warding off or curing disease. As late as the 1770s a Bavarian priest attracted a tremendous following when he proclaimed that illness was a result of demonic possession and should be treated therefore by exorcists rather than doctors. Thousands waited upon his ministrations, and although his movement died with him, the popular conviction that he had been a legitimate healer remained. Not without reason was it said that some islands in the Caribbean became, after the arrival of the Europeans and the subsequent introduction of African slaves, one hundred percent Catholic as well as one hundred percent voodoo. Confessors despaired of persuading Italian women not to mark their bodies with texts from the Bible in order to keep themselves healthy. In eastern France pilgrimages to a wooded shrine, where mothers sought relief for their sick children from a saint who also happened to have been a dog, continued into the latter part of the nineteenth century. In southern Germany a book appeared in 1771 (and promptly went into ten editions) that precribed as treatment for a sick (and therefore bewitched) cow a dose of blessed salt or bread and forced inhalation of smoke from a fire of blessed sulphur or palm branches. Young men who succeeded in leaping unscathed across a bonfire lit on the vigil of the feast of St. John the Baptist (June 24) were guaranteed good health through the following year. Seers and wizards could be found trudging along every road, ready to cure sprains, burns, or scrofula by a combination of ancient herbal remedies and pseudo-Christian incantations. One French peasant treated rheumatism by applying the bodies of boiled cats to the painful joints, all the while mumbling a set number of paters and aves. Prayer to St. Apolline, who had been martyred by having her teeth torn out, together with signs of the cross traced on the sore jaw, was the sure way to get rid of toothache. A pilgrim who had gone to the shrine of St. Hubert in the Ardennes could cure rabies by using a key obtained there combined with certain prayers and sacred gestures. At the end of the seventeenth century, Naples was reputed to have eleven miracle-working statues of the Virgin Mary.[55]

The survival of so much superstition among the masses of tridentine Catholics appears, at first glance, to have confirmed the strictures of Protestant polemicists upon the intrinsically idolatrous character of Catholicism. The truth, however, is considerably more complicated. Certainly the melding into bizarre combinations of crude rural nostrums with pagan ritual and Christian symbol (or vice versa) was commonplace, no less in Catholic Europe than in the mission lands, and it persists to this day. The fact is that tridentine Catholicism, imbued with the principle of immanence, was peculiarly vulnerable to popular cults that involved distorted sacramental acts. The difference between the institutional church—which recommended veneration of relics, blessings for animals, and rogation-day processions to seek divine aid for the bounty of the seasons, to say nothing of the formal ritual grounded in oil and bread—and a populace that invoked age-old rites and incantations, more or less Christianized, to ward off evil was a difference of *degree,* not of a kind. The parish priest, fresh from a tridentine seminary, might disapprove of what he conceived to be the excesses of his people in, say, mixing herbal potions with prayers to the Virgin or seeking cures from a wandering seer with talismans pinned to his hat. But the sin lay in exaggeration, overindulgence, and extravagance, not in the use of physical things for sacred purposes. Neither the priest nor his hierarchical superiors were prepared to deny the reality of an interventionist God who sanctified the Christian people through ritual observance, who, within the confines of the village church, worked the physical miracle of changing bread into Christ's body every morning. And, in any case, how far removed was the average parish priest, despite his time in the seminary, from the tribal instincts of the people from whom he had been taken and to whom he had now returned?[56]

He often found himself hard put to rein in the enthusiasms of his people, especially because he was not totally out of sympathy with those enthusiasms. He faced a dilemma. On the one hand, he risked the outbreak of anticlericalism within the parish if he resisted too forcefully the importunities of his people to grant his official sanction to their enterprises; on the other, he risked the wrath of his relatively sophisticated bishop—particularly from the eighteenth century onward—if he encouraged or winked at the lighting of bonfires on St. John's eve. Most of the time he evaded as best he could the unpleasant choices and hoped no one would ask him how the relief offered to the sick by extreme unction differed from boiled cats applied to rheumatic joints.

To understand the ambivalence tridentine Catholicism experienced in this regard, one must very often remind oneself of the commitment made at Trent to the instrumental function of physical things in the process of justification. The great breach within western Christendom at the time of the Reformation turned indeed upon differing opinions about the value of "faith" and "works" to the Christian man or woman seeking salvation. "Works," so said the fathers of Trent, played an integral part of that process, and they included in the meaning of the word the intrinsic soundness of the material. Matter participated in the divine. Material things therefore were genuine conduits of grace and capable of sharing in the supernatural order. The primacy belonged not to the word alone, but to the Word made flesh. Here was a difference in kind that separated Protestant from Catholic, an irreconcilable difference that no amount of effort has ever managed to solve. The trouble on the Catholic side was that Trent could not, simply by denouncing it, eliminate the manipulative interpretation of its doctrine. Unlettered people stubbornly held to the view that sacramental action had to be automatic in its results, a species of magic. Perhaps it was too much to ask a person writhing in pain that he remember that all ritual acts were at root not demands, not bargains, but petitions.

A solution of sorts to this problem was worked out during the last phase of the tridentine epoch, from the mid–nineteenth century to the mid–twentieth. It did not stem from a flagging of interest among Catholics in extra-medical treatment of sickness. Indeed, it is ironic that the great flowering of pilgrimage devotion should have occurred just at the moment when scientific medicine was embarking upon its dramatic advancement. What led to the solution was the curious combination of two typically modern developments. First was the swift and unprecedented growth of centralization within the Catholic church. The arm of Rome had never been so long as it was during (and since) the pontificate of Pius IX (1846–1878). The relative independence of diocese and parish, at least on a day-to-day basis, was virtually swept away during the eras of the French Revolution and Napoleon. The papal bureaucracy, of which the bishops increasingly became mere agents, kept a stern eye upon the exuberances of local piety.[57] Simultaneously, new modes of mass communication and transport made it easy for people to learn about and travel to glamorous centers of devotion which they quickly came to esteem more than the humdrum ones closer to home.

The miraculous shrines of La Salette and Lourdes (in France), of St. Ann de Beaupré (Canada), of Knock (Ireland), of the Virgin of

Guadalupe (Mexico), and of Fatima (Portugal), their walls festooned with the crutches of the cured, have all been preempted by the institutional church. The hierarchy has taken great care to avoid what might be called a peasant reputation from attaching itself, for example, to the healing capacity of the waters of the fountain at Lourdes, where of the thousands of pilgrims who have claimed healing, only sixty-four have been "certified" by ecclesiastical authority. No doubt this exercise of control has helped the church maintain its hold upon at least a portion of its people—during the early 1980s three million pilgrims visited Lourdes each year—culturally uprooted by industrialization and prone to alienation from religion by the whole complexus of modernity.[58] But it has also managed thereby to minimize the tridentine dilemma by insisting upon the petitionary character of these devotions and by formally granting the distinction between public and private revelation: Even the most fervent devotee of the cult of Lourdes must admit that no Catholic is bound to believe that Bernadette Soubirous really saw a lady in a dump outside that Hautes-Pyrénées town in 1858 or that the waters of her fountain have cured anybody of anything.

But in the end all cures fail; the most skilled physician gives way at last to the power of death, and even God does not intervene forever. Bernadette Soubirous, who never washed in the waters she had discovered, died after hideous suffering of bone cancer at the age of thirty-five (1879), and the funeral mass was chanted over her wasted body, as it was over countless other tridentine Catholics less brave and holy than she. It was a somber affair, this rite of farewell, filled with stern reminders that "while we lament the departure of our sister, thy servant, out of this life, we know that we are most certainly to follow her." The amount of pomp depended often upon the social standing of the deceased; a rich man might be buried with a solemn high mass—a priest, assisted by a deacon and a subdeacon—or, in Poland, with three masses going on simultaneously. Nothing was more bleak than a pauper's funeral, no one more abject than he who had no money to leave behind him for masses to be offered for his swift deliverance from purgatory. The village church was in any case suffused in gloom, the priest dressed in black vestments, the hymns sung without accompaniment. The theme was not so much the resurrection as the judgment. *Dies irae, dies illa,* the choir sang: "O day of wrath, that dreadful day. Deliver me, O Lord, from everlasting death on that day of terror, when the heavens and the earth will be shaken, as thou comest to judge the world by fire."

Yet tridentine Catholics did their best to believe what they recited each Sunday in the creed, that they belonged to the communion of saints, that life for them was destined not to be taken away, but only changed. So however sad or fearful they may have felt, they listened with bounding hope to one of the most beautiful of the Gregorian chants, sung as the corpse was carried slowly out of the church to the cemetery: "May the angels take thee into paradise; may the martyrs come to welcome thee on thy way, and lead thee into the holy city, Jerusalem. May the choir of angels welcome thee, and with Lazarus who once was poor may thou have everlasting rest."[59]

Caring and Curing

One of the most striking features of Martin Luther's preaching was the insistence that the loftiest Christian "calling" was to be lived out in the world, not within the confines of a remote monastery or convent.[60] This represented not only a repudiation of Luther's own monastic background, but also of the whole notion of a hierarchically structured spiritual experience to which the church gave witness. The old tradition was that certain individuals were called by God to live in a "higher" state than their fellows, to be guided by the evangelical counsels over and above the observance of the commandments required for everybody, to withdraw from the world and its concerns and its pomps, and to formalize all this by taking upon themselves (as parish priests did not do) the vows of poverty, chastity, and obedience. Predictably, the Fathers of Trent rejected Luther's egalitarianism and maintained that the so-called religious orders of monks, nuns, and friars, although in some instances in need of internal reform, did in fact enjoy a higher than ordinary calling and were essential to the full flowering of the church's life.

Among the evangelical counsels were the admonitions to "visit the sick" and to "bury the dead."[61] It was natural that such works of charity, to the extent that they took on an organized form, should have come to be associated with religious whose vocation demanded a more elevated level of response to cries of distress than that of the average Christian. Thus the *medicina clericalis* that flourished during the early middle ages simply meant the free medical care offered by monks to their tenants and to others living in the neighborhood of their monasteries. Various orders of men dedicated themselves to alleviating, as far as they could, the sufferings of galley slaves, lepers, Christians captured by Moslem pirates, or even foot-sore travellers. Some brothers practiced in-home nursing, others maintained pesthouses in the towns. The Alexian Brothers began their corporate existence in the Netherlands and Rhenish Germany as buriers of victims of the plague and evolved into an order that specialized in operating insane asylums and, in nineteenth-century England at least, hospices for alcoholic priests.[62]

Trent, the council of "good works," supported these endeavors and others like them. But there remained much more sickness and misery than it was possible to deal with. That is why the intervention of Vincent de Paul in the seventeenth century was of such monumental importance.

Vincent de Paul (1580–1660) did more than any other individual to rationalize and institutionalize Catholicism's commitment to caring for the sick. Through his various foundations, and particularly through the Sisters of Charity (whom he recruited indifferently among ladies of the highest rank and among pink-cheeked country girls), he brought intense, organized charitable activity to the Paris slums and to blighted country districts. The precedent had been set for a system that was destined to be imitated everywhere and to affect profoundly the tridentine church as well as society at large. And a revolutionary precedent it was, because prior to the time of the Sisters of Charity, nuns were invariably cloistered, always prohibited from working in the world. Vincent de Paul and his colleagues opened a huge reservoir of feminine energy and talent, all the more so because the older orders of women tended to expand into activist roles, and the scores of orders founded after de Paul's death followed with few exceptions the Vincentian model. But it was the Sisters of Charity themselves who provided in their garb a universal symbol of gentle healing.

> There was no idea of giving them a special habit. Like women of the people they were dressed in a simple drab-colored dress, with their hair stuffed into a cap. In the course of time this dress developed. A coif was allowed to those sisters who found too great discomfort in the exposure of their faces to the cold air; then, for uniformity, the coif became obligatory for all. It was made originally of unstiffened white linen and hung down over the shoulders on either side of the face. Then the two side pieces were slightly raised; to keep them in position they were starched. Finally, with this stiffening the two sides were made to project like wings. The Sisters of Charity thus have wings to fly to the help of the sick and the poor. In this way there gradually developed that religious habit which is known the world over as the emblem of French charity.[63]

By the eve of the Revolution (1789), there were 426 houses of the Sisters of Charity in France alone.[64] A few years later the order was introduced by Elizabeth Ann Seton into the United States, where it operated under diocesan rather than more centralized management.[65] This administrative detail mattered little; what counted was that new orders continued to spring up under the same inspiration, even if the women who joined them did not wear the fabled winged coif. Simple black and white was the garb of the Dominican Sisters of the Sick–Poor, founded by Nathaniel Hawthorne's daughter Rose, a convert to Catholicism, while in Brittany in the 1840s. The Little Sisters of the Poor wore black and brown when they started their worldwide apostolate to the aged.[66] One order of nuns dedicated itself exclusively to caring for patients terminally ill with cancer, that they might die in dignity.

The first nursing sisters were not nurses in the modern professional sense of the term. They "visited" the sick, by which they meant they brought their concern and willingness to alleviate what sufferings they could by keeping the patient clean, decently fed, and as physically comfortable as possible. But at the same time they were beginning the evolutionary process that led by the early twentieth century to the thousands of hospitals, dispensaries, and asylums all over the world where scientific medicine was practiced with nursing nuns as full partners in the enterprise. The most spectacular example was the association of Dr. William J. and Dr. Charles H. Mayo with the Franciscan nuns of Rochester, Minnesota. On 1 November 1887, the doors of St. Mary's Hospital were opened for the first time, with a staff of five nursing sisters under the direction of the Mayo brothers. The nuns, by scrimping and saving, had raised all the money themselves and thus took the initial step leading to the development of one of the greatest medical complexes of all time. They opened a nursing school as well and even enrolled in it themselves in order to refine their skills. The Doctors Mayo (who were not Catholics) took a dim view of this latter idea. "Dr. Charlie and I," Dr. Will observed, "had always done our surgical work with the sisters' help, and we were much concerned as to whether any one could be taught, even by the sisters themselves, to perform the duties of the nurse as well as they. We had absolute confidence, then as now, in this group of women who have no thought outside their duty to the sick."[67]

The achievement at Rochester was in many ways typical of tridentine Catholicism in its American manifestation. The church in the United States, which produced few remarkable thinkers or artists, continued well into the twentieth century to depend upon European models for ideas and ideals. But at the same time, American Catholics revealed a striking ability to institutionalize and organize, and, most visible of all, to express their ethos in brick and mortar. Poor immigrants and their children built great churches and a vast system of schools. They raised unprecedented amounts of money to take on an enterprise so colossal in scale that nothing like it had been seen by any Catholic community anywhere in the world at any time. When the fathers gathered for the second Council of the Vatican—at the end of the tridentine era—there were in operation 950 Catholic hospitals in the United States, with a bed capacity of 156,000, serving sixteen million patients a year. Nearly all of these were the work of religious orders of women, as were the 376 homes for the aged and the 337 nursing schools.[68] A peculiarly

American drive to excel, combined with a predictable tridentine exclusivity, led to the foundation of medical schools under Catholic auspices, to the formation of associations of Catholic doctors and nurses, and the provision of learned journals for them to read.

But even thus professionalized, the sisters and their institutions of healing clearly gave priority to cure of soul over cure of body. They acted out of no mere humanitarian impulse, but out of the conviction that performing the corporal works of mercy was a primary means of securing salvation for those who performed them, as well as an occasion of supernatural grace to those for whom they were performed. These were "good works" in the tridentine sense, sacramental as well as ameliorative.

The same point of view suffused that other great tridentine movement, the missions outside Europe.[69] From the century of the Reformation onward the Roman church, to misappropriate George Canning's famous aphorism, "called the new world into existence to redress the balance of the old." Even before the first session of the Council of Trent, missionaries were following in the footsteps of explorers and conquerors into Asia and the Americas. They were predominantly members of religious orders of men, chiefly Franciscan friars and Jesuits. (Religious women did not come to the missions in any numbers before the mid–nineteenth century.) Medical activities were always considered part of the missioners' apostolate, but curing illness was never their first objective. They used medical skills as an entree so that their spiritual message would be listened to. Those skills, while perhaps not significant in an absolute sense, were nevertheless impressive to a backward clientele, and they did in fact relieve much suffering.

The last phase of European colonialist expansion, that into Africa in the latter part of the nineteenth century, coincided with rapid advances in scientific medicine, and the medical component of Catholic missionary activity predictably displayed from that time on a new sophistication.[70] Even so, the old priorities did not change. (Twenty years ago I knew an aged nun, retired in Ireland, who had served around the turn of the century as a nurse in a hospital in Nigeria; her greatest boast was that she had baptized fifteen hundred dying infants who, she said proudly, were now in heaven praying for her.) The tridentine church was remarkably consistent in resisting the allure of humanitarian theory, so that its last great spokesman, Pope Pius XII (1939–1958), could write more than four hundred years after the missionary movement had begun: "We wish to pay the highest tribute to the care taken of the sick [in] hospitals, leprosaria, dispensaries, homes for the aged and for new mothers, and orphanages. Such works of charity are undoubtedly of the highest efficacy in preparing the souls of non-Christians and in drawing them to the faith and to the practice of Christianity."[71]

Tridentine Ethics

Out of the Council of Trent and tridentine theology came a strong confirmation of the ancient *jus naturale,* the natural law, which was less the Pauline "law written in men's hearts"[72] and more the expression of the classical view of nature as essentially changeless reality. "Human nature" is understandable, not so much through historical processes as through the constant functioning of the various human faculties. The concept of God's sovereignty was thus adhered to by attributing to every human act a goal or purpose in harmony with God's own intention and revealed by the very "nature" of the act. So, for example, sexual intercourse was clearly (physically) designed to produce offspring, and therefore any attempt to frustrate that object (except by a periodic abstinence which took advantage of the "natural" rhythms of a woman's reproductive system) was unnatural and wrong.

This static view of natural law had immense consequences not only for tridentine Catholicism's judgments about sexual morality, but also for its attitude toward the whole field of medical ethics.[73] Masturbation and homosexual activity (as distinguished from homosexual orientation) were always and under all circumstances sinful, because they involved the obvious misuses of human organs. But what about medical procedures—amputation, for example, or the administration of mood-altering drugs—which just as obviously interfered with the discernibly ordinary course of nature? What about the prolongation of life beyond what nature apparently intended? And, the largest question of all, how did the tridentine Catholic square the advances of medical science with his or her notion of the redemptive character of pain?

The answers to these and related questions were determined—the word is not too strong—by the application of the theory of natural law. So long, for instance, as anesthetic did not permanently impair the proper functions of the human body, its use was deemed permissible. "Ordinary" means must be employed to sustain life, "extraordinary" ones need not be. As for amputations, a corollary of the natural law, the so-called "principle of totality," could be invoked whereby the destruction of a particular limb was permitted for the sake of preserving the "natural" body as a whole.

Roman Catholic medical and sexual ethics adhered consistently to the natural-law model from the Council of Trent to the 1960s. There were, however, considerable differences in the application of principles between pre-industrial and industrial societies. The rapid development of a sophisticated, scientific medicine from the middle of the nineteenth century, and the discovery of cheap and virtually fool-proof methods of contraception in the middle of the twentieth, put an enormous strain on the conceptual system—or at least on the consensus about it—and eventually broke it apart. But before that, the application was relatively simple, because the societal conditions were relatively simple. The questions raised by the primitive medical ethics of Paul Zacchia (1621) and Michael Boudewyns (1666) form a curious hodgepodge by contemporary standards: Is a doctor permitted to pray for illness in order that he will have patients? May a magistrate allow a Jew to practice medicine in his jurisdiction? May a doctor ever prescribe masturbation?[74] The eighteenth and early nineteenth centuries witness no significant advance over such preoccupations. The *medicina clericalis* that survived into the nineteenth century was much less concerned with adumbrating the moral norms for medical practice—they seemed clear enough—than with instructing the parish clergy in fundamental skills to serve people in rural areas who were more often than not without the regular services of a physician. The genre, its name changed to *pastoral medicine,* has not been unknown in the twentieth century, when it has tended to concentrate on psychological matters rather than anatomical. A harbinger of the future has been the relatively recent emphasis Catholic thinkers have given to a theology that questions the notion of body as instrument and instead stresses physical and emotional wellness as an essential aspect of the redemptive process. "Holiness is Wholeness," was Joseph Goldbrunner's celebrated expression of this view.

A not unrelated phenomenon was the willingness of Catholics to adopt twentieth-century categories with regard to mental illness; even to embrace, albeit gingerly, at least some of the principles put forward by the likes of Freud and Jung. The analogy between sacramental confession and psychotherapy was often pointed out, and Catholics, once confident enough to reject what they conceived to be the overstated sexual component of Freudianism, appeared to have no fear of terms like *ego, id,* and *unconscious.* But the tridentine church until its very last days remained faithful in this regard to its clerical ethos: The key question raised during the 1950s, in Germany first and then elsewhere, was how the parish priest might contribute to the spiritual well-being of his people by a proper and faith-informed application of the insights of psychology—application to himself no less than to those with whom he had professional dealings.[75]

The rapid advance of scientific medicine gave rise to a Roman Catholic medical ethics as such; to an avalanche of works in all languages, all departing sharply from the concerns of pastoral medicine and all, until very recently, representing the natural-law tradition.[76] The moral theologians in this area have been extremely sophisticated, and they have not feared to tread into questions involving highly complex therapeutic procedures. They have carried with them, until very recently, their natural-law baggage, and at the risk of oversimplifying, it might be said that they have approached every problem of medical morals from the vantage point of the principle of double effect.

This notion, also called the indirect voluntary, was developed during the period immediately after the Council of Trent and received definitive expression from Jean Jury in the mid–nineteenth century.[77] The principle has been succinctly stated by Gerald Kelly:

> The principle of double effect, as the name itself implies, supposes that an action produces two effects. One of these effects is something good which may be legitimately intended; the other is an evil which may not be intended. . . . An action is permitted, in accordance with the principle, if these conditions are fulfilled: 1) the action considered by itself and independently of its effects must not be morally evil; 2) the evil effect must not be the means of producing the good effect; 3) the evil effect is sincerely not intended but merely tolerated; 4) there must be a proportionate reason for performing the action in spite of its evil consequences.[78]

This principle appeared to Catholic moralists as widely applicable in medical matters, because every treatment, every act of surgery or dispensation of drugs, was seen to be in one way or another an intervention in the "natural" functioning of the human person. So even when in a particular case the four conditions of double effect did not fully apply, the assumptions on which it rested remained at the top of the mind of the Catholic ethicist.

Perhaps the most common example of the double effect in recent times has had to do with instances of surgical sterilization. A cancerous uterus may be removed because the act itself falls under the principle of totality (as described earlier), because the evil effect (loss of fertility) does not cause the good effect (removal of a tumor), because (presumably) the woman does not desire the evil effect, and, finally, because the woman's health is a proportionate price to pay for her henceforth sterile condition. Conversely, if a woman's heart condition would make childbirth mortally dangerous for her, a hysterectomy would *not* be justified by double effect, because the good effect (health) would be *caused* by the bad effect (loss of fertility).

Much of Catholic medical ethics over the last generation or so has dealt with biosexual matters. The natural-law position has been advocated with force and, until recently, with virtual unanimity by the church's hierarchy, especially by the prolific Pope Pius XII (d. 1958); supported, again until recently, by most theologians and spiritual writers. Contraception provided the dramatic and controversial instance of this teaching, but it should be borne in mind that what appeared at issue was the conviction that the precepts of the natural law formed a seamless robe; if one of them were ripped away, the whole fabric would unravel.

If contraception were allowed, it would mean that no rational opposition could be mounted to abortion, homosexual activity, or even bestiality, artificial insemination, genetic engineering, or indeed a host of medical procedures within the capacity of doctors and hospitals. The static concept of *nature* had to be *consistently* applied, or it fell away to nothing. The papal magisterium, grown so powerful since Trent, maintained its consistency, and when Pope Paul VI issued his encyclical *Humanae Vitae* (1968) confirming the ban on artificial contraception, he provoked the most severe crisis of authority within the church since the Reformation.[79] Just as the genius of the natural law tradition informed all Roman Catholic thinking about ethics in medicine and about the mysteries of birth and sexuality, so the collapse of it promises to dominate discussions and decisions for the unforseeable future.[80]

Since Vatican II

That future is now twenty years old, and, besides the virtual disappearance of the formerly confident arguments based upon the ethics of the natural law, there are plenty of signs that Roman Catholics have indeed entered a new era in their corporate history and have left the tridentine days behind. The liturgy, the common prayer of ordinary people, has been drastically altered. Fish on Friday is only a memory. The sacramental principle itself has come under review by hard-eyed German, Dutch, and Peruvian theologians. Penance has given way to the sacrament of reconciliation, and the old confessional box gathers dust. Extreme unction is now called the anointing of the sick. The funeral mass has become a joyous proclamation of the resurrection rather than a somber reminder of the day of judgment—the vestments all white, the pascal candle glittering at the head of the casket, and the choir singing "Alleluia" rather than "Dies irae." Who, in the western world at least, has gained an indulgence lately?—the issue that ignited the tragic quarrel of the sixteenth century.

The time of Catholic exclusivity has passed away. No more are there flourishing associations of Catholic doctors or Catholic nurses, no more journals strictly for Catholic health practitioners. Catholic hospitals now depend upon public monies and are hardly distinguishable from those operated under Protestant or secular auspices. The nursing sister is a rarity now, and Viaticum is dispensed not by a priest garbed in full regimentals accompanied by bell and candles, but by a member of the ecumenical ministry team who casually carries the Host round the hospital corridors in his (or her) pocket.

The second Council of the Vatican (1962–1965) formally repudiated none of the decisions reached at Trent and indeed claimed many of those decisions as its own. Nevertheless, it did express itself in personalist and historical categories considerably different from the scholastic and legalistic modes of thinking familiar to the sixteenth century. Since the council adjourned, sharp divisions have arisen among Catholic thinkers, and indeed among the Catholic populace at large, as to whether the teaching of Vatican II represents an organic development of the teaching of Trent (as Trent, it would be argued, grew out of soil prepared at Lateran IV in the thirteenth century or even at Nicea in the fourth); or whether Vatican II, particularly its "spirit" or its "thrust," marks a severe break with the past and a radically new orientation of the church, making it more directly relevant to the problems and opportunities of the modern world. The quarrels on this point continue; any description therefore of a contemporary "Catholic position" with regard to health care or anything else remains, within certain broad parameters, necessarily tentative.

There has been a wrenching character to all of these developments, at least for those Catholics born and raised under the tridentine dispensation. Their gravest obligation has become not to romanticize, and therefore trivialize, the church of their youth and, even as they hold fast to the timeless values of their faith, not to indulge in feckless nostalgia which in fact demeans the accomplishments of their forebears. *Ecclesia semper reformanda est;* the church *always* has to be reformed. No believer need fear genuine reform, nor legitimate change. Indeed, "in a higher world it is otherwise; but here below to live is to change, and to be perfect is to have changed often."[81]

Notes

1. Hubert Jedin, *Geschichte des Konzils von Trient,* 5 vols. in 4 (Freiburg, 1951–1975). First two vols. trans. by Ernest Graf (St. Louis, 1949; London, 1961).
2. Robert Bellarmine, *Opera,* 7 vols. (Cologne, 1617–1620), 6:206.
3. See Theodore Casteel, "Calvin and Trent: Calvin's Reaction to the Council of Trent in the Context of his Conciliar Thought," *Harvard Theological Review* 63 (1970):91–117.
4. Vincent Schweitzer, ed., *Concilii Tridentini Tractatuum Collectio,* 12 vols. (Freiburg, 1965–1980), 12:134–144.
5. Quoted by Jedin, *Trent* (Eng. trans.), 2:26.
6. Thomas Stapleton, *Speculum pravitatis haerecticae* (Douay, 1580), in *Opera Omnia,* 4 vols. (Paris, 1620), 2:394.
7. See Marvin R. O'Connell, *Thomas Stapleton and the Counter Reformation* (New Haven, CT, 1964), pp. 65–67.
8. Philip Hughes, *The Church in Crisis* (Garden City, NY, 1961), pp. 309–313.
9. Henry Denzinger, *Enchiridion Symbolorum Definitionum et Declarationum de rebus Fidei et Morum,* 28th ed. (Freiburg, 1952), pp. 321–323.

10. *Catechism of the Council of Trent for Parish Priests,* trans. John A. McHugh and Charles J. Callan (New York, 1954), pp. 307–311.
11. Epistle of James 5:14–15.
12. Denzinger, *Enchiridion,* p. 322.
13. *Catechism,* p. 315.
14. Guy E. Swanson, *Religion and Regime* (Ann Arbor, MI, 1967), esp. pp. 3–43. For sharply dissenting views, see the symposium published in *The Journal of Interdisciplinary History,* 1 (1971), 381–446.
15. H. Outram Evennett, *The Spirit of the Counter-Reformation* (Cambridge, 1968), pp. 43–66.
16. C.S. Lewis, *English Literature in the Sixteenth Century Excluding Drama* (Oxford, 1964), esp. pp. 3–9.
17. John Henry Newman, *Tract Seventy-one* (London, 1839), p. 17. Emphasis added.
18. See Marvin R. O'Connell, *The Counter Reformation, 1559–1610* (New York, 1974), p. 102.
19. Ludwig von Pastor, *The History of the Popes,* 40 vols., trans. Ernest Graf et al. (London, 1891–1952), 16:85–89.
20. See Pierre Pourrat, *Father Olier, Founder of St. Sulpice,* trans. W.S. Reilly (Baltimore, 1932).
21. Fernand Braudel, *Le Méditerranée et le monde méditerranéen à l'époque de Philippe II,* 2 vols. (Paris, 1966), 1:387, 379.
22. Philip Hughes, *The Reformation in England,* 3 vols. (New York, 1951–1954), 3:335–373.
23. Compare Thomas N. Tentler, *Sin and Confession on the Eve of the Reformation* (Princeton, 1977), pp. 95–104.
24. Ellsworth Kneal, *Medical Practice by the Clergy* (Rome, 1967), pp. 23–39.
25. Quoted in ibid., pp. 52–57.
26. Francis Cangiamila, *Embryologia Sacra* (Ieper, 1745).
27. *The Arte of Dyeing* (London, 1621).
28. Francis de Sales, *Introduction to the Devout Life,* trans. John K. Ryan (New York, 1950), p. 83.
29. Henry Boudon (1624–1702), *Le Chemin royal de la sainte croix,* in *Les grands auteurs spirituels* (Montreal, 1945), pp. 20–23.
30. *Colossians* 1:24.
31. John Vianney (Curé of Ars), *Sermons for the Sundays and Feasts of the Year* (New York, 1901), pp. 56–66. (Originally preached in the 1850s).
32. Owen Chadwick, *The Popes and European Revolution* (Oxford, 1981), p. 6.
33. First Epistle of Peter 5:8–9.
34. Among the multitude of studies, see the perceptive piece by Lawrence Stone, "The Disenchantment of the World," *New York Review of Books,* 17 (December 2, 1971):17ff.
35. *Collectio Rituum* (Milwaukee, WI, 1964), pp. 280–283.
36. Hermann Buzembaum, *Medulla Theologiae Moralis* (Rome, 1844), pp. 583–589 (Original printing 1648).
37. Denzinger, *Enchiridion,* p. 321.
38. Charles Billuart, *Summa Summae S. Thomae, vel Compendium Theologiae,* 3 vols. (Venice, 1787), 3:319–320 (Original printing 1754).
39. In the famous phrase of Thomas Hobbes (1588–1679), *Leviathan* (London, 1651).

40. Peter Canisius, *Ane Catechisme* (Paris, 1588), fol. 102–104.
41. Buzembaum, *Medulla,* pp. 172–174.
42. Thomas Tamburnini (1591–1675), quoted in John Noonan, *Contraception* (Cambridge, MA, 1965), p. 407.
43. Thomas Doughty, *The Practice How to Finde Ease* (Douay, 1618), fol. 122f.
44. Buzembaum, *Medulla,* pp. 390ff.
45. The Archbishop of Mechlin [Engelbert Sterckx], ed., *Instructiones SS. Caroli Barromaei [et al.] de recta Administratione Sacramenti Poenitentiae* (Mechlin, 1850), pp. 25–28.
46. Quoted in Noonan, *Contraception,* p. 449.
47. See Tentler, *Sin and Confession,* pp. 162–232.
48. Jerome Noldin, *De Sexto Praecepto,* 2nd ed. (Oeniponte, 1900), pp. 28ff.
49. *Catechism,* pp. 343ff.
50. *Genesis* 38:9–10. The sin of Onan was not simply masturbation, but rather his refusal to raise up children for his deceased brother.
51. See Noonan, *Contraception,* pp. 368–403.
52. Elizabeth Longford, *Queen Victoria* (New York, 1966), p. 270.
53. Fernand Braudel, *The Structures of Every Day Life,* trans. Sian Reynolds (New York, 1981), pp. 187ff.
54. Carlo M. Cipolla, *Faith, Reason and the Plague in Seventeenth Century Tuscany* (Ithaca, NY, 1979), esp. pp. 50 ff.
55. See Chadwick, *Popes,* pp. 3–47; Jean-Claude Schmitt, *The Holy Greyhound* (Cambridge, 1983), pp. 171–178; Thomas A. Kselman, *Miracles and Prophecies in Nineteenth Century France* (New Brunswick, NJ, 1983), pp. 12–36; and Alain Molinier, "Curés et parpoissiens de la contre-réforme," in Jean Delumeau, ed., *Historire vécue de peuple chrétien,* 2 vols. (Paris, 1979), 2:67–91.
56. S.J. Connolly, *Priests and People in Pre-famine Ireland, 1780–1845* (New York, 1982), pp. 74–134.
57. See Marvin R. O'Connell, "Ultramontanism and Dupanloup: The Compromise of 1865," *Church History,* 53 (June 1984):200–217.
58. See Kselman, *Miracles,* esp. pp. 141–188.
59. *Collectio Rituum,* pp. 375–405.
60. Max Weber, *The Protestant Ethic and the Spirit of Capitalism,* trans. Talcott Parsons (New York, 1958), pp. 79ff.
61. For the "corporal works of Mercy," see *A Catechism of Christian Doctrine,* revised ed. of the *Baltimore Catechism* (Paterson, NJ, 1949), pp. 152–154.
62. Christopher J. Kauffman, *Tamers of Death* (New York, 1976), esp. pp. 199–210.
63. Jean Calvet, *Vincent de Paul,* trans. Lancelot C. Sheppard (New York, 1951), p. 111.
64. Mrs. Jameson, *Sisters of Charity, Catholic and Protestant, and the Communion of Labor* (Boston, 1857), p. 66.
65. Joseph B. Code, "Bishop John Hughes and the Sisters of Charity," (Louvain, 1949), pp. 1–48.
66. *Heroines of Charity* (New York, 1860), pp. 225–260.
67. Helen Clapesattle, *The Doctors Mayo* (Minneapolis, 1941), pp. 242–267, 499.
68. *The Catholic Directory* (New York, 1964), Statistical recapitulation.

69. Georges Goyau, *L'église en marche: études d'histoire missionaire,* 5 vols. (Paris, 1928–1936).
70. See Joseph Mullin, *The Catholic Church in Modern Africa* (London, 1965).
71. *Evangelii Peaecones,* June 2, 1951, in *The Papal Encyclicals, 1939–1958,* ed. Claudia Carlen (New York, 1981), pp. 196–197.
72. *Romans* 2:15.
73. See David F. Kelly, *The Emergence of Roman Catholic Medical Ethics in North America* (New York, 1979), esp. pp. 149ff. and 244ff.
74. Paul Zacchia, *Quaestiones medico-legales,* new ed. (Lyons, 1701); and Michael Boudewyns, *Ventilabrum medico theologicum* (Antwerp, 1666).
75. Joseph Goldbrunner, *Holiness is Wholeness and Other Essays,* trans. Stanley Godman (Notre Dame, IN, 1964), esp. pp. 3–29; and *Cure of Mind and Cure of Soul* (New York, 1958), pp. 12ff.
76. See the bibliography in Kelly, *Medical Ethics,* pp. 460–511.
77. J. Ghoos, "L'Acte á double effect: étude de théologie positive," *Ephemerides Theologiae Lovanienses* 27 (1951):30–52.
78. Gerald Kelly, *Medico-moral Problems* (St. Louis, 1958), pp. 12f.
79. Text of *Humanae Vitae,* July 25, 1968, in *The Papal Encyclicals,* ed. Carlen, pp. 223–236.
80. Daniel Callahan, ed., *The Catholic Case for Contraception* (London, 1969), esp. pp. 67–70.
81. John Henry Newman, *An Essay on the Development of Christian Doctrine,* 7th ed. (London, 1890), p. 40.

CHAPTER 5

The Eastern

Orthodox

Tradition

Stanley Samuel Harakas

Eastern Orthodox Christianity conceives of itself as the mother-church of Christendom, as being identical in all essentials with the undivided church of the first eight centuries. This sense of an unbroken continuity and identity with the early church is one of its strongest characteristics. It expresses itself in all aspects of Eastern Orthodox life and thought: in its faith, organization, liturgical life, and theological teaching.

The source of Eastern Orthodox doctrinal teaching is the divine revelation embodied in Holy Scripture and Holy Tradition, which fulfill, interpret, and authenticate each other. The most important expressions of Holy Tradition are the doctrinal decrees of the Seven Ecumenical Councils and the writings of the major fathers of the church. Since the Seventh Ecumenical Council, held in 787, numerous other councils of lesser stature have served to express the "mind of the church" on many matters. Orthodox Christians affirm the Nicene-Constantinopolitan creed, formulated in the fourth century. Their faith is based on the doctrine of the Holy Trinity, the teaching regarding the divine–human nature of

146

Jesus Christ, the sacramental life, and their understanding of the nature of the church.

Historically, liturgically, doctrinally, and canonically, the Orthodox Church is organized around the office and person of the bishop. As head of the local church, that is, the diocese, the bishop embodies in his person the full life of the church. All bishops are fundamentally equal, yet some have been accorded honors of primacy over large areas, the first being the five patriarchates of Rome, Constantinople, Alexandria, Antioch, and Jerusalem.

The one, holy, catholic, and apostolic church of Christ was essentially without major division until a series of events caused the "Great Schism" between eastern and western Christianity. The division, based on numerous cultural, political, liturgical, and doctrinal factors, took place over a period of several centuries, marked by three periods of intense conflict. Beginning in the ninth century, Constantinople (present-day Istanbul) and Rome suffered a brief severance of relations resulting from competing claims to previously non-Christian areas (Illyricum). Additional conflicts occurred in 1054, producing mutual excommunications. Finally, the sack and temporary control of Constantinople by the Fourth Crusade in 1204 sealed the division of East and West.

The fall of Constantinople to the Moslem Turks in 1453 ended the over one-thousand–year history of the christianized eastern Roman Empire known as Byzantium. Greek and Arab Orthodox Christians became subject peoples, while Eastern Orthodoxy spread and flourished in Russia. During the four-hundred–year period of domination by the Moslems, Orthodox Christianity fought a survival struggle made more difficult by the prosyletizing efforts of both Protestant and Roman Catholic missionaries, especially during the late eighteenth and nineteenth centuries.

During the period of the demise of the Moslem Ottoman Empire in the nineteenth and early twentieth centuries, during which numerous modern nation–states were established in eastern Europe, the Orthodox in many of those nations formed autocephalous (self-governing) and autonomous (partially dependent) local churches. Thus, today, in addition to the four ancient Patriarchates of the East, there are four modern patriarchates, four autocephalous churches, and three autonomous churches, as determined by the Ecumenical Patriarchate of Constantinople. Many of these churches are national or cultural in character, such as the churches of Greece, Russia, Romania, Yugoslavia (Serbia), and Finland. A twentieth-century phenomenon of major proportions is the spread of Eastern Orthodoxy to all of the world's continents, forming an "Orthodox Diaspora." Statistics are very hard to come by in the Orthodox Church, especially because of the political situation. Estimates vary greatly. It would appear that there are approximately 150 million Orthodox Christians throughout the world and about one and a half million in the Americas. Since the inception of the ecumenical movement, the Orthodox Church, under the leadership of the Ecumenical Patriarchate of Constantinople, has actively participated in such organizations as the World Council of Churches.

Orthodox life focuses upon worship, particularly the Eucharist, which is the sacrament of Holy Communion conducted in a service known as the Divine Liturgy. The worship life of the church embodies all of its faith, value system, doctrinal formulations, church organization, and ethical teaching. The exposition of the faith in propositional form, however, belongs in the province of theology, which draws its teachings and perspectives from the total ethos of the church: scripture, ecumenical and regional synods, patristic writings, liturgy, hymnology, hagiology, canon law, pastoral practice, penitential discipline, monastic spirituality and discipline, ecclesiastical archeology, architecture, and iconography. All these witness to a tradition of life and teaching that reaches back to the very beginnings of Christianity in unbroken continuity.

Eastern Orthodox Christianity views every good thing in this world, including human art and science, as a creation and gift of God.[1] The story of the relationship of the Orthodox Church to issues of health and medicine is complex, not alone because it encompasses twenty centuries, but also because it expresses itself historically in many different ways. Further, the story is complicated by variation of practice and thought, especially in reference to the efficacy and value of the medical profession as compared to spiritual means of healing. Nevertheless, the history of interactions between the Orthodox Christian faith and the human quest for health forms a cohesive, if still developing, unity.

The Formative Years (to 324)

Converts brought many of their attitudes and practices regarding health and medicine with them when they entered the Christian life. This occurred in part because of an affinity between some of the attitudes of classical Greek and Roman culture and Christian teachings. But it also resulted because Christians expected that old attitudes would have to be changed by a slow process of growth through Christian nurture. The classic tradition praised the concept of *philanthropia,* that is, concern for the welfare of the suffering.[2] Among the Greeks, there was widespread respect for the medical profession, which embodied many of the nobler philosophical values of the Greek tradition.[3]

Early Christians also drew on the Old Testament, which described God as the source of both sickness (for example, as a punishment for sins) and health. Old Testament writers described God's healing power as a sign of his love for his People of Israel (*Dt.* 7:15) and taught that pious living and obedience to the Lord led to well-being and health (*Is.* 58:8), while sinfulness produced ill-health and disease (*Jer.* 30:12–17).

In the later Jewish deuterocanonical writings, which are included in the Orthodox Church's official Greek Septuagint version of the Old Testament but not in the Hebrew version, the healing power of the Lord is exalted above the medicinal practices of men: "For it was neither herb, nor mollifying plaster that restored them to health: by thy word, O Lord, which healeth all things. For thou hast the power of life and death" (*Wis.* 16:12–13).[4] Nevertheless, the physician is to be honored, "for the Lord has created him" (*Eccl.* 38:1). In the deuterocanonical tradition, prayer to God and recourse to the physician are not contradictory, but supplementary practices, providing the normative foundation for the Eastern Orthodox Church regarding the relationship of faith and medicine. This relationship is illustrated in the advice found in *Ecclesiasticus* 38:9–15:

> My son, in thy sickness be not negligent: but pray to the Lord, and he will make thee whole. Leave off from sin, and order thy hands aright, and cleanse thy heart from all wickedness. Give a sweet savour, and a memorial of fine flour; and make a fat offering. Then give place to the physician, for the Lord hath created him: let him not go from thee, for thou hast need of him. There is a time when in their hands there is good success. For they shall also pray unto the Lord, that he would prosper that which they give for ease and remedy to prolong life. He that sinneth before his Maker, let him fall into the hands of the physician.

The themes of this passage—the primary reliance on God, the emphasis on moral, spiritual, and physical health, the encouragement of liturgical approaches to healing, the approval of the medical profession—appear repeatedly in the subsequent history of the Orthodox Church, although alternate views were often vigorously promoted.

The New Testament accounts of Christ's compassionate healing ministry, indicative of his divine power, created a climate in which sickness was readily seen as something to be healed.[5] Yet, the New Testament writers also viewed suffering, including illness, as potentially redemptive. For example, Jesus, speaking of the illness of his friend Lazarus, articulated what would become a distinctly Christian perspective: "This illness is not unto death; it is for the glory of God, so that the Son of God may be glorified by means of it" (*Jn.* 11:4).

The *Acts of the Apostles* presents the disciples as continuing the healing ministry of Christ.[6] They not only prayed for the healing of the sick, but instructed the faithful to do so as well (*Acts* 28:8). Prayer for the sick as advocated in *James* 5:13–18 became institutionalized in what the Eastern Orthodox Church came to call the sacrament of prayer-oil (unction). This same passage, however, intimately connected the sacramental cure of illness with the spiritual and moral condition of the believers and with the intercessory prayers of acknowledged saintly figures, a relationship that also prefigured subsequent practice in the Eastern Orthodox Church.

Given these intertwined sources, differing approaches to sickness and health inevitably evolved within the broad context of the church's life. On the personal level, health was to be safeguarded by personal purity, righteousness, devotion to God, prayer, and clean living. On the ecclesiastical or institutional level, the prayers of the church members for one another and for nonbelievers and the official prayer of the church for members prepared the ground for a sacramental approach to illness on the one hand and for the cult of the intercession of the saints for healing on the other.

Justin Martyr (ca. 100–165), an early church writer, spoke of Christian healing in the name of Jesus Christ. Tertullian (ca. 160–ca. 220) referred to healing as a clerical function, although in reference to heretical groups. According to some researchers, "the earliest blessing over oil is probably found in the Coptic fragment of the *Didache*" (ca. 150) which may well have been for the purpose of healing. Hippolytus, in his *Apostolic Tradition* (ca. 215), included a prayer for the blessing of oil: "Sanctify this oil so that it may give strength to all that taste of it and health to all that use it."[7]

The personal, ecclesiastical, and social approaches to health and healing at times coexisted comfortably in the life of the church, sometimes with a measure of conflict, and sometimes in unresolved tension, each claiming a justification for its existence in the scriptural and traditional sources of authoritative revelation.[8]

Evidence of appreciation of much of the cultural heritage of the past appears in the influential writings of Clement of Alexandria (ca. 150–ca. 215), who taught that the sciences were "kindled of God," because God the Holy Trinity was the author of all creation, especially humanity. In his writings he freely used medical examples and metaphors, and expressed appreciation for the work of physicians: "a good doctor, in dealing with diseased bodies, uses poulticing for some, rubbing for others; some he cuts with a knife, others he cauterizes, and in some cases he even amputates, if by any means he can restore the patient to health by removing some part or limb."[9]

At the same time, other leaders in the early church took quite negative stands, sometimes not consistently, toward secular culture. One scholar has described Tatian the Syrian (ca. 160) in his book *The Discourse to the Greeks* as betraying "a determined hatred of all that belongs to Greek civilization, art, science and language. His character was so inclined to extremes that in his mind Christianity did not go far enough in its rejection of contemporary education and culture."[10] This negative attitude never prevailed in the later history of the church, but it existed and at times informed the attitudes of some Orthodox Christians toward medicine, particularly in the cult of the healing saints and in some expressions of monasticism. The ascetic attitudes of monasticism sometimes led monks to disregard their own physical infirmities because they tended to see illness either as a "thinly-disguised metaphor for sin" or as "a means of spiritual and moral testing." In fact, it became common, in a paradoxical dualistic fashion, for the ascetic tradition to equate bodily illness with spiritual health. Yet this formula generally did not apply to the illnesses of others. Early monastics, aided and abetted by their holiness, used the panoply of prayer together with their medical skills, folk wisdom, and herbal lore to cure the ills of others, believing that the "care of others was a significant part of the ascetic's career, particularly care for the sick."[11]

This concern for the sick manifested itself in the early church's general life as well. Reflecting the values found in both the Old and New Testaments, early Christians concerned themselves with the care of the sick long before they were legally able to establish formal institutions. About the year 203 a great pestilence fell upon the city of Alexandria. The Christian bishop of the city, Dionysios (d. ca. 264) described the differing attitudes and behaviors of pagans and Christians in the face of this disaster.

> The most of our brethren were unsparing in their exceeding love and brotherly kindness. They held fast to each other and visited the sick fearlessly, and ministered to them continually, serving them in Christ. And they died with them most joyfully, taking the affliction of others, and drawing the sickness from their neighbors to themselves and willingly receiving their pains. And many who cared for the sick and gave strength to others died themselves, have transferred to themselves their death . . . . Truly the best of our brethren departed from life in this manner, including some presbyters and deacons and those of the people who had the highest reputation; so that this form of death, through the great piety and strong faith it exhibited, seemed to lack nothing of martyrdom.[12]

The Early Byzantine Period (324–Eighth Century)

Until recent times, historians often maligned the early Byzantine period as a time of compromise and betrayal of the Christian life and of scientific decline.[13] Modern studies in Byzantine history have provided a more balanced view: In addition to its failings, shortcomings, and problems, the officially Christian Roman Empire supported a wide array of noble embodiments of Christian values, including some related to the maintenance of and the practice of medicine.[14] According to historian

Demetrios J. Constantelos, "The Byzantines loved man and expressed this love or philanthropia in active efforts to alleviate his miseries, to prolong his life, to guide him into the certainties of faith, and to orient him to a purposeful life."[15]

This approach to the human condition reflected not only the ethical teachings of Christianity regarding *agape* (love), but also the Eastern Orthodox doctrines regarding human nature that consistently linked the physical, mental, and spiritual into an interpenetrating and interrelated whole. This view appeared in many writings from the period. Gregory of Nyssa (ca. 330–395), in his treatise *On the Making of Man*, clearly distinguished among the corporeal, spiritual, and rational dimensions of human nature, but tied them closely together into a single unity, dominated by the rational nature of man. His contemporary Gregory of Nazianzus (329–389), in speaking of the creation of humanity, similarly described a human being as the totality of reality "writ small,"

> as a kind of second world, a microcosm; another kind of angel, a worshipper composed of a blended nature, a full initiate of the visible creation, but a mere neophyte, in respect of the intelligible [spiritual] world combining in the same being spirit and flesh. . . . Thus he is a living creature under God's providence and in process of deification by reason of his natural tendency towards God.[16]

In the last decade of the fourth century, Nemesius, Bishop of Emesa, also wrote on the unity of human nature, in a work entitled *Of the Nature of Man*.[17] Schooled both in philosophy and Greek medicine, Bishop Nemesius saw humankind as a composite of soul and body that linked the physical and the spiritual elements. In his work he discussed the physiology of the body; the material elements from which it is formed; the senses of perception, sight, feeling, taste, hearing, and smell; and the psychology, philosophy, and morality of the human condition. Although his discussion presupposed a Christian theological framework, its tone was not primarily theological, but rather, objective, descriptive, even scientific. Nemesius presented human biology as subject to its own laws, but he did not accord it total autonomy as far as human nature, purpose, and ethics were concerned.

These themes were integrated in the eighth century in St. John of Damascus' (ca. 675–749) great summary of patristic doctrine, *An Exact Exposition of the Orthodox Faith*,[18] which was part of a larger encyclopedic compendium of knowledge, *The Fount of Wisdom*.[19] John incorporated the physics and biology of his day into his teaching regarding human nature, subsuming both to a Christian theological perspective.

Such writings indicate that there was no essential sense of conflict in Eastern Christian theology between science and philosophy on the one hand and the affirmations of faith on the other. The institution of clergy–physicians, in which fathers of the church, bishops, priests, deacons, and monks frequently studied medicine as part of their general education and in conjunction with their spiritual ministrations often practiced medicine, also testified to this basic harmony.[20]

The convergence of the spirit of philanthropy with an appreciation for medicine led to the widespread establishment of hospitals in Byzantium.[21] Early Byzantium also boasted such well-known and innovative physicians as Oribasius (ca. 325–ca. 400); Caelius Aurelianus (fifth century); Aetius of Amida (fl. ca. 550), perhaps a court physician to the Emperor Justinian, whose Christian faith reportedly played an important part in his treatment of disease; Alexander of Tralles (525–605); and Paul of Aegina (fl. ca. 640 in Alexandria). The latter's work *Epitome* "remained the principal medical text of Byzantium until the end of the empire. It emphasized the practical aspects of medicine, and its surgical section became celebrated not only in Byzantium but among Western and Arab doctors as well."[22]

The organization of the medical profession into various ranks of healers during this period coincided with the development of hospitals.[23] The most famous of these early hospitals was found in the philanthropic center known as the Basilias, established by St. Basil the Great in the mid–fourth century outside Caesarea of Cappadocia, in Asia Minor; but there were many others scattered throughout Byzantium. St. John Chrysostom (354?–407), Patriarch of Constantinople, established several of them in the Byzantine capital, staffed by clergymen as directors, and hired physicians, cooks, attendants, and nurses. According to one historian, the "presence of physicians implies that rational medical procedure played a central role in ministering to the patients."[24]

By the time of the reign of Justinian (527–565) in the sixth century, imperial legislation governed the place of physicians in hospitals. However, with the inroads of the barbarian tribes and the decline in the fortunes of the empire in the seventh century, many Byzantine hospitals were forced into decay or were destroyed. About the same time "the medical profession in Byzantium temporarily lost its social standing; in any case the society became luke warm and negligent toward medical doctors." The people turned instead to the healing powers of the saints. In the words of one commentator, hagiography waged "a sharp war against secular physicians and scold[ed] the greediness and incompetence of the medical doctor." This rather negative view of medicine remained strong until the twelfth century.[25]

The apparent antagonism between physicians and healing saints often resolved itself into an arrangement that acknowledged the complementarity of these healing methods. Scholars have found the medieval "lives of saints" to be important sources of knowledge about the details of Byzantine life and, in particular, attitudes regarding social relationships. This has been especially true regarding the study of the interactions of the Eastern Christian religious experience with the sphere of health and healing.[26]

Hagiographical records often describe saints and physicians as competitors who frequently denigrated the work of each other. Thus St. Theodore of Sykeon is described as saying "Have done with doctors. Don't fall into their clutches; you will get no help from them. Be satisfied with this prayer and blessing and you will be completely restored to health."[27] Such sentiments typify the hagiography of the sixth and seventh centuries in which medical doctors are described repeatedly as "loaded with ignorance and avarice and . . . unable to vie with the healer-saints."[28] However, by the middle Byzantine period this antagonism had softened.

Occasionally physicians expressed disdain for the medical powers of "holy men." Thus the *Miracles of Saints Cosmas and Damian* tells of a woman suffering from cancer who decided to go to the shrine of the "holy unmercenaries" after physicians were unable to heal her without radical surgery. Her physicians predicted that "You will go there, and you will return because your cancer will worsen."[29] However, as Harry J. Magoulias has warned, such accounts describe "the conscience of the people, an attitude of the religious-minded Byzantine, and not the official stand of the Byzantine Church. The Church did not combat the physician."[30] Many literary sources support this perspective; additional evidence is provided by the continuing establishment of hospitals by the church during this period, the appointment of clergy and monks as administrators of such institutions, and the tradition of the cleric–physician.

Either before they consulted physicians or after physicians had failed to cure them, the people of the Byzantine Empire sought healing from living holy persons, as well as from shrines and churches dedicated to healing saints, where relics were frequently kept.[31] The reported healings follow no routine or definable pattern. The holy man might pray for the sufferer, give him or her a special article of clothing to wear, administer some sacred dust, prescribe medicine, perform minor surgery, or give instructions on how a physician should heal the patient. For example, after the earlier-mentioned woman suffering from cancer of the breast went to the Church of Sts. Cosmas and Damian seeking a cure, "the doctor-saints appeared in a vision—not to the sick woman, but to her regular physician—and advised him" regarding the treatment, including surgical as well as pharmacological procedures.

Thus, even the cult of the "holy unmercenary healing-saints" gives evidence of a cooperative relationship between religious and medical practice. Moreover, the hostile comments about medicine were often tempered in the same documents by statements of appreciation for the physician and his art. A saint such as Theodore of Sykeon, despite his negative attitude toward medical doctors, prescribed medicines himself, referred sick persons to surgery, and even recommended which doctors ill persons should consult.[32]

Not infrequently, hospitals and shrines of the healing saints were located side by side. Some patients would go to the hospital first, where physicians might refer them to the saints; others would go to the church first and then, at the urging of the saints, to the hospital. More often than not, the healing of the pilgrim involved some kind of action or unusual "medical practice" ordered in a dream by the saint–healer.[33]

This attitude toward medicine was exemplified by St. Basil, who considered sickness and healing of the body as most important in their providing an analogy for the care and cure of the soul, thus accepting both in his *Larger Rule*.[34] In his sermon on the "Forty Martyrs," he advocated personal prayers for recovery from illness as well as prayers to "be made with martyrs," soliciting the intercession of the saints.[35] In view of such examples, one should neither discount, nor overestimate, the pious rejection of the medical arts by the Christian faithful.

During the early Byzantine period, in both the East and West, there is evidence—for example, in the fourth-century writings of Aphaates the Syrian—that oil was blessed for physical healing. St. Athanasius, in his fifth *Encyclical Letter to the Bishops,* tells that priests healed the sick, and St. Ambrose indicates the same in his work on *Penance.* In the early fifth century, Sozomen, in his *Ecclesiastical History,* and St. Gregory of Nazianzus, in his *Theological Orations,* suggest that Christians expected healing. In the West, Pope Innocent I (416) described the norm in a letter: "the faithful who are sick can be anointed with the holy oil of unction, which has been prepared by the bishop and which not only priests but all Christians may use for anointing, when their own needs or those of their family demand."[36] From the fourth-century *Sacramentary of Serapion,* it would appear that no separate service for the blessing of the oil existed, but that a prayer, essentially the same one used by the Eastern Orthodox and Coptic Churches to this day, was inserted into the eucharistic celebration for this purpose. In part it reads:

we pray Thee to send down from the heavens of thy Only-begotten a curative power upon this oil, in order that to those who are anointed . . . , it may become a means of removing "every disease and every sickness," of warding off every demon, of putting to flight every unclean spirit, of keeping at a distance every evil spirit, of banishing all fever, all chill, and all weariness; a means of grace and goodness and the remission of sins; a medicament of life and salvation, unto health and soundness of soul and body and spirit, unto perfect well-being.[37]

It appears that there was much flexibility in the administration of the sacrament, as indicated by Pope Innocent's letter. However, in the West, beginning in the fifth century and continuing to the eighth century, clerical anointing almost completely died out, with lay anointing becoming very popular. Possibly this change reflected a tendency in the West to divide spirit and body rather than to unite them.[38] Christians in the East, both lay and clerical, continued the practice of blessing the oil at the Eucharist, indicating that the sacrament of prayer oil remained an important means in the life of the Eastern Church for healing spirit, soul, and body.[39]

The concerns of the church, especially its moral values, were little by little incorporated into the law of the Byzantine Empire. Nevertheless, the tone was not legalistic. "One gets the impression," observes Constantelos, "that the Byzantines believed much more in the love of God than in His judgment or justice."[40] Often, changes in the law from pagan customs and toward Christian values were characterized in the text itself with the words "for the sake of greater philanthropy."[41] This was the rationale given for the regulation of medicine in the Justinianic corpus, which accorded honors to physicians, stipulated the treatment to be given to lepers, and so forth.[42] Church or canon law also addressed issues of health and medicine. Thus, for example, in the fourth century, the fifty-seventh of the so-called Apostolic Canons condemned and punished those who ridiculed disabled persons, such as the blind or the crippled.

Concern for the poor and their health was a significant priority in Byzantine society during this period. Christians established the first hospitals primarily for the poor, who could not afford regular physicians,[43] but by the fifth century middle-class persons were being admitted as well. In later centuries the rich, even emperors, sometimes patronized hospitals.[44] In times of epidemics, the churches were mobilized to care for the sick.[45] During this period, a lay institution made up of upper–middle-class and wealthy Christians came into existence. Known by the name *philoponoi* ("friends of those who suffer"), these Christians banded into voluntary organizations to care for the poor sick at night, without charge, after their daily work was over.

The protection of human life also concerned the early church, which consistently condemned abortion. Thus, St. Basil wrote:

The woman who purposely destroys her unborn child is guilty of murder. With us there is no nice enquiry as to its being formed or unformed. In this case it is not only the being about to be born who is vindicated, but the woman in her attack upon herself; because in most cases women who make such attempts die. The destruction of the embryo is an additional crime, a second murder, at all events if we regard it as done with intent.[46]

Among the Romans it was not uncommon to abandon unwanted new-born children, who then died of exposure and starvation, or were eaten by animals, or were found by child abusers who exploited them for economic gain, as beggars or prostitutes. The earliest writings of Christian churchmen condemned such practices, as well as all sorts of sexual sins. Both canon and civil law recognized marriage as the only appropriate place for sex. In spite of an appreciation for virginity and celibacy, the Byzantines honored marriage and condemned such practices as castration.[47]

Care of the aged also fell within the philanthropic purview of Byzantine society. The church in particular established and maintained numerous old-age homes *(gerokomeia)*. Theologically, Eastern Christianity viewed death as an enemy, a consequence of the Adamic sin, and therefore a condition to be struggled against.[48] The Eastern Christian emphasis on the saving work of Jesus Christ as victor over death, sin, and evil, strong themes in the Gospel of John, joined with a sense of God-granted eternal life through Christ's resurrection to help overcome the terror and fear of death.

Rejecting the pagan practice of cremation out of a respect for the body as the temple of God, Christians buried their dead in anticipation of the general resurrection at the expected second coming of Jesus. The body would be washed, clothed in a shroud, placed on a litter, and taken to the church, accompanied by the singing of psalms. By the fifth or sixth centuries, fixed funeral services consisted primarily of psalms, New Testament passages focusing on the resurrection, hymns, and prayers by the priest for the forgiveness of the sins of the deceased and for the soul to find a "place where there is no pain, sorrow, or suffering." Then, again accompanied by the singing of psalms, the deceased would be taken to the place of burial.[49] The Christians viewed death as a "falling asleep" of the body in expectation of the coming resurrection, which would be an "awakening."[50] Mourning for the dead was not condemned by the fathers of the church during this period; rather, they viewed it as a duty. However, such fathers as Chrysostom, Ambrose, and Jerome did condemn excessive mourning and displays of grief as inappropriate to the Christian understanding of death and faith in Jesus Christ as victor over death.[51]

The Middle Byzantine Period (Ninth–Twelfth Centuries)

The subsequent history of the Orthodox Church in Byzantium continued to reflect the basic trends articulated for the previous two periods. Orthodoxy prided itself on its continuity with the past—not a static and merely repetitive continuity, but one that fostered a growth and development.[52]

The ninth century found the Byzantine Empire vigorous and strong, rebounding from the earlier attacks of the barbarians and asserting temporal and spiritual authority northward into the Balkans and Kievan Russia. Constantinople, the capital, was a truly international power. However, by the end of the twelfth century its influence had been severely curtailed, resulting from extensive Moslem conquests to the south and demands for independence from the nations to the north. Not unexpectedly, the decline of the Byzantine Empire influenced the relationship of the Orthodox Church to issues of health and medicine. Our knowledge of hospitals during this period, especially to the eleventh century, is very limited; nevertheless, we know that in the tenth and eleventh centuries some "homes for the sick" and church-related hospitals were erected under the royal patronage of such emperors as Romanos Lecapenos, Constantine IX, and Nicephoros Botaneiates.[53]

In spite of the declining fortunes of the empire (or perhaps because of them) the twelfth century exhibited a most remarkable medical establishment under Emperor John II Comnenos, at the great monastery of the Pantokrator in Constantinople. Among the complex of philanthropic institutions at the Pantokrator was a medical center that "provided preventative as well as therapeutic care [including] a general hospital, a home for the aged . . . and what we would term outpatient service."[54] The treatment offered at the Pantokrator included drugs, physical therapy, special diets, surgery, and emergency care. The hospital was organized into five main clinics, one of which was devoted to the specialized treatment of eye diseases and intestinal sickness, another to the treatment of women. The clinic had a staff of thirty-five doctors, including some women physicians. Connected with the hospital was a chapel with a full-time staff of two priests and two preachers and a program of pastoral care.[55] Emperor Isaac II Angelus (reigned 1185–1195, 1203–1204) did much philanthropy; in fact, he supported hospitals so enthusiastically it affected the economy of the empire. Historical evidence also indicates the establishment of hospitals in Thrace and in Antioch during this period.[56]

Recourse to healing saints remained strong in this period as well. A study of the hagiographical literature shows a fluctuation in attitudes toward "rational medicine" by those who trusted the saints more than physicians. In the eighth and ninth centuries, accounts of the lives of the healing saints tended to ignore physicians rather than attack them, a common practice earlier. At worst, these accounts contrasted the ineffectiveness of physicians to the success of the saints. However, by the end of the tenth century, antagonism increased and acquired "a particular sharpness." The eleventh century showed a mixed attitude of appreciation for the medical art and disapproval of the medical practitioner's alleged avarice and inhumanity. The twelfth-century life of St. Meletios the Younger and Prodromus' *Executioner or Doctor* both distinguished "good doctors" from "bad doctors," praising the former and ridiculing the latter. By the twelfth century, concludes one historian, the physician had become "respected, although mocked time and again by a society that started to care for its health more than for its salvation."[57] It is in the twelfth century, significantly, that physicians assumed administrative control of the hospital system in Byzantium, supplanting monastics and clergy in this role.[58]

Concurrently, some sentiment appeared against the study and practice of medicine by clergy. Patriarch Lukas Chrysoberges issued an encyclical requiring that clergy cease studying and practicing medicine, not because medicine and theology were essentially incompatible, but because "he considered it improper for persons of the cloth to change into medical robes." Yet, in the judgment of a student of the period, "despite the patriarch's ruling, it is doubtful whether physicians were excluded from the priesthood."[59] Nevertheless, both religious and secular leaders continued to contrast the limitations of the best physicians to "God's almightiness."[60]

A balanced attitude toward medicine and religion is also found in a work entitled *Concerning the Construction of Man,* produced during this period by Meletios the Monk.[61] Its extensive biological description of the human body and its organs went beyond the ancient authors and betrayed a physician's experienced eye. It was, by and large, an objective work that defined human beings in scientific, not theological, terms. Nevertheless, Meletios placed his work in a theological context by emphasizing the uniqueness of human life, as compared to that of animals. In the end, all of his description pointed to the fact that "Only human beings, distinguished from the other animals, are made worthy of the providence and care of the Creator so that you might reverence the Lord's provident care for you, and that you may stand in awe of the work."[62] Thus, Meletios remained in full harmony with the Orthodox tradition that saw science and medicine as valuable and true, but placed them within the larger framework of faith in God, his care, and his love for humanity.

As in previous times, medical care fostered by the church continued to be directed primarily toward the poor, but did not exclude the middle class. In many ways, the Byzantine church and its institutions "were not remote from the spiritual, psychological, or temporal needs of its people. The clergy in general were the apologists for the lower classes and often assumed a healthy paternalism over the persecuted, the destitute and the poor."[63] This concern for the downtrodden also expressed itself in the church's canon law, which accorded punishments for malfeasance and malpractice on the part of physicians and pharmacists.[64]

Various manuscripts from the middle period mention the sacrament of prayer oil, described in the previous section. One late eleventh- or early twelfth-century source called for seven priests to conduct the service, which now involved the saying of seven prayers, the familiar passage from the *Book of James,* and the anointing of the ill person and family members. A later manuscript specified that the ill person was to lie on a cot in the church during the service; then, after the anointing, to return home with his relatives. There, the priests anointed the bed, house, and doors before concluding the service by reading the passage in *Luke* 19 describing Christ's visit to the home of Zacchaeus. These and other manuscripts of the period betray a fluidity of service structure, in which it appears that the church was beginning to respond to a need to assert more strongly its concern for healing—a development perhaps related to its having given up control of the hospitals to the physicians.

The Late Byzantine Period (Thirteenth to Fifteenth Centuries)

The last period of Byzantine history was one of decline. The misfortunes of the empire—political, military, social, and economic—were instigated in part by the increasing influence of the Venetian and Genoese traders and by the sack of Constantinople during the Fourth Crusade in 1204. The intellectual life of the late Byzantine period was marked by an increasing, although certainly not dominant, secularization, represented by the philosopher Gemistos Pletho and the Emperor Theodore Lascaris. Although thirteenth-century literature mentions the establishment of hospitals by churchmen, no presently existing evidence indicates that hospitals were founded outside Constantinople in the fourteenth and fifteenth centuries. Existing hospitals often became schools of medicine for the training of physicians. The last major figure in Byzantine medicine was the mid–fourteenth-century court physician of Emperor Andronikos III, John "Aktouarios" who wrote important medical treatises on medical method, urine, and psychology.[65] The subsequent decline occurred rapidly, but Byzantine medicine lived on as scholars from the East moved westward to help ignite the Renaissance.[66]

Not surprisingly, the cult of the healing saints continued unabated during these times. For example, the biography of Athanasios I, Patriarch of Constantinople, born in the early 1230s, contains numerous descriptions of healing miracles by him. Physicians are condemned for such practices as misleading the sick in order to extract money from them and for not telling the truth about their inability to heal until after their patients' funds had been exhausted. In contrast, the saint's center of activities is praised as "a place of free healing." When medicine was used philanthropically to benefit humanity, it and its practitioners were accepted and praised; when it was perceived as exploiting the sick, it was condemned.[67]

With the decline of the empire and its ability to support social services, including the institutional care of the sick, a great need for alternative, or at least supplementary, care developed. Perhaps in response to this situation, the sacramental approach to healing became stronger and more defined during the final days of the empire. Patriarch Nicephoros of Constantinople (1260–1261) recorded that his predecessor, Patriarch Arsenios Autoreianos (1255–1260), had ordered that the sacrament of prayer oil be conducted by seven priests, defined seven prayers for the service, and added five readings from scripture to the existing two, for a total of seven. Some scholars believe that this same Arsenios wrote a canon of hymns especially for the service of the prayer oil. Among the last Byzantines to contribute to the formation of the sacrament was Symeon, Archbishop of Thessalonike (1410–1429), who was a prolific author of liturgical and doctrinal works, including prayers and acts connected with the forgiveness of sins prior to the anointing with the healing oil.[68] On the eve of the fall of Constantinople in 1453, a fully developed liturgical healing service was thus ready for use by the Orthodox, who were destined for the next four centuries to live under the domination of a theocratic Islamic state in the role of second-class citizenship.

Under the Turks (1453–1850)

The Turkish system for governing minorities under the dominion of the Ottoman Empire permitted the church to continue all kinds of philanthropic endeavors, but under new forms, because the existing institutions, in particular those under imperial or private patronage, lost their previous support. Under the new Moslem form of government, called the "millet" system, the Turks considered the leaders of each religious group in the empire to be the ethnic as well as spiritual leaders of their respective peoples. Thus, the Patriarch of Constantinople was perceived to be the leader in all things pertaining to the inner life of the subjected Orthodox peoples, regardless of their ethnic backgrounds. Needless to say, this arrangement produced many shortcomings and failures. Nevertheless, these peoples survived for four hundred years and eventually reestablished their national identities on the basis of heritages preserved primarily through the care, influence, and protection of the Orthodox Church.

The Turks allowed the subjected people to reestablish their own social institutions. Because of their education and willingness to engage in activities such as the professions of medicine and business, which the Turks disliked, the Greeks in particular were invited into careers in government, or chose careers in medicine, business, and the trades. Although always at the mercy of the capricious will of the overlords, the subject population enjoyed a measure of economic well-being. This, coupled with the Byzantine tradition of philanthropy, allowed the "millet" to develop a new, yet much more modest, system of philanthropic institutions, including hospitals, and to train persons to staff them.[69] Sixty-four years after the fall of Constantinople, the first new Orthodox Christian hospital was established there, and two centuries later three more were founded. In 1794 the Patriarchate united them into one institution and dedicated the income from the Monastery of the Life-Giving Fountain in the Baloukle section of the capital for its funding. The Hospital of Baloukle, rebuilt in 1836, remains to this day an institution of the church. Through the years, the church established in Constantinople, as well, specialized medical institutions for lepers and the mentally ill.

Similar facilities, under the direct inspiration and control of the church, and often well regarded for their advanced scientific methods, came into being in the Patriarchates of Alexandria and Jerusalem. Following the Byzantine tradition, nearly all of these were associated with monasteries, such as the Monastery of St. Menas, outside of Cairo, famous for its therapeutic center, hostelry, and baths; and the Monastery of St. George the Great Martyr in Jerusalem. In the provinces, generous individuals and church leaders often collaborated to establish, fund, staff, and maintain hospitals and clinics—from Epiros at the northern boundaries of modern Greece to the Mediterranean islands of Crete and Chios and throughout the Balkans, most notably among the Vlachs and in Moldavia of modern-day Romania. These therapeutic establishments were often found in the numerous monasteries that flourished throughout the Ottoman Empire. The tradition of the cleric–physician continued into the period of the Turkish domination.[70] Educational opportunities for Christians within the Ottoman Empire were severely limited. Elementary education was available in "secret schools," usually associated with churches and monasteries, which taught reading, writing, and religion. The few advanced schools rarely provided more than training for the clergy. During the seventeenth and eighteenth centuries, Italy became an important center of education for Christians from the Ottoman Empire, especially in medicine. According to one historian,

> Boys who felt no special religious vocation gravitated towards [Padua's] famous medical schools. Medicine offered a promising career in the Ottoman Empire; for few Turks would demean themselves to do the hard work that a medical training involved, and thus became dependent upon Greeks and Jews for their physicians; and the Greeks soon discovered how influential a family doctor can become.[71]

Many Christians studied both theology and medicine with a sense of their ready compatibility. Such theologian–physicians were far from unusual during this period. One of the best known was Eustratios Argenti (1687–1757), who began practicing medicine in Chios in 1720 and continued to do so for a quarter of a century. His biographer noted that

> the Greek Orthodox Church has never regarded theology as a specialized matter of concern only to the clergy, but has a long and honourable tradition of 'lay-theologians.' Those who combined medicine and theology were known as 'doctor-philosophers' < *'iatrophilosophoi'*>, a name used by Eustratios on the title-pages of several of his books.[72]

The tradition of prayer for the sick continued during the period of the Ottoman Empire. In addition to a collection of various prayers for the sick that were included in the *Service Book,* Orthodox Christians used the sacrament of prayer oil. Among the Greek Orthodox, this essentially private service took on a public role when it began to be practiced in liturgical services on Holy Wednesday. Because Protestants rejected it as a sacrament, and Roman Catholics, following the Council of Trent, restricted it to the dying, only the Orthodox maintained the earlier tradition of the sacrament as an agent of healing—a source of controversy among the three groups during the sixteenth and seventeenth centuries. The differences in belief and practice regarding unction became topics for theological treatment in the various "Confessions" of faith issued by the Orthodox during this period.[73]

Pilgrimages to monasteries for healing and the veneration of miraculous icons at shrines of special importance continued the tradition of holy healers. Persons who experienced healing began the practice of placing a bas-relief silver replica of the healed limb or organ, such as an eye, on the icon of the saint as a sign of gratitude and a symbol of the pledge or promise that they made in exchange for the healing.

The Russian Experience

The history of healing in Russia paralleled the Byzantine experience with the exception that Russians imported scientific medicine from the West. With the introduction of Christianity in the tenth century, the now-familiar pattern of monastic healing—the founding of hospitals attached to monasteries—appeared in Old Russia. By the twelfth century, an independent medical establishment had come into being. Nevertheless, the tradition of the cleric–physician persisted in Russia at least to the fourteenth century, when Alexei, Metropolitan of Moscow, "enjoyed the reputation of being a good ophthalmologist."[74] After the fall of Constantinople and the establishment of Russia as the only free Orthodox nation, the Russians increasingly turned to the West for medical expertise, as they did in so many other cultural areas. In 1707 Tsar Peter I (1689–1725) established and funded a general military hospital and surgical school in Moscow, importing a director from Leiden University. By and large, the state controlled the education and employment of physicians. In 1722 a Table of Ranks with fourteen levels of status for public service was established by the state, providing, as the years went on, a system of rewards and privileges, and the possibility for commoners to advance socially. Medicine attracted lower-class persons, including churchmen and, significantly, the children of priests. Nancy Frieden, a historian of Russian medicine noted,

> By the end of the eighteenth century, sons of the clergy predominated in the motley assortment of medical students. The regime, unable to find suitable recruits elsewhere, turned to seminarians, whose curriculum included Latin, the language of learned Europe for theology and medicine. Medical administrators in the Medical Collegium (1722–1763) regularized the bond with the seminary by enlisting the state's authority to designate a specified number of seminary graduates to become surgical candidates every year.[75]

Many children of clergy were accepted to study for medical careers, and chose to do so in large numbers as the only way they were able to raise their social standing, even though the nobility by and large avoided the profession and considered it beneath their dignity.

Tzar Nicholas I (1825–1855) upgraded the education of physicians and established uniform standards for medical practice. In the thirty years from 1840 to 1870, the number of physicians in the Russian Empire almost doubled, and the quality of training substantially improved. This eventually led to the development of a professional consciousness among physicians which came into conflict with the direct control of the profession by the state. Privileges and an advanced social class for physicians was accorded by the reforms enacted into law in 1849, but the Crimean War (1853–1859) brought all of this down with the influx of only partially trained physicians into military service.[76]

In the 1870s and 1880s, a new system of health care came into being, based on prevention and sanitation. Known as Zemstvo medicine, it was a free rural health program, which had elements of idealism, social sensitivity, and service orientation closely related to the practice of medicine. The physicians were employees of the organizations of Zemstvo committees. As the physicians became more and more professionally competent, the attraction to the field increased and it became a boast at a medical conference in Moscow in 1891 that medical students no longer had to be recruited from the seminaries. The next year a huge cholera epidemic served not only to challenge the abilities of the medical profession but also to renew, in a totally different context, the negative attitudes of some church people to medicine. Some priests called on their parishioners to resist all official measures designed to limit the effect of the epidemic because they perceived it to be punishment for sins. Rather, they organized processions of icons to ward off the effects of the disease.[77] Nevertheless, in characteristic fashion, the clergy continued to send their children to medical schools in large numbers. Thus, almost twenty-six percent of all medical students in Russia in 1880 were the children of clergy, and more than half of all Russian Orthodox Christians in Russian universities were in medical schools. Clearly, the Russian Orthodox did not have many doubts about the appropriateness of "rational medicine" in the life of the believer.[78]

The present-day church in the Soviet Union is prohibited by law from establishing hospitals or engaging in any kind of philanthropy, even hospital visitation by clergy. Nevertheless, a vigorous liturgical and sacramental life for healing continues. For example, the Orthodox Church in Russia ends each Saturday-night vigil service by anointing the worshippers with oils from the vigil lights of the icons of the saints.[79]

The Modern Era

Nearly all of the traditions described in the preceding sections have survived through to the nineteenth and twentieth centuries into the modern era. The Orthodox Church still encompasses within it—without a sense of contradiction—the theologically trained physician, respect for scientific medicine, trust in the healing power of God, the appeal to the saints, belief in the miraculous, the routine offering of prayers for the sick, and the sacrament of healing.

The existence of the clergy–physician continues, although given the expanded professional training normally required for both, the numbers are very few in the present era, the most notable being an archbishop in the Church of the Diaspora. Although secularization has, without doubt, influenced the relationship of medicine and religion, so that many in the medical communities of ostensibly Orthodox nations such as Greece retain little or no contact with the Orthodox church, many physicians are part of worshipping parishes. This is particularly true in the Orthodox Diaspora, where the physicians are always honored persons in the Orthodox Christian community, frequently holding positions of leadership among the laity in the life of the church.

In the ethical teaching of the Orthodox Church there is a continuing and sustained teaching of Christian responsibility for health care. Thus in a standard seminary text, used at the Ecumenical Patriarchate during the first three decades of this century, there are to be found separate treatments on the topics of "diet, life and health, abuse and excess, sins against one's own life and health, sickness and death, and public health."[80] A similar textbook, used during the same period at the University of Athens School of Theology, treats similar subjects, but evidences a certain dualism that is not traditional.

> That persons should attend to their health when they become ill is self-evident. One seeks healing by having recourse to scientific physicians and using the means of scientific medicine. Seeking divine grace and assistance is equally necessary, in that it strengthens the believer, inspiring him with aid and comfort, that he may bear the pains of the illness uncomplainingly. He should not however, depend for his healing only upon prayer or religious means, expecting that divine power will create a miracle in him, utterly rejecting scientific means. Much less should he seek healing by using magical charms and incantations, and other such superstitions.[81]

In an ethics textbook used at the School of Theology at the University of Thessalonike in the 1970s, sections are dedicated to respect for the health of the neighbor, the health of the body, and sickness.[82] Some criticism of the dualistic dimensions illustrated by the older quotation above, however, have appeared among Orthodox ethicists. For instance, George Mantzarides, Professor of Orthodox Christian Ethics at the University of Thessalonike, is not so ready to separate scientific medicine and the spiritual dimensions of life and health.[83] In the graduate Orthodox seminaries of the United States, courses are offered in bioethics where this same wholistic perspective is taught.[84]

Consequently, the contemporary faithful Orthodox Christian has no religious scruples in consulting a physician in time of illness. Yet, in conformity with this perspective, frequently, priestly ministrations are also sought. The nature of these ministrations is of interest. In a study of the expectations of both clergy and laity of the priestly role, based on an ecumenical and wide-ranging survey sponsored by the Association of Theological Schools, a characteristic Orthodox stance was revealed.[85] Neither Orthodox laity nor clergy had significant expectations of the Orthodox priest in many ways as a counselor. Thus, the Orthodox were lowest of forty-seven American and Canadian denominations in expecting the priest to be proficient in such things as perceptive and enabling counseling. In contrast, "the Orthodox clergy and laity both accord more importance to the dimension entitled 'Sacramental-Liturgical Ministry' than do all other responding groups."[86] This has its application to the present-day ministry of the Orthodox church to the sick. The approach is strongly liturgical. The priest's main function is to offer liturgical prayer and sacramental ministrations for the sick. In the public realm, this is most strongly exemplified by the services offered for the sick in the church building. In several of the Orthodox jurisdictions, for example, the Sacrament of Holy Unction is offered as part of the regular Holy Week services. Many come for anointing, and nearly all take oil home with them in order to anoint the family members unable to attend. Another popular service in cases of distress, including illness, is the Supplicatory Service to the Theotokos, sung in most Greek Orthodox churches during the first two weeks of August. Both these services, however, are also conducted privately. Needless to say, Holy Communion has always had a healing character, and frequently, persons planning to be hospitalized will receive Holy Communion after a period of abstinence from certain foods, as a way of preparing physically and spiritually for medical treatment.

In the United States, regular hospital visitations are a requirement for the priest. For example, the official guidebook for priests of the Greek Orthodox Archdiocese specifically instructs that the priest is to "visit the sick in the hospitals and in the home."[87] The laity normally welcome and expect the visitation of their pastor. Although unction or Holy Communion may be administered, it is more usual for the priest to read a liturgical prayer from the *Service Book.*

Notes

1. Kallistos Ware, "The Value of the Created Universe," *Sobornost,* Series 6, no. 3 (Summer 1971):154–165.

2. Demetrios J. Constantelos, *Byzantine Philanthropy and Social Welfare* (New Brunswick, NJ, 1968), pp. 3–11. See also A.R. Hands, *Charities and Social Aid in Greece and Rome* (London, 1968), chs. 6, 9.

3. Ludwig Edelstein, "The Professional Ethics of the Greek Physician," *Bulletin of the History of Medicine* 30 (1956):391–419; and Edelstein, "The Distinctive Hellenism of Greek Medicine," ibid. 40 (1966):197–225.

4. Deuterocanonical quotations are from *The Septuagint Version of the Old Testament and Apocrypha,* trans. Sir Launcelot Lee Brenton (London, 1851; reprinted Grand Rapids, MI, 1980).

5. For example, *Matthew* 12:13, 15:31; *Mark* 5:34; *Luke* 4:10, 6:18, 7:21; *John* 5:6–15.

6. For example, *Acts* 4:14, 30, 5:16, 14:19.

7. Justin Martyr, *2nd Apology,* ch. 6 in *The Ante-Nicene Fathers,* eds. Alexander Roberts and James Donaldson (Grand Rapids, MI, 1956), p. 190; Tertullian, *On the Prescription of Heretics,* 41 in *The Ante-Nicene Fathers,* vol. 3, p. 263; Coptic Fragment, 10, 3b-12, 2a, in Paul F. Palmer, *Sacraments and Forgiveness: History and Doctrinal Development of Penance, Extreme Unction and Indulgences* (Westminster, MD, 1959), p. 277; Gregory Dix, *The Treatise on the Apostolic Tradition of Hippolytus* (Cambridge, 1924), vol. 5, p. 10.

8. For an explication of these dimensions of church life, see Stanley S. Harakas, "Greek Orthodox Ethics and Western Ethics," *Journal of Ecumenical Studies* 10 (Fall, 1973):728–751.

9. *Stromata,* VI, xvii in *Ante-Nicene Fathers,* II. p. 517; *Exhortation to the Greeks,* in *Clement of Alexandria,* Loeb Classical Library (Cambridge, MA, 1982), ch. 1, p. 13; ch. 10, pp. 213, 235; ch. 1, p. 21.

10. Johannes Quasten, *Patrology* (Utrecht-Antwerp, 1966) vol. 1, p. 221.

11. Susan Ashbrook Harvey, "Physicians and Ascetics in John of Ephesus: An Expedient Alliance," in *Symposium on Byzantine Medicine,* ed. John Scarborough, vol. 38 of the *Dumbarton Oaks Papers* (Washington, DC, 1984), pp. 87–93. Professor Harvey graciously shared her work for use in this chapter, prior to its publication. I am indebted to Professor Peter Topping of Dumbarton Oaks for permission to quote from this, and other papers, noted later, in advance of the publication of the volume.

12. Eusebius, *Church History,* Book VII, ch. 23 in *The Nicene and Post-Nicene Fathers,* eds. Philip Schaff and Henry Wace (Grand Rapids, MI, 1979) 2nd Series, vol. 1, p. 307.

13. Edward Gibbon's *The Decline and Fall of the Roman Empire* (1776–1788) is the classic exposition of this understanding of Byzantium. For a similar perspective on Byzantine medicine, see Benjamin Lee Gordon, *Medieval and Renaissance Medicine* (New York, 1959), ch. 3.

14. For the general inclusion of Christian values in Byzantium, see Panagiotes Demetropoulos, *He Pistis tes Archaias Ekklesias hos Kanon tes Zoes kai ho Kosmos* (Athens, 1959); Pericles-Pierre Joannou, *La Legislation Impériale et la Christianisation de l'Empire Romain (311–476)* (Rome, 1972). For more balanced assessments of Byzantine medicine, see Demetrios Constantelos' articles on "Medicine, Byzantine," and "Hospitals, Byzantine," in the forthcoming *Dictionary of the Middle Ages,* which he has generously shared with me prior to their publication. Also, Phaidon Kukules, *Byzantinon Bios kai Politismos,* 6 vols. (Athens, 1947–1957), 6:9–43; Aristotles C. Eftychiadis, *He Askesis tes Byzantines*

Iatrikes Epistemes kai Koinonikai Epharmogai Autes kata Schetikas Diataxeis (Athens, 1983).

15. Demetrios J. Constantelos, *Byzantine Philanthropy and Social Welfare* (New Brunswick, NJ, 1968), p. 66.

16. *Oration* 45:8, 9, in Henry Bettenson, ed., *The Later Christian Fathers: A Selection from the Writings of the Fathers from St. Cyril of Jerusalem to St. Leo the Great* (New York, 1970), pp. 101–102.

17. *Cyril of Jerusalem and Nemesius of Emesa*, trans. William Telfer, vol. 4 of *The Library of Christian Classics* (Philadelphia, 1955).

18. John of Damascus, *An Exact Exposition of the Orthodox Faith*, in *Nicene and Post-Nicene Fathers*, 2nd Series, vol. 9.

19. St. John of Damascus, *Fount of Knowledge, On Heresies, The Orthodox Faith*, trans. Frederick H. Chase, Jr. (Washington, DC, 1958).

20. Mary Emily Keenan, "Gregory of Nazianzus and Early Byzantine Medicine," *Bulletin of the History of Medicine* 9 (1941):8–30; Keenan, "St. Gregory of Nyssa and the Medical Profession"; ibid. 15 (1944):150–161; Darrel W. Amundsen, "Medicine and Faith in Early Christianity," ibid. 56 (1982):326–350; Demetrios J. Constantelos, "Physician–Priests in the Medieval Greek Church," *Greek Orthodox Theological Review* 14 (1967):141–153; and Constantelos, "Clerics and Secular Professions in the Byzantine Church," forthcoming. I am grateful to Professor Constantelos for sharing this article with me prior to its publication.

21. Constantelos, *Byzantine Philanthropy*, ch. 11; Timothy S. Miller, "Byzantine Hospitals," in *Symposium on Byzantine Medicine*, ed. Scarborough, pp. 53–63; and Miller, *The Birth of the Hospital in the Byzantine Empire* (Baltimore, MD, 1985).

22. Deno John Geanakoplos, *Byzantium: Church, Society, and Civilization Seen Through Contemporary Eyes* (Chicago, 1984), p. 430. See also Gordon, *Medieval and Renaissance Medicine*, p. 51.

23. See Kukules, *Byzantinon Bios kai Politismos* 6:13; Miller, "Byzantine Hospitals."

24. Miller, "Byzantine Hospitals," p. 55.

25. Alexander Kazhdan, "The Image of the Medical Doctor in Byzantine Literature of the Tenth to the Twelfth Centuries," in *Symposium on Byzantine Medicine*, ed. Scarborough, pp. 43–52. I am grateful to the author for sharing this paper with me prior to its publication.

26. Examples of this recent scholarship include Sergei Hackel, ed., *The Byzantine Saint* (London, 1981), especially E.G. Hunt, "Traffic in Relics: Some Late Roman Evidence," pp. 171–180; the essays in Scarborough, ed., *Symposium on Byzantine Medicine;* Peregrine Horden, "Saints and Doctors in the Early Byzantine Empire: The Case of Theodore of Sykeon," in *The Church and Healing*, ed. W.J. Sheils, vol. 19 of *Studies in Church History* (Oxford, 1982), pp. 1–13; Harry J. Magoulias, "The Lives of the Saints as Sources of Data for the History of Byzantine Medicine in the Sixth and Seventh Centuries," *Byzantinische Zeitschrift* 57 (1964):127–150.

27. A-J. Festugière, *Vie de Théodore de Sykeon*, 2 vols. (Brussels, 1970), quoted in Horden, "Saints and Doctors," p. 1. See also Magoulias, "The Lives of Saints," pp. 128–131.

28. Kazhdan, "The Image of the Medical Doctor," p. 45.

29. Described by Magoulias, "The Lives of the Saints," pp. 110–141.

30. Ibid., p. 132. Magoulias continues: "The Church did not combat the physician—with one exception. The Church refused to allow Christians to be doctored by Jews."

31. Gary Vikan, "Art, Medicine, and Magic in Early Byzantium," in *Symposium on Byzantine Medicine,* ed. Scarborough, pp. 65–86. I am grateful to the author for sharing his paper with me prior to its publication.

32. See Horden, "Saints and Doctors," p. 1, for a startlingly irenic quotation from the *Vita.*

33. For example, Magoulias, "The Lives of Saints," is full of such illustrations; see pp. 135–136 and footnote 38.

34. St. Basil, *Ascetical Works,* trans. Monica Wagner (Washington, DC, 1950), Question 55, pp. 330–337.

35. J. P. Migne, *Patrologia Graeca,* vol. 31, p. 523.

36. References to be found in Palmer, *Sacraments and Forgiveness,* p. 278.

37. Ibid., p. 280.

38. This view is held by Henry S. Kryger, "The Doctrine of the Effects of Extreme Unction in its Historical Development" (Ph.D. diss., Catholic University of America, 1949).

39. Reginald Maxwell Woolley, *Coptic Offices* (London, 1930); Vasileios Kostin, *He Koptike Latreia en Syngkrisei pros ten Latreian tes Orthodoxou Ekklesias* (Athens, 1972), pp. 83–84; Panagiotes N. Trembelas, *He Akolouthia tou Euchelaiou* (Athens, 1948); Trembelas, *Mikron Euchologion,* 2 vols. (Athens, 1950, 1955), vol. 1, pp. 99–191; Paul F. Palmer, *Sacraments and Forgiveness* (Westminster, MD, 1959), pp. 273–320; Palmer, *Sacraments of Healing and of Vocation* (Englewood Cliffs, NJ, 1963); Morton T. Kelsey, *Healing and Christianity in Ancient Thought and Modern Times* (New York, 1973), ch. 8; Casimir A. Kucharek, *The Sacramental Mysteries: A Byzantine Approach* (Allendale, NJ, 1976), ch. 21.

40. Constantelos, *Byzantine Philanthropy,* p. 39.

41. In addition to Constantelos, *Byzantine Philanthropy,* see Constantelos' articles on "Byzantine Philanthropy" and "Poor Relief, Byzantine" in the forthcoming *Dictionary of the Middle Ages;* and Panagiotes Demetropoulos, *He Pistis tes Archaias Ekklesias hos Kanon tes Zoes kai ho Kosmos* (Athens, 1959). For extensive bibliographies on the topic of Eastern Christian social concern, Stanley S. Harakas, *Let Mercy Abound: Social Concern in the Greek Orthodox Church* (Brookline, MA, 1983), ch. 1.

42. Kukules, *Byzantinon Bios kai Politismos,* 6:25–41.

43. Magoulias, "Lives of Saints," p. 131.

44. For a full treatment of this issue, see Miller, *The Birth of the Hospital.*

45. Magoulias, "Lives of Saints," p. 137.

46. "To Amphilochios, concerning the Canons," Letter 158, 2 in *Nicene and Post-Nicene Fathers,* vol. 8, p. 225. See Michael J. Gorman, *Abortion and the Early Church* (New York, 1982).

47. Kukules, *Byzantinon Bios Kai Politismos,* 6:19; Harvey, "Physicians and Ascetics," pp. 87–93.

48. John Romanides, *To Propatorikon Hamartema* (Athens, 1959); Jaroslav Pelikan, *The Christian Tradition: A History of the Development of Doctrine,* vol. 1, *The Emergence of the Catholic Tradition* (Chicago, 1974), pp. 153–154, 164–165, 272–273, 284–286.

49. *Constitutions of the Holy Apostles,* Book VI, 30, in *Ante-Nicene Fathers,* vol. 7, p. 464.

50. *Matthew* 27:52; *John* 11:11–13; *Acts* 7:60, 13:36; 1 *Corinthians* 7:29, 11:30, 15:6, 15:18–20, 15:51; 1 *Thessalonians* 4:13–15; 2 *Peter* 3:4, where the Greek for "to fall asleep" is used for "death."

51. Philotheos Faros, *To Penthos: Orthodoxe, Laographike kai Psychologike Theorise* (Athens, 1981), pp. 152–155.

52. For a theological expression of this perspective on Holy Tradition, see Georges Florovsky, "Patristic Theology and Ethos of the Orthodox Church," in his collected works, vol. 4, *Aspects of Church History* (Belmont, MA, 1975), pp. 11–30; and George S. Bebis, "The Concept of Tradition in the Fathers of the Church," *Greek Orthodox Theological Review* 15, (1970): 22–55.

53. Constantelos, *Byzantine Philanthropy,* pp. 170–171.

54. Geanakoplos, *Byzantium,* p. 314.

55. Constantelos, *Byzantine Philanthropy,* pp. 171–179.

56. Ibid., pp. 180–181, and Miller, "Byzantine Hospitals."

57. Kahzdan, "The Image of the Medical Doctor."

58. Miller, "Byzantine Hospitals."

59. Constantelos, "Clerics and Secular Professions," pp. 15–16.

60. Ibid.

61. *Patrologia Graeca,* vol. 64, pp. 1075–1310. The work is variously dated as from the eighth, ninth, or tenth centuries.

62. Ibid., 1277D.

63. Constantelos, "Clerics and Secular Professions," p. 18.

64. Theodore Balsamon, *Ekklesiastikon Diataxeon Sylloge, Patrologia Graeca,* vol. 138, p. 1245.

65. Constantelos, "Byzantine Medicine," in *Dictionary of the Middle Ages,* forthcoming. See also *Megale Hellenike Enkyklopaideia "Pyrsos"* (Athens, 1933), vol. 13, p. 367; *Nea Hellenike Enkyklopaideia* (Athens, 1972), vol. 14, p. 470.

66. Deno John Geanakoplos, *Byzantine East and Latin West* (New York, 1966); Harry J. Magoulias, *Byzantine Christianity: Emperor, Church and the West* (Chicago, 1970); Speros Vryonis, *Byzantium and Europe* (London, 1967).

67. Alice-Mary Talbot, *Faith Healing in Late Byzantium* (Brookline, MA, 1983), pp. 82, 84, 88, 90, 108, 110, 116.

68. Trembelas, *Mikron Euchologion,* vol. 1, pp. 109–113; John M. Fountoulis, *To Leitourgikon Ergon to Symeonos Thessalonikes* (Athens, 1966).

69. I. Alexiou et al., *It Prosphere Ho Christianismos? vol. 3, Koinonike Merimna sten Tourkokratia* (Athens, 1980).

70. A. Gkiala, *He Hellenike Iatrike kai oi Hellenes Iatroi apo tes Aloseos mechri tes Ethnegersias* (Athens, 1979).

71. Runciman, *The Great Church,* p. 213.

72. Timothy Ware, *Eustratios Argenti: A Study of the Greek Church Under Turkish Rule* (Oxford, 1964), pp. 45–47.

73. Ioannes N. Karmires, *Ta Dogmatika kai Symbolika Mnemeia tes Orthodoxou Katholikes Ekklesias* (Athens, 1953), vol. 2, ch. 4.

74. Franz Dorbeck, "Origin of Medicine in Russia," *Medical Life* 30 (1923):223–233.

75. Nancy Mandelker Frieden, *Russian Physicians in an Era of Reform and Revolution, 1856–1905* (Princeton, NJ, 1981), p. 24.

76. Ibid., ch. 3.
77. Ibid., ch. 4.
78. Ibid., ch. 9.
79. I was a witness in 1982 to the eagerness with which the faithful received this anointing, as well as to the devotion of pilgrims to various holy shrines in Kiev, Moscow, and Leningrad.
80. Vasileios Antoniades, *Encheiridion kata Christon Ethikes* (Constantinople, 1927), sec. 27, 40, 43, 44, 45, 46.
81. Chrestos Androutsos, *Systema Ethikes,* 2nd ed. (Thessalonike, 1964), p. 197.
82. Panagiotes X. Demetropoulos, *Orthodoxos Christianike Ethike* (Athens, 1970), pp. 239 ff., 158 ff., 185 ff.
83. George I. Mantzarides, *Christianike Ethike,* 2nd ed. (Thessalonike, 1983), p. 331.
84. Stanley S. Harakas, *For the Health of Body and Soul: An Eastern Orthodox Introduction to Bioethics* (Brookline, MA, 1980); Harakas, *Contemporary Moral Issues Facing the Orthodox Christian* (Minneapolis, MN, 1982), Part III.
85. David S. Schuller, Merton P. Strommen, and Milo L. Brekke, eds., *Ministry in America* (New York, 1980).
86. Stanley S. Harakas, "Orthodox Church," in *Ministry in America,* p. 343.
87. *Hodegos Hiereos: A Ceremonial Guide for Celebrants* (New York, 1969), p. 4.

CHAPTER 6

The Lutheran

Tradition

CARTER LINDBERG

In spite of Martin Luther's (1483–1546) insistence "that people make no reference to my name; let them call themselves Christians, not Lutherans," the churches rooted in the Reformation initiated by this German monk usually identify themselves as Lutheran. However, some Lutheran churches, mainly those outside of North America, refer to themselves as "evangelical" or "of the Augsburg Confession" to indicate their allegiance to Luther's interpretation of the gospel as set forth by his followers in the city of Augsburg in 1530. Titles aside, the history of the Lutheran tradition clearly shows the strong impress of Luther and the Lutheran Confessions. Luther's collected writings (parts of which are now available in nearly every major language) total over 100 volumes, and more has been written about him than any other figure in church history. Although they are found in practically every country of the world, today's approximately eighty million Lutherans reside largely in their traditional strongholds of Germany, Scandinavia, and North America.

Lutherans have always shared with all Christians the ecumenical affirmations of the Apostles' and Nicene Creeds, as well as professed their Lutheran identity through subscription to the Augsburg Confession. The latter's Article Seven states that "it is sufficient" for the unity of the church "that the Gospel be preached in conformity with a pure understanding of it and that the sacraments be administered in accordance with the divine word." Although this allowed considerable latitude in faith and life, ecclesial polity, and worship, the controversies of the Reformation period soon required further elaborations. In 1580, these were collected in the *Book of Concord,* which continues to be widely accepted as authoritative for the faith and life of the Lutheran churches. It includes Luther's *Large* and *Small Catechism* (1529), which have remained central to Lutheran religious and moral education. Even today, Luther's explanations of the Ten Commandments, the Apostles' Creed, and the Lord's Prayer are studied and memorized by many catechetical students.

This emphasis upon catechetical instruction, plus the important place of the sermon in worship, has maintained distinctive elements in the Lutheran churches. We list these here in anticipation of their later elaboration and application. The foundation upon which the church stands or falls is the emphasis upon the good news (gospel) of God's unconditional promise of salvation. In opposition to the medieval Roman Catholic position that salvation was partly contingent upon a person's good works, Luther asserted that salvation, the triumph over sin, death, and the devil, is entirely the work of God. The shorthand for this is the formula "justification by grace alone through faith alone." A second distinctive is that the life of the Christian is an ongoing struggle between faith and doubt, forgiveness and sin, life and death, wellness and illness. This is expressed by Luther's formula of the theology of the cross and by the teaching that the Christian is simultaneously saint and sinner, that is, always a forgiven sinner. Lutherans have understood Good Friday and Easter to mean that death and its various penultimate forms are not vanquished, but only strengthened, by denial and repression. This means that the cross and the simultaneity of sin and righteousness point to life and health as gifts rather than as achievements. A third distinctive is the "this-worldliness" or materiality of the Christian faith. This affirmation of God's presence in, with, and under nature is linked to Luther's sacramental understanding that the finite is capable of bearing the infinite. In the celebration of the sacraments of baptism and the Lord's Supper, Lutherans understand that God's activity in the life, death, and resurrection of Jesus continues to be materially communicated by water, bread, and wine. Related to this is a fourth distinctive: that Scripture is the bearer of God's word of judgment and promise.

But there is diversity as well as strong confessional loyalty and identity in the Lutheran tradition. This diversity reflects not only differing cultural and historical contexts ranging from European state and folk churches to Third World indigenous churches, but also such variables as sex, race, education, and socioeconomic status.

Lutheran history is often divided into the Reformation era (sixteenth century), Orthodoxy (roughly the seventeenth century), Pietism (late seventeenth and eighteenth centuries), and the modern period. The Reformation arose out of Luther's religious struggle for certainty of salvation in the midst of the crises of the late Middle Ages. The first Lutheran generations struggled with the challenges of both the Roman

Catholic Counter Reformation and rival Protestant churches. From this struggle arose the drive for theological and institutional consolidation known as Lutheran Orthodoxy. Although frequently viewed pejoratively, this emphasis upon theological and ecclesial system building should not be understood merely in terms of intellectual gymnastics or an edifice complex, but rather as a response to challenges to clarity of faith and commitment. While the careful doctrinal formulations by Orthodox Lutheran theologians on the basis of Aristotelian argumentation were not infrequently polemical, they also took on a profoundly moving form in the hymnody and music of the time.

The tragedies of the Thirty Years' War (1618–1648), the culmination of decades of religious strife in Europe, gave impetus to the reaction to Orthodoxy known as Pietism. Understanding themselves as completing the Reformation begun by Luther, the Pietists attempted to carry out the program set forth by their acknowledged leader, Philip Spener (1635–1705), in his famous *Pious Desires* (1675). Christian experience and lifestyle were emphasized in contrast to the perceived overemphasis by the Orthodox on correct doctrine. Although the Pietists held that social change depended upon the conversion of individuals, they responded to the issues of the day by establishing orphanages, schools, hospitals, and missions, the last of which contributed to the spread of the Lutheran churches beyond their original Germanic and Scandinavian concentration.

Major European emigrations as well as foreign missions planted Lutheran churches throughout the world in the eighteenth and nineteenth centuries. For the immigrants, Lutheran identity went hand in hand with ethnic and linguistic identity so that in America, for example, there were Swedish, Norwegian, Danish, and German Lutheran churches. In the twentieth century, these "hyphenated" churches, although still concerned with preserving their Lutheran identity, became increasingly Americanized. Most of the ethnic Lutheran churches have united into two major church bodies: the American Lutheran Church (ALC, 1960), and the Lutheran Church in America (LCA, 1962). The other large Lutheran church in America, the Lutheran Church–Missouri Synod (LC–MS, name adopted in 1947), theologically conservative in comparison to the ALC and LCA, suffered severe doctrinal controversy during the 1970s that prompted a number of pastors and congregations to withdraw and form the Association of Evangelical Lutheran Churches (1976). The ALC, LCA, and AELC have committed themselves to form a new Lutheran church to be constituted in 1988. The LC–MS declined to join this merger. In general, the European and American Lutheran churches have been largely middle class and have reflected most of this class's customs, mores, and attitudes.

The scholarship of the nineteenth century and the intense Reformation research of the twentieth (ecumenical in scope) have contributed a profound awareness to contemporary Lutheran churches of their identity and heritage. This, in turn, has become a major resource in their struggle with the issues of the present. This complex of heritage and contemporary challenge, especially during the two world wars, led to a global Lutheran self-consciousness that produced the Lutheran World Federation (1947), an involvement in the World Council of Churches, and national and international dialogues with nearly every non-Lutheran church. In all of this, Luther's expression of the gospel has continued to be a major resource for the Lutheran tradition's unity in its own historical and cultural diversity, as well as its impetus and contribution to an ecumenical orientation of reconciled diversity among all churches.

Dividing Lutheran history into the Reformation, Orthodox, Pietistic, and modern periods is useful for discussing the tradition's medical history because each period gave rise to distinctive attitudes and activities. Of course as the Lutheran tradition developed, it became increasingly complex; thus our simple divisions may distort some aspects even while clarifying others. We need to bear in mind, for instance, that particular emphases did not abruptly end as one major orientation gave way to another and that there was personal as well as chronological overlapping. It is clear, however, that both Luther and the Lutheran Confessions run like a red line through the tradition.[1]

The Reformation Era

In many ways Luther was, as the nineteenth-century Danish Lutheran Søren Kierkegaard said, "A patient of exceeding import for Christendom." What Kierkegaard had in mind was Luther's well-known struggle with illness, out of which he found the resources to deal forcefully with the issues of sickness and health. Luther was perpetually in ill health. He suffered throughout his reforming career from attacks of vertigo; severe and sometimes incapacitating headaches; hemorrhoids; constipation; and stones of the urinary tract, kidneys, and bladder; in later life he suffered from an ulcerated leg, heart problems, sinus infections, colds, and a middle-ear infection. Throughout his life he also experienced *Anfechtungen,* severe assaults—temptations is too weak a translation—upon his faith, which he attributed to the devil and even to God.[2] Thus Luther was no stranger to personal, physical, psychological, and spiritual suffering. He also lived in a time when persons were old if not dead by their forties, illness was endemic, and the ravages of disease were sudden and swift.

His primary response to personal and social suffering was to proclaim God's forgiveness of sinners. This did not mean either escaping from suffering or trivializing of it, but rather trusting that in some way suffering was linked to God's choice to redeem persons and the world through Christ's death on the cross.[3] This "theology of the cross" served as an epistemological and theological principle for Luther.[4] Although the whys and wherefores of illness and death were frequently not clear to him, he remained confident of never being deserted by Christ. After an illness so severe that even his basic life signs were not detectable, Luther gave poetic expression to his consciousness of having been in the battlefield between God and Satan in his chorale "A Mighty Fortress Is Our God," which concludes:

> God's Word forever shall abide,
> No thanks to foes, who fear it;
> For God himself fights by our side
> With weapons of the Spirit.
> Were they to take our house,
> Goods, honor, child, or spouse,
> Though life be wrenched away,
> They cannot win the day.
> The Kingdom's ours forever![5]

"The Kingdom's ours forever!" was Luther's poetic assertion of the central Reformation doctrine of justification by grace alone. He succinctly stated that God's unconditional gift of salvation was not the goal of life, but its presupposition:

> The gospel commands us to look, not at our own deeds or perfection but at God himself as he promises, and at Christ himself, the Mediator. . . . And this is the reason why our theology is certain: it snatches us away from ourselves and places us outside ourselves, so that we do not depend on our own strength, conscience, experience, person, or works but depend on that which is outside ourselves, that is, on the promise and truth of God, which cannot deceive.[6]

Luther's understanding of justification by grace alone rejected all human claims to be salvatory whether they were religious, social, political, or medical. That is to say, the burden of proof for salvation and well-being rests upon God, not upon persons. To the achievement-oriented Middle Ages (as to our own), this was a radical shift of perspective.

But this reorientation did not lead Luther to spiritualize illness and suffering. To the contrary, in earthy humor he could say in light of his bouts with constipation, diarrhea, and urine retention due to stones (once for eight days!) that one's rear has its own rules, which are not sufficiently esteemed. Luther respected doctors—indeed, his son Paul studied medicine and served as court physician to the Electors of Saxony and Brandenburg—but his faith convinced him that they did not have the last word. Luther expected doctors to seek and treat the natural causes of illness with medical remedies. Yet he also believed that illness was not just an external invasion of the body. He said that when Satan instigates a disease, then a "higher medicine, namely, faith and prayer," must be applied. He continued, "I have nothing but praise for the physicians who adhere closely to their principles. But they should not take it amiss if I do not always agree with them. . . ."[7]

Luther's view of human nature did not allow a separation of faith and medicine. His understanding of the relationship was grounded in his theology of justification by grace alone—the whole person, body and soul, flesh and spirit, is unconditionally accepted by God—and its corollary, that the Christian is simultaneously sinner and righteous, sick and convalescent. If the only way a person may be justified is by God's unconditional forgiveness and mercy, then sin involves more than merely breaking commandments. To Luther, sin disrupts the relationship between God and the person, and between one person and another, not because it breaks rules, but because it is egocentricity. The good news, Luther never tired of proclaiming, was that in spite of being a sinner, the person was accepted by God. Trust in this good news allowed God to be God and the sinner to be what he or she was intended to be—human. The sinner, Luther said, was not called to try to be like God—a supremely egocentric task—but to trust in his or her God-given righteousness. The Christian was thus "at the same time a sinner and a righteous person; a sinner in fact, but righteous by the sure imputation and promise of God that he will continue to deliver him from sin until he has completely cured him. And thus the person is entirely healthy in hope, but in fact is still a sinner. . . ."[8]

Luther therefore viewed wellness and illness in terms of the simultaneity of God's caring and curing process, which excluded neither medical assistance nor prayerful trust in God. Luther urged a close working relationship between doctor and pastor in care of the sick. He knew that people all too often viewed illness as a punishment from God. As a pastor, he addressed this in his tract "Whether One May Flee from a Deadly Plague," where he pointedly rejected suffering and disaster as simply God's punishments. This idea would lead, he said, to the absurd notion that drugs and doctors were unnecessary because all illnesses came from God.[9] Indeed, he regarded carelessness with regard to health as a form of suicide. "God created medicine and provided us with intelligence to guard and take care of the body so that we can live in good health," he wrote.[10]

Luther did not imply, however, that once the sinner accepted and trusted God, his or her life would be smooth sailing into eternity. To the contrary, Luther opposed this naive triumphalism (he called it a "theology of glory") by realistically describing life as a continual struggle from birth to grave. Luther did not think suffering good in itself nor something to be sought for self-improvement, but when encountered it could be the locus of wellness. As one scholar has observed, "Luther found healing precisely in his sickness not in escape from it."[11] The theology of the cross was Luther's expression of the good news that God chose to meet and redeem his creation in the midst of its limitations, breakdowns, and failures rather than demanded that his creation achieve perfection in order to be redeemed. The "voice of illness" therefore addressed the perennial Promethean delusion of humankind that it can secure its own present and future.

Because Luther saw all human efforts to distance oneself from suffering, illness, and death as defense mechanisms with no possibility of long-term success, he stressed prophylactic as well as therapeutic responses to illness. In his "Sermon on Preparing to Die," he counseled reflection on sickness and death in times of health so that illness would not catch one unprepared. He saw the fellowship and faith of the church as crucially supportive:

> . . . in the hour of his death no Christian should doubt he is not alone. He can be certain, as the sacraments point out, that a great many eyes are upon him: first, the eyes of God and of Christ himself, for the Christian believes his words and clings to his sacraments; then also, the eyes of the dear angels, of the saints, and of all Christians. There is no doubt, as the Sacrament of the Altar indicates, that all of these in a body run to him as one of their own, help him overcome sin, death, and hell, and bear all things with him. In that hour the work of love and the communion of the saints are seriously and mightily active.[12]

Preparation for sickness and death, however, involved social as well as pastoral activities. Here Luther's emphasis upon personal ethics and the vocation of serving neighbors as a "little Christ" widened into social ethics and concern for justice. The clearest example of this was the Reformation effort to establish public-welfare institutions which rapidly became part of the Church Orders ("constitutions" governing the community) in the cities where the Reformation took root.[13] Believing that the Christian was responsible not only for alleviating suffering, but for preventing it, Luther urged the establishment of public hospitals with government support. He also urged commonsense public instruction in health care and sanitation. Of course, Luther was not unique in advocating such reforms. In fact, on his 1510 journey to Rome he had observed the operation of pre-Reformation Italian hospitals.[14]

It may be argued that Luther's greatest contribution to science and medicine was not these specific contributions, but the initiation of a new era in thinking, what one scholar has termed a "paradigm shift."[15] This shift was from the medieval epistemology based on deduction from textual authorities to an epistemology of induction and experience. Of course, Luther's opposition to Aristotle and scholastic method was in the context of philosophy and theology. He expressed this succinctly when he said, "It is not by understanding, reading, or speculation that one becomes a theologian, but through living, dying, and being damned."[16] He made the same point less dramatically when he said, "None of the arts can be learned without practice. What kind of physician would that be who stayed in school all the time? When he finally puts his medicine to use and deals more and more with nature, he will come to see that he hasn't as yet mastered the art."[17] That Luther facilitated a "paradigm shift" from deduction to induction was recognized by his contemporaries who said of the maverick physician Paracelsus (1493–1541) that he was "the Luther of the physicians." The point was not that Paracelsus followed Luther's theology, but that he shared Luther's view of authority. The historian of medicine Owsei Temkin wrote, "Just as with Luther, the unity of the Catholic Church is decisively broken, so with Paracelsus—the 'Lutherus medicorum'— the unity of Galenism is destroyed."[18] Similarly, the non-Lutheran English scientist Francis Bacon (1561–1626) expressed a very "Lutheran" attitude when he compared Aristotle to Antichrist and indicted Greek philosophers for conjuring scientific knowledge out of their heads instead of seeking it in nature.[19]

The doctrine of justification by grace alone apart from works also contributed to the development of science and medicine because it liberated human energy from the medieval preoccupation with other-worldly pursuits for this-worldly activities. At the University of Wittenberg, Luther and his colleague Philip Melanchthon (1497–1560) were instrumental in increasing the size of the medical faculty. Melanchthon's son-in-law Caspar Peucer (1525–1602) was both theologian and physician and taught in both fields as well as serving as personal physician to the Elector August of Saxony. The largest section of Peucer's library was his medical collection. Among the contemporary authors in Peucer's collection were works of innovative physicians such as the anatomist Vesalius (1514–1564) and the theorist of contagious disease Fracastoro (?1483–1553). Medical students at Wittenberg were being acquainted with new developments in the field.[20] By the seventeenth century, the University of Wittenberg had a renowned medical faculty and was firmly established in anatomical studies through the work of Salomon Alberti (1540–1600). The turn away from Aristotle toward the study of nature also stimulated a long line of distinguished botanists.[21]

One of the most important doctrinal contributions to this shift from otherworldly to this-worldly concerns resulted from Luther's under-standing of vocation. Up to the time of the Reformation era, vocation or calling was understood in the narrow confines of priesthood and monastery. The highest vocation was dedication to the church. Through the doctrines of the universal priesthood of all believers and vocation, Luther argued that all areas of life, all forms of honest work, are avenues for obedience to God's command to serve the neighbor. This not only gave a new dignity to secular work, but also imbued it with a theological–ethical dimension. The Bible, wrote Luther,

> has been put into your workshop, into your hand, into your heart. It teaches and preaches how you should treat your neighbor. Just look at your tools. . . . Nothing that you handle every day is so tiny that it does not continually tell you this, if you will only listen. Indeed, there is no shortage of preaching. You have as many preachers as you have transactions, goods, tools, and other equipment in your house and home. All this is continually crying out to you: "Friend, use me in your relations with your neighbor just as you would want your neighbor to use his property in his relations with you."[22]

Nowhere was this understanding of vocation applied more explosively to medieval life than in the area of sex and marriage. "No institutional change brought about by the Reformation was more visible, responsive to late medieval pleas for reform, and conducive to new social attitudes than the marriage of Protestant clergy," writes the historian Steven Ozment. "Nor was there another point in the Protestant program where theology and practice corresponded more successfully."[23] The Reformers vigorously criticized priestly and monastic vows of celibacy because they removed men and women from service to the neighbor, contravened the divine order of marriage and family, and denied the goodness of sexuality. The Reformers viewed marriage not just as the legitimation of sexual fulfillment, but above all as the context for creating a new awareness of human community. "Marriage does not only consist of sleeping with a woman—anybody can do that— but keeping house and bringing up children," declared Luther.[24] The Reformation brought to marriage a new, indeed joyous, appreciation for the created sexual drive and a new respect for women as companions. Luther was fond of extolling marriage as a "gift of God," "superior to any celibacy," for "the companionship of husband and wife is a marvelous thing."[25]

The Lutheran Reformers also emphasized coeducational, universal education—not just for the sake of preparing a learned ministry and a Christian community able to read and understand the Scriptures, but as a means of serving society by preparing educated public servants, doctors, and lawyers. The mid–sixteenth-century explosion of manuals and pamphlets on home remedies, such as herbal medicines, as well as more technical scientific and medical treatises must be seen against this background.[26]

On the personal, pastoral level, Luther responded to sickness by prayer and counseling. One of his most startling uses of prayer occurred during the apparently mortal illness of his friend and colleague Philip Melanchthon. Finding Melanchthon on his deathbed, Luther demanded God to restore his health. "I need him for my work, and since my work is your work, God, you must help me!"[27] But Luther rarely resorted to such demands or to exorcism by prayer. Usually he petitioned "thy will be done," adding in crisis situations the phrase from Psalm 31:5, "Into thy hand I commit my spirit; thou hast redeemed me, O Lord, faithful God." Luther's customary request for prayers (*ora pro me*—"pray for me") was not an empty formula, but expressed his conviction that God is the Lord of life and death and that prayers are efficacious.

Most scholars agree that pastoral care and counseling of the sick took root in the Reformation.[28] But they often overlook that in this developing of the office of pastor as *Seelsorger* (spiritual advisor), Luther contributed an earthy common sense and humor rooted in his conviction that to "let God be God" allowed persons to be human. For example, with regard to depression Luther recommended not only Scripture and prayer, but good company, good food and drink, music, laughter, and, if necessary, fantasies about the other sex! "When you are assailed by gloom, despair, or a troubled conscience you should eat, drink and talk with others. If you can find help for yourself by thinking of a girl, do so."[29] Thus Luther related physical and mental health, commenting at one point: "Our physical health depends in large measure on the thoughts of our minds. This in accord with the saying, 'Good cheer is half the battle.'"[30]

For the most part, Luther took his own advice seriously. In spite of perpetual illness, he gave himself unstintingly to pastoral and academic responsibilities as well as to public issues. His last days were devoted to mediating a dispute between the two Counts of Mansfeld. It was one of the forms of ministry he believed he was made for; as he explained, "A cow does not get to heaven by giving milk, but that is what she is made for."[31] Following the resolution of the dispute, he suffered an angina attack. During the evening of 17 February 1546, Luther complained of severe chest pains. He died sometime after midnight. His last prayer expressed his certainty that nothing could tear him out of God's hands.[32]

Luther's astonishing energy in the midst of opposition and illness was not the result of being some sort of superman, but was rooted in his faith that "the righteous shall live by faith" (*Rom.* 1:17). And to Luther, this "living" was not to be put off until heaven. His legacy was to reverse the medieval warning of death, "in the midst of life we are surrounded by death," making it a call to life: "In the midst of death we are surrounded by life."[33]

The Age of Orthodoxy

The age of Orthodoxy, which coincided roughly with the seventeenth century, sought to conserve and reinforce the contributions of the Reformation. Like Calvinists, Lutherans were stimulated by the Roman Catholic Counter Reformation and the need to define their church in the context of the widespread wars of religion and the political atmosphere of the post-Reformation period. Legal recognition of the church within territories and nations depended on its exact definition. The concern for order on every level of life, including the theological and ecclesial, was further heightened by the last major religious war in Europe. The Thirty Years' War (1618–1648), fought between Catholics and Protestants, resulted in social chaos, unspeakable suffering, and a massive loss of life (estimated at nearly one-third of the German population) and induced a profound feeling of gratitude among survivors to any government able to create a minimum of order. In this light, one might regard the Orthodox emphasis upon order in all areas of life as a form of social caring. Unfortunately, Luther's joy in the goodness of the created order, his dynamic proclamation of the gospel, and his understanding of vocation and ethics in terms of faith active in love now began to recede behind an increasingly restrictive emphasis upon right belief and right action.

It is not surprising in this context that Orthodox Lutherans in universities and churches were convinced that one of the most important results of the Reformation was the purification of Christian doctrine. They proceeded to protect this heritage by constructing lengthy discourses on doctrine not infrequently characterized by dogmatic rigidity and polemical attacks on Catholic and Calvinist opponents. The theological absolutism of Orthodoxy fit in well with the developing political absolutism of the seventeenth century. Church life suffered not only from this dogmatic orientation, but also from the fact that the clergy frequently were perceived as being out of touch with the common life and serving a government-maintained church.

The Orthodox never denied that "faith without works is dead," but their emphasis upon pure doctrine left them open to the charge of passivity in social ethics. Their printed sermons, writes the historian Jaroslav Pelikan, suggest that "the type of preaching to which the people were being exposed was unproductive of religious, spiritual, or ethical power."[34] A major reason for this was the Orthodox preoccupation with the study of philosophy, especially Aristotle's, which based ministry upon dogmatic speculation rather than interpretation of Scripture. As a consequence of this orientation, theological debate displaced ministering to the people, apathy toward missionary work abounded, and ethics became separated from theology.[35] The neglect of ethics in theory was all too often matched by a neglect of ethics in practice.

However, even in this confused period of war and its aftermath, when church authority shifted largely into the hands of the "Christian prince," leading Lutheran theologians did not entirely overlook pastoral care. Johann Valentin Andreae (1586–1654) advocated pastoral guidance and the discipline of evildoers in his 1619 publications, *The Good Life of an Honest Servant of God* and *Christianopolis,* a celebrated utopia. Among the writings of Johann Gerhard (1582–1637), the "archtheologian" of Orthodoxy, was a work on mystical theology, which in 1615 was translated into English as *The soules watch, or a day-booke for the devout soule.* Johannes-Andreas Quenstedt (1617–1688), sometimes known as the bookkeeper of Lutheran Orthodoxy, recommended devotional books to his students and set forth his ethical concerns in his *Pastor's Ethics and Pastoral Instruction* (1678). Nevertheless, this was an age of pastoral decline. As one scholar has written,

> The cure of souls was much neglected and largely confined to a limited amount of visitation and the rather mechanical practice of private confession . . . for which a fee (the *Beichtpfennig*) was paid to the pastor. . . . Critics revived a saying of Sarcerius [1501–1559]: "The binding key is quite rusted away while the loosing key is in full operation."[36]

The theological controversies endemic to Orthodoxy contributed indirectly to scientific and medical studies by prompting more than one theological student to change vocational plans when confronted by what Melanchthon late in life called the "rabies theologorum" (the madness of the theologians). A good example is Johannes Kepler (1571–1630), who was refused ordination after his theological studies because his theology of the Lord's Supper was not regarded as orthodox. He then became an assistant to the Danish Lutheran astronomer Tycho Brahe (1546–1601). In spite of his disappointment over rejection for the ministry, Kepler wrote in his first publication, "I wanted to become a theologian. For a long time I was restless. Now, however, observe how through my efforts, God is being celebrated in astronomy."[37] Kepler went on to influence Newton and contribute to the triumph of the Copernican over the Ptolemaic theory of planetary motion.

Pietism

The Thirty Years' War and the confessional–dogmatic battles of Orthodoxy had a sobering effect upon Lutherans and contributed to the reaction to Orthodoxy known as Pietism. Pietism is difficult to define because it emerged as a transnational and transdenominational movement in the late seventeenth century. Lutheran Pietists protested against what they saw as the Orthodox displacement of Luther's living faith by dogma. Slogans such as "life vs. doctrine," "Holy Spirit vs. the office of ministry," and "reality vs. the appearance of godliness" frequently appear as clues to the Pietist position. In important respects, Pietists emphasized ethical renewal of the individual in opposition to what they perceived as the spiritual and ethical lassitude of Orthodoxy. The elements of what later came to be known as the "Protestant ethic"— thrift, honesty, and diligence in work—were actively fostered by Pietism.

The leadership of Philip Spener, "the Father of Pietism," promoted a notable revival in pastoral care as well as in other areas of the church's life. His program of edifying members through small group discussions of the Bible drew on Luther's understanding of the priesthood of all believers and the centrality of the Scriptures to Christian faith and life. In his programmatic work, *Pious Desires* (1675), Spener wrote: "What did our sainted Luther seek more ardently than to induce people to a diligent reading of the Scriptures? . . . it was one of the major purposes of the Reformation to restore to the people the Word of God." The purpose of these study groups, he explained, was to impress on the people "that it is by no means enough to have knowledge of the Christian faith, for Christianity consists rather of practice." A few paragraphs later Spener set forth both the individualistic introspection and diligence in charity for which Pietism came to be known: "They must become accustomed not to lose sight of any opportunity in which they can render their neighbor a service of love, and yet while performing it they must diligently search their hearts to discover whether they are acting in true love or out of other motives."[38]

Spener's friend and follower August Hermann Francke (1663–1727) gave institutional shape to the Pietist goal of changing the world by changing individuals. Francke, a professor of theology at the University of Halle, made that institution a center of Pietist education and mission. In 1695 he established a school for poor children, and then in quick succession added other institutions—a common school, an orphanage, a teacher training school, and a high school—which became world famous. He also established a printshop, book store, and a pharmacy, the last of which served an educational purpose in training aspiring pastors. Ministerial students at Halle acquired a rudimentary knowledge of medicines and served internships in the sick wards of local hospitals.

The program at Halle stimulated the development elsewhere of institutions for the physically and mentally handicapped, refugees, and prisoners.

The 1699 typhus epidemic ravaged the orphanage and spurred a search for a curative medicine. Francke gave this task to the young physician Christian Friedrich Richter (1676–1711), who had studied medicine and theology at Halle. Richter, also known as a Pietist hymnwriter, labored intensively in the pharmacy and in 1701 produced his *Essentia dulcis* (basically a colloidal gold solution), which became widely used as a cure "discovered by God's blessing." This medicine stood in the old tradition of the alchemical search for a "universal medicine" that preceded the early Reformation urging by Paracelsus for a chemical treatment for disease. The influence of alchemy may also be seen in the effort to incorporate gold, the perfect metal, into medicine in order to release its properties in the body, and in the perspective that only a changed person can change material into medicine.[39]

The promotion of the *Essentia dulcis* reflected Francke's understanding of miracle that corresponded more to the changing intellectual situation than did that of the Orthodox. Francke saw medicine within the scope of special divine providence. Effective medicine was the miracle of God's love experienced in life. The Orthodox understood medicine as an expression of God's general grace (the sun shines on the just and unjust alike), but not as a divine confirmation of the pharmacist's work. Richter's conviction was that "our pharmacy must be conceived as none other than God's revealed treasure chest wherein the miserable and sick might know and love God as good and comforting through the splendid power of the medicines given according to his goodness and mercy."[40] Francke's and Richter's understanding of miracle foreshadowed by almost a century the view of the "father of liberal theology," Friedrich Schleiermacher, who wrote in 1799:

> Miracle is simply the religious name for event. Every event, even the most natural and usual, becomes a miracle, as soon as the religious view of it can be the dominant. To me all is miracle. . . . The more religious you are, the more miracle would you see everywhere.[41]

The Orthodox understanding of miracle in terms of transcendent power intervening in nature impeded their contributions to science. But Pietists such as Francke and Richter saw God at work in nature and medicine as the stimulant restoring natural bodily functions. Once again, pastor and physician could be partners in God's activity in the world.

One avenue of partnership envisioned by Francke was education for renewal of church and body. A simple but important example was education in hygiene. Well before the acceptance of the germ theory of disease (1861), Francke was teaching separate laundering of clothes, linens, and towels for the sick; isolation of the very sick; and regular hygiene habits including brushing teeth. He also developed clinical instruction for physicians, and in 1717 the orphanage clinic was connected to the medical faculty. Halle became the first German university to have a practical institute for medical studies. The first professors of medicine at Halle University (founded in 1694) were Friedrich Hoffmann (1660–1742) and Georg Ernst Stahl (1660–1734), who are regarded to have been among the founders of medicine in Germany. According to Richter, the University clinic was to educate theological students in ministry to the sick, and medical students in medical and surgical praxis. Other universities followed the Halle model; for example, the Halle-trained physician Friedrich Wendt founded in 1779 the "Erlangen Institute for the Practical Training of Young Doctors and for the Gratuitous Healing of the Poor."[42]

The University of Halle also became a great missionary center, sending out Pietists who struggled to serve soul and body by preaching to the poor, feeding the hungry, and healing the sick.[43] From Halle, preachers and teachers went throughout the world, while at the same time many foreign students came to Halle. Two of the more famous missionaries from Halle were Bartholomaeus Ziegenbalg (1682–1719), who went to India, and Henry Melchior Muhlenberg (1711–1787), the "Patriarch of American Lutheranism."

Muhlenberg, although not a physician, was one of the first Lutheran medical missionaries. Like most of the Halle graduates, he had worked on the local sick wards. Describing Muhlenberg's training, John N. Ritter has written:

> How well Muhlenberg learned that every fact of a patient's life had to be taken into account to understand the soul's need! He patiently wrote out many cases as a task in psychiatric casuistry. That was a scientific duty required of all Halle men. He believed that in order to cure the soul a pastor had to be able to cure the body, or at best understand the disfunctions of the body. . . .[44]

Once in America, Muhlenberg attracted not only many patients, but also physicians who came to him for advice.

The conversion of individuals was the great motivating force behind Pietism's charitable works. But in spite of the Pietists' widespread establishment of orphanages, hospitals, educational institutions, and missions, their individualism hindered development of a social ethic.

On the one hand, their struggle against personal ethical laxity may have contributed to wellness by emphasizing a pure mind and a pure body. On the other hand, Pietism courted indifference, if not antagonism, to the world—so much so that it has been dubbed "monasticism outside the monastery." According to Franklin Sherman, "Smoking and drinking were disapproved of; dancing, card-playing and theatre-going were prohibited; and frivolity in general was frowned upon. Sexuality was viewed with suspicion, and even within marriage its expression was to be characterized by sobriety and restraint."[45] Pietist attitudes of asceticism became widespread and left a permanent mark on the Lutheran churches of the world.

The Modern Period

In Europe, rationalism and the Enlightenment corroded the life of the churches in more significant ways than by their critical attacks on faith. Luther's understanding of the church as community, already undermined by the Orthodox emphasis upon correct doctrine and the Pietist tendency to withdraw into conventicles of true Christians within the church, was further debilitated by rationalism. The congregation, earlier understood as a caring and curing community focused on the Word of God and the sacraments, now tended to become a meeting hall for lectures to the neglect of Scripture and sacraments. In the nineteenth century these challenges were further sharpened by the rapid growth of industrialization and urbanization. The Lutheran churches responded with a mix of creativity and defensiveness.

A pioneer in the Lutheran response to the social issues of the day was Johann Friedrich Oberlin (1740–1826), after whom a city and college in Ohio were named. As pastor of the remote and barren area of Walderbach in the Vosges mountains of Alsace for 59 years, he transformed the impoverished villages of the area into prosperous communities. He engaged in every area of life, establishing schools, roads, bridges, banks, stores, agricultural societies (which introduced potato cultivation), and industries. His nursery schools *(kindergartens)* were imitated in many areas through "Oberlin Societies."

Germany experienced a religious awakening in the aftermath of the struggle against Napoleon. One of the leaders in this revival was Klaus Harms (1778–1855), known among other things for his sharp attack on rationalism in his "Ninety-Five Theses" delivered on the 300th anniversary (1817) of Luther's similarly named protest. The controversies generated by his address led him further in the direction of emphasizing pastoral care. He himself desired to be a "psychic physician" and to have ministers trained in "psychiatry."[46] Other reformers who followed his lead inaugurated two of the more creative and influential developments of the nineteenth century: the Inner Mission and deaconess movements. These movements, soon interrelated, addressed themselves to all aspects of wellness and illness.

Johann Hinrich Wichern (1808–1881), the "Father of Inner Missions," gained a vivid awareness of urban poverty from visiting student homes while a teacher in Hamburg.[47] This motivated him to establish rescue homes for neglected children. His prototype, the *Rauhe Haus* (literally, the "Rough House"), opened in 1833 in a suburb of Hamburg. It not only emphasized education and job training in the context of the gospel of God's forgiving grace, but also included time for leisure and sports. Wichern enlisted and trained capable assistants, thus becoming a forerunner in the movement to prepare deacons and deaconesses. In 1844 he began publishing an influential newspaper, which aroused the social conscience of his time. Concerned that both the future of Christianity and society were being jeopardized by the growing alienation among the urban masses from a seemingly uncaring church, in 1848, soon after the appearance of Karl Marx's "Communist Manifesto," he issued a "Protestant Manifesto."

He delivered this long, gripping speech at the Wittenberg *Kirchentag*, an annual mass assembly of Protestant laity that had recently begun to meet. Here he proclaimed that "love no less than faith is the church's indispensable mark." He saw the dawn of a new future in the church if it would incarnate the deeds of God in Inner Mission.[48] His forceful speech led to the formation of the Central Committee for Inner Missions of the German Evangelical Church.

The concept of the Inner Mission included the transformation of the church from an authoritarian establishment into a fellowship, in which the laity would rediscover its mission as the universal priesthood. All the various organizations and charities that were only loosely connected with the church were to be united into a single, church-sponsored home mission organization to respond to the spiritual and social plight of society. For Wichern, the revitalization of Luther's emphasis on "faith active in love,"

> brought forth from the bosom of the divine community of life, draws wider and wider rings with the staff of faith. Its provinces are at the cradle of the infant, with the games of tender children. . . . It eases the pain and wounds at the sickbed, comforts the dying, fights vice and disgrace. . . . The chasms of physical distress and moral corruption with their hundreds of branches and shapes in the low and high places of society do not terrify this love, but rather summon it to even greater courage, even more shining deeds.[49]

The chief aims of the Inner Mission initially included reclaiming those who had left the church and assisting the needy, sick, and poor.

Later they were broadened to embrace prison reform (Wichern himself became a special counselor in the Prussian Ministry of the Interior in charge of prison and welfare work), as well as care for the homeless, the mentally and physically handicapped, immigrants, and seamen. The Inner Mission soon spread from Germany to other European countries and to America. It eventually became an umbrella for a wide variety of activities including social-welfare work and services for the elderly, children, families, and the sick. The American Lutheran churches used the term *Inner Mission* for a time, but eventually substituted such phrases as *Christian social welfare* and *social services.*

The diaconal movement (from the word *diakonia,* meaning faith active in love and service to all) in the Lutheran churches was also rooted in Luther's understanding of vocation and the universal priesthood. By the beginning of the modern period, congregations in the state churches of Europe had relinquished most social-welfare responsibilities to the state and had limited *diakonia* mainly to an expression of individual Christian piety. The revival of Christian service in connection with the congregation, and separate from, though cooperative with, the government, came not only through the Inner Mission, but also through the development of the deaconess movement by the German Lutheran pastors Theodore Fliedner (1800–1864) and Wilhelm Loehe (1808–1872), who among others greatly desired the renewal of a women's ministry in the church.

One of the important precursors of the deaconess movement was Amalie Sieveking (1794–1859), who in 1823 began developing a sisterhood analogous to the Roman Catholic Sisters of Charity. During the 1831 cholera epidemic in Hamburg, she appealed to others of like mind to join her in nursing the sick. Undeterred by the lack of response, she worked on her own and soon became superintendent of the cholera hospital. In 1832 she organized a women's society for the care of the sick and poor in her native Hamburg, which served as an inspiration to Fliedner.[50]

Fliedner's own first steps toward the development of the female diaconate began with his work on behalf of prisoners, which was inspired by the English Quaker Elizabeth Fry (1780–1845) and the Mennonite deaconess movement he had observed in Holland. The cradle of the institutions he founded at Kaiserswerth was the small garden summer house attached to the parsonage, where he and his wife in 1833 lodged a discharged woman prisoner who had come to them for help. Others soon followed. As the number of deaconesses in Kaiserswerth increased, so did their field of labor. Soon they were not only helping released women prisoners, but also serving the sick, orphans, and the morally outcast. The deaconesses soon felt the need for a structured environment of mutual support. Thus in 1836 the Fliedners established the first deaconess motherhouse, in Kaiserswerth, and organized the Rhenish–Westphalian Deaconess Association. Dozens of these centers soon sprang up throughout Europe. In his short history of Lutheran deaconesses, Frederick Weiser summarizes this rapid growth:

> By 1884 there were fifty-six deaconess communities which had a total of 5653 deaconesses. The most outspokenly Lutheran of these was at Neuendettelsau, a small peasant village in Franconia near Nuremberg, at which Pastor Wilhelm Loehe (1808–1872) had invested his community with rich liturgical life and lively confessional commitment. The largest single group of deaconesses came to be the one at Bethel near Bielefeld in Westphalia. After 1872 its leader was Pastor Friedrich von Bodelschwingh (1831–1910). Ministry to vagrants and to epileptics there caught the imagination of all Germany.[51]

Primarily known for nursing, the deaconesses fostered many other facets of Christian service as well.

In addition to deaconesses, the Fliedners also trained salaried Christian nurses. In 1851, the pioneer English nurse Florence Nightingale (1820–1910) went to Kaiserswerth for training and later, in 1860, opened her own school of nursing. By that time deaconesses from Kaiserswerth were serving hospitals in England, America, Jerusalem, Constantinople, Smyrna, and Alexandria. The historian of medicine Harry Wain states: "Thus modern nursing schools can trace very definite lines back to Kaiserwerth [sic] and the Fliedners."[52]

Loehe's establishment of a deaconess motherhouse in Neuendettelsau in response to the crying needs of the people manifested his concern for transforming the church into an instrument of service. Loehe himself felt a strong loyalty to the Lutheran Confessions and a deep appreciation of the significance of the liturgy and sacraments as the source of the life of the church. "A really Christian congregation, he thought, would be a fellowship of brethren gathered around the Lord's table, edified and nourished by Word and Sacrament, and led by a true shepherd of souls, a bishop in the New Testament sense of the term."[53]

His contributions flowed from these convictions. In 1849 he organized the "Society for Inner Missions in the Sense of the Lutheran Church" as the confessional counterpart to Wichern's movement and as part of his long struggle in Bavaria for a clear confessional basis for the church. He was particularly concerned about foreign missions, and from 1841 on he sent hundreds of pastors to North America to serve the German immigrants and to evangelize the Indians. In this work he was instrumental in establishing the Missouri and Iowa Synods in America. The Neuendettelsau Foreign Mission Society also trained ministers to serve German immigrants in Australia and Brazil. In the midst of all this work, Loehe also organized hospitals and, true to Luther's pastoral concern, continued to visit the sick in his village three times a day.[54]

Neuendettelsau remained influential in missionary and diaconal work into the twentieth century. In 1954, it challenged women to give one year of service to the physically and mentally ill. Similar "diaconic year" programs developed elsewhere, including many Third World countries. By the 1980s, Lutheran deaconesses were involved in ecumenical ministries and frequently belonged to the ecumenical International Federation of Deaconess Associations, called "Diakonia." A contemporary formulation of diaconal mission from the Evangelical Church in Germany reads:

> The Church has the mission to bear witness to God's love to the world in Jesus Christ to all persons. *Diakonia* is a form of this witness which cares for persons in bodily need, spiritual affliction, and who live in unjust social relationships. It also seeks to remove the causes of these afflictions. It addresses in ecumenical breadth individuals and groups, those near and far, Christian and non-Christian. Because alienation from God is the deepest affliction of persons and because salvation and well-being belong indivisibly together, *diakonia* takes place in word and deed as wholistic service to persons.[55]

It was reported in 1960 that there are approximately 60,000 deaconesses worldwide, the majority of whom are Lutheran. The 1978 statistics of the Lutheran deaconesses in West Germany list 95 motherhouses and 24,347 deaconesses.[56]

Although the Inner Mission and diaconal movements were not always concerned directly with health and medicine, they clearly saw that sickness and health were related to economic and social conditions, including work environments, discrimination, and joblessness. The conservative Lutheran tradition, which through the doctrine of the priesthood of all believers had stressed the vocation of the individual to serve the neighbor, gradually rediscovered Luther's awareness of the need to address social and political structures in terms of ethics and justice. By the late nineteenth century, there existed in some quarters the conviction that individual needs could not be separated from social structures and environmental conditions.

The politicization of Lutheran social programs in Germany resulted from the work of Adolf Christian Stoecker (1835–1909), who in the course of various pastoral responsibilities realized that the Inner Mission methods were not succeeding in bringing the laboring classes back into the church. Firmly grounded in Lutheran confessionalism, Stoecker argued:

It is essential that Christians carry the vision of the Kingdom of God into the world, working and struggling, so that as much as possible will be glorified in the light of Christ. Christians, then, cannot just authorize but must be engaged in the practice of Christian morality in the world, in order to win others and to endeavor to shape this world by the ideal of the Kingdom of God.[57]

For these reasons, as well as because of his patriotic reaction against the Marxists and Social Democrats, he organized in 1878 the Christian Socialist Workers Party. The party's program to renew and reform society called for obligatory pensions for widows, orphans, invalids, and the elderly, and the protection of workers from unsafe and unhealthful working conditions. Both in and out of the pulpit, Stoecker vigorously advocated his conviction that the causes of human misery must be addressed and changed.

His political party, however, soon foundered on the rocks of Marxist ridicule and the opposition of landowners and industrialists. To make matters worse, his close identification of the Christian faith with German nationalism had an ugly consequence in his anti-Semitic opposition to Jews as representatives of radical liberalism. "While seeking to Christianize politics," explains one author, "he had merely politicized Christianity."[58]

Another Lutheran pastor who entered politics to promote social reform was Friedrich von Bodelschwingh (1831–1910). Unlike Stoecker, however, Bodelschwingh believed that there could be no such thing as a "Christian state"; thus, he disapproved of organizing a "Christian Socialist" party. The death of his four children within two weeks in 1869 determined the future course of his life. In 1872 he accepted the directorship of the Rhenish-Westphalian home for epileptics and its small affiliated deaconess home. Named Bethel after the first building erected there in 1873, the center grew to include a training school for deacons, a theological school, and a nearby home for destitute workers. His view of suffering, strongly influenced by Luther's theology of the cross with its emphasis on unselfish love, and his concern for rehabilitation of the sick and the outcast led him to enter politics. Elected to the Prussian Diet in 1903, he secured passage of a law in 1907 that provided for homes for itinerant workers. By this time the government was favorable to such measures as possible means to undermine the socialist movement. Earlier Bismarck himself had said, "Give the working man the right to work as long as he is healthy, assure him care when he is sick, and maintenance when he is old. . . . If the state will show a little more Christian solicitude for the working man, then the socialists will sing their siren song in vain."[59]

Bodelschwingh's son, by the same name (1877–1946), succeeded him as administrator of Bethel. Under the younger Bodelschwingh's leadership the home was further enlarged, its medical facilities improved, and its research into treatment of epilepsy expanded. At the beginning of the German church struggle (the opposition to Hitler's effort to assimilate the church into the Nazi state), he was elected national bishop—only to have the election nullified by the Nazi state. He and his friends later led out in opposition to the Nazi proposal to destroy all "life that was not worthy of living" and thereby protected not only the physically and mentally handicapped residents of Bethel, but those of other institutions as well.[60]

Since World War II, Bethel has expanded to include a staff of nearly 3,000 responsible for over 4,000 sick, elderly, and physically and mentally handicapped persons. Wholistic service is pursued through the use of therapeutic teams comprised of physicians, teachers, pastors, physical and speech therapists, and psychologists who work with individuals and small groups including the families of the patients. The traditional Bethel ministry to epileptics has continued (some twenty-five percent of the residents and patients are epileptics). Over 300 scientific publications on epilepsy have come out of the clinical research at Bethel. The partnership of physicians and pastors in therapeutic teams extends to "open evenings" with patients and their families that provide forums for discussing issues of living, working, education, and sexuality. For these comprehensive rehabilitative activities, Bethel has frequently been characterized as an ecumenical, educational, and therapeutic model.[61]

The nineteenth-century European concern for institutions of mercy also found expression among Lutherans in America. In the United States, however, the church's charitable enterprises acquired a different flavor, because not only were church and state legally separate, but the American Lutherans were often foreign-speaking immigrants concerned mostly with taking care of their own. Wave after wave of immigration put added pressure on existing Lutheran institutions.[62] The foremost exponent of social concern among nineteenth-century Lutherans in America was the Pennsylvania pastor William Passavant (1821–1894), who, according to one source, has "the distinction of establishing the largest number of orphanages, hospitals, homes for the aged, and other institutions of mercy among Lutherans in America."[63] In 1849 he opened the first Lutheran hospital in America, in Pittsburgh; later he founded similar institutions in Milwaukee; Chicago; and Jacksonville, Illinois. Three years after visiting Kaiserswerth in 1846, he brought the deaconess movement to America. However, American deaconesses did not become popular until the mid-1880s, when seven German deaconesses joined the staff of the German (later, Lankenau) Hospital in Philadelphia, where the first motherhouse was established.

The Philadelphia Motherhouse of Deaconesses, patterned on the German Inner Mission institutions, created a hospital, home for the aged, children's hospital, girls' school, and kindergarten. Although the different Lutheran bodies in America established other deaconess motherhouses, usually in conjunction with hospitals, the diaconate never effectively took root. Reasons for this included financial exigencies and relative lack of structural support in America as compared to Europe; for example, the churches were not committed to the promotion and maintenance of this form of ministry until nearly the turn of the century. Furthermore, it had been stipulated in Europe that a deaconess remain unmarried in order to give full service to the church. European social restrictions reinforced this and also presented the diaconate as a respectable and honored vocation for women (who outnumbered men). American society almost from the beginning was less restrictive. Thus when Loehe sent some deaconesses to Iowa, they all soon married and he concluded that this was not an appropriate field for his deaconesses. In the twentieth century, increased opportunities of education, work, and social freedom have provided other vocational possibilities for women besides the diaconate.[64]

In the late nineteenth and early twentieth centuries, numerous Lutheran hospitals related to the deaconess movement appeared in areas with strong Lutheran communities. Institutions with a specific focus such as Ebenezer Mercy Institute in Brush, Colorado (1905) and Bethphage Mission in Axtell, Nebraska (1913) modeled their ministry to retarded and epileptic persons on the work of Bethel in Germany. It would take too much space to detail contemporary American Lutheran health care facilities. However, Martin Marty provided a helpful overview when he wrote:

> Annual volumes of the *Lutheran Health and Welfare Directory* canvass these agencies and suggest something of the scope of involvement. A code at the beginning of the volume points to the variety of services: six types for "services to the aging"; thirteen for "child welfare"; five for "family welfare"; three for "health services," including "general" and "special" hospital and "mental health clinic"; four services to handicapped adults; and many kinds of settlement and resettlement agencies. These codes connect with hundreds of identified institutions in North America. Those institutions do not begin to suggest the dimensions of care in modern Lutheranism. Congregations also may generate their own.[65]

The question of Lutheran identity for hospitals, however, became a critical one in the twentieth century. With the decline of the diaconate, rising costs for health care, and in many cases tenuous relationships to the churches stemming from the factors mentioned earlier and the fact that the original Lutheran immigrant communities once served had now dispersed by moving and assimilation, the validity as well as the viability of church-owned hospitals became more uncertain. In the late 1950s, Dr. Fredric Norstad, a Lutheran expert on hospitals, stated: "I no longer believe in Church-owned hospitals. I don't see that they are any different from any other hospital."[66] Indeed, many of the surviving Lutheran hospitals took on an increasingly ecumenical orientation.

The recent history of Lutheran involvement in health care reflects a deep-seated ambivalence. On the one hand, contemporary American Lutherans such as Granger Westberg and David Belgum have been in the forefront of modern contributions to the development of hospital chaplaincy, stressing the importance of medical and pastoral teamwork and the incorporation of multidisciplinary perspectives in caring and curing.[67] On the other hand, the Pietist legacy of an individualistic ethic positing social change through individual conversion has left a neurotic aversion to involving the church in political and legislative processes as well as a quietistic if not legalistic ethic.[68] As one of Lutheranism's more socially concerned educators said in 1919, "For Christians the stomach is always secondary to the soul."[69] Although this Pietist orientation has been overcome in much of contemporary Lutheranism, it still has a noteworthy if uncharacteristic expression among many Lutheran laypersons and in the present Lutheran charismatic movements.

A recent social research survey of Lutheran laity and clergy indicated both the continuing Pietist orientation of Lutherans and the differences in attitudes between laity and clergy. On the question of faith, 40 percent of the laity and 74 percent of the clergy understood faith as trust in God's grace, while 27 percent of the laity and 10 percent of the clergy associated faith with doing right. On personal and so-cial–ethical issues, the following percentages indicate, respectively, the lay and clergy responses of "always wrong" to: homosexual relations— 66 and 50 percent; premarital sexual intercourse—47 and 36 percent. On abortion, however, roughly 50 percent of both laity and clergy said it depends on the situation as to whether it is right or wrong. The research indicated a different picture on a major social issue: 73 percent of the laity and 85 percent of the clergy "favor" to "strongly favor" a "national program to improve health-care services and curtail rising health-care costs."[70]

In an essay interpreting these social research data, Timothy Lull wrote:

> But the meaning of our human sexuality is something that cries out for fresh interpretation and for relation to the fundamentals of our faith. Lutherans are rarely willing to say that God's laws must be obeyed blindly

and without understanding. Our hope rather is that one can come to see the reason for rules. . . . What is less clear is that any specifically Christian or even Lutheran response is being formulated to help persons deal with their own sexuality and with the issues that touch almost every family.[71]

It must be granted that Lutheran theological scholarship has not produced many substantive studies on sexuality and the family. Furthermore, significant studies such as Helmut Thielicke's *The Ethics of Sex* (1964) or William Lazareth's *Luther on the Christian Home* (1960) are not readily accessible to a lay readership.[72]

This perceived lack of Lutheran guidance has impelled minority Lutheran conservative groups to step into the breach with their own moral absolutes. One such group is the recently formed (1983) Fellowship of Evangelical Lutheran Laity and Pastors. Their "Affirmation of Faith" details what they stand against:

> . . . we stand against . . . the expression of ethical relativism within our churches, colleges, seminaries, social service agencies, and auxiliaries. We stand against the fruits of ethical relativism and call for specific discipline of those church leaders and agencies who condone and promote homosexual behavior, advocate abortion on request, approve and promote immoral sexual behavior and deny the biblical challenge to lead the new life in Christ.[73]

Equally controversial today has been the introduction of faith healing, previously a peripheral phenomenon in the Lutheran tradition, by Lutheran charismatic movements. (A notable exception to the church's traditional antipathy toward faith healing was the movement and center founded by Johann Christoph Blumhardt at Bad Boll, Germany, as the result of a famous exorcism and consequent religious revival in 1845.) The Lutheran charismatic leader Larry Christenson proclaims that "Though human reason cannot encompass its working, a simple believer can obediently bring the sick to the Lord—and they will experience God's healing power."[74] Despite their positive emphasis upon the relationship of healing to salvation, such claims upon God's power can induce confusion, guilt, and despair in those who expect healing directly, but do not receive it.[75]

On all levels of the church today, there is increased sensitivity to the issues of health and medicine. On the congregational level, where worship and pastoral visitation form the core expressions of the faith, there is a growing openness to ecumenical resources for caring and curing.[76] Congregations have more and more access to programmatic assistance ranging from printed materials to regional health mission projects.[77] The important role of the liturgy is exemplified in the new *Occasional Services* book (1982), issued by the American Lutheran churches, which includes psalms, prayers, and lessons not only for the traditional passages of life such as birth, baptism, marriage, and death, but also for such life crises as addiction, stillbirth, surgery, and sickness. "The occasional services provide more than helpful and even necessary forms for ministerial acts," explains one Lutheran. "Properly understood and employed, the services provide an entire course in pastoral theology . . . and a comprehensive expression of the church's care to those who are the recipients of the ministry which they embody."[78]

On the national level, Lutheran bodies have undertaken study projects and formulated statements on a variety of issues related to health and medicine. The Lutheran Church in America alone has, since its organization in 1962, issued statements on capital punishment, aging and the older adult, sex, marriage and the family, and ecology, to name but a few topics.[79] Its "Man, Medicine and Theology" series of pamphlets includes such titles as "Replacement Therapy," "Drug Use and Abuse," "The Ethics of Conception and Contraception," "The Problem of Abortion," and "Christian Faith and the Dying Patient." Its book *Health Care in America: A National Illness* (1974), as well as *A Study of the Healing Church and Its Ministry: The Health Care Apostolate,* by Ralph E. Peterson, indicates that the quietism so long associated with Lutheranism is being tempered by the recognition that social ethics and justice are crucial elements in the provision of health care. At the denomination's recent conference on health, healing, and health care, the conferees stated:

> As the church addresses faith questions it addresses societal issues. Health is not just the health of a whole person but of the whole society. Health is a part of the mending of creation, but it must always be seen in the larger context of justice. There will never be health or the right distribution of health care in the world without justice. Questions of employment, of economics, of distribution of resources, of war and peace, of participation in society must all be addressed in order to address the issues of health and health care.[80]

We began by emphasizing the strong and continuing influence of Luther and the Lutheran Confessions upon the faith and life of the Lutheran churches. This impact has been both nuanced and challenged by historical and cultural change, but remains a strong "feeling tone" among Lutherans. At their best, Lutherans have put a high premium on their tradition as a resource for the present. We have seen that the long suit of the Lutheran tradition has been in the areas of caring, curing, and life passages. Here the high priority that Lutherans have traditionally placed upon Scripture and sacraments, pastoral visitation, and mutual consolation through living the universal priesthood of all believers is clearly visible. The short suit of the Lutheran tradition has been in the realm of social ethics and justice. As impressive as the mission and service work of Pietism and the Inner Mission were, they had difficulty moving beyond responding to symptoms to addressing the root causes of those symptoms. This is not to gainsay the heroic efforts present in the Lutheran tradition, but to confess that it is mainly in our own time that the church has begun to take the vocation of doing justice as seriously as it has always taken caring and curing. Lutherans have learned and continue to learn from others in this area. They are also rediscovering their own Reformation roots for a faith active in justice as well as love. It is appropriate that the self-study conducted by the Lutheran World Federation related to this rediscovery is titled: *The Identity of the Church and Its Service to the Whole Human Being*.[81]

Notes

1. See, for example, Jaroslav Pelikan, ed., *Interpreters of Luther: Essays in Honor of Wilhelm Pauck* (Philadelphia, 1968); Walther von Loewenich, *Luther und der Neuprotestantismus* (Witten, 1963); and Heinrich Bornkamm, *Luther im Spiegel der deutschen Geistesgeschichte* (Göttingen, 1955).
2. Carter Lindberg, "Mask of God and Prince of Lies: Luther's Theology of the Demonic," in *Disguises of the Demonic: Contemporary Perspectives on the Power of Evil*, ed. Alan M. Olson (New York, 1975), pp. 87–103; and Eric W. Gritsch, *Martin—God's Court Jester: Luther in Retrospect* (Philadelphia, 1983), pp. 155–158.
3. See Aarne Siirala, *The Voice of Illness: A Study in Therapy and Prophecy* (Philadelphia, 1964).
4. Walther von Loewenich, *Luther's Theology of the Cross*, trans. Herbert J. A. Bouman (Minneapolis, 1976), pp. 17ff.
5. *Lutheran Book of Worship* (Philadelphia, 1978), hymn number 228; and see Helmar Junghans, "Luther in Wittenberg," in *Leben und Werk Martin Luthers von 1526–1546*, ed. Helmar Junghans (Berlin, 1983), p. 19.
6. Helmut T. Lehmann and Jaroslav Pelikan, eds., *Luther's Works*, 55 vols. (Philadelphia, 1955), 26:387.
7. Theodore Tappert, ed., *Luther: Letters of Spiritual Counsel* (Philadelphia, 1955), pp. 46–47.
8. *Luther's Works*, 25:260.
9. Ibid. 43:124–125.
10. Ibid. 43:131.
11. Siirala, *The Voice of Illness*, p. 130.
12. *Luther's Works*, 42:101–102, 112.
13. Carter Lindberg, " 'There Should Be No Beggars Among Christians': Karlstadt, Luther, and the Origins of Protestant Poor Relief," *Church History* 46 (1977):313–334; see also George Rosen, *Madness in Society: Chapters in the Historical Sociology of Mental Illness* (New York, 1969), pp. 142, 159–160.

14. *Luther's Works,* 54:296; Edward P. de G. Chaney, " 'Philanthropy in Italy': English Observations on Italian Hospitals, 1545–1789," in *Aspects of Poverty in Early Modern Europe,* ed. Thomas Riis (Stuttgart, 1981), pp. 183–217.

15. See Thomas S. Kuhn, *The Structure of Scientific Revolutions* (Chicago, 1970).

16. *D. Martin Luthers Werke* (Weimar, 1883), 5:163.

17. *Luther's Works,* 54:50–51; see also Lewis W. Spitz, *The Renaissance and Reformation Movements* (Chicago, 1971), p. 582; and Harold J. Grimm, *The Reformation Era, 1500–1650* (New York, 1973), pp. 476–480.

18. Owsei Temkin, *The Double Face of Janus and Other Essays in the History of Medicine* (Baltimore, 1977), p. 74.

19. Joseph Needham, "The Pattern of Nature–Mysticism and Empiricism in the Philosophy of Science," in *Science, Medicine and History: Essays on the Evolution of Scientific Thought and Medical Practice written in Honor of Charles Singer,* 2 vols., ed. E.A. Underwood (London, 1953), vol. 2, p. 382.

20. See Robert Kolb, *Casper Peucer's Library: Portrait of a Wittenberg Professor of the Mid–Sixteenth Century* (St. Louis, 1976), pp. 2, 5, 12–13.

21. See Werner Elert, *Morphologie des Luthertums,* 2 vols. (Munich, 1931), vol. 2, pp. 407–408.

22. *Luther's Works,* 21:237.

23. Steven Ozment, *The Age of Reform 1250–1550: An Intellectual and Religious History of Late Medieval and Reformation Europe* (New Haven, CT, 1980), p. 381.

24. *Luther's Works,* 54:441.

25. Rudolf Thiel, "The Truth About Luther's Marriage," trans. Gustav K. Wiencke, *Lutheran Church Quarterly* 19 (1946):167–174, quotation on p. 174. See also, William Lazareth, *Luther on the Christian Home: An Application of the Social Ethics of the Reformation* (Philadelphia, 1960).

26. See Miriam Usher Chrisman, *Lay Culture, Learned Culture: Books and Social Change in Strasbourg, 1480–1599* (New Haven, CT, 1982); and Kenneth Thibodeau, "Science and the Reformation: The Case of Strasbourg," *Sixteenth Century Journal* 7 (1976):35–50.

27. Ernst Walter Schmidt, "Luther und das Bittgebet: Ein Beitrag zur Phänomenologie und Theologie des Gebets," *Luther* 40 (1969):1–12, account on pp. 1–4.

28. John T. McNeill, *A History of the Cure of Souls* (New York, 1951), p. 163.

29. *Luther's Works,* 54:17–18.

30. Tappert, *Luther,* p. 17.

31. Roland Bainton, *Here I Stand: A Life of Martin Luther* (New York, 1955), p. 299.

32. Vilmos Vajta, "Luther als Beter," in Junghans, *Leben und Werk,* pp. 279–295, p. 294.

33. See Heiko A. Oberman, *Luther: Mensch Zwischen Gott und Teufel* (Berlin, 1982), p. 344.

34. Jaroslav Pelikan, *From Luther to Kierkegaard: A Study in the History of Theology* (St. Louis, 1963), p. 80.

35. Ibid., pp. 78–79; James A. Scherer, . . . *that the Gospel may be sincerely preached throughout the world: A Lutheran Perspective on Mission and Evangelism in the 20th Century* (Geneva, 1982), pp. 16–19.

36. McNeill, *A History of the Cure of Souls*, p. 182.

37. Bruce Wrightsman, "Lutheranism and the Protestant Synthesis: Religion and Science in America," in *The Lutheran Church in North American Life*, ed. John E. Groh and Robert H. Smith (St. Louis, 1979), pp. 59–97, quotation on p. 66.

38. George W. Forell, ed., *Christian Social Teachings: A Reader in Christian Social Ethics from the Bible to the Present* (Minneapolis, 1971), pp. 262–264.

39. Eckhard Altmann, *Christian Friedrich Richter (1676–1711): Arzt, Apotheker und Liederdichter des Halleschen Pietismus* (Witten, 1972), p. 46.

40. Ibid., p. 43.

41. Friedrich Schleiermacher, *On Religion: Speeches to its Cultured Despisers*, trans. John Oman (New York, 1958), p. 88; and *idem, The Christian Faith*, eds. H.R. Mackintosh and J.S. Stewart (New York, 1963), pp. 71–73, 178–184.

42. Altmann, *Christian Friedrich Richter*, p. 135.

43. Hans-Werner Gensichen, " 'Dienst der Seelen' und 'Dienst des Leibes' in der frühen pietistischen Mission," in *Der Pietismus in Gestalten und Wirkungen: Martin Schmidt zum 65. Geburtstag*, ed. Heinrich Bornkamm, et al. (Bielefeld, 1975), pp. 155–178.

44. John N. Ritter, "Muhlenberg's Anticipation of Psychosomatic Medicine," *Lutheran Church Quarterly* 19 (1946):181–188, quotation on p. 186; and Ronald L. Numbers and Ronald C. Sawyer, "Medicine and Christianity in the Modern World," in *Health/Medicine and the Faith Traditions*, eds. Martin E. Marty and Kenneth L. Vaux (Philadelphia, 1982), p. 141.

45. Franklin Sherman, "Secular Calling and Social Ethical Thinking," in *The Lutheran Church Past and Present*, ed. Vilmos Vajta (Minneapolis, 1977), pp. 185–205, quotation on p. 201.

46. McNeill, *A History of the Cure of Souls*, pp. 186–187; Julius Bodensieck, ed., *The Encyclopedia of the Lutheran Church*, 3 vols. (Philadelphia, 1965), vol. 2, p. 984.

47. See J.F. Ohl, *The Inner Mission* (Philadelphia, 1911), pp. 65ff.

48. See Gerald Christianson, "J. H. Wichern and the Rise of the Lutheran Social Institution," *Lutheran Quarterly* 19 (1967):357–370.

49. Ibid., p. 369.

50. Ohl, *The Inner Mission*, p. 60.

51. Frederick S. Weiser, *1884–1984: To Serve the Lord and His People: Celebrating the Heritage of a Century of Lutheran Deaconesses in America* (Gladwyne, PA, 1984), p. 51.

52. Harry Wain, *A History of Preventive Medicine* (Springfield, IL, 1970), p. 213.

53. *Encyclopedia of the Lutheran Church*, 2:1332; see Hans Rössler, *Unter Stroh- und Ziegeldächern: Aus der Neuendettelsauer Geschichte* (Neuendettelsau, 1982).

54. McNeill, *A History of the Cure of Souls*, p. 187.

55. Hans Christoph von Hase, "Arbeitsfelder heutiger Diakonie," in *Theologische Realenzyklopädie*, vol. 8 (Berlin, 1981), pp. 660–679, quotation on p. 660.

56. Ibid., pp. 674–677; *Encyclopedia of the Lutheran Church*, 1:664.

57. Ronald L. Massanari, "Christian Socialism: Adolf Stoecker's Formulation of a Christian Perspective for Social Change for the Protestant Church in Nineteenth Century Germany," *Lutheran Quarterly* 22 (1970):185–198, quotation on p. 185.
58. *Encyclopedia of the Lutheran Church,* 3:2267.
59. Ibid., 3:2202.
60. Bernhard Gramlich, *Friedrich von Bodelschwingh: Werk und Leben* (Stuttgart, 1981), pp. 41, 76.
61. Ibid., pp. 12–14, 32, 44, 52–54, 70.
62. See F. Dean Lueking, *A Century of Caring: The Welfare Ministry Among Missouri Synod Lutherans 1868–1968* (St. Louis, 1968).
63. August R. Suelflow and E. Clifford Nelson, "Following the Frontier, 1840–1875," in *The Lutherans in North America,* ed. E.C. Nelson (Philadelphia, 1975), pp. 147–251, quotation on p. 197.
64. Weiser, *1884–1984,* pp. 12, 14, 26–27.
65. Martin E. Marty, *Health and Medicine in the Lutheran Tradition* (New York, 1983), p. 79; see also Ross T. Wilbur and Helen T. Novak, eds., *Lutheran Health and Welfare Agencies and Institutions* (New York, 1976).
66. Lawrence Holst, "25 Years: Chance or Destiny? Luck or Grace?" *Chronicle of Pastoral Care* 3 (1983):3–5; Kenneth L. Vaux, *Lutheran General Hospital: An Institution Intent on a Moral Purpose* (Park Ridge, IL, 1980), pp. 15ff.
67. David A. Buehler, "Caring, Curing, Calling: The Minister and the Ministry of Healing," *LCA Partners* 3 (1981):7–9, 25.
68. Ulrich Duchrow, ed., *Lutheran Churches—Salt or Mirror of Society?* (Geneva, 1977), pp. 243–252; Merton P. Strommen, ed., *A Study of Generations* (Minneapolis, 1972); Roger A. Johnson, ed., *Views from the Pews: Christian Beliefs and Attitudes* (Philadelphia, 1983).
69. Fred Meuser, "Facing the Twentieth Century, 1900–1930," in Nelson, *The Lutherans in North America,* pp. 359–449, quotation on p. 419.
70. Johnson, *Views from the Pews,* pp. 224, 237.
71. Ibid., p. 140.
72. Helmut Thielicke, *The Ethics of Sex,* trans. John W. Doberstein (New York, 1964); William Lazareth, *Luther on the Christian Home.*
73. Fellowship of Evangelical Lutheran Laity and Pastors, 1200 69th Avenue North, Brooklyn Center, MN 55430.
74. Larry Christenson, *The Charismatic Renewal Among Lutherans* (Minneapolis, 1976), p. 104.
75. See Marty, *Health and Medicine,* pp. 86–97; Carter Lindberg, *The Third Reformation? Charismatic Movements and the Lutheran Tradition* (Macon, GA, 1983), pp. 231ff.; and Hubert Kirchner et al., eds., *Charismatische Erneuerung und Kirche* (Neukirchen-Vluyn, 1984), pp. 163–168.
76. Andre Birmele, ed., *Local Ecumenism* (Geneva, 1984). See also F. Dean Lueking, "The Congregation: Place of Healing and Sending," in Marty and Vaux, *Health/Medicine,* pp. 273–291.
77. See, for example, H. Jill Westberg, *Starting a Health Cabinet in Your Church: A Challenging Approach for Revitalizing the Healing Ministry of the Congregation* (Hinsdale, IL, 1981); Frederick J. Schenk and J.V. Anderson, *Aging Together, Serving Together: A Guide to Congregational Planning for the Aging* (Minneapolis, 1982); Floramae Geiser, "A Healthy Difference," *The Lutheran* (June 19, 1985):12–14.

78. Philip Pfatteicher, *Commentary on the Occasional Services* (Philadelphia, 1983), pp. xii–xiii.

79. Available from the Division for Mission in North America of the Lutheran Church in America, 231 Madison Avenue, New York, NY 10016.

80. "Findings: The LCA Conference on Health, Healing, and Health Care" (New York, n.d.), p. 1; Harold C. Letts, ed., *Health Care in America: A National Illness* (New York, 1974); Ralph E. Peterson, *A Study of the Healing Church and Its Ministry: The Health Care Apostolate* (New York, 1982); Ulrich Eibach, *Medizin und Menschenwürde: Ethische Probleme der Medizin aus christlicher Sicht* (Wuppertal, 1976).

81. *The Identity of the Church and Its Service to the Whole Human Being,* 2 vols. (Geneva, 1977). See also John Reumann, ed., *The Church Emerging: A U.S. Lutheran Case Study* (Philadelphia, 1977).

CHAPTER 7

The Reformed

Tradition

JAMES H. SMYLIE

The World Alliance of Reformed Churches (Presbyterian and Congregational) numbers within its membership 157 different bodies found in over eighty countries and claims an estimated membership of seventy million people. The Alliance, organized in 1875, represents the spread of the Reformed tradition around the world and offers an opportunity for member churches to discuss and act upon matters of mutual and global interest.

As indicated by the number of members of this body, the Reformed tradition is a complex one. While those in the tradition identify themselves as Christians who confess with the major Christian communions that the church of Jesus Christ is "one, holy, catholic, and apostolic," this particular family of Christians traces its origins to the European Reformation in the sixteenth and seventeenth centuries. Unlike the Lutheran movement before it and the Wesleyan movement afterward, those who identify themselves with the Reformed tradition acknowledge a number of important persons and experiences as part of this Reformation legacy. John Calvin (1509–1564), however, was the single most important figure in the Reformed tradition. Calvin's impact was through his personality, his large correspondence, his many commentaries on the Bible, his *Institutes of the Christian Religion* (1536), and his concern for the reform of life in Geneva. The Reformed movement spread widely in Europe to France, Germany, Holland, Hungary, Poland, England,

Scotland, Ireland, and to America, represented by New England Puritans, Presbyterians, and the Dutch Reformed. Moreover, Calvinists, as the Reformed are often called, produced a number of doctrinal statements to express their beliefs and attitudes toward life, for example, the Gallican Confession (1559), the Scots Confession (1560), the Heidelberg Catechism (1563), the Belgic Confession (1574), and the Westminster Confession and Catechisms (1648), the latter of which had the most widespread influence in Scotland and the United States.

Although this variety of Reformed experiences points to richness of confessional expressions, those in the Reformed tradition have been known for emphasizing several important aspects of Christian belief. They are Trinitarians who have stressed the belief that all things, whether in the natural world or in human affairs, are governed by God's creative and providential powers, that the whole of human life should be brought under the subjection of God's sovereign will, and that there is no genuine health or freedom unless God's reign is fulfilled and manifest. With regard to subjection to God's will, those in the tradition have also placed an emphasis upon the person and work of Christ in the redemptive process. God, according to Calvinists drawing upon the Hebrew and Christian Scriptures, has entered into covenants with human beings. One covenant was with Adam. This was a covenant of works and the law which· men and women have broken and continue to break; the other covenant is one of grace under Jesus Christ who has, through his life and person, restored human beings freely to a right relationship with God. The nature and manner of this restoration has been interpreted in different ways throughout Reformed history according to the variety of images in the Scriptures. Calvinists have also stressed that the Scriptures referred to here are the supreme rule of faith and life for the Christian when God's Spirit witnesses to those things that have to do with law, grace, the restoration of our right relationship with God, and responsibilities to the neighbor. Thus, all formulations of worship and Reformed life are subject to this standard and to Jesus Christ, who is witnessed to in the Scriptures. Moreover, those in the Reformed tradition have also stressed the vocation of the Christian to bring all personal and public life into obedience to God's will for "God's glory and the common good," according to the Westminster Confession of Faith.

Calvinists have also made much of the importance of the Christian church, under Jesus Christ who is the head, confession of whom provides for the church's continuity, together with the interpretation of the Bible and the administration of the two sacraments of Baptism and the Lord's Supper. The Triune God calls the church into existence and makes it faithful and visible. While believing in the priesthood of all Christian believers, those in the tradition organized the church in various ways, but primarily under the offices of pastors, teachers, elders, and deacons, and also under councils of the congregations and of presbyteries, synods, and general assemblies, which include representatives of clergy and laity. Elders and deacons are laity who have responsibility for governance in the church and physical as well as spiritual care of congregations. While some in the Reformed tradition have allowed the episcopal office and others have been congregational in polity, most have governed themselves under a representative system. There has always been a strong sense of the one holy, catholic, and apostolic church, and the Reformed have been leaders in the modern ecumenical movement. Various Reformed bodies have developed numerous agencies for educational, mission, and charitable purposes, including hospitals, retirement homes, and orphanages, for example.

As already indicated, the Reformed family is located in many countries around the world. In the United States, the largest members of the World Alliance of Reformed Churches are the Presbyterian Church, formed by the union of the United Presbyterian Church in the United States of America and the Presbyterian Church in the United States, with a membership of 2,342,441; the United Church of Christ (which traces its ancestry through the Congregationalists and the Puritans of New England and the Evangelical and Reformed Church), with 1,716,723 members; and the Reformed Church of America, Dutch in ancestry, with a membership of 346,293 (figures from the *Yearbook of American and Canadian Churches, 1984*).

In 1960 the General Assembly of the United Presbyterian Church in the United States of America adopted a major report entitled "The Relation of Christian Faith to Health." Written by pastors and physicians, the report opens with these affirmations:

> The redemption which God in Jesus Christ brings to the world through his Church is sufficient for the ultimate conquest of every evil. . . . Among the evils from which God in Christ is able to redeem man are the myriad forms of physical and mental illness. It is plainly the understanding of the New Testament that health in body, mind and spirit is the ultimate will of God. To be sure, God can use any untoward circumstance for man's spiritual upbuilding and his own glory. But the consistent attitude of Jesus Christ and the apostles toward illnesses is one of positive conquest. The conquest of various diseases and infirmities is one of the chief evidences given in the New Testament for believing that God in Christ is overcoming the power of evil. . . . The Church of Jesus Christ has a ministry to the sick which cannot be compartmentalized or delimited. Our ministry is not to "souls" in abstraction; our ministry is to men in their totality as creatures whose lives need to be filled with the power of God.[1]

In these affirmations and in the historical portions of the study, Presbyterians illustrate the way in which communicants in the Reformed tradition confess God revealed in the Hebrew and Christian Scriptures and in Jesus Christ, and identify with his Apostles. While it is essential to remember that those in the Reformed tradition think of themselves as a part of the larger Christian family, the "one, holy, catholic, and apostolic church," they have been and may be considered as distinct members of that family.

In terms of this historical analysis, the Reformed tradition and those in it who are often called Calvinists may be considered in two ways. First of all, the tradition may be seen as one that has some distinctive traits, influenced by Calvin, yet nevertheless a very complex one because of the number of places to which this tradition spread and the variety of ways in which those in the tradition expressed their Christian faith and life. John T. McNeill indicated this in his volumes on *The History and Character of Calvinism* (1954), and more to the point, in *A History of the Cure of Souls* (1951), in which he places variations of the Reformed tradition in the whole context of Christian history.[2] While aware of this way of identifying the Reformed tradition and alert to some of its most influential thinkers from Calvin to Karl Barth in the twentieth century, Kenneth L. Vaux suggests a second approach in *Health and Medicine in the Reformed Tradition* (1984). Using the typology of H. Richard Niebuhr, Vaux suggests that those in the tradition have a view of nature and grace that allows Calvinists to look at the subject of health and healing in a dynamic manner and in terms of God's call to Christians to a ministry of reconciliation and the transformation of the world as responsible human beings.[3] In this study, we shall keep in mind various ethnic and confessional lines as well as this theological insight of Vaux. Moreover, we shall refer most frequently to American Presbyterians to illustrate some of the continuities and continuing debates within the Reformed faith about health and healing. Because Calvinists think of themselves as Christians first, and identify themselves with the ideas and endeavors of other Christians, it is sometimes difficult to sort out what is distinctive in terms of this subject.

We shall look first at the way in which the early Reformed thought of God as the Great Physician from whom all healing comes, and who has provided through Jesus Christ teachings about life, victory over death, and means to care for and cure one another in times of sickness. In subsequent sections we shall deal with certain Reformed emphases that emerge in the history of the tradition and also of medicine: the quest for longer life through healing vocations and institutions, and the moral uses of suffering; the search for an abundant life through self-acceptance, shepherding, and sexual fulfillment. We shall then conclude by reviewing certain affirmations about some of the problems of health that have arisen in our time with the development of medical technology, including a holistic approach to the subject and the attempt to distribute health care in a just manner.

God the Physician: Death, Life, and the Use of Means

The formative period of the Reformed tradition stretched from the earliest years of the sixteenth century, covering the life and work of Calvin and his earliest followers, to the middle of the seventeenth century, when the Westminster standards, so important to American Presbyterians, took shape. During these years, death swallowed up many in war, disease, and pestilence. The mortality rate was high. Although medical knowledge and practice were still primitive by modern criteria, the scientific revolution that occurred along with the spiritual revolution of the period foreshadowed profound changes for the future. While it is dangerous to generalize about so diverse a tradition as the Reformed, we may discern several important dimensions of the relation between faith and health that Calvinists shared in common: God is the Physician who heals our infirmities. Health involves the whole of life shaped by the hope that God has given through Christ's victory over death. Moreover, health is an aspect of life together in the body of Christ, by the ministry of the Word of preaching and sacraments, by the disciplined life, and by the means of medical science.

John Calvin emerged as the theologian of the sovereignty of God. Only when human beings know God as Creator, Provider, Redeemer, Sanctifier, Judge, and Victor do they know themselves and the covenants that God has made with them and in which God has called them to live as responsible creatures.[4] In his *Institutes,* Calvin called attention to human dependence upon God and to God as the source of health:

> Now the great thing is this: we are consecrated and dedicated to God in order that we may thereafter think, speak, meditate, and do nothing except to his glory . . . . We are God's: let us therefore live for him and die for him. We are God's: let his wisdom and will therefore rule all our actions. We are God's: let all the parts of our life accordingly strive toward him as our only lawful goal. O, how much has that man profited who, having been taught that he is not his own, has taken away dominion and rule from his own reason that he may yield it to God! For, as consulting our self-interest is the pestilence that most effectively leads to our destruction, so the sole haven of salvation is to be wise in nothing and to will nothing through ourselves to follow the leading of the Lord alone.[5]

Calvin taught that God's creation is good. God created us, male and female, in God's image, and called us good. Moreover, God is a God of order, not of chaos. Calvin took sin, personal and corporate, seriously, and he related suffering and ill health to idol-making and self-interest contrary to God's covenants with creatures.[6] While Calvin was too good a biblical interpreter and theologian to blame God or human sinfulness as the direct cause of afflictions, he did hold that ultimately afflictions are related to breaking covenants that God has made with human beings. No affliction, however, is beyond God's concern or desire to heal. God uses affliction to chastise us, to make us depend upon him, and to bring us back to his will and ways. As Calvin observed, "The heavenly physician treats some more gently but cleanses others by harsher remedies, while he wills to provide for the health of all, he yet leaves no one free and untouched, because he knows that all, to a man, are diseased."[7]

In Calvin's writing, God appears as the Great Physician. Through Jesus Christ, the Genevan wrote, God gives human beings one who shares afflictions of flesh and blood, gives signs of God's desire for our good health, reconciles to God, and calls persons to be reconciled in love with one another. Through Jesus Christ, God gives victory over sin and death through Christ's resurrection and the promise of the coming and presence of God's kingdom, where there will be no mourning, or crying, or death.[8] The Reformed, therefore, gave thanks to God, as did the writers of the Heidelberg Catechism in their very first question:

Q. What is your only comfort, in life and in death?

A. That I belong—body and soul, in life and in death—not to myself but to my faithful Saviour, Jesus Christ, who at the cost of his own blood has fully paid for all my sins and has completely freed me from the dominion of the devil; that he protects me so well that without the will of my Father in heaven not a hair can fall from my head; indeed, that everything must fit his purpose for my salvation. Therefore, by his Holy Spirit, He also assures me of eternal life, and makes me wholeheartedly willing and ready from now on to live for him.[9]

Christians learn of this health through the Scriptures, which teach how to live and die in Christ's comfort, how great is sin, how believers are freed from sins and their "wretched consequences," and how they are to thank God for such a redemption.[10] Then, as the first words of the Westminster Catechism put it, life's chief end is to "glorify God and enjoy Him forever."[11]

Calvinists stressed life within the Christian community, the body of Christ, as a means of health. In the church, people meet Christ, the Word, witnessed to by the Holy Spirit in the Scriptures and in preaching. In the church, people receive the benefits of the sacraments of Baptism and the Lord's Supper. In the church, people learn discipleship, and how to bear one another's burdens. First of all, Calvin felt that health, physical and spiritual, is shaped by the believer's hearing and receiving the Word. He made preaching one of the marks of the Christian community. At the time of the Reformation, Calvinists rediscovered and reenvisioned Christian salvation and life through studying and interpreting the Scriptures. Furthermore, Calvin considered the proper administration of the sacraments as a mark of the church, although he rejected the Roman Catholic inclusion of confirmation, marriage, penance, ordination, and extreme unction as among them. About the latter, Calvin said that presbyters had an obligation to pray over the sick in such a way as to indicate that healing is a gift, that it comes from God, and that such prayer has to do with "forgiveness of sins and easing of bodily sickness, not the salvation of the soul at death," as Roman Catholics contended.[12] In Baptism, which embraces children as well as adults in Christ's covenant, Christians die and are raised with Christ and share in the benefits of Christ's body. At the Eucharist, or Lord's Supper, always to be accompanied by the preaching of the Word, Christ comes to dwell in the believer and the believer in Christ by the power of the Holy Spirit. Such dwelling-in and in-dwelling of the Word are the true sources of our health. Reflecting on the importance of the preached word and the sacraments, John Knox of Scotland, Calvin's contemporary and friend, spoke of the Lord's Supper as "a singular medicine for all poor sick creatures, a comfortable help to weak souls; and that our Lord requireth no other worthiness on our part, but that we unfeignedly acknowledge our sinfulness and imperfection."[13]

That Calvin and his followers took seriously the relationship between the total outlook of the Christian and health may be seen in directions found in the "Ecclesiastical Ordinances" (1541) of Geneva. The city magistrates declared that the sick should go no longer than three full days without calling upon a pastor for consolation. Yet they admonished that the sick should call for the minister at times when they would not "distract him from that office in which he and his colleagues serve the Church in common."[14] Thus, while ministers were to show concern for the afflicted, they were responsible for contributing to the health of all through the ministry of the Word.

Discipline also contributed to health. Christians, Calvinists believed, are to encourage one another to live according to God's laws, found in nature and also in the Ten Commandments. While Calvin taught that God used the law as a means of judgment and for bringing us to Christ, he also believed that the law is God's gift and continues to be essential for the Christian life of freedom and responsibility.[15] Discipline, or disciplining, was not considered a mark of the true church in all Reformed communities, but discipline was exercised in churches where Calvin's influence was felt. It was considered an aspect of the healthy life lived to God's glory. Discipline by church authorities, pastors in cooperation with elders, was exercised by visitation and by appearance before and examination by these officials. While discipline may have been abused at times, it was supposed to contribute to the health of the Christian and of the church. Calvin taught his disciples to interpret commandments having to do with our duties to God, to the neighbor, and to ourselves, negatively, in terms of what is prohibited, and positively, in terms of what is required of us. Requirements of the commandment "Thou shall not kill," as interpreted in the Westminster Larger Catechism, are instructive. The emphasis is on the respect for life, avoidance of temptation, advocacy of temperance, and the fruits of the Holy Spirit for the enhancement of life. Calvinists are required

> to preserve the life of ourselves and others, by resisting all thoughts and purposes, subduing all passions, and avoiding all occasions, temptations, and practices, which tend to the unjust taking away the life of any; by just defense therefore against violence; patient bearing of the hand of God; quietness of mind, cheerfulness of spirit, a sober use of meat, drink, physic, sleep, labor, and recreation; by charitable thoughts, love, compassion, meekness, gentleness, kindness; peaceable, mild, and courteous speeches and behavior; forbearance, readiness to be reconciled, patient bearing and forgiving of injuries, and requiting good for evil; comforting and succoring the distressed, and protecting and defending the innocent.[16]

Here Christians are warned against gluttony, drunkenness, addiction, even skewing life's rhythms by extremes of work and play.

In the treatment of the commandment about adultery, the authors of the Larger Catechism affirmed sexual drives as good gifts of God. Although Calvinists denied that marriage is a sacrament, they considered it God's high calling for clergy as well as for laity. They warned against the lust of body and the eye as dangerous to one's health. God gives man and woman to one another not merely for the purposes of procreation, but for cohabitation and conjugal love, according to the early teaching of Calvinists. Realistic about sexual power and perversion, Calvinists considered a wholesome sexual relationship an aspect of good health, the "chaste love of matrimony" as a second kind of virginity. Calvinists stressed moderation as an aspect of good health primarily because improper attachment to and love of the things of this world constitute idolatry and a source of affliction in this life.[17]

Calvin joined other Reformers in dignifying lay as well as clerical vocations, underscoring the usefulness in God's sight of many callings. Having given to us the good gift of creation, God calls those made in the divine image to participate in creative activity. In this connection, Calvin expressed thanks to God for all means by which Christians deal with suffering, especially through physicians and physic. Christians should not "cease to take counsel," he wrote, "nor be sluggish in beseeching the assistance" of those who "have means to help us."

Christians are to consider "whatever creatures are capable of furnishing anything to us as offered by the Lord" and as "lawful instruments of divine providence."[18] Calvin attacked those who spread the untruth that physicians and medicine come from evil spirits. Anyone with an "ounce of brains," even a pagan, he wrote, knows that these are gifts of God.[19] Like the writer of *Ecclesiasticus* (38:1–15) in the Apocrypha and Paul, who honored Luke (*Col.* 4:14), Calvin honored those who studied medicine and dispensed physic. In Geneva he encouraged the upgrading of medical care in the hospitals, which were supported at city expense so that even the poor might receive treatment. Pastors visited the sick and drew lots for the chaplaincy of those with contagious diseases. The city magistrates exempted Calvin from this latter duty because of his importance to the welfare of the whole city. His letters indicate the breadth of his sympathies. Deacons, assisted by women, took over the service of the sick, which had been interrupted when the religious orders were dissolved because of the hostility toward Roman Catholic institutions.[20]

Because life for most people was hard and short during these centuries, Calvinists emphasized the importance of a Christian death and triumph over the last enemy. According to the instructions in *The Directory for the Worship of God* (1644) of the Westminster Assembly, ministers have a duty to "admonish" Christians "in time of health to prepare for death."[21] Presbyterians and Puritans in the British Isles and in New England took this seriously. Richard Baxter (1615–1691), for example, a pastor who dispensed medical advice, instructed all ministers to preach as a dying man to dying men. He gave extensive "Directions for the Sick" in the *Christian Directory.* He encouraged the sick to seek out the best of physicians, as God's appointed "means of life," yet also to be prepared to meet incurable diseases and to face mortality. He was especially concerned for sinners whose ignorance and unbelief made sickness a "dungeon of darkness." He encouraged faith, repentance, humility, and hope in Christ so that Christians may die well. He gave instructions on how the sick might instruct the well, and the well may minister to the sick, giving sensitive consideration to the circumstances in which people find themselves during affliction. Baxter discussed also what he called "melancholy and overmuch sorrow," sorrow, even for sin, that may swallow a person up. He prescribed, among other things, comfort for the spirit and medicine, including a special diet for the body. This Puritan clergyman counseled those suffering from melancholy to remember above all things that "God's goodness is equal to his greatness," that God is "essentially love itself."[22]

Cotton Mather (1663–1728), Baxter's younger contemporary, also practiced some medicine, in New England. Mather gained a reputation in the Old World as well as the New for advocating inoculation for smallpox during an epidemic and for encouraging and supporting the physician Zabdiel Boylston in carrying out an early and successful experiment in immunization. While the population and other physicians abused him and Boylston for this experiment, the clergy of New England supported him.[23] Mather also wrote *The Angel of Bethesda,* the first book of medicine written on this side of the Atlantic, but published posthumously in the twentieth century. God is the Great Physician, Mather proclaimed. Sin is the ultimate cause of sickness and disease, and affects both body and soul. Health involves caring for both. Temperance, according to Mather, appealing to ancient Christian traditions, is the best way to stay well. Mather knew *Ecclesiasticus* and underscored the fact that God has given means for spiritual and physical health. While he wrote of health and healing, he knew about the precarious conditions of life, and also about the uncertain and contradictory advice of physicians who often do not know what they are doing. Therefore, Mather cautioned all Christians to look in faith and hope to God:

> O *Thou afflicted,* and under Distemper, Go to *Physicians* in *Obedience* to God, who has commanded the *Use of Means.* But place thy *Dependence* on God alone to Direct and Prosper them. And know, that they are all *Physicians of no* Value, if He do not so. Consult with *Physicians;* But in full Perswasion *[sic],* That if God leave them to their own *Counsels,* thou shall only *Suffer many Things from them;* They will do thee more *Hurt* than *Good.* Be Sensible, *Tis from God, and not from the Physician, that my Cure is to be Looked for.*[24]

Despite this caution, Mather gave impetus to the development of medical science by encouraging scientific observation and experimentation with the means of nature that God has given for health and healing and by blessing those called to practice medicine.[25]

Christians are to call upon God in afflictions and in the shadow of death, the sting of which is sin. "God of all comfort!" Calvin urged his followers to pray,

> We commend to thee those whom thou art pleased to visit and chasten with any cross of tribulation; the nations whom thou dost afflict with pestilence, war, or famine; all persons oppressed with poverty, imprisonment, sickness, banishment, or any other distress of body or sorrow of mind: That it may please Thee to show them thy fatherly kindness, chastening them for their profit; to the end that in their hearts they may turn unto thee, and being converted, may receive perfect consultation, and deliverance from all their woes.[26]

God may "chasten some with harshness," to use Calvin's words. Therefore, Christians must learn the meaning of suffering. Samuel Rutherford,

Scottish Presbyterian, counseled a bereaved mother with a succinct approach to such an experience and the meaning of suffering:

> This school of all suffering is a preparation for the King's higher house; and let all your visitations speak all the letters of your Lord's summons. They cry—1. "O vain world!" 2. "O bitter sin!" 3. "O short and uncertain time!" 4. "O fair eternity, that is above sickness and death!" 5. "O kingly and princely Bridegroom, hasten glory's marriage, shorten time's short-spun and soon broken thread, and conquer sin!" 6. "O happy and blessed death, that golden bridge laid over by Christ my Lord, between time's clay-banks and Heaven's shore! And the Spirit and the Bride say, 'Come!' and answer ye with them, 'Even so, come, Lord Jesus! Come quickly!' "[27]

So God, the Great Physician, gives health with the final victory over death and the establishment of God's kingdom where there will be no tears and no death.

Longer Life: Vocations, Institutions, and the Moral Use of Suffering

In the eighteenth century and well into the nineteenth century, those in the Reformed tradition (along with other people) were still preoccupied with death, and Calvinists still found much comfort in the words of a Puritan like Baxter. At the end of the eighteenth century, American Presbyterians recognized in a prayer recommended for use in congregations that sin is the "procuring cause of all the calamities which come upon us," that God gives life, continues life, takes life, and uses affliction for our correction. Christians are to commit themselves and the sick to God, so that if we as human beings live, we may live unto God; that if we die, we may die to God; that whether we live or die we may belong to God—echoing Calvin's earlier expression about our dependence upon God. In the nineteenth century, people thought more and more about life. The median age of Americans began to rise especially after 1820. In that year the census noted a slight change from sixteen to sixteen and a half. Thereafter, the median age moved up steadily to nineteen by 1850, twenty by 1870, twenty-five by 1920, and thirty by 1950.[28] Those in the Reformed tradition contributed to this extension of life in various ways.

In general, Calvinists, with a traditional concern for learning, contributed to the development of scientific medicine, and helped to explore pathways to better health and healing. In his intellectual history entitled *A Brief Retrospect of the Eighteenth Century* (1803), Samuel Miller, a Presbyterian pastor in New York City, spoke with approval of a Baconian age in medical science as he reviewed some of the remarkable achievements in the field in the century about which he wrote. Francis Bacon, a seventeenth-century Christian layman, wrote about scientific method, and how induction from the facts of experience rather than deduction was the pathway to truth about the creation. This method proved very helpful to Calvinists who wished to be faithful Christians, but who wanted to participate in the scientific quest of the modern age.[29] The age of Bacon, as Miller put it, extended into the nineteenth century as those in the health field developed the germ theory, immunology, anesthesia, antiseptic surgery, X-ray, and other breakthroughs that curbed suffering and began to prolong life.

Life was prolonged more, however, through changes in standards of living and lifestyles and also through public health measures. Those in the Reformed tradition continued to think of the unity of the body and the spirit; to encourage proper eating, drinking, and dressing; and to explore environmental aspects of health. In the reformist and perfectionist ethos of the nineteenth century, heirs of Calvin participated in the fight against the misuse of alcohol, for example, although they tended to stress temperance rather than total abstinence. One Presbyterian suggested that while he thought temperance was appropriate, he would not sign a pledge to give up alcohol altogether. It was neither biblical nor necessary for his piety, sobriety, or for the reformation of society. Sylvester Graham, an ordained Presbyterian minister and maverick and a temperance lecturer, became known for his "graham crackers" and for his views on sexuality as he explored the relation of the right food and proper sex behavior to health. He sounded the new note against death in his book entitled *Lectures on the Science of Human Life* (1839). A Presbyterian layman by the name of Robert M. Hartley campaigned for the public health movement during the century.[30] While those in the Reformed tradition thought about health and healing in a number of ways, here we shall stress how they encouraged the professionalization of ministry and medicine; supported hospitals, medical education, and research; and explored the "moral use" of suffering in the pursuit of longer and healthier life.

First, heirs of Calvin, continuing the Reformation emphasis on the importance of callings, contributed to the professionalization of those who entered the caring and curing vocations. Through the preceding centuries, pastors and physicians often cooperated in their work. As has already been noted, Baxter and Mather belonged to a breed of pastor-physicians who practiced medicine. John Redman, a Philadelphia layman whose long life spanned parts of the eighteenth and nineteenth centuries, also served as a physician-pastor. He attended the academies of Presbyterian clergy, studied medicine in Edinburgh and Leyden, built up a sizable practice in Philadelphia, and taught his knowledge and skills to persons such as Benjamin Rush. So great was his reputation that he long served as president of the College of Physicians of Philadelphia. He treated the physical complaints of his patients and counseled them when they were under emotional and spiritual stress, visiting them several times a year even when they were not sick. He reminded the young Rush when the latter was in Scotland to gain knowledge to qualify as a physician, but also to seek the one thing needful—the knowledge of God. Although Redman was a pious Presbyterian, his colleagues complained that he did not add enough to medical knowledge, a complaint that pointed to a growing competition between the responsibilities of the physician to the soul and the physician to the body.[31] While some evidence suggests that Calvinists tried to speak for the wholeness of the person, they may have contributed to a division by the tendency to separate the body and the spirit theologically. The emphasis upon the validity of vocations in God's sight and professionalization may have added to this development.

As theological seminaries emerged to offer better training, ministers were introduced in a more systematic way to pastoral theology and the ways in which clergy should minister to the sick in their congregations. Samuel Miller, now at Princeton Theological Seminary, addressed his *Letters on Clerical Manners and Habits* (1827) to ministers who spent much time in the preparation of their sermons, yet little time in preparing to visit and speak to those who were afflicted and dying. Many volumes gave ministers in the Reformed tradition considerable instruction on the preaching of the Word and the administration of the sacraments, indicating the importance of these ministrations for the health of the entire Christian community.[32]

James Spencer Cannon (1776–1852) taught at the Reformed Dutch seminary in New Brunswick. He published *Lectures on Pastoral Theology* (1853), a weighty volume that illustrates this emphasis on pastoral care for the whole congregation and includes, it should be noted, instruction from the Heidelberg Catechism. In a short section of the book, Cannon offers help on visiting families and individuals when they are well and when they are sick, in speaking with persons who are troubled in mind and sick in body. Pastors are not to wait to visit the sick until they are called. They are to use visitations as an opportunity to speak the truth of the gospel to those confined and exposed to death. The good pastor will know something about the patient and remember that the circumstances of sickness may impose certain restraints on the visitor. Visits and conversations should not be loud or long. Nevertheless, the pastor is constrained by his calling to speak a word of truth on such visits to the irreligious and the ignorant as well as to those who are truly pious. Such a word should be tender and affectionate or, as Congregationalist Washington Gladden put it some years later, "heart to heart," as the minister summons the sick to believe the gospel and rest in God's promises in sickness and in death. While some manuals insisted that every pastoral visit should be a sincere confrontation of souls in the presence of mortality, later pastoral guides cautioned against such an invasion of the privacy of the sick.[33] Presbyterians Ezra Stiles Ely in *Visits of Mercy* (1829) and Ichabod S. Spencer in *A Pastor's Sketches* (1851, 1853), which recorded case studies of the afflicted, shared their insights and indicated a more Baconian, that is, inductive, approach to the subject of pastoral care.[34]

The education of doctors grew more scientific and also more systematic in the nineteenth century. In their addresses to physicians about their God-given vocations, clergy in the Reformed tradition urged them to be good doctors and good Christians at the same time. The Presbyterian minister E.R. Beadle provides an interesting example. He addressed the students of medical schools in Philadelphia on "The Sacredness of the Medical Profession" (1865) and "The True Physician" (1874), taking as his texts "Luke, the Beloved Physician" (*Col.* 4:14) and "Heal the Sick" (*Mt.* 10:8). Beadle held that the physician, like Luke, had to be a preacher as well as a practitioner to be truly godly. He made a close connection between the ills of the body, of the emotions, and of the mind. As Christ's servants, physicians had to deal with the soul as well as the body. They had to take responsibility for the preservation of life and human welfare in general. Medicine is "progressive," Beadle suggested, and the good doctor must press on to unlock the secrets of nature and to uncover agents for the alleviation and cure of sickness. But the Christian physician, confronted with the call to prolong life against fearful odds, needs the faith and hope of the Christian so as not to be discouraged.[35] Another clergyman, John M. Krebs of New York, spoke of the mutuality of the clerical and medical professions, and urged cooperation. Devout doctors, while not excluding ministers from the sickroom, should speak a word of comfort to their patients, and clergy, while not pretending to be physicians, should encourage Christians to seek out well-trained doctors for assistance. Such clergy stressed the importance of true piety for the medical profession and often reminded physicians that they too were sinners, mortals, and needed the comforts of religion.[36]

Undoubtedly, many Reformed physicians kept the faith and fought the good fight as Christians. They could think of medicine as an aspect of what has been called "doxological science," through which they glorified God. Surgeon Hugh Hodge, brother of the famed theologian Charles Hodge, thought that the Christian should be the "world's Bible," and the surgeon D. Hayes Agnew, another Presbyterian layman, was praised in his death for his "moral symmetry," his "purest kindliness," his "devout piety," his settled "faith and convictions," and his "broad catholicity of spirit"—characteristics his pastor thought a doctor should have. J. Marion Sims of New York was deeply pious, while the chemist–doctor–librarian Lewis Henry Steiner collaborated in publishing an edition of the Heidelberg Catechism for the German Reformed Church. Others, raised in Reformed homes, sometimes by minister fathers, went to medical school for the education that ministers urged and were transformed into skeptics, a turn of events that some ministers feared. Thus ministers may have helped to widen the gap between professions that they described as closely related.[37] In this connection, when Presbyterian Abby Woolsey took up the task of upgrading the care of patients through nursing, she wrote in *A Century of Nursing* (1876) that while work "done to the Lord, and not to men, ought to be the best work," the "spirit in which work is done must not be confounded with technical proficiency." She gave expression not only to her piety, but also to the extent to which medical care had been professionalized.[38]

During the nineteenth century, most caring and curing of the afflicted took place in homes and not in hospitals, and medical education was often carried out without systematic clinical training. In order to gain more control and to provide better care for patients and training of doctors, those concerned for health began to build hospitals with the help of philanthropists. While those in the Reformed tradition did not follow any one strategy with regard to such institutions, some philanthropists organized and built hospitals, many of which developed connections with medical schools. The Presbyterian Hospital and the Columbia-Presbyterian Medical Center of New York provide a good illustration of what was involved. In the 1860s, Presbyterian James Lenox wanted to sponsor a hospital where Presbyterians especially might find care. Soon after the hospital was founded, however, its sponsor broadened the concept of service: "For the Poor of New York without Regard to Race, Creed, or Color." The institution would be, according to Lenox, "Presbyterian in its burdens," because Presbyterians would bear the costs, and "undenominational in its benefits," because of the admission of patients on the basis of need. Later, other Presbyterian philanthropists, Mrs. Stephen V. Harkness and her son, Edward, supported the development of the Columbia-Presbyterian Medical Center. In describing the purposes for his support, Edward Harkness wrote that he wanted to contribute to the prevention as well as the curing of disease. He saw the hospital and the medical school as interdependent, the latter supplying the physicians of the future, the former supplying the "material" for study and scientific research which might contribute to the prevention of sickness. The use of the word *material* to describe patients may be seen as an unintended illustration of the tendency of the modern hospital to depersonalize caring and curing. Harkness' intention was to alleviate human ills.[39] Physician Louise J. Lyle, a Presbyterian minister's daughter and minister's wife, founded the Louise Lyle Hospital, which became the Presbyterian Hospital of Pittsburgh, to carry on the "work of Christ for suffering humanity" of "every creed and nationality." Like the New Yorkers, the Pittsburgh Presbyterians joined their institution with the Medical Department of the University of Pittsburgh to develop a teaching hospital.[40] Presbyterians supported hospitals in Baltimore, Charlotte, Chicago, Philadelphia, Detroit, and Hollywood, among other places. As an expression of Christian concern for the sick, the agencies in charge of home missions also supported medical care for persons for whom it was not readily accessible.[41]

Almost from the beginning of the "Great Century," Reformed concern for health manifested itself throughout the world in missions. Beadle urged students at the medical college in Philadelphia to follow Luke in choosing medical missions as a career. Peter Parker, one of the early missionaries sent out by the American Board of Commissioners for Foreign Missions, supported by Congregationalists, Presbyterians, Dutch Reformed, and others, established an eye clinic in Canton, China. Medical missionaries, men and women, became heroes and heroines of the cause, and American philanthropists satisfied charitable impulses by funding this kind of work.[42] Missionaries went out to fulfill the "Great Commission" (*Mt.* 28:16–20): "Go therefore and make disciples of all nations, baptizing them in the name of the Father, and of the Son and of the Holy Spirit, teaching them to observe all that I have commanded you. . . ." The practice of medicine was a means to help in the evangelization of the world. Missionary concern for the health of people grew until medical missions obtained a more independent role in missions as an expression of Christian love, even though it remained subordinate to bringing the world to a saving knowledge of Christ. Mary H. Fulton intimated the growing importance of visiting and healing the sick when she entitled the autobiography of her life and work in China *"Inasmuch"* (n.d.), a reference to the "Great Judgment" (*Mt.* 25:40), in which Jesus admonished his followers to care for the afflicted in his name and as unto him.[43]

At first, missionaries who were not physicians often dispensed medicine and developed hospitals, sometimes offering care not much better than medicine practiced in the host country. As Western medicine developed, however, trained physicians heard the call and replaced those whose education and experience were inadequate. This professionalization process sometimes caused tension within the missionary community, which tended to treat health care as only a means of extending Christ's influence. W.J. Wanless, a medical missionary to India, supported both evangelism and professional developments in this field in *The Medical Mission: Its Place, Power and Appeal* (1911).[44]

While medicine was used to spread the good news about Jesus Christ, the good news of medicine was not generally withheld from those who needed treatment, whether or not the patients became members of the church. Medical missions became a sizable part of the work of the foreign mission boards of Reformed churches.

In addition to emphasizing healing vocations and institutions, Reformed attitudes reflected a theological shift during the nineteenth century, when knowledge of health and healing was expanding. Some Calvinists began to place less stress on God's sovereignty and more on the love of God made known in Jesus Christ, less stress on dying and more on life, less stress on the vain world and more on the "moral" use of suffering in life. Horace Bushnell (1802–1876), Congregationalist of Connecticut, heir of the Puritans such as Baxter and Mather, reflected on the "mystery of suffering" as it was often referred to in his day, and represents this tendency.[45] Bushnell preferred to speak of Christ as the Healer rather than God as a Physician because this seemed biblically appropriate. He noted the close relations between the body and the spirit. Ill health, Bushnell argued, is caused by sin, the "condition of general intemperance," which does its work in the world by "poisoning all the roots of health and making visible its woes, by so many woes of disease and death." What a "hospital the world is!" he sighed. Bushnell believed that Christ vicariously takes upon himself the burden of sickness as well as our sin, revealing the "Gethsemane hid in all love." He described how Jesus healed:

> Sometimes he appears to have operated for the soul through the body, and sometimes for the body through the soul, contriving in what manner to elicit faith before the cure and assuming, evidently, that fact of a reciprocal action and reaction operating naturally between them—the healing of the body helped by the faith of the soul and the faith of the soul by the healing of the body. In the large view his operation is but one, and life, complete life, is or is to be the result.

Pain and suffering, according to Bushnell, operate as "God's mute prophet in the body," as a "kind of general sacrament of the world," not only to help deal with sin, but also to motivate to bear one another's burdens. Those who learn how to suffer will gain the "highest of mortal victories."[46]

Henry Ward Beecher (1813–1887), another Congregationalist, also spoke of the uses of suffering. Beecher was one of the most popular preachers of the age. The Boston physician Oliver Wendell Holmes, revising the remark of Richard Baxter, spoke of Beecher as one who preached as "living man to living men." Suffering, Beecher held, was an "unfolding process" and, in the nature of things, a "passage from a lower to a higher stage" of life. Referring to Christ, he maintained that all human suffering is in the hands of the Sufferer, and while it may be a "rod to Chastise," it may also be a "scepter to empower." Beecher called his hearers to "Rule in it, and rule over it. So God rules in you."[47] While neither Bushnell nor Beecher treated suffering lightly, they appeared positive about how it might be used in this life rather than as a preparation for death.

During these years, Calvinists reflected on the nature and efficacy of prayer, and recalled neglected liturgical traditions. American Presbyterians, for example, began to recover such resources of the Reformation to help minister to the sick. Concerned about the proliferation of faith-healing groups, A.A. Hodge, Princeton theologian, thought it helpful to remind people in an essay on "Prayer and the Prayer-Cure" of some things about Reformed belief about prayer. Hodge held that while in general sickness is a consequence of sin, all sickness is not the immediate punishment for some particular sinful act or state of some persons; that for Christians, sickness is a matter of God's chastisement, not of anger or displeasure; that Christians cannot demand the cure of disease in every case unconditionally and without proper submission to God's laws; and that Christians should use God's appointed means to secure health. Not to pray for God's blessing upon means of healing represents a spirit of "restless disobedience." Like the Reformers, Hodge continued to hold that God worked miracles only in Christ's day and for special purposes, arguing that God should not be expected to perform such "upon our call" in our day.[48] Prodded by John W. Nevin, Presbyterian-turned-German-Reformed, and Philip Schaff, Calvinists also began to give the Lord's Supper the importance that Calvin gave to it, providing forms for communion services to the sick. In the nineteenth century, Presbyterian clergy and laity produced books of worship that included prayers for the sick, those afflicted by plagues and pestilence, and the dying. This movement culminated for Presbyterians in the adoption of a *Book of Common Worship* (1906) for "voluntary use."[49] Those in the Reformed tradition prayed for health, just as they encouraged healing vocations and institutions in an era in which life was being prolonged gradually and death was less of a specter than it had been in earlier centuries. The *Book of Common Worship* of 1906 contained this prayer:

> O Lord our God, who art the Physician of our souls and our bodies; who chastenest and again Thou healest; We beseech Thee mercifully to regard Thy servant, N., for whom we pray that *his* life may be spared, and *his* strength restored. O Thou, who didst give Thy Son to bear our sicknesses and carry our sorrow; for His sake deal compassionately with this Thy servant, and send upon *him* Thy healing power and virtue, both in *his*

body and in *his* soul and spirit. Into Thy hands we commit *him;* unto Thy gracious mercy and protection we commend *him* as unto a faithful and merciful Savior. *Amen.*[50]

An incident relating to the opening of the Johns Hopkins Hospital in the 1890s suggests something of what was happening in terms of the relations between faith and health. The hospital administration caused considerable consternation among some Christians when it opened the facility without the benefit of prayer. In order to ease the discomfort of people in the city, especially Presbyterians, it permitted the placing of a Bertal Thorwalsen statue of "Christus Consolator" in the lobby in 1896 to remind people of the centrality of Christ as the source of all health and healing. Presbyterian layman and philanthropist William Wallace Spence paid for the sculpture. The statue may have satisfied the faithful. The event itself perhaps points up an unintended consequence of Reformed concern for Baconism, that is, for scientific medicine, for professionalization, and for the hospital as a center for medical care and experimentation. Some physicians may have been preoccupied with the pursuit of scientific medicine to the neglect of the relations between Christian faith, health, and healing.[51]

The Abundant Life: Self-Acceptance, Shepherding, and Human Sexuality

Years of development in medical science, depersonalization in health-care delivery, and controversy among Christians about the relation of faith and health helped shape the way in which those in the Reformed tradition approached health and healing in the twentieth century and the adaptation of the tradition itself. Undoubtedly, some thought that no conflict existed between the medical culture that was prolonging life and personal and communal needs and aspirations. But the persistence and popularity of "faith-healers" and "positive thinkers," persons whom A.A. Hodge addressed, pointed to something amiss. Benjamin B. Warfield, heir of Calvin and of the Westminster Confession, expressed concern about the heresy of a simplistic approach to health when he delivered his lectures on *Counterfeit Miracles* (1918). The Princeton theologian mused over the visit of Mary Baker Eddy, the prophetess of Christian Science, to a dentist and her use of anesthesia to kill pain during the extraction of an aching tooth. He did not see how the tooth, the toothache, and the suffering could be dismissed as illusion. Repeating the earlier Reformed position that miracles of healing were confined to the early church, Warfield stressed, as did Calvin before him, that God gives us the means of medical science to deal with illness, disease, and pestilence. Famed physician William Osler was of the opinion, Warfield reminded his readers, that the "prayer of faith neither sets a broken thigh nor checks an epidemic of typhoid fever." Warfield may not have gauged accurately the yearning of his generation for some fresh spiritual perspective on the subject and for help for the "wilderness" of loneliness, doubt, darkness within, as Mrs. Eddy put it in *Science and Health with Key to the Scriptures* (1875).[52] While Calvinists continued the quest for a longer life, they also sought a better understanding of the inner self in the age of Freud, more helpful means of "shepherding" by the whole Christian community, and a healthier approach to human sexuality. In a word, they engaged in a quest for an abundant life.

Despite some tendency in Calvinism to separate body and spirit and to accentuate that separation through the professionalization of the vocations of ministry and medicine, Calvinists in general have continued to recognize the unity of the whole person and the reciprocal relationship between the health of body and the health of the spirit. Calvin did. Redman did. Jonathan Edwards did in the eighteenth century when he wrote about "religious affections" and reflected on the behavior of those who suffered from "melancholy."[53] So did Bushnell. The development of psychology and psychiatry illuminated the whole context of discussion of the inner self.

Anton T. Boisen (1876–1975), Presbyterian–Congregationalist, pioneered in the psychology of religion and offered his reflections in *The Exploration of the Inner World* (1936). On several occasions he suffered emotional disorder and confinement. Out of his own experiences, recovery, and reflection, he concluded that crises in the religious life may contribute to the reordering of the person's inner self and social relations. Boisen thought it important to include in the study of the relation between faith and health "living human documents" and the experiences of men and women made in the image of God. As a result of his own hospitalization, he concluded that the gap between professionals had widened in the twentieth century. He set in motion a movement of clinical training and case study that would bring together pastors and physicians in a common enterprise that would deal more effectively with those who may be afflicted emotionally as well as physically.[54] Karl A. Menninger (b. 1893), a Presbyterian layman, agreed with Boisen, although he approached faith and health from the perspective of a psychiatrist and not a clergyman, and as one of the founders of the Menninger Foundation in Topeka, Kansas. In *Man against Himself* (1938), for example, he analyzed the self-destructiveness of human beings, while in *Love against Hate* (1942), written with his wife, Jeanetta L. Menninger, he affirmed the power of love as an essential element of health. Thus in the language of his vocation, he gave expression to dimensions of the human condition that reflect the Reformed tradition and that have to do with health. He emphasized the need for some integrative view of life in *The Vital Balance* (1963).[55] Like Boisen, Menninger encouraged pastors and physicians to overcome unhealthy compartmentalization in the health field.

The focus on the inner self and the importance of psychotherapy has suggested to some that many have moved from an emphasis on divine redemption to self-realization, as though a healthy integration could be achieved by human beings alone. Norman Vincent Peale, Methodist turned Dutch Reformed, has been accused of oversimplifying the relationship between Christian faith and health by preaching *The Power of Positive Thinking* (1952), which made him one of the most popular figures in American life.[56] Others have taken an appreciative but critical view of the movement represented here by Boisen and Menninger. Robert Bonthius, for example, in *Christian Paths to Self-Acceptance* (1948) suggested that the exploration of the inner world has helped Calvinists see the Reformed heritage in a different light by allowing an accent on the theme of human responsibility. Calvin's stress on our complete dependence on God in the *Institutes,* Bonthius argued, made the Reformed too authoritarian in thinking about matters of faith and health. The author asserted that insights from psychotherapy permit an expression of dependence upon God in a way that fosters sound self-acceptance, strengthens persons in the use of personal resources for choosing values and making decisions, and encourages responsible community life.[57] In a similar manner, David Roberts explored some of the same themes in *Psychotherapy and a Christian View of Man* (1950). As a Calvinist, he tried to show how psychotherapeutic theory could deepen understanding of theological confessions. It gives a better understanding of sin, thereby undermining Pelagianism, which stressed human ability, and reinforcing Augustinian insights, which stressed God's activity. Moreover, by helping explore the meaning of healing in personal attitudes and interpersonal relations of acceptance and trust, it provides a better perspective on divine initiative and human responsiveness.[58] Persons such as Bonthius and Roberts demonstrated how such theory could enrich theology, and vice versa.

In fact, this discussion about the inner world and self-acceptance gave impulse to continue to consider health not simply in terms of self-realization and the individual person, but holistically in terms that involve all of life and all of the caring professions in the service of a longer and fuller life. Seward Hiltner (1909–1984), friend of Boisen and Menninger, worked at the center of this movement, and shaped Reformed thinking through his teaching and numerous writings, first as secretary of the "Committee on Religion and Health" of the Federal Council of Churches (1938) and later as professor at the University of Chicago and Princeton Theological Seminary. Although a Presbyterian, he had an ecumenical impact by stimulating and guiding the pastoral-care and counseling movements among many religious groups over the years. In his first book, *Health and Healing* (1943), he focused on problems that are still being discussed: the integrity of the patient, the treatment of the whole person, and the necessity and means of promoting spiritual and psychological growth as important to physical health. Hiltner gave attention to themes important to Calvinists, such as salvation. He claimed that sin is for the Christian a decisive aspect of health, and that health must be thought of in terms of the "psyche" (inner self) as well as the "soma" (body) and in terms of cosmic wholeness, not simply in individualistic terms. He also cautioned against an unbiblical preoccupation with personal health. In *Preface to Pastoral Care* (1958), he set out to deliver the pastoral-care and counseling movements from their overdependence on the scientific world view and place them in the context of a responsible Christian community and its total ministry. In his study, Hiltner adopted the word *shepherding* as an appropriate term to describe Christian responsibility. By *shepherding* he did not mean to suggest the Roman Catholic image of the ruler over a flock. Instead, he meant a whole ministry of healing, sustaining, and guiding by the use of skilled organization and communication within the Christian family.[59] In this approach, he touched base with his Reformed tradition in which, ideally, health has been a result of life together within the community of faith, love, and hope.

This brings us to the report of the United Presbyterian Church on *The Relation of Christian Faith to Health* (1960), with which we began this essay. Hiltner had much to do with this paper. Among others, Pastor Bonthius and Doctor Menninger contributed to it also. Presbyterians also rooted this study in the Scriptures, in *Ecclesiasticus,* in Christian history, in Reformed tradition, reaffirming in this ecumenical context some of the emphases that have already been mentioned in this essay. This report refers to "salvation" in the New Testament as a deliverance from sin, death, and the destructive powers of the world, but it also includes deliverance from physical and mental evil. While the authors recognize that mortality and Christian health are ultimately related to hope in the resurrection, the emphasis in this report is upon Jesus Christ, who came that human beings might have life "and have it abundantly" (*Jn.* 10:10), here as well as hereafter. God is the source of health and healing. Health is a dynamic process that involves the condition of the body, mind, and spirit. It is a social matter that includes not only those in the health professions, but those who take thought for the physical and psychical conditions in which people live. Illness is an evil which God intends should be overcome. However, God is recognized as the giver of life for which human beings have responsibility, whether sick or in good health, while they work and wait for the redemption of the whole person and whole created order.

In this study, Presbyterians expressed thanks for the scientific break-throughs in medicine and for medical institutions. They also deplored the compartmentalization of life as illustrated in the field of health. The Christian church has a responsibility to provide for the "integrating principles" that make for health, and for communicating "God's gift of a meaningful life in Christ" as its continuing contribution to the "total health of man." Pastors, physicians, and others who provide professionally for health are urged to work cooperatively, remembering God's high calling, preparing well for vocations, understanding both limitations and contributions that they can make to the healing process. Professionals are to remember the need people have for acceptance in the conflicts in which they may be caught, the need for confession and the assurance of forgiveness, and the need for recognizing the presence and power of God. Such a ministry by pastors, physicians, and others should not be performed in a mechanical manner, in predetermined patterns, but with sensitivity as circumstances indicate. The study holds that all members of the Christian family are ministers to those who are ill. Moreover, the church is responsible for strengthening the home through worship, education, counseling, and in other ways that con-tribute to the health of all, and which may be considered discipline— or discipling in the best sense. The study concludes with ways by which these affirmations about faith and health may be implemented in the church, for example, by supporting those called to be pastors and physicians, and by supporting Presbyterian seminaries and hospitals dealing with faith and health issues and the ministry to the physically and mentally ill. All Christians are called to be priests to one another in bearing one another's burdens.[60] Presbyterian institutions attempted to implement suggestions in this paper.

At the same time that American Presbyterians were preparing this study on the relationship of faith and health, Calvinists were struggling with the sexual revolution stimulated by Alfred Kinsey's reports on human sexual behavior, the *Playboy* mentality, and the development of the pill as an effective means of contraception. Whereas people in the nineteenth century seemed to talk much about death and whispered about sex, in the middle of the twentieth century people seem to whisper about death and talk much about sex. Those in the Reformed tradition did not deny death. Indeed, they tried to remind people of finitude. They did talk much about sex. Seward Hiltner was one of the first to respond to Kinsey, whose family was connected with the Pres-byterian church in Indiana, and who gave a statistical and descriptive account of the varieties of sexual experiences and behavior. Hiltner questioned the scientist's naturalistic bias, yet urged that his findings be seriously considered by Christians for understanding human sexuality. Others explored history and asked, as did Congregationalist–Quaker Roland Bainton in *What Christianity Says about Sex, Love, and Marriage* (1957).[61] In papers on marriage, on the nature and purpose of human sexuality, and on homosexuality, Presbyterians gave serious attention to this aspect of the abundant life of our time. The whole discussion has taken place within the broader context of the Reformed confession of God's good work in creating us, male and female, of God's reconciling work in Jesus Christ, and of the covenants that God has made with responsible sexual beings, as did Calvin and the authors of the Westminster Larger Catechism. Sex, to be sure, may become an idol, a bondage, or a manifestation of sinfulness and not of Christian liberty. Because sexual relationships are a profound way of knowing and communicating with one another within the marital bond, they may be enjoyed in both their procreational and recreational aspects. While not a sacrament, marriage is a reminder of God's presence in our common life. In earlier years, those in the Reformed tradition discouraged the use of contraceptive devices. Recently, however, these have been accepted as a means to more satisfying sexual partnerships and planned parenting,[62] a position consistent with the Calvinist emphasis on the legitimate use of the developments in medical science.

Calvinists have offered members education on healthy family life, affirmed the celibate life as a rewarding psychological and spiritual experience, and expressed pastoral concern for homosexuals and their civil rights. While some congregations of the Universal Church of Christ have ordained homosexuals to the ministry, generally speaking, Calvinists have not approved of the homosexual lifestyle as a Christian manifestation of human sexuality. With regard to this matter, discussion continues among Calvinists in reference to the nature and cause of homosexuality. The church as a shepherding community has a responsibility for encouraging healthy sexual relations, and for discouraging the immoderate attachment to and the idolization of the sexual self, which makes it a curse rather than a blessing.[63] Concerns about life, death, and sex came into focus in the debate over abortion. In the past, those in the Reformed tradition condemned infanticide and abortion when practiced in the United States and in mission fields. Presently, abortion is not seen to be a desirable solution to any problem. However, Calvinists recognize the possibility of abortion in some cases, and the need for responsible choice in the context of pastoral counseling about the value of life. Some Presbyterians, including the late theologian Francis A. Schaeffer and physician C. Everett Koop, think that other Calvinists are less guarded on this issue than they should be, given the Reformed tradition's emphasis on the respect for life.[64]

In their continuing quest for the longer and fuller life, Calvinists tapped not only the Reformed tradition, but other Christian traditions for help in dealing devotionally with matters of faith and health. For example, Carl J. Scherzer, chaplain of the Protestant Deaconness Hospital, Evansville, Indiana, offered aids for ministry in *Ministering to the Physically Sick* (1963) and *Ministering to the Dying* (1963), ecumenical in spirit and content. Scherzer also published a historical survey of the Christian approach to health entitled *The Church and Healing* (1970), in which he touched upon some aspects of the Reformed tradition's approach to this subject.[65] In this connection, Presbyterians urged the use of Bible reading, prayer, and communion with the sick as important aspects of shepherding. Moreover, they took another look at New Testament practices of anointing with oil and laying on of hands. Calvinists, in general, have not used these, especially because anointing has been associated with the sacrament of extreme unction. But Presbyterians now recognize that these practices have had a long and honored use in the history of the Christian family, and allow their use if people are properly prepared and do not consider the oil and the touching as medicinal and as substitutes for medical care. Such practices should be used as signs of "God's redemptive presence at work" in the body and the mind.[66] Paul W. Pruyser, a psychologist of the Menninger Foundation, has urged that Christians recover the use of the blessing by touching as a symbolic way of overcoming some of the drawbacks of a secularized medical system and a way of affirming that all things, even the medical system, exist for a divine purpose and proceed from God's hand. Just as in the case of the ministry of word and sacraments, so the blessing may be helpful therapeutically to reinforce belief that God is the true physician and healer. It should be noted that in his book on "faith-healing" in 1956, Wade Boggs made the useful suggestion that Christians stop quarreling over the use of the word *miracle* in the healing process. Because Calvinists believe all healing is divine, discussion should not be about supernatural and natural, but about familiar and unfamiliar procedures of healing, a point confirmed by Pruyser in his suggestion about God's blessing.[67]

Calvinist concern for a fuller life for all may be seen in the way in which they have expanded subjects of prayers in the *Worshipbook* (1970). They now pray not only for the sick and the dying, but also for a wider range of the afflicted—for those who are mentally distressed, handicapped, addicted, or sexually confused. Thus in prayer the shepherding community has expanded its sympathies and its sense of responsibility for the health of all.[68]

God and Health: Wholeness, Justice, and Finitude

In this historical review of the Reformed tradition, emphasis has been on God as the Great Physician and healer, the goodness of creation and life, the use of means and the importance of healing vocations and institutions, a holistic approach to health, and the responsibility that the Christian community has in dealing with matters of faith and health. Moreover, following Kenneth Vaux, we have suggested that Calvinists have approached matters of health and healing in dynamic terms. They have participated in the various transformations in the field of health care over the centuries. Calvinists today employ insights from the past to deal with problems raised by advances in medical technology, questions of medical ethics, a holistic and just approach to health and health care, and the debates over the meaning of life and death as Calvinists continue to be realistic about finitude and the need for hope in our human situation.

The growth of modern medicine has heightened the debate over ethics in the field. This, in turn, has pressed those in the Reformed tradition to assess theological affirmations about God in their approach to the decisions that those in healing vocations must make in offering medical services to persons in need. Willard Sperry, Congregationalist minister and dean of Harvard Divinity School, pioneered in this field when he published *The Ethical Basis for Medical Practice* (1950), an attempt to build religious bridges to physicians to whom he was speaking as a Christian about ethical matters.[69] More recently, James Gustafson (b. 1925) has been explicit in emphasizing what may be considered Reformed emphases in his work on *The Contributions of Theology to Medical Ethics* (1975). Gustafson, a minister of the United Church of Christ who teaches at the University of Chicago, suggests that it is essential to consider all questions of medical ethics by drawing inferences, as did the writers of Scripture, from experiences with the ultimate power Christians call God. First, God wills the well-being of the creation and human beings in relation to the creation. Second, God, by His power, presence, and activity, seeks to preserve and sustain life, and opposes that which does not value human life. Third, God creates conditions for new possibilities in which different decisions and actions are required for preserving and sustaining life. Drawing insight from Karl Barth about idolatry, Gustafson prefers to speak about our respect for life rather than a reverence for life, in order to avoid giving absolute value to human existence. He recognizes, as did Sperry before him, the ambiguities in all ethical decisions made by finite human beings who also are sinners. While he does not hold that we are reduced to complete relativism in matters of life, death, and health, he does suggest that people who deal with such matters must be self-critical and modest in terms of moral values, judgments, and certitude. Human beings should be humble in the presence of the creation and life of which God has made them stewards. Gustafson distinguishes himself from some ethicists, notably Roman Catholics, by suggesting that he thinks of the created order in more dynamic and less static terms, and that he is more open to the future.[70]

Adding to Gustafson's insights, the Presbyterian ethicist Kenneth Vaux argues in *Biomedical Ethics* (1974) that the Christian's eschatological vision of the future helps us to persevere with patience in our witness to the Kingdom of God, where death shall be no more and there will be no more pain or crying (*Rv.* 21:4). This kingdom vision also underscores the value of life, according to Vaux, and stimulates us in the quest for the longer and more abundant life. Moreover, the vision is a warning against utopianism, yet places under judgment all that dehumanizes.[71] Thus in recent years, heirs of Calvin have reaffirmed some of the progenitor's basic theological emphases in dealing with persons and the relation between faith and health.

While some Calvinists have been giving considerable attention to dealing with faith and health in terms of ethical dilemmas, others have asked about the nature of health itself. They have suggested that health must be considered not simply in terms of personal need, however essential, but in a holistic way. Calvin and his contemporaries thought of health in terms of total existence in relationship to God, to one another, and to the whole of creation. Swiss Reformed physician Paul Tournier has written in the twentieth century about health in these terms, and he has been read widely among American Calvinists.[72] The Office on Health Ministries of the United Presbyterian Church stated this approach in contemporary terms in a statement entitled "Health Ministries and the Church" (1978). In this statement, the agency called upon Presbyterians to ameliorate suffering and to promote "health and well-being on the broadest possible scale," not simply in times of personal and corporate crisis. "The love of life," the paper suggests, "not the fear of death, is the church's primary and empowering motivation." Jesus' ministry is directed toward the good health of humankind, not only in a hereafter, but in the here and now. The Bible knows nothing of a truncated salvation in which people's souls are saved and their bodies are neglected, or of individuals apart from their biological, economic, and political existence. The office held that health care, a constant concern of members of the human race, means the positive support of life:

> Health care is a theological matter involving spiritual, physical, and social factors because the biblical vision sees not only healthy individuals but a celebrating and healing community in the present and coming kingdom. In

fact, the healthy individual is the person whose life is significant and meaningful insofar as it becomes a contribution to the ultimate fulfillment of life in God's kingdom. Life lived to the glory of God is life lived for the coming of that kingdom—hence the care of life means concern for and participation in the promise for a full life for all—the care and healing of society. Individual life and death finds its meaning in that total vision—a theo-centric and not ego-centric vision. . . . Such social concern is signified in the central sacrament of the Christian community—the Lord's Supper.[73]

So Calvinists have concerns, many of which were expressed in the sixteenth and seventeenth centuries, about health in terms of the wholeness of God's creative work and God's wisdom and will for all his creation and creatures. Reformed concern for the peace of the world in recent years may be considered as an aspect of this holistic approach to faith and health.[74]

Calvinists have continued to struggle with the problem of healthcare delivery, how it may best be done. But they have become advocates of a more equitable distribution of the benefits of modern medicine. In sixteenth-century Geneva, the Reformed operated hospitals for all. In the nineteenth century, Calvinists founded hospitals to provide Presbyterians and others who came with medical services. So under new circumstances in the twentieth century, Calvinists believe that medical care belongs to all. As early as 1946, American Presbyterians began to study the merits of compulsory health insurance. In 1971 they strongly advocated a national policy leading to a "comprehensive system of health care," a system "accountable to the general public," with services available to "all persons in the United States" and "administered by a single national health agency with power to enforce standards to provide the highest quality health care possible." The biblical basis of this concern is Jesus' declaration "I have come that men may have life, and may have it in all its fullness" (*Jn.* 10:10 NEB). The theological basis is that "God's holy purpose for mankind is to be of worth and be well, and to be in health and nurturing health for one another, in institutions and with the whole world." Presbyterians acknowledge "a commitment under God, to exercise public compassion and justice for all citizens of our land, and therefore, to increase the public well-being." Health is everybody's business, a mutual enterprise. Therefore Christians must cooperate not only with one another, but with international organizations, such as the World Health Organization, in finding ways to deal with the world's afflictions.[75]

The Reformed discuss the basis of this concern today. For example, physician John Bryant has turned to the theory of rights and contract and to John Rawls' (b. 1921) *A Theory of Justice* (1971) to deal with fairness in the delivery of health care. In a study for the World Council of Churches, Bryant writes from Rawls' perspective that "Whatever health services are available should be equally available to all. Departures from equality of distribution are permissible only if those worse off are made better off." While this approach is attractive to some and has its merit, William F. May of Southern Methodist University warns about the pressures of life that often tempt us to abandon the approach of rational self-interest and contract. In his work *The Physician's Covenant: Images of the Healer in Medical Ethics* (1983), he urges Christians to approach this matter from the perspective of covenant responsibilities and not simply rights, because such a covenantal dimension takes into consideration the communal aspects of our relations with one another. While such statements of the churches and by Reformed authors are supported by numerous pastors and physicians, many others in the Reformed churches in the United States would be suspicious of any system that looked like "socialized" medicine.[76]

Because the number of older people in the population has grown dramatically in recent years, those in the Reformed tradition have tried to help the elderly think of this time as "bonus years." Suffering and death persist, despite all efforts to conquer them. Those in the Reformed tradition from Calvin's day to the present take suffering and death seriously. Their persistence continually reminds us, as H. Richard Niebuhr wrote, of the "exhibition of the presence in our existence of that which is not under our control, or of the intrusion into our self-legislating existence of an activity operating under another law than ours." Suffering and death "cut athwart our purposive movements" and frustrate our "movement toward self-realization or toward the actualization of our potentialities."[77] Suffering and death intrude into life in new ways since modern technology has curbed much suffering and prolonged life, even though life may be reduced to mere existence on machines and may be very costly. Difficult questions arise about whether some people should continue to live or should be allowed to die.

The General Assembly of the Presbyterian Church in the United States adopted a paper on "The Nature and Value of Human Life" (1981), returning to the Scriptures of the Old and New Covenants for insight. God affirms life, this paper suggests, through the life and ministry of Jesus Christ. God gives us insights into how we should show respect for life in the commandment against killing (*Ex.* 20:13). The commandment helps today as it helped the Reformed in the sixteenth and seventeenth centuries. This commandment requires that Christians do no harm. Yet in terms of the life-and-death decisions that must be made in connection with contemporary technology, the requirement that we do no harm may come into conflict at times with the obligation to protect and preserve life. In some cases it is conceivable that taking life may be justified as more consistent with the respect for life. In the case of euthanasia, for example, Presbyterians make a distinction between "active" euthanasia, where death may not be assumed, and "passive" euthanasia, where death is predictable and depends on whether medical interventions are made and continued. They do not rule out either active or passive euthanasia in every case, but in all cases, for example, such as abortion or cancer, decisions must be made in terms of the value God places on life and the respect that Christians should have for life, and with pastoral concern for those making decisions about life and death.[78] Here Donald Shriver, Reformed ethicist and theologian of Union Theological Seminary in New York, warns about idolatry with regard to health and medical science. Life is a pilgrimage of suffering, suffering unto death. In our struggles for the longer and fuller life, physicians ought to remember that they too are human, and patients ought not to expect of physicians more than they have any right to expect. Pastors, physicians, and patients need to remember their finitude. Although dying may have its sting, it is, from the Christian perspective, as Rutherford saw many years ago, not the last word about the value of life.[79]

In matters of faith and health, the followers of John Calvin in the Reformed tradition have believed and taught that Christians are called upon to bear one another's burdens, following Paul's admonition, "Bear one another's burdens, and so fulfill the law of Christ" (*Gal.* 6:2). William B. Oglesby suggests in his book *Biblical Themes for Pastoral Care* (1980) a return to the Bible for the insights that will help Christians confront sin, sickness, suffering, and death and participate in a ministry of reconciliation.[80] Reconciliation is another way in which those in the Reformed tradition have thought of that "redemption which God in Jesus Christ brings to the world through his Church" which is "sufficient for the ultimate conquest of every evil," to return to words with which we began this study. The Reformed recognize the promise of reconciliation, although the victory is not yet. Thus Christians pray for one another:

> By your great power, great God, our Lord Jesus Christ healed the sick and gave new hope to the hopeless. Though we cannot command or possess your power, we pray for those who want to be healed (especially for ___). Close wounds, cure sickness, make broken people whole again, so they may live to rejoice in your love. Help us to welcome every healing as a sign that, though death is against us, you are for us, and have promised renewed and risen life in Jesus Christ the Lord. Amen.[81]

Notes

1. United Presbyterian Church in the United States of America [hereafter UPCUSA], *The Relation of Christian Faith to Health* (New York, 1960), p. 9.
2. See John T. McNeill, *The History and Character of Calvinism* (New York, 1954); McNeill, *A History of the Cure of Souls* (New York, 1951), pp. 192–217.
3. Kenneth L. Vaux, *Health and Medicine in the Reformed Tradition* (New York, 1984), pp. 21–23; H. Richard Niebuhr, *Christ and Culture* (New York, 1951), pp. 190–229.
4. John Calvin, *Institutes of the Christian Religion*, 2 vols., trans. Ford Lewis Battle (Philadelphia, 1960), 1:35–39.
5. Calvin, *Institutes*, 1:690.
6. Ibid., 1:99–102, 383–388.
7. Ibid., 1:706. See bk. 3, ch. 8, for cross-bearing as medicine.
8. Heinrich Quistorp, *Calvin's Doctrine of Last Things*, trans. Harold Knight (Richmond, 1955), pp. 34–51.
9. "The Heidelberg Catechism" (1563) in Philip Schaff, *The Creeds of Christendom*, 3 vols. (New York [1877], 1919), 3:307–308. See also UPCUSA, *Book of Confessions* (Philadelphia, 1970), 4.001–4.002.
10. Schaff, *The Creeds*, 3:676; *Book of Confessions*, 7.001.
11. "The Westminster Shorter Catechism" (1647), Schaff, *The Creeds*, 3:676.
12. Calvin, *Institutes*, 2:1467–1469.
13. See Charles W. Baird, *Eutaxia, or the Presbyterian Liturgies: Historical Sketches* (New York, 1855), p. 123. This publication represents renewed interest in pastoral and liturgical concerns of the past.
14. *The Register of the Company of Pastors of Geneva in the Time of Calvin*, ed. and trans. Philip Edgecumbe Hughes (Grand Rapids, MI, 1966), p. 46.
15. See Edward A. Dowey, Jr., *The Knowledge of God in Calvin's Theology* (New York, 1952), pp. 221–238.
16. See "The Larger Catechism" (1647), in *The Constitution of the Presbyterian Church in the United States of America* (Philadelphia, 1956), pp. 157–158.
17. See Derrick Sherwin Bailey, *The Man–Woman Relation in Christian Thought* (London, 1959), pp. 169–179, 180, 182; Roland Mushat Frye, "The Teachings of Classical Puritanism on Conjugal Love," in *Studies in the Renaissance*, ed. M.A. Shaaber, 21 vols. (New York, 1955), 2:148–159; Edmund S. Morgan, "The Puritans and Sex," in *Procreation or Pleasure: Sexual Attitudes in American History*, ed. Thomas L. Altherr (Malabar, FL, 1983), pp. 5–16; Morgan, *The Puritan Family* ([1944] rev. ed., New York, 1966). See also "The Larger Catechism," pp. 160–162.
18. Calvin, *Institutes*, 1:221–222.
19. John Calvin, *Treatises Against the Anabaptists and Against the Libertines*, ed. and trans. Benjamin Wirt Farley (Grand Rapids, MI, 1982), pp. 178–181, 244–245, 320–324.
20. Alexander M. Zeidman, "The Care of the Poor and Indigent in Geneva in the Latter Half of the Sixteenth Century" (Th.M. Thesis, Knox College, Toronto), pp. 56–84; Leon Gautier, *La Médecine a Geneve Jusqu'a La Fin Du XVIIme Siecle*, in *Memoires et Documents* publies par La Societe D'Histoire et D'Archeologie (Geneve, 1906), pp. 1–169.

21. *A Directory for the Public Worship of God* . . . [1644], in Bard Thompson, ed., *Liturgies of the Western Church* (Cleveland, 1961), pp. 354–371; McNeill, *Cure of Souls*, pp. 247–278.

22. "Directions for the Sick," *The Practical Works of Richard Baxter,* 4 vols. (London, 1854), 1:522–547. Baxter, "The Cure of Melancholy and Overmuch Sorrow, By Faith and Physic," in *Puritan Sermons,* 6 vols. (Wheaton, IL, 1981), 3:253–292. See also David E. Stannard, *The Puritan Way of Death: A Study in Religion, Culture, and Social Change* (New York, 1977).

23. Otho T. Beall, Jr. and Richard H. Shryock, *Cotton Mather: First Significant Figure in American Medicine* (Baltimore, 1954); Cotton Mather, *The Angel of Bethesda,* ed. Gordon W. Jones (Barre, MA, 1972), pp. xi–xxxv.

24. Mather, pp. 5–38, 186–191.

25. See Beall and Shryock, *Cotton Mather,* for Mather's contribution.

26. See Baird, *Eutaxia,* p. 41. For Calvin's letters of consolation to the afflicted, see John Calvin, *Letters of John Calvin Compiled from the Original Manuscript and Edited with Historical Notes by Jules Bonnet,* trans. David Constable et al., 3 vols. (Philadelphia, 1858), 1:331–335; 2:217–223.

27. *Letters of the Rev. Samuel Rutherford,* ed. Andrew A. Bonar (New York, 1866), pp. 488–489.

28. "The Directory for the Public Worship of God," in *A Draught of the Form of the Government and Discipline of the Presbyterian Church in the United States of America* . . . (New York, 1787), pp. 49–143; David Hackett Fischer, *Growing Old in America* (New York [1977], 1978), pp. 26–27, 102–103.

29. Samuel Miller, "Medicine," in *A Brief Retrospect of the Eighteenth Century,* 2 vols. (New York, 1803), 2:201–326. Miller expressed his gratitude to a "medical friend" for assistance in writing this chapter. The friend may have been his brother.

30. For an understanding of the ethos and campaign for temperance (which featured persons such as Benjamin Rush and Lyman Beecher), see Charles I. Foster, *An Errand of Mercy* (Chapel Hill, NC, 1960); Charles E. Rosenberg and Carroll S. Rosenberg, "Pietism and the Origins of the American Public Health Movement: A Note on John H. Griscom and Robert M. Hartley," *Journal of the History of Medicine and Allied Sciences* 23 (1968):16–35; Stephen Nissenbaum, *Sex, Diet and Debility in Jacksonian America: Sylvester Graham and Health Reform* (Westport, CT, 1980).

31. Whitfield J. Bell, Jr., "John Redman, Medical Preceptor, 1722–1808," *Pennsylvania Magazine of History and Biography* 81 (1957):157–169; William C. Lehmann, *Scottish and Scotch-Irish Contributions to Early American Life and Culture* (Port Washington, NY), pp. 65–209; Richard Harrison Shryock, *Medicine and Society in America, 1660–1860* (Ithaca, NY, 1960).

32. Samuel Miller, *Letters on Clerical Manners and Habits* (Philadelphia, 1852), pp. 150–152. See A. Vinet, *Pastoral Theology,* trans. and ed. Thomas H. Skinner (New York, 1953); Heman Humphrey, *Thirty-Four Letters to a Son in the Ministry* (Amherst, MA, 1842); James M. Hoppin, *The Office and Work of the Christian Ministry* (New York, 1869); William S. Plumer, *Hints and Helps in Pastoral Theology* (New York, 1874); Theodore L. Cuyler, *How to be a Pastor* (New York, 1890).

33. James Spencer Cannon, *Lectures on Pastoral Theology* (New York, 1853), esp. pp. 522–584; Washington Gladden, *The Christian Pastor and the Working Church* (New York, 1898), pp. 186–193.

34. See Ezra Stiles Ely, *Visits of Mercy,* 2 vols. (Philadelphia, 1827); Ichabod S. Spencer, *A Pastor's Sketches: . . . First and Second Series* (Philadelphia [1851, 1853], 1900, 1906).

35. E.R. Beadle, *The Sacredness of the Medical Profession* (Philadelphia, 1865); Beadle, *The True Physician* (Philadelphia, 1874).

36. John M. Krebs, *The Reciprocal Relations of Physicians and Clergymen* (New York, 1847); also see Joel Parker, *A Sermon on the Moral Responsibility of Physicians* (Philadelphia, 1848); E.P. Rogers, *The Medical Profession and the Duties of its Members* (Northampton, MA, 1850); Duncan Kennedy, *A Clergyman's Idea of a Model Physician* (Albany, NY, 1858).

37. See A.A. Hodge, *The Life of Charles Hodge* (New York, 1880), p. 542; also Edward Miller, *Medical Works . . .,* ed. Samuel Miller (New York, 1814); J. Howe Adams, *History of the Life of D. Hayes Agnew* (Philadelphia, 1892), pp. 288–297; J. Marion Sims, *The Story of My Life* (New York, 1889); "Lewis Henry Steiner," *Dictionary of American Biography,* 22 vols. (New York, 1928), 17:562–563. For physicians who grew up in Reformed households but who seemed to have changed course, see Wade W. Oliver, *The Man Who Lived for Tomorrow: A Biography of William Hallock Park* (New York, 1941); Simon Flexner and James Thomas Flexner, *William Henry Welch and the Heroic Age of American Medicine* (New York, 1941); Alice Hamilton, *Exploring the Dangerous Trades* (Boston, 1943); William Sharpe, *Brain Surgeon* (New York, 1952). Also see Charles E. Rosenberg, "The Therapeutic Revolution: Medicine, Meaning, and Social Change in Nineteenth-Century America," *Perspectives in Biology and Medicine* 20 (1977):485–505.

38. [Abby Howland Woolsey], *A Century of Nursing* (New York, 1876), p. 37; Anne L. Austin, *The Woolsey Sisters of New York* (Philadelphia, 1971). For nursing by religious orders, see Ann Doyle, "Deaconesses, 1855–1928," *American Journal of Nursing* 29 (1929):1331–1343.

39. Albert R. Lamb, *The Presbyterian Hospital and the Columbia-Presbyterian Medical Center, 1868–1943* (New York, 1955), pp. 11, 75–78; Charles E. Rosenberg, "Inward Vision and Outward Glance: The Shaping of the American Hospital, 1880–1914," *Bulletin of the History of Medicine* 53 (1979):346–391.

40. Ruth Maszkiewicz, "The Presbyterian Hospital of Pittsburgh: From Its Founding to Affiliation with the University of Pittsburgh" (Ph.D. diss., University of Pittsburgh, 1977).

41. See files of National Presbyterian Health and Welfare Association, Presbyterian Historical Society, Philadelphia, PA, and Office of Health Ministries, Presbyterian Church (U.S.A.), New York. See, for a contemporary example, Edwin W. Stock, Jr., "The Role of the Church in the Inception and Survival of the Appalachian Regional Hospital" (D. Min. Thesis, Louisville Theological Seminary, 1979).

42. Edward Vose Gulick, *Peter Parker and the Opening of China* (Cambridge, MA, 1973). See also Robert E. Speer, *The Hakim Sahib, The Foreign Doctor: A Biography of Joseph Plumb Cochran, M.D., of Persia* (New York, 1911); Speer, *A Missionary Pioneer in the Far East: A Memorial*

of *Davie Bethune McCarter* (New York, 1922); Speer, *Lu Taifu: Charles Lewis, M.D., a Pioneer Surgeon in China* (New York, 1930).

43. Mary H. Fulton, *Inasmuch: Extracts from Letters, Journals, Papers, Etc.* (West Medford, MA, n.d.); and also Sara Tucker, "A Dual Calling: John Glasgow, M.D., and the Changing Patterns of Presbyterian Missionary Medicine at Canton, 1854–1901," unpublished manuscript, 1983.

44. W.J. Wanless, *The Medical Mission: Its Place, Power and Appeal* (Philadelphia, 1911); Edward M. Dodd, M.D., *Our Medical Task Overseas* (New York, 1934); The Board of Foreign Missions of the Presbyterian Church in the U.S.A., *Our Medical Task Overseas* (New York [1950]).

45. See, e.g., T.B. Kilpatrick, "Suffering," in *Encyclopedia of Religion and Ethics,* ed. James Hastings, 13 vols. (New York, 1922), 11:1–10.

46. Horace Bushnell, "Of Physical Pain," in *Moral Uses of Dark Things* (New York [1867], 1910), pp. 95–119, and *passim* on plagues and insanity. Also for other works, H. Shelton Smith, ed., *Horace Bushnell* (New York, 1965), pp. 246–247, 279–283, 289–293.

47. Henry Ward Beecher preached on suffering numerous times. See for examples: "Sources and Uses of Suffering," *Plymouth Pulpit* (New York, 1892), pp. 155–174; Beecher, *Plymouth Pulpit,* 9 vols. (New York, 1893), "Suffering, The Measure of Worth," 1:324–339; "The Worth of Suffering," 7:313–328; Beecher, "The Ministration of Suffering," in *Sermons,* 2 vols. (New York, 1969), 2:263–278.

48. Archibald Alexander Hodge, *Popular Lectures on Theological Themes* (Philadelphia, 1887), pp. 94–116.

49. See Jack Martin Maxwell, *Worship and Reformed Theology* (Pittsburgh, 1976); Julius Melton, *Presbyterian Worship in America* (Richmond, 1967); and *The Book of Common Worship* (Philadelphia, 1906), pp. 127, 139, 140.

50. *Book of Common Worship,* p. 139.

51. Nancy McCall, "The Statue of the Christus Consolator at the Johns Hopkins Hospital: Its Acquisition and Historic Origins," *Johns Hopkins Medical Journal* 151 (1982):11–19.

52. Benjamin B. Warfield, *Counterfeit Miracles* (New York, 1918), pp. 229–230; Mary Baker Eddy, *Science and Health with Key to the Scriptures* (Boston, 1875), p. 597.

53. Gail Thain Parker, "Jonathan Edwards and Melancholy," *New England Quarterly* 41 (1969):193–212.

54. See Anton T. Boisen, *The Exploration of the Inner World* (Chicago, 1936), and Boisen, *Religion in Crisis and Custom* (New York, 1945). Also see Glenn H. Asquith, Jr., "Anton T. Boisen and the Study of 'Living Human Documents,'" *Journal of Presbyterian History* 60 (1982):244–265.

55. Karl A. Menninger, *Man Against Himself* (New York, 1938); Menninger, with Jeanetta L. Menninger, *Love Against Hate* (New York, 1959); Menninger, with Martin Mayman and Paul Pruyser, *The Vital Balance* (New York, 1963). See also Menninger, *Whatever Became of Sin?* (New York, 1973); Paul W. Pruyser, "Religio Medici: Karl A. Menninger, Calvinism and the Presbyterian Church," *Journal of Presbyterian History* 59 (1981):59–72.

56. See E. Brooks Holifield, *A History of Pastoral Care in America: From Salvation to Self-Realization* (Nashville, 1983); see also Donald Meyer, *The Positive Thinkers* (New York, 1965).

57. Robert H. Bonthius, *Christian Paths to Self-Acceptance* (New York, 1948), pp. 1–38, 185–191, 201–215.

58. David E. Roberts, *Psychotherapy and a Christian View of Man* (New York, 1950); see also Daniel Day Williams, *The Minister and the Care of Souls* (New York, 1961).

59. Seward Hiltner, *Religion and Health* (New York, 1943); Hiltner, *Preface to Pastoral Theology* (Nashville, 1958), pp. 43–51, 70–85, 18–29; Hiltner, "Christian Understanding of Sin in the Light of Medicine and Psychiatry," *Medical Arts and Sciences* 20 (Second Quarter, 1966):35–49; Hiltner, "Salvation's Message about Health," *International Review of Missions* 57 (1968):157–174. See also William B. Oglesby, Jr., ed., *The New Shape of Pastoral Theology: Essays in Honor of Seward Hiltner* (Nashville, 1969).

60. *The Relation of Christian Faith to Health,* in which the authors deal with Scripture, history, and current challenges.

61. Seward Hiltner, *Sex Ethics and the Kinsey Reports* (New York, 1953); Hiltner, *Sex and the Christian Life* (New York, 1957); Roland H. Bainton, *What Christianity Says About Sex, Love and Marriage* (New York, 1957). See also Otto Piper, *The Biblical View of Sex and Marriage* (New York, 1960).

62. *Responsible Marriage and Parenthood* (New York, 1962); *Sexuality and the Human Community,* UPCUSA study paper (New York, 1970); Presbyterian Church in the United States [hereafter, PCUS], *Marriage: A Theological Statement* (Atlanta, 1980); PCUS, *The Nature and Purpose of Human Sexuality* (Atlanta, 1980). See Donald G. Dawe, "A Look at 'Sexuality and the Human Community,'" *Presbyterian Outlook* 152 (October 19, 1970), 5–6.

63. UPCUSA, *The Church and Homosexuality* (New York, 1978); PCUS, *The Church and Homosexuality: A Preliminary Study* (Atlanta, 1977).

64. PCUS, *Abortion,* study paper (Atlanta, 1973); UPCUSA, *Covenant and Creation: Theological Reflections on Contraception and Abortion* (New York, 1983). See Francis A. Schaeffer and C. Everett Koop, *Whatever Happened to the Human Race?* (Old Tappan, NJ, 1979); Koop, *The Right to Live; The Right to Die* (Wheaton, IL, 1976).

65. Carl J. Scherzer, *Ministering to the Physically Sick* (Englewood Cliffs, NJ, 1963); Scherzer, *Ministering to the Dying* (Englewood Cliffs, NJ, 1963); Scherzer, *The Church and Healing* (Philadelphia, 1950).

66. *The Relation of Christian Faith to Health,* pp. 48–50.

67. Paul W. Pruyser, "The Master Hand: Psychological Notes on Pastoral Blessing," in Oglesby, *New Shape,* pp. 352–365; Wade H. Boggs, Jr., *Faith Healing and the Christian Faith* (Richmond, 1956), pp. 53–54.

68. *Worshipbook* (Philadelphia, 1970), pp. 32–33, 181–185.

69. Willard L. Sperry, *The Ethical Basis of Medical Practice* (New York, 1950), esp. pp. 51–55 on conscience, and pp. 160–173 for reverence for life.

70. James M. Gustafson, *The Contributions of Theology to Medical Ethics* (Milwaukee, 1975), pp. 18–19, 70–75, and *passim.*

71. Kenneth Vaux, *Biomedical Ethics* (New York, 1974), pp. 24, 112–113.

72. See, e.g., Paul Tournier, *Guilt and Grace: A Psychological Study,* trans. Arthur W. Heathcote (New York [1958], 1962); *The Whole Person in a Broken World,* trans. John and Helen Doberstein (New York [1947],

1964). Tournier has written on loneliness, fatigue, and the "seasons of life."

73. UPCUSA, *Health Ministries and the Church,* (New York, 1978), pp. 6–7 and *passim.*

74. See UPCUSA, *Peacemaking: The Believers' Calling* (New York, 1980) and PCUS, *Peacemaking* (Atlanta, 1981) for pastoral summons to consider peace as discipline of the faithful.

75. See "Toward a National Policy for the Organization and Delivery of Health Services," *Minutes,* General Assembly, UPCUSA, 1971 (Philadelphia, 1971), pp. 585–595, for a statement and review of positions.

76. John Bryant, "Principles of Justice as a Basis for Conceptualizing a Health Care System," mimeo, 1973; William F. May, *The Physician's Covenant: Images of the Healer in Medical Ethics* (Philadelphia, 1983), pp. 124–127. See also J.M.T. Finney, *A Surgeon's Life* (New York, 1940), pp. 377–381, for a Presbyterian physician's approach to the doctor's responsibility and for an example of opposition to "socialized medicine"—even though Calvin encouraged a form of it in Geneva.

77. See Thomas Bradley Robb, *The Bonus Years: Foundations for Ministry with Older Persons* (Valley Forge, PA, 1968). Robb now directs the Presbyterian Office on Aging in Atlanta. Also see Robert W. McClellan, *Claiming a Frontier: Ministry and Older People* (Los Angeles, 1977); James A. Thorson and Thomas C. Cook, Jr., *National Intra-decade Conference on Spiritual Well-being of the Elderly* (Atlanta, 1977); H. Richard Niebuhr, *The Responsible Self: An Essay in Christian Moral Philosophy* (New York, 1963), p. 60.

78. PCUS, *The Nature and Value of Life* (Atlanta, 1981), pp. 4–10, 16–19.

79. Donald Shriver, Jr., "The Interrelationships of Religion and Medicine," in Shriver, ed., *Medicine and Religion: Strategies of Care* (Pittsburgh, 1980), pp. 21–45.

80. William B. Oglesby, Jr., *Biblical Themes for Pastoral Care* (Nashville, 1980), pp. 39–40. In 1967 the UPCUSA adopted a contemporary statement of faith entitled the "Confession of 1967" based upon 2 *Corinthians* 5:18–20 and the theme of reconciliation. This became a part of a *Book of Confessions,* which included several Reformation credal statements cited in this essay.

81. *Worshipbook,* p. 183.

CHAPTER 8

The Anglican

Tradition

JOHN E. BOOTY

The distinctive Anglican (or English) tradition officially began in 1534 when an act of Parliament established the supremacy of the crown, initially of King Henry VIII, over the church in England, thus renouncing the "supremacy" of the pope in Rome. The causes for this action were manifold, including the growth of English patriotism, the persistence of Lollard heretical teachings, the advent of the teachings of Martin Luther, the advancing influence of Christian humanism amongst the intelligensia in the Universities of Oxford and Cambridge, and the king's frustration at being denied the divorce he sought from Catherine of Aragon in order to marry Anne Boleyn. Along with the renunciation of papal authority there came the dissolution of the monasteries in England by 1539, partly due to lust for monastic wealth and partly due to the erosion of piety in many of the religious houses. A Bible in English was officially published in 1539; officials of Protestant, reformist, and humanist backgrounds were appointed to key offices; and liturgical reform was begun under Thomas Cranmer as Archbishop of Canterbury; but the king's basic conservatism was asserted toward the end of his reign. His preference was for the maintenance of traditional doctrine and worship.

King Henry VIII died in 1547 and he was succeeded by a son who was still a minor in the eyes of the law. King Edward VI ruled through his uncle, the Protector Somerset. During Edward's short reign, the

Reformation in England advanced rapidly. The first *Book of Common Prayer* was published in 1549 and was followed by a more Protestant edition in 1552. The prayer book, largely produced by Cranmer, was influenced by the continental Reformation. It was, however, traditional, recognizing the authority not only of Scripture, but of the early church, and maintaining continuity with medieval worship, chiefly through the influence of the Sarum (Salisbury) Use. During the reign of Edward VI, the *First Book of Homilies* was published, containing teachings of the Reformed church in England. Such teachings were also buttressed by the promulgation of forty-two Articles of Religion, strongly influenced by Lutheran articles, and by the publication of the works of many of the reformers. Through visitations—national and local—the official teaching was enforced and elaborated throughout the country, eventually affecting every parish church.

The progress of reform was halted by the death of Edward in 1553 and the accession of his half-sister Mary, the daughter of Henry VIII and Catherine of Aragon. Mary restored the English church to papal allegiance and began the process whereby the religious orders were to be revived. She married King Philip of Spain and restored Spanish influence in the royal court. Some of the reformers were tried and executed for heresy, including Thomas Cranmer; others escaped to Europe and awaited a turn in the events. Mary's success in restoring the medieval church in England was doomed by the resistance of Protestant sympathizers and by nobility and gentry who benefited from the seizure of monastic wealth. It was also doomed by her failure to produce a male heir before she died in 1558.

Mary was succeeded by her half-sister, who became Queen Elizabeth I and reigned until 1603. Elizabeth was the daughter of Henry VIII and Anne Boleyn and was raised by persons who are justly described as Protestant humanists. Those who had been in exile on the continent during Mary's reign returned determined to restore the English church to the position it held under Edward VI. In the Parliament of 1559, royal supremacy over the Church of England was restored, but whereas her father was declared "head" of the church, Elizabeth was named its "governor." The *Book of Common Prayer* was restored by means of a uniformity act. It was the second, more Protestant book of 1552, but with enough conservative amendments to indicate that the queen would not give the exiles all that they demanded. There were further indications that she intended to steer something of a middle course between Rome and Geneva, between papists and Puritans, as the most devoted of the reformers were to be known. Such indications were to be seen in amended Articles of Religion, now thirty-nine in number, and a *Second Book of Homilies.* But chiefly, her position was declared by her growing opposition to the Puritans who opposed Episcopal government in the church, which is to say government by bishops, priests, and deacons, rather than pastors, elders, teachers, and deacons, and the *Book of Common Prayer,* which Puritans characterized as a "dungheap full of popish abominations."

Out of this beginning in England, the Anglican communion developed. It is a worldwide fellowship of independent churches sharing a common heritage derived from the Church of England in the sixteenth and following centuries. There are forty-eight provinces, located on every continent, with 414 dioceses, and approximately sixty-three million members. While independent, its member churches acknowledge a common heritage, involving the *Book of Common Prayer*, the Thirty-nine Articles, and the threefold ministry of bishops, priests, and deacons. The bishops meet every ten years in the Lambeth Conference, held at the residence of the Archbishop of Canterbury. Cooperation is assisted by the Anglican Consultative Council and Regional Councils. The Communion is committed to the reunion of all churches and in 1888 adopted a quadrilateral as its basis for reunion, affirming (1) that the Holy Scriptures contain all that is necessary to salvation and are the rule and ultimate standard of faith; (2) the Apostles' Creed, as "the Baptismal Symbol," and the Nicene as "the sufficient statement of faith"; (3) Baptism and the Lord's Supper, "ministered with unfailing use of Christ's words of institution, and of the elements ordained by him"; and (4) "The Historic Episcopate, locally adapted in the methods of its administration to the varying needs of the nations and peoples called of God into the Unity of His Church."

The Episcopal Church, the American branch of the Anglican Communion, has approximately three million members in eight thousand parishes and missions, with thirteen thousand clergy. In 1789, after the American Revolution, the Church of England in the colonies became an independent church, determined to preserve its Anglican heritage, but committed to American ideals, such as separation of church and state. This church established a polity bearing resemblance to the Articles of Confederation, in which the democratic, lay-dominated structures of the church were set in tension with aristocratic, episcopally dominated structures of government. A General Convention, to meet triennially, was established, composed of a house of bishops and a house of clerical and lay deputies. The subsequent history of the Episcopal Church is largely that of expansion, with the growth of the United States in territory and population, and of revisions of polity, laws, and liturgy. The church's missionary commitments led to the founding of the Domestic and Foreign Missionary Society in 1820. Its president was the Presiding Bishop, the senior bishop in the House of Bishops. This marked the beginning of a permanent national executive for the Church. A 1919 General Convention created the National Council, changed to "the Executive Council," which absorbed the Missionary Society and other societies for educational and social concerns. The *American Book of Common Prayer*, created in 1789, has been revised, principally in 1892, 1928, and most recently in 1979 with the provision of a new *Book of Common Prayer*. The all-male ordained ministry has been enlarged to include women.

The newest prayer book and the ordination of women to the priesthood caused some members to leave the church, beginning around 1976. Ordination of women was objected to on biblical and theological grounds.

The 1979 prayer book was rejected by many as being too great a departure from the traditional *Book of Common Prayer* as well as being theologically suspect. The Episcopal Church has been actively engaged in ecumenical efforts, largely through the National and World Councils of Churches and Churches of Christ Uniting (COCU). It has participated in conversations with other churches, principally the Presbyterians, Roman Catholics, Orthodox, and Lutherans.

It should be noted that the Episcopal Church is in part characterized by a tension, sometimes disruptive but often creative, between the various parties and points of view: for instance, the Evangelicals with their emphasis on the authority of Scripture; High Churchmen, emphasizing tradition; Anglo-Catholics with their concern for ritual and sacramental theology; Broad Churchmen, who have traditionally emphasized human reason and freedom; Liberals, concerned for the untrammeled pursuit of truth and for social action; Low Churchmen, emphasizing simplicity and charity; and various combinations of all of these. Such diversity makes it difficult for the Episcopal Church to speak with one voice on any issue of consequence in the areas of health and medicine.

The history of health and medicine in the Anglican tradition began in the sixteenth century, when the tradition started to take shape with the reform of the ancient *ecclesia Anglicana,* the rejection of papal control, and the assertion of royal supremacy over the church. These reforms coincided with the age of rational inquiry and critical judgment, associated with the Northern Renaissance. Within the church, the simple mass priest gave way to the literate and learned preacher. But popular supernaturalism remained widespread among the common folk and continued to influence the lives of the gentry and the nobility. In preaching before Queen Elizabeth I, John Jewel (d. 1571), the Bishop of Salisbury, denounced magic and necromancy, demanded the death penalty for all practitioners of the black arts, and identified Lord Robert Dudley, the queen's favorite, as one of those practitioners. Yet the queen herself was known to consult the astrologer John Dee for aid in making decisions, and kings and queens down to Queen Anne (d. 1714) were believed to possess miraculous powers of healing. In London, single-sheet publications, known as broad-sheets, pandered to the public's curiosity about strange events, explaining birth defects, such as a ruff of flesh around the neck of a newborn baby, as having been caused by the sins of its parents or the apostasy of the society as a whole. Sixteenth-century writers attributed madness to the work of Satan or the warfare of demons struggling against the good spirits in the minds of the mentally ill.

The Formative Period

It is well to keep this tension between the natural and the supernatural, rationalism and credulity, in mind as we turn to the formularies, in particular to *The Book of Common Prayer,* for evidence concerning attitudes toward health and medicine in nascent Anglicanism. The sixteenth-century prayer books reflected the influence of popular religion in England.

The Book of Common Prayer, first crafted in 1549 by Thomas Cranmer, Archbishop of Canterbury, and his associates, was perfected by revisions made in 1552 and 1559. The first two books were short-lived, but the third, the *Elizabethan Prayer Book* of 1559, remained in use until 1662, when a new edition appeared. *The Book of Common Prayer,* especially the revisions of 1559 and 1662, has been *the* book of Anglicanism, exercising great influence on the development of Anglican tradition, as well as being influenced by external and internal developments in church and state. It has provided the regular public services of worship in all Anglican churches, including the Episcopal Church in the United States of America, from the sixteenth century to the present age.

During the sixteenth and seventeenth centuries, the English were forced by law to use *The Book of Common Prayer* and no other order of worship. We know, however, that some of those discontented with the official book used a modified, "further reformed," order of worship attached to the Geneva Bible of 1583, while other discontented churchmen used Puritan books. The 1559 Act of Uniformity also enforced attendance in the parish church on Sundays and other holy days, on pain of censure and the payment of a fine of twelve pence, collected by the churchwardens for the relief of the poor.[1] Thus, with few exceptions, the people of England, from infancy to death, were exposed to the influence of *The Book of Common Prayer* and its attitudes and teachings concerning sickness and health.

A.L. Rowse speaks as a modern historian of Tudor England when he says: "It is impossible to over-estimate the influence of the Church's routine of prayer and good works upon Elizabethan society: the effect upon the imagination and conduct of the liturgy with its piercing and affecting phrases, repeated Sunday by Sunday."[2] The Holy Bible, translated into English during the reign of Henry VIII (1507–1547), also assumed great importance, but much of its influence on the ordinary people came through the prayer book, which provided for the regular reading of the Scriptures and which was itself largely biblical in content. Furthermore, through the years the prayer book served as a standard for doctrine and belief among Anglicans; thus its various editions, revised in response to cultural changes, reveal fundamental convictions concerning health and medicine at different times and in different places.

The sixteenth-century prayer book, issued during the formative age of the Anglican tradition, provided for the sanctification of life from birth to death. Each newborn child was baptized in the name of the Father, the Son, and the Holy Spirit and signed with the sign of the cross "in token that hereafter he shall not be ashamed to confess the faith of Christ crucified, and manfully to fight under his banner against sin, the world, and the devil, and to continue as Christ's faithful soldier and servant unto his life's end."[3] To the sixteenth-century mind, baptism in the triune Name with the sign of the cross guarded against the assaults of Satan and his hosts, although it was acknowledged that the Christian was willfully to resist temptation.

Having given birth and having seen to the baptism of her child, the mother went to the church for the service called "The Thanksgiving of Women after Childbirth, Commonly called the Churching of Women." There she gave thanks for safe deliverance from "the great pain and peril of childbirth."[4] The first prayer book (1549) described the service as a rite of purification, based upon the conviction that the new mother was unclean. In 1552 purification was dropped in favor of thanksgiving, indicating a shift of focus from uncleanness associated with copulation to thanksgiving that the woman had survived the pains and perils of childbirth.

The sixteenth-century prayer book also provided for the "Solemnization of Holy Matrimony," noting at the outset the traditional purposes of marriage in Western society: procreation, the provision of "a remedy against sin, and to avoid fornication," and "mutual society, help, and comfort."[5] Although the first and second were the dominant reasons for matrimony in the sixteenth century, the third was also taken seriously, especially by those influenced by Reformation theology. The earthiness and the physical nature of marriage were emphasized in the words spoken by the man as he put a ring on the fourth finger of the woman's left hand: "With this ring I thee wed: with my body I thee worship. . . ."[6] Richard Hooker (1544–1600), the greatest of the sixteenth-century Anglican theologians, commented on this with reference to 1 *Corinthians* 7:4:

> The apostle [Paul] doth so expreslie affirme that parties married have not anie longer intire power over them selves but ech hath interest in others person, it cannot be thought an absurd construction to saie that worshipping with the bodie is the imparting of that interest in the bodie unto another which none before had save onlie our selves.[7]

In writing about sex and marriage in early modern England, Lawrence Stone has noted "the dominance of a religion—Christianity—which has always been more or less hostile to sex as pleasure or play, and anxious to confine its legitimacy to the functional purpose of procreation."[8] *The Book of Common Prayer,* in its marriage service, did emphasize procreation, but, as Stone suggests, there were powerful forces in sixteenth- and seventeenth-century England running counter to the church's condemnation of sex as pleasure or play. Beyond the influence of the Church of England, sex and play were conjoined in much of the popular literature of the time. This is evident in some of the verse of Ben Jonson (d. 1637), who wrote, "Come my Celia, let us prove,/While we may, the sports of love." John Wilmot, Earl of Rochester (d. 1680), expressed similar feelings:

> Naked she lay, clasped in my longing arms,
> I willed with love, and she all over charms;
> Both equally inspired with eager fire,
> Melting through kindness, flaming in desire.

Such lines are secular, not religious. Church court records, which surely expose but the "tip of the iceberg," reveal in endless detail the ways in which people, high and low, disregarded the church's admonitions concerning sex as pleasure or play. The courts proved unable to suppress or eradicate what was then called fornication.[9]

John Donne (d. 1631) wrote secular love poetry as a young man but turned to sacred verse as a mature poet, priest of the church, and dean of St. Paul's Cathedral, London. In his maturity he celebrated marriage as a condition of joy and fulfillment. With reference to sexual intercourse in marriage, he wrote:

> By this act of these two Phenixes
> Nature againe restored is,
> For since these two are two no more,
> Ther's but one Phenix still, as was before.[10]

In at least three sermons, Donne waxed eloquent concerning the importance and sacred character of marriage, which he viewed as a sacrament, *"bonum sacramenti,* a mysticall representation of the union of two natures in Christ, and of him to us, and to his Church."[11] Donne strove to combat the idea that the joining of two persons, body and soul, in matrimony was inferior, unworthy, or unclean.

Some practices were considered dishonorable by both the church and society at large. Church court records report cases of rape, incest, coition with animals, and mutual male and mutual female masturbation.[12] Anglican moral theology disapproved of any form of masturbation, but books on childraising remained silent on the subject. Some medical practitioners in seventeenth-century England condoned male masturbation, perhaps believing that good health required occasional evacuation of superfluous body fluids.[13]

In this early period there were no efficient means of birth control other than coitus interruptus, and the effectiveness of that method could not be guaranteed. Pregnancy and childbirth were thus the usual results of sexual intercourse, and childbirth, as Stone says, "was a very dangerous experience, for midwives were ignorant and ill-trained, and often horribly botched the job, while the lack of hygienic precautions meant that puerperal fever was a frequent sequel."[14] This reality greatly influenced thinking about sex and marriage in early modern England.

However much the society's attitudes toward sex and marriage may have been changing, the old views, fundamentally conservative, were preserved in popular devotions and in pious guides to conduct. One of the latter was the popular and influential *Rule and Exercises of Holy Living* (1650) by Jeremy Taylor (1613–1667), Bishop of Down and Connor. Concerning matrimony, Taylor wrote:

> Although in this, as in eating and drinking, there is an appetite to be satisfied, which cannot be done without pleasing that desire, yet since that desire and satisfaction was intended by nature for other ends, they should never be separate from those ends, *with a desire of children*, or *to avoid fornication*, or *to lighten and ease the cares and sadnesses of household affairs*, or *to endear each other;* but never with a purpose, either in act or desire to separate the sensuality from these ends which hallow it. Onan did separate his act from its proper end, and so ordered his embraces that his wife should not conceive, and God punished him.[15]

The end of life was marked by a formal service for the burial of the dead. Because rites of burial seemed to perpetuate superstition, at least through the ritual associated with them in the late Middle Ages, as well as through popular understandings of purgatory, some Puritan Anglicans expressed displeasure. But the sixteenth-century prayer book retained a simple liturgical form. Richard Hooker, defending the burial service against the objections of the Puritans, wrote:

> The ende of funerall duties is first to show that love towardes the partie deceased which nature requireth; then to doe him that honor which is fitt both generallie for man and particularly for the qualitie of his person; last of all to testifie the care which the Church hath to comfort the living, and the hope which wee all have concerning the resurrection of the dead.[16]

The burial service was not the only place in the prayer book emphasizing death and dying, however. Services for the Visitation of the Sick and Communion of the Sick were conducted throughout with the purpose of assisting those who were ailing in preparing for imminent death. The second of Taylor's guides for living the Christian life, *The Rule and Exercises of Holy Dying* (1651), dealt with sickness in great detail as a preparation for dying. This emphasis on preparation for dying derived from the service of visitation in the Sarum *Manual,* the medieval source from which Cranmer worked as he fashioned the English service for the 1549 prayer book. During the Middle Ages the practice of anointing the sick with oil, so widespread in the early church of the first five centuries, became the sacrament of dying, or "Extreme Unction," ministered to those on the verge of death. Thus in the 1549 book, the visitation of the sick, which included anointing, was regarded as a preparation for dying. The governing statement read: "vouchsafe for his [God's] great mercy (yf it be his blessed will) to restore unto thee thy bodely helth, and strength, to serve him, and send thee release of al thy paines, troubles, and diseases, both in body and minde."[17] This was deleted from the 1552 book, being regarded as a nonessential practice associated with Roman Catholic ritual, and, although unction appeared in the Latin book of 1560, designed for use in the universities of Oxford and Cambridge, it was rarely performed until the nineteenth and twentieth centuries.

Devoid of the positive influence of anointing, as understood in the early church, the prayer book provisions for ministry to the sick emphasized the causal relationship between sin and sickness. In the face of certain death, it exhorted repentance: "know you certainly, that yf you truely repent you of your sinnes, and beare your sickness paciently . . . it shall turn to your profit."[18] In suffering patiently, the sick were being "made lyke unto Christe. . . . So truely oure waye to eternall ioye is to suffre here with Christ."[19] For centuries this mood of resignation prevailed among the leadership of the Church of England.

The prayer book understanding was reflected in other writings of the time. The "Prayer for Them that are Sick," written by Thomas Becon (1512–1567) and published around 1538, stated plainly that those who broke God's laws were, for the sake of their salvation, visited with sickness. The prayer urged repentance: "Make whole so many as acknowledge their miseries, repent them of their sinful manners. . . ."[20] In 1563, Alexander Nowell (1507–1602), dean of St. Paul's Cathedral, London, wrote a sermon, given official status by the queen, entitled "An Homily concerning the Justice of God, in punishing impenitent sinners, and of his mercies towards all such as in their afflictions unfeignedly turn unto him. Appointed to be read in the time of sickness."[21] The "Great Litany" published in 1544 and included in the prayer book, ended with a prayer to be used "In Time of Any Common Plague or Sickness," containing these words: "Have pity upon us miserable sinners, that now are visited with great sickness and mortality, that like as thou didst command thy angel [in the time of David and the plague of pestilence] to cease from punishing, so it may now please thee to withdraw from us this plague and grievous sickness. . . ."[22]

In view of the weight of such conviction, the relative ineffectiveness of medical science at this early date, and the fact that much healing, whether medical or spiritual, was in the hands of clerical amateurs, it is understandable that early modern Anglicans saw an equation between sin and sickness, health and repentance. Also understandable is the emphasis on death in a society where plague and sickness periodically swept away large segments of the population, and death during childbirth and infancy was commonplace.

Both the teachings of the church and the ever-present reality of death encouraged early Anglicans to meditate upon "Last Things," including their own deaths and the judgment to come. In time of plague, corpses sometimes seemed to be everywhere, and the bodies of executed criminals were displayed for all to see. John Donne, in telling of hearing the church bell toll, the passing bell marking the death of some man or woman, mused, "Now, this bell tolling softly for another, says to me: Thou must die."[23] In response to such conditions there appeared a steady flow of books teaching readers how to die well *(ars moriendi).* As Bettie Anne Doebler says, "The Christian is told to consider every day as the day of death and to reckon with himself as on the last day."[24]

Anglican divines may have sought to arouse fear of death and judgment, but, as Richard Hooker taught, "feare worketh noe mans inclination to repentance, till somewhat else have wrought in us love alsoe."[25] Hooker directed attention to the goodness of God and the promise of eternal life for those who loved him. In an exhortation "Agaynste the Feare of Deathe" (1574), we read that

> bodily death is a door or entering unto life; and therefore not so much dreadful, if it be rightly considered, as it is comfortable [strengthening] . . . leading us, not to mortality, but to immortality, nor to sorrow and pain, but to joy and pleasure, and that to endure for ever; if it be thankfully taken and accepted as God's messenger, and patiently borne of us for Christ's love, that suffered most painful death for our love, to redeem us from death eternal.[26]

There thus existed a tension between fearing death and welcoming it as the door to eternal life and joy.

Practitioners of healing in the seventeenth century came from a variety of pursuits and professions. The historian Michael MacDonald, writing of psychological healing, describes a rich mixture of scientific, religious, and magical elements that applies to bodily healing as well:

> Mentally disturbed people were treated with drugs and therapeutic regimens to restore the balance of their humours, with religious counsel and prayer to ease their spiritual afflictions, and with amulets, charms, and exorcisms to protect them against the malignancy of demons and witches. The kinds of healers were as diverse as the remedies for mental maladies: physicians, astrologers, folk magicians, clergymen, and lay adepts all treated psychological disturbances.[27]

It was expected that the clergy would minister to those who were sick, whether physically or mentally or both. George Herbert (1593–1633), priest and poet, wrote of "The Parson Comforting," which meant strengthening or encouraging: "The Country Parson, when any of his cure [parish] is sick, or afflicted with losse of friend, or estate, or any ways distressed, fails not to afford his best comforts, and rather goes to them, then sends for the afflicted."[28] The most conscientious clergy of the Church of England also cared for the health and welfare of the community at large. For example, Godfrey Goodman (d. 1656), while parson of Stapleford Abbots in Essex, aimed through preaching, administration of the sacraments, and the discipline of the church to maintain a healthful, orderly, peaceful, and prosperous community.[29]

The clergy at their best served as community leaders, which often involved the practice of medicine. John Favour, Vicar of Halifax (d. 1623), started a grammar school, encouraged the cloth-making industry in his parish, and made himself available to his people as both their physician and their lawyer. He tells of being busy "preaching every Sabbath . . . exercising justice in the commonwealth, practicing physic and chirurgery [medicine and surgery] in the great pensury and necessity thereof in the country where I live."[30]

One of the most colorful clergymen-physicians was the orthodox Anglican priest Richard Napier, alchemist, astrologer, physician, and incumbent of Great Linford, Buckinghamshire (d. 1634), who claimed to be in constant communication with the angel Raphael. Napier, who was licensed to practice medicine, treated as many as two thousand patients a year. As MacDonald says:

> Napier treated between five and fifteen patients a day, repeating with each one of them a ritual of interrogation and annotation that invoked axioms of astrological medicine. Napier began every consultation with a fixed litany of questions. Who is the patient? Where does he live? How old is he? . . . When the precise coordinates of the patient's identity had been recorded,

the astrologer noted the time and date and drew a cross-hatched box on the page. Deciphering the ephemeris at his elbow, he mapped the heavens at that moment, positioning the symbols of the planets and the signs of the zodiac along the celestial frame.

Napier thus located the patient in the cosmos, presuming that bodily and mental illnesses were "mirrored in the motions of the stars, and the horoscope was an aid to discovering their nature and origins." On the basis of such analysis, he selected "remedies possessing the appropriate celestial and medical virtues."[31] Anglicanism was on the whole strongly opposed to astrology, but Napier, whose patients included John Williams, Bishop of Lincoln, could take comfort in the knowledge that even Archbishop William Laud showed an interest in astrology and that Puritans, not Anglicans, were his chief critics. The Church of England, at least prior to the Civil War, was actively concerned with the practice of medicine, played a role in the licensing of medical practitioners, and in its clergy provided many of those practicing medicine and surgery in the country. It is equally evident that not all combined astrology with medicine as did Napier, but the degree of interest in astrology during the sixteenth and seventeenth centuries in England has been revealed by modern scholars such as Keith Thomas, the author of *Religion and the Decline of Magic.*

The Eighteenth Century

The tradition of clergymen-physicians continued into the eighteenth century. Thomas Secker (1693–1768), who became Archbishop of Canterbury, studied human anatomy under William Cheselden, a surgeon; materia medica under Bakewell, an apothecary; and surgery and obstetrics at the Hôtel Dieu, a hospital in Paris. Secker took his medical degree at Leyden in 1721, writing for his thesis "a work of theoretical physiology concerned with perspiration."[32] As rector of Houghton-le-Spring (1724–1727), Secker practiced medicine among his parishioners; in fact, he continued throughout the rest of his life offering medical advice and ministering to physical as well as spiritual needs. His sermons "On the Duties of the Sick" reflected medical as well as theological expertise.[33]

Samuel Seabury (1729–1796), the first bishop of the newly formed Protestant Episcopal Church in the United States of America, and the first Bishop of Connecticut, was born into a family of clergymen-physicians. He studied first under his physician father and then in Edinburgh, Scotland. Ordained to the priesthood, he practiced physic among the people of his congregation. The ministry, however, remained his chief occupation, except during the Revolutionary War. As a loyalist priest, he sought refuge with the British in New York, where in order to earn a living he practiced medicine and served as physician to an almshouse.[34]

It is evident from these examples that while clergymen might still seek to qualify as physicians, their training in medicine was becoming more and more taxing as the subject became more and more scientific. Indeed, during the seventeenth and eighteenth centuries, Anglicanism itself felt the impact of rationalism and the Enlightenment. Many Anglicans relegated miracles to the past as they grew increasingly skeptical. The naturalist John Ray (1627–1705), a priest until the Restoration of the English monarchy in 1660, attributed much of what was formerly thought to be miraculous to the working out of God's will through natural causes, and his point of view was adopted by increasing numbers of the literate during the eighteenth century. Of course "popular supernaturalism" did not disappear altogether. The common folk retained their belief in the causal relationship between the natural and the supernatural, sometimes in relation to God's wrath aimed at sinners who had sold out to the vanities of this world, sometimes in relation to the work of Satan in causing mental and physical illnesses. The practice of the healing arts by those not trained in scientific medicine and properly licensed became more and more the occupation of persons outside of the established church.

The Anglican priest John Wesley (1703–1791), who founded Methodism, criticized modern medical practice and the scientific outlook on life and health. According to one scholar,

> Wesley's collection of remedies was certainly a bizarre mixture of commonsense health advice; harmless if not beneficent medicaments; and folk medicine sometimes verging on magic. His famous electric shock treatment can be cited as evidence of modernity, but it was used more like a quack's panacea. Some remedies have predictably figured in modern dismissals of the book. There is our old friend the powdered toad; a live puppy on the belly for the 'iliac passion'; cowdung plaster; breathing into a hole in the ground for consumption; a relic of the 'doctrine of signatures' in celandine for jaundice.[35]

Some medical practitioners and many Anglicans, chiefly priests and bishops, denounced Wesley for his "enthusiasm," his medical advice, and his belief in witches. But many laity, including some Anglicans, were attracted to the healing practices of such dissenters as the Methodists. "John Wesley claimed that hundreds of humble folks flocked to the dispensaries he had established to receive medicine and spiritual solace."[36] As the gap between the erudite, privileged upper class, and the common laborers in the new urban industrial centers grew, it threatened the peace and stability of the nation. Among the working classes in cities such as Sheffield, the Methodists often enjoyed greater success than the Church of England. The French Revolution at the end of the eighteenth century so alarmed the English that it brought about a conservative reaction, as well as concern for justice that helped to heal the ruptures in the social fabric. In the more stable conditions that emerged, the growth of industrialism was promoted as was the climate needed for the development of scientific medicine in England.

Reformers and Missionaries in the Nineteenth Century

By the nineteenth century, the Anglican Communion was taking shape. Beginning with the age of exploration and the establishment of colonies in North America during the fifteenth and sixteenth centuries, the British established outposts in various regions of the world. By the nineteenth century they had penetrated every continent and subcontinent, and worship according to *The Book of Common Prayer,* by then most often the 1662 revision, was found around the earth. At the start it was clearly a case of the cross following the crown; clergy accompanying explorers, settlers, and military units. When such clergy began reaching out to indigenous people, they did so as representatives of his majesty's government. In time missionary societies, such as the Society for Promoting Christian Knowledge (1698), the Society for the Propagation of the Gospel in Foreign Parts (1701), and the Church Missionary Society (1799), took over the support of foreign missions. In the nineteenth century, the great age of missions, former colonies of Great Britain, such as the United States, began sending out missionaries of their own through such agencies as the Domestic and Foreign Missionary Society (1820). As missions became more and more the concern of voluntary societies, the national identity of the missionaries decreased in importance.

Medical missions and missionaries did not play a significant role until the latter part of the nineteenth century. This resulted from two factors. First, medicine was developing professionally during the nineteenth century. By 1840, as the medical historian John Pickstone says,

All but the oldest regular practitioners would now have some kind of diploma, probably a License of the Society of Apothecaries or a Membership of the Royal College of Surgeons, or both. These testified to attendance at lectures and at teaching hospitals in addition to medical apprenticeship. In a city like Manchester most of the practitioners would have attended one or other of the local proprietary medical schools.[37]

Prior to this, it had been more difficult to distinguish professional medical personnel from ecclesiastics performing healing ministries. Thus there would seem to be little reason to identify medical missions and missionaries as such. Second, until the latter part of the century Anglicans showed little if any interest in providing medical assistance as part of foreign missions. The emphasis fell rather on converting non-Christians than on healing them of their physical ills. As late as 1861, Henry Venn (1796–1873), secretary of the Church Missionary Society, advised against the plans of a potential missionary to seek training in medicine: "It very seldom answers any good purpose."[38] If medical personnel did accompany missionaries, it was largely to serve them and their families. If they ministered to others, their activities might be explained in terms of helping to woo people to the church and making them available for conversion, the main purpose of Christian missions.

The situation did not change significantly until the appearance of a new motivating principle. In 1884, William Gray, the Church Missionary Society secretary, argued that healing was an aspect of evangelism and not just an aid or instrument. The principle inherent in this view was that of benevolence, earlier enunciated in the United States by the Calvinist Samuel Hopkins. As the historian C. Peter Williams has explained,

> This was not quite the case that was developed later, that Christ was as concerned with the body as the soul, but rather that his concern for the body was an appropriate model for his nineteenth century disciples committed both to saving souls and to humanising culture by demonstrating "that industrial, domestic life which is the product of Christianity."[39]

This principle helps to account for the growth in the number of European, including Anglican, medical missionaries from thirteen in 1852 to six hundred and fifty in 1900. Along with the increased number of medical missionaries went the founding of hospitals, many of which became, in time, major medical centers. Bishop Channing Moore Williams, an American who arrived in Japan in 1873, founded hospitals in China and Japan, with St. Luke's Hospital in Tokyo achieving considerable importance during the twentieth century. The expertise with which this was done was based upon experience in England and the United States where the church had long taken responsibility for providing health-care facilities. Under the aegis of American Episcopal missionaries, hospitals and other health-care institutions were begun far and wide, from the Yukon in Alaska to Bontoc in the Philippines. Writing in 1964, Raymond Albright said that

> the Episcopal Church from the beginning has been a leader among American churches in building hospitals and providing medical services and eleemosynary services. Although hospitals and many other similar institutions of the church have been merged with community institutions, the church still maintains throughout the world sixty-eight hospitals and convalescent homes, eleven residences and rest homes, eighty-three institutions and agencies for the care of the aged, and an even larger number for children and youth.[40]

By the twentieth century, the provision of medical missionaries and related institutions and facilities formed a major element in Anglican church life.

Changing Attitudes

In 1789 the American Episcopal Church adapted the English *Book of Common Prayer* to the circumstances of a new and independent nation. An 1892 revision of that book omitted all controversial innovations resulting from the Anglo-Catholic movement. In 1928 a revision provided greater flexibility in the use of the prescribed services, added prayers for all occasions, and enriched the liturgy as a whole. Shortly thereafter the General Convention of the Episcopal Church established a permanent liturgical commission, which began working toward a much more comprehensive revision, indeed a new *Book of Common Prayer.* The resultant 1979 book maintained continuity with the prayer books from 1549 to 1928, yet declared its independence of them, attempting to adjust Anglican worship to the secular and religious realities of the late twentieth century. Some of those changes reflected a modern understanding of health and medicine, not only in the U.S. Episcopal Church, but in Anglicanism almost everywhere. In parts of Asia, Africa, and the Pacific basin, however, native cultures modified Anglican views—and will do so more and more as the administration of churches in such areas becomes the responsibility of indigenous leaders.

First and foremost, the new prayer book revealed considerable change in the way modern Anglicans viewed sickness. One Episcopal commission described the change thus:

> Our attitudes toward sickness in the twentieth century have changed greatly from those of earlier periods. The grim view of illness as punishment for

sin and the concept of the 'visitation' [of the sick] as a preparation for death no longer are sound in the light of the advances of medical knowledge and techniques, particularly in the last fifty years, nor has such an approach any foundation in Scripture.[41]

The following prayer from the 1979 book illustrates the modern outlook:

Strengthen your servant *N.,* O God, to do what *he* has to do and bear what *he* has to bear; that, accepting your healing gifts through the skill of surgeons and nurses, *he* may be restored to usefulness in your world with a thankful heart; through Jesus Christ our Lord.[42]

The "Ministration of the Sick" called for repentance—but only when the patient's conscience was troubled. No longer was sickness viewed as chastisement for sin.

Unlike the 1928 book, which provided a prayer and a form for use in the anointing or laying-on-of-hands for healing but made no provision for blessing the oil, the 1979 book provided for Holy Unction—no longer "extreme" Unction—with the laying-on-of-hands and anointing with oil as a means of healing. This service, an integral part of the "Ministration of the Sick," consisted of a prayer for blessing the oil, an anthem, forms for the laying-on-of-hands and for anointing with oil, a final prayer, and a benediction.

The revival of spiritual healing in the course of the twentieth century undoubtedly contributed to these changes. The revival in England was controversial but steady.[43] In the United States the Episcopal Church was prompted by Christian Science to reconsider the relationship between religion and health. In 1906, Elwood Worcester, an Episcopal clergyman, started a healing ministry at Emmanuel Church, Boston, that evolved, with the aid of psychiatrists and other medical doctors, into the Emmanuel Movement. Worcester acknowledged the primacy of mind over body and believed that through prayer one could draw upon divine resources for healing. According to one church historian,

The efforts of Dr. Worcester, who had earned a doctorate in psychology in Germany, were most successful in dealing with persons afflicted with functional nervous disorders, although he and the staff did not neglect alcoholics and drug addicts. The physicians examined all patients, detailed records were kept, and individual therapy was usually followed by moral and spiritual re-education in the church where regular meetings with periods of prayer were conducted.[44]

This was a beginning. More recently, the International Order of St. Luke the Physician, associated with the names of John Gaynor Banks, a clergyman, and Agnes Sanford, has become the most prominent advocate of spiritual healing in the Episcopal Church.

A careful study presented to the Joint Commission on the Ministry of Healing to the General Convention of the Episcopal Church in 1964 defended the revival of spiritual healing, but recognized that the ministry of healing was not to be narrowly understood:

> The theology of the Church's ministry of healing must steadfastly assert the truth that all healing is of God. It is God the Holy Spirit Who gives effectiveness, and power, and salvation, to all ministry. Possibly one of the reasons the spiritual power of the Church is not as vigorous as it could and should be, is the lack of devotion and response to the Holy Spirit. Healing is the work of God the Holy Spirit, Who uses Sacraments, the Laying-on-of-Hands, the priest, the healer, the physician and surgeon, nurses, psychiatrists and psychologists—indeed, the Church herself, the blessed company of all faithful people—as agents through whom He achieves His will to heal.[45]

While some in the church may have over-emphasized spiritual healing to the neglect of modern medicine, the official view of the church remained holistic, including every legitimate means of health care and healing. The chief concern was stated in a committee report to the Lambeth Conference of bishops of the Anglican Communion in 1930:

> The Church must sanction methods of religious treatment of bodily disease, but in doing so must give full weight to the scientific discoveries of those who are investigating the interrelation of spirit, mind, and body. . . . No sick person must look to the clergyman to do what it is the physician's or surgeon's duty to do.[46]

More problematic was the revival of exorcism. The Exeter Commission in England in 1971 defined Christian exorcism as "the binding of evil powers by the triumph of Christ Jesus, through the application of the power demonstrated by that triumph, and by his Church."[47] Concerning the revival in this century, Robert Mortimer, Bishop of Exeter wrote:

> In countries with a long Christian tradition the need for exorcism to find a place in the regular ministry of the Church is not, perhaps, very urgent or evident. In countries which were, comparatively recently, pagan or primitive the urgency has been only too apparent, and the place of exorcism in the regular ministry of the Church has been taken for granted. In Western countries today, the widespread apostasy from the Christian Faith, accompanied by an increasing recourse to black magic and occult practices, is revealing the presence and the power of evil forces and the contaminating influence of an evil atmosphere in particular places and environments. The

need, therefore, for the restoration of the practice of exorcism to its proper place is becoming more urgent and more evident.[48]

Not every Anglican would agree with the Bishop of Exeter. Indeed, there is no consensus on exorcism in Anglicanism; many would support the seventeenth-century ban on exorcism by the clergy, and most would approve of the fact that the 1979 book has no rite of exorcism.

The 1979 prayer book also contains evidence of changes in attitude toward sex and marriage. In the marriage rite, the emphasis shifted from procreation and the avoidance of sin to the expression of love and fidelity and the enacting of a community compact. The Standing Liturgical Commission, in preparing the new rite, described marriage as "a solemn act, the creation of a new family within the larger family of mankind, of which the Christian community is a part. It is the highest expression of love between a man and a woman."[49] In 1958 a committee of Lambeth Conference on "The Family and Contemporary Society" emphasized the reproductive purpose of marriage, but then went on to say:

> The Biblical revelation, however, does not limit the function of sexuality and the family to the reproductive purpose. Equally deep-rooted in Genesis is the reflection of a second factor—the need of man and woman for each other, to complement and fulfil each other and to establish a durable partnership against the loneliness and rigour of life.[50]

The change in emphasis was necessitated by the emergence of industrial society, new insights into personal and family life, and the development of contraceptive devices and techniques. The Lambeth committee recognized in the light of these developments that the two most pressing issues were family planning and the permanence of the marriage bond.[51] Without idealizing "indissolubility" in a legal sense, they emphasized the need for responsible procreation and for depth and permanence in family ties.

The 1979 prayer book changed the order and thus the emphasis on the purposes of marriage in the statement made by the priest at the beginning of "The Celebration and Blessing of a Marriage," with procreation, which formerly came first, now coming last:

> The union of husband and wife in heart, body, and mind is intended by God for their mutual joy; for the help and comfort given one another in prosperity and adversity; and, when it is God's will, for the procreation of children and their nurture in the knowledge and love of the Lord.[52]

The clause "when it is God's will" allows for families in which there will be no children, considering the lack of children no barrier to the marriage contract.

In 1979 the Standing Commission on Human Affairs and Health of the General Convention of the Episcopal Church issued a report that declared that the

> purposes of human sexuality are to contribute to human welfare, pleasure, family procreation, social order and a more abundant quality of life for all. More specifically, sex should be used as a means of achieving such purposes and should be under the guidance and expression of the kind of love taught by Jesus and revealed by God through Christ.[53]

The use of the word *pleasure* in an official report clearly signaled a change in attitude. According to the commission, most Anglicans agreed "that sex is more good than bad, and that it is a volatile and pervasive power that therefore needs control and direction." However, differences appear when one attempts to "deal with specific means of dealing with sex and when one renders value and moral judgments about particular acts of sex."[54] There was, in fact, much difference among Anglicans on the subject.

The Lambeth Conference addressed the issue of family planning in a reply to the papal encyclical *Humanae Vitae.* The reply, dated 6 August 1968, stated the Anglican view:

> The Conference believes that the responsibility for deciding upon the number and frequency of children has been laid by God upon the consciences of parents everywhere: that this planning, in such ways as are mutually acceptable to husband and wife in Christian conscience, is a right and important factor in Christian family life and should be the result of positive choice before God. Such responsible parenthood, built on obedience to all the duties of marriage, requires a wise stewardship of the resources and abilities of the family as well as a thoughtful consideration of the varying population needs and problems of society and the claims of future generations.[55]

The prayer book statement "and, when it is God's will, for the procreation of children" should be understood in the light of such thinking.

The moderate revision of the burial service in 1979 was designed to emphasize triumph rather than defeat, to comfort rather than to condemn. The Standing Liturgical Commission of the Episcopal Church stated: "The Order [of Burial] attempts to strike a dominant note of joy in the faith that we shall rise again through the power of Christ's resurrection, rather than that of a penitential and mournful contemplation of death, without, however, ignoring the latter's stark reality."[56]

One of the suggested collects or prayers in the 1979 prayer book struck the keynote:

> O God, who by the glorious resurrection of your Son Jesus Christ destroyed death, and brought life and immortality to light: Grant that your servant *N.*, being raised with him, may know the strength of his presence, and rejoice in his eternal glory; who with you and the Holy Spirit lives and reigns, one God, for ever and ever.[57]

In recent years Anglicanism has also taken into account the increasing numbers and the growing plight of elderly persons. The Lambeth 1958 report on "The Family in Contemporary Society" recognized the seriousness of the problem in the twentieth century, especially the abandonment of the aged, produced partly by the industrial and social change that separated the young from their parents. "In the face of these situations the Church must constantly teach the integrity of the family and the mutual responsibility for each other of young and old," the report urged. It also recognized that the church has a responsibility to improve the social conditions of the aged, to provide adequate housing and centers for fellowship and recreation.[58] In the United States the Episcopal Society for Ministry on Aging, an official agency of the church, championed the cause of the elderly.

Facing the Future: Issues and Debates

Anglicanism involves a great variety of people. It began in England, but is now found all around the world. There are Anglicans of every race, from a multitude of nations, with widely differing political and economic systems. There are conservative Anglicans and liberal Anglicans: Evangelicals, Anglo-Catholics, and Broad Churchmen and women. They do not agree on every issue. In the recent past their disagreements have tested and on occasion shattered the unity of the Anglican Communion. In the Episcopal Church in the United States, the church's approval of the ordination of women (1976) and its provision of a new prayer book by the General Conventions of 1976 and 1979 caused many members to break away and form new church bodies or to join more conservative churches with which they were in agreement.

When it comes to difficult questions concerning medical ethics and human welfare, virtually every possible point of view can be found somewhere in Anglicanism. The first problem, an issue for generations, concerns the way in which the church arrives at a decision on any controverted issue: Who speaks for the church? There are two possible answers: the Lambeth Conference of Bishops, which meets every ten years and has no authority to legislate for any part of the Anglican Communion; and provincial synods, such as the General Convention of the Episcopal Church, which does have legislative power over the church in the United States. Thus decisions are reached through certain councils of the church, which are representative but seldom capable of speaking for every point of view or of legislating in such a way that everyone is included in every legislative decision. The conciliar mode necessitates ample discussion and debate, a large measure of patience, and a willingness to compromise. To compound the difficulty, the church encourages individuals to come to their own conclusions, in responsible relationship to God and to others in the communion, a matter that is taken seriously. Rights of conscience are protected so long as the bonds of love in communion are not violated.

An issue of considerable importance for the contemporary church concerns medical technology. The church's reaction to technological achievements and forecasts has been a mixed one of hope and fear. In 1967 the Joint Commission on the Church in Human Affairs of the Episcopal Church pointed to the possibility "of manipulating hereditary factors; to the decisions surrounding artificial insemination and abortion; to test-tube experiments with human ova and sperm; to the prolongation of life in terminal illness, or, following irreparable brain damage; to the modification of human personality by the use of drugs and electrical stimulation; and to more uncertain possibilities."[59] The commission spoke of the "need for moral criteria for human experimentation": "Man is now confronted with an inescapable new freedom. Nature alone does not supply categorical answers to all his questions, and the traditional resources for moral judgment in these matters are becoming increasingly inadequate."[60] The commission, therefore, asked that the Executive Council of the church be "instructed to carry out a study of the moral issues raised by medical technology, with the participation of scientists and theologians."

The results of this study were presented to the 1970 General Convention. The report positively recognized "the varied and innovative technological advances made by the health scientists" and encouraged further exploration. But the commission lamented the "morass of facts, figures, and statistics" rapidly engulfing medical personnel and their patients, arguing that this "threatens to remove from man both his appreciation for his real position in creation and his ability to determine the direction in which to turn for help, thus immobilizing him in decision making." An examination of the medical and technological problems facing Christians revealed a common concern for and appreciation of the fullness of life. Such concern may not produce satisfactory solutions to all problems, but it establishes a basis for the development of answers.

The commission emphasized the unity and continuity of human experience, the importance of external influences on the ability to develop and fulfill individual humanness, and the necessity of "sharing in the decision making process" if persons were to participate in "the total process of creation." The report stated that "one of man's greatest qualities, in which he participates with God to a limited extent, is his awareness of himself, and his relationship with others like him, and with God."

Believing that human beings derived fulfillment from assuming responsibility for their own situations, the commission argued that the health community should share its knowledge with patients and provide an environment "in which learning, decision-making, and participation with others" could take place. The commission insisted that it is

> the responsibility of society to provide for all men, of whatever station, economic level, ability, or talent, those opportunities for proper growth and development that will allow each man to exercise and celebrate his individuality within the community of man, to his and its corporate good. From a medical point of view, as well as from others this imperative implies, and we vigorously support, provision of high-quality medical care for all persons and the assurance of each individual's right to claim it; the provision of a high nutritional level for all men and the assurance of their inalienable right to call for it; and the highest possible degree of freedom in the exercise of individual conscience, in company with others, in the determination of a life-style, functional identity, and participation in the fullest expression of individual life, including choices surrounding his death.[61]

Thus the commission raised the banner of humanity in the face of a technology that, in spite of its contributions to the well-being of society, could lead to the realization of George Orwell's *1984.*

The emphasis upon individual rights in the commission's report was derived in part from the Renaissance humanism present in the formation of Anglicanism and from the revival of emphasis on the doctrine of the Incarnation in nineteenth-century English theology. William Temple, the great English theologian and ecclesiastical statesman, who became Archbishop of Canterbury in 1942, considered the ways in which God becoming a man in Jesus Christ reflected basic truths about individual human beings in society. Among those truths is the belief that because God dwells in persons they are "capable of apprehending universal principles and absolute values." They are not, however, automatons, for even as empowered images of God "the free choice of the individual remains." They are free to choose or not to choose to love God. Their tendency is to turn from God. To save humanity from this fatal tendency, God became man in Jesus Christ.

From Him a new influence goes forth, the attractive power and compelling appeal of perfectly holy love, expressed in the human fashion that calls forth sympathy. This power is none other than the divine potency in men that urges them to progress; but it is its perfect counterpart. In the response of love which the human being makes, he is at once free and enslaved; he is the willing slave, as the lover is the willing slave of his mistress. This was the one way by which God could draw men to Himself without overpowering their freedom.[62]

It was on the basis of such teaching that Temple and others like him insisted upon the freedom and the rights of the individual. Temple baldly asserted: "the Church must make respect for freedom its most fundamental principle of action."[63] It was not surprising that those studying the technological advances of modern society, and in particular some aspect of medical technology, with the theological point of view that Temple espoused should have warned against the loss of freedom and supported only that which advanced human freedom as well as human welfare.

In recent years Anglicans have engaged in an ongoing discussion of artificial insemination or "surrogate parenthood." In 1973 the Joint Commission on the Church in Human Affairs condoned the use of artificial insemination, provided only that the sperm of the husband and the ova of the wife were involved. Use of the semen of a donor or of a host uterus was seriously questioned on the basis of the Christian understanding of the family and the danger that human beings may be used as mere objects.[64] In 1982 the Joint Commission on Human Affairs and Health recognized the complex issues and hazards involved in surrogate parenthood, but nevertheless gave its cautious approval to surrogate parenthood involving childless couples. The commission condemned surrogate parenthood for single persons, arguing that "On the whole this action appears to us to be in the mainstream of American narcissism and self-indulgence."[65]

Although the General Convention of the Episcopal Church has urged the repeal of statutes banning abortion performed by licensed health personnel and has condoned abortions under emergency conditions, in 1973 the Joint Commission of the Church in Human Affairs stated that it felt compelled to "reject the concept of abortion as a legitimate method of birth control."[66] The 1976 General Convention concurred, pointing out that because new life is a gift of God, procreation should not be undertaken "unadvisedly or lightly." This position recognized the necessity for responsible birth control. The 1976 convention supported abortion where "the physical or mental health of the mother is threatened seriously, or where there is substantial reason to believe that the child would be born badly deformed in mind or body, or where the pregnancy has resulted from rape or incest." In cases involving termination of pregnancy for other causes "members of this church are urged to seek the advice and counsel of a Priest of this Church, and, where appropriate, Penance." Furthermore, the resolution of 1976 urged that alternatives to abortion in such other cases be seriously considered. The convention resolution ended with a statement opposing legislation on the part of national or state governments limiting or denying "the right of individuals to reach informed decisions in this matter and to act upon them."[67] The debate on abortion did not end in 1976.[68] As long as the issue remains alive in contemporary society, it will be a matter of concern to the church.

The Episcopal Church, as well as worldwide Anglicanism, has tended to reject euthanasia involving "the deliberate use of means for the termination of life decided upon and prescribed by the physician in charge."[69] However, the church has adopted a more tolerant attitude toward "the deliberate withholding or withdrawal of available clinical means for the prolongation of life of a patient for whom there is little or no hope of recovery or survival." Church leaders have argued that the physician in charge must reach his or her decision in this matter in consultation (where possible) with the patient, relations, clergy, and others close to the patient. "Such decisions must be made, under God, with deep concern for the value of each human life, but without the morbid concern to deny mortality and the ultimate facing of death." The report of the 1973 Joint Commission ended with a statement that conflicted with the sentiment of most people in modern society and of many in health-care facilities:

> Our emphasis would be on the treatment of death as a normal event in the whole of life, in contrast to the regarding of it as an unintended catastrophe, and on the right of every person to prepare for and experience his own death. It is natural for some to insist on the use of heroic methods for prolonging life when there is essentially no clinical value indicated for their use. Against this, it must be admitted, also, that others might give up too easily. In the tension between these two poles, the ultimate decision must be left to the corporate conscience of all parties under God, including the patient himself, and the guidance of . . . Christian principles. . . .[70]

Human sexuality, in particular homosexuality, has lately received increasing attention in the Episcopal Church. As early as 1967 General Convention expressed its concern for careful study of the matter.[71] In 1976 General Convention affirmed "that homosexual persons are children of God who have a full and equal claim with all other persons upon the love, acceptance, and pastoral concern and care of the Church."[72] The issue generated heated debate when homosexual persons and their supporters urged the church to ordain those who openly acknowledged their homosexuality. After a lengthy period of study, the Standing Commission on Human Affairs and Health in 1979 concluded that where homosexual behavior is regarded by most Christians "as abnormal, immoral, and/or anti-social," it "constitutes a disqualification for ordination." The commission's concern focused on whether or not any priest, homosexual or heterosexual, could live and would live "a life which is a wholesome example to Christ's flock." If a homosexual met this criterion, the commission saw no barrier to ordination. The commission concluded that clergy were to treat homosexual persons with compassion but "not to promote or foster a homosexual adaptation as a generally-acceptable alternative for Christians." Finally, it argued that the General Convention "should enact no legislation which singles out a particular human condition and makes it an absolute barrier to ordination, thus depriving Bishops and Commissions on Ministry of the proper exercise of their discretion in the particular cases for which they are responsible."[73] The end result of the commission's deliberations pleased neither homosexual persons seeking full approval nor those who would bar them altogether from the ordained ministry, but it pointed in a direction that for many provided a viable way of handling an admittedly difficult problem.

The Underlying Point of View

In its 1973 report, the Joint Commission on the Church in Human Affairs identified "common threads" running through its deliberations on health and medicine in contemporary society. These principles included an insistence upon the worth and dignity of human existence, the right of each individual to exercise choice in issues determining life and death, and the assurance that each person shall "be guaranteed the right of survival (the provision of adequate nutritional levels) and the right of protection from attack by others (high quality medical care for protection against disease or disability; and the protection of one man against the unwarranted or constraining action of his neighbors)." Human beings, said the commission, were not to be used as mere objects, whether in research or elsewhere, without their "informed consent and knowledge of the consequences" of their decisions.[74]

This report echoed a statement made on "The Christian Doctrine of Man" at the Lambeth Conference in 1948, which endorsed "every claim that can rightly be made for man." Christianity, it was claimed, recognizes "the Divine Spirit" in everything that raises human beings above the animals:

In Christ all humanity is ennobled, for He shows us what God intends man to be. All that makes for man's true fulfillment and enrichment is the friend of Christianity, all that thwarts or coarsens it is its enemy. This fundamental respect for human dignity, this vivid concern for all human decencies, which are the root of Christian civilization and are today so seriously endangered, spring from the central Christian dogma called the Incarnation.[75]

This doctrine, which has been closely associated with Anglicanism from Richard Hooker to William Temple, respects the material presuppositions of the good life. "As the religion of the Word made Flesh," declared the Lambeth report, Christianity "regards the material as instrumental to the cause of spiritual personality, made for eternity."[76] Furthermore, human beings were acknowledged to be the children of nature and as such are rightly "regarded as the object of scientific inquiry." Anglicans thus welcomed "the findings of scientific investigation" while insisting that science could never present an adequate account of human nature.

In dealing with moral issues, modern Anglicanism, like the moral theologians of the seventeenth century, has inclined to be pastoral rather than dogmatic and legalistic. The Joint Commission in its report of 1973 stated:

Anglican tradition has traditionally been more interested in and has manifested its concern with, the problems that man's increasing knowledge exposes him to by a stance of pastoral rather than juridical posture. That is, the Church has tended to deal with these problems in terms of a pastoral concern from the pulpit and in personal counseling rather than in terms of reliance upon dogmatic statement based on juridical principles. It does this because of the obvious difference between concern for the individual in trouble and the concern for the whole of mankind in trouble.[77]

According to this understanding, both the individual and the world community must be respected. The rightness of an individual's action was not to be judged in terms of immediate circumstances alone, but "in relation to the facts as they can be known at any time and with proper regard for the quality of life possible for all mankind at all times." The effort to judge the rightness of an individual's action, however, seems to have resulted in more problems than answers.

The Cartesian tendency to demand proofs for each and every problem in a logical progression of research has rapidly engulfed both the medical technological worker and those who are recipients of his labor in a morass of facts, figures, and statistics. This threatens to remove from man both his appreciation of his real position in creation and his ability to determine the direction in which to turn for help, thus immobilizing him in decision making.[78]

The challenge to the church has been to support persons in the pursuit of responsible decision making, assisting them in what is admittedly a most difficult task. As the Joint Commission concluded, "Ultimately, each man makes his own decisions, and the Church can only provide the support necessary to allow him to arrive at those decisions in keeping with his informed conscience with the least possible civil constraint consistent with the peace and safety of all people."[79]

As we have seen, attitudes toward sickness and death, sex and marriage, and health and healing have changed as Anglicanism has evolved from its period of formation in the sixteenth and seventeenth centuries to the twentieth. Continuity has been maintained through a persistent respect for the interrelationship of body and spirit, spiritual healing and medical science, and the individual and the community. The Anglican tradition has displayed a high regard for human nature as part of God's good creation while recognizing the finitude and sin that limit the realization of humanity's potential. Realism has been an important element in what might justly be called the Christian humanism of the tradition. This view of humanity as flawed but nevertheless essentially of infinite worth has been transmitted from age to age through an ever-changing liturgy and through the works of theologians such as Richard Hooker at the beginning and William Temple in the recent past. Both Hooker and Temple qualified and strengthened humanism by reference to the Incarnate One, the God–Man, sacrificed for the sake of humanity, and by the contrition and renewal which that reference arouses in the hearts and minds of the faithful. The best of Anglicanism has thus been supportive of all that medical science has done on behalf of humanity and critical of all that it has done to limit or destroy humanity's true nature.

Notes

1. Henry Gee and W.J. Hardy, eds., *Documents Illustrative of English Church History* (London, 1914), pp. 460–463.
2. A.L. Rowse, *The England of Elizabeth* (New York, 1966), p. 433.
3. *The Book of Common Prayer 1559: The Elizabethan Prayer Book*, ed. John E. Booty (Charlottesville, VA, 1976), p. 275. I use the 1559 prayer book because it was the book used in England from the time of Queen Elizabeth to the Restoration in the seventeenth century.
4. *Book of Common Prayer 1559*, p. 283.
5. Ibid., pp. 290–291.
6. Ibid., p. 293.

7. Richard Hooker, *Of the Lawes of Ecclesiastical Polity*, book 5, ch. 73, sec. 7, The Folger Library Edition, ed. W.S. Hill (Cambridge, MA., 1977–), 2:405.

8. Lawrence Stone, *The Family, Sex, and Marriage in England, 1500–1800* (New York, 1977), pp. 490–491.

9. Paul Hair, ed., *Before the Bawdy Court: Selections from Church Court and Other Records Relating to the Correction of Moral Offences in England, Scotland and New England, 1300–1800* (London, 1972), p. 233. See also Ralph Houlbrooke, *Church Courts and the People During the English Reformation* (Oxford, 1979).

10. *The Complete Poetry of John Donne*, ed. J.T. Shawcross (Garden City, NY, 1972), p. 177. Written for Elizabeth, daughter of James I, and Frederick, Elector of Palatine, married February 14, 1613.

11. *The Sermons of John Donne*, eds. G.R. Potter and E.M. Simpson, 10 vols. (Berkeley and Los Angeles, 1955), 2:340.

12. Hair, *Bawdy Court*, pp. 238–239.

13. See Stone, *Family, Sex, and Marriage*, pp. 491–493, 512–513.

14. Ibid., pp. 238–239.

15. Jeremy Taylor, *The Rule and Exercises of Holy Living* (Boston, 1864), p. 103.

16. Hooker, *Lawes*, 5.75.2; 2:409.

17. *The First and Second Prayer Books of Edward VI*, Everyman's Library (London, 1949), p. 264.

18. Ibid., p. 418, from the Second Prayer Book (1552).

19. Ibid., p. 419.

20. Thomas Becon, *Prayers and Other Pieces*, ed. John Ayre (Cambridge, 1844), pp. 31–32.

21. *Liturgies and Occasional Forms of Prayer set forth in the Reign of Queen Elizabeth*, ed. William Keatinge Clay (Cambridge, 1847), p. 491.

22. *Book of Common Prayer 1559*, p. 76.

23. John Donne, *Devotions Upon Emergent Occasions* (Ann Arbor, MI, 1975), p. 107.

24. Bettie Anne Doebler, *The Quickening Seed: Death in the Sermons of John Donne* (Salzburg, 1974), pp. 106–107.

25. Hooker, *Lawes*, 6.3.3; 3:9.

26. *Certain Sermons or Homilies* (London [1864]), p. 96.

27. Michael MacDonald, "Religion, Social Change, and Psychological Healing in England, 1600–1800," in *The Church and Healing*, ed. W.J. Sheils, *Studies in Church History* vol. 19 (Oxford, 1982), p. 101.

28. *The Works of George Herbert*, ed. F. E. Hutchinson (Oxford, 1941), p. 249.

29. See S.I. Soden, *Godfrey Goodman, Bishop of Gloucester 1583–1659* (London, 1953), pp. 64–66.

30. Rowse, *England of Elizabeth*, p. 431.

31. Michael MacDonald, *Mystical Bedlam: Madness, Anxiety, and Healing in Seventeenth Century England* (Cambridge, 1981), p. 26.

32. John R. Guy, "Archbishop Secker as a Physician," in *The Church and Healing*, p. 133.

33. Ibid., p. 135.

34. See Bruce E. Steiner, *Samuel Seabury, 1729–1795* (n.p. [1971]), pp. 44–50.

35. Henry D. Rack, "Doctors, Demons and Early Methodist Healing," in *The Church and Healing,* p. 144.
36. MacDonald, "Religion, Social Change, and Psychological Healing," p. 117.
37. John V. Pickstone, "Establishment and Dissent in Nineteenth Century Medicine: An Exploration of Some Correspondence and Connections Between Religious and Medical Belief-Systems in Early Industrial England," in *The Church and Healing,* p. 172.
38. C. Peter Williams, "Healing and Evangelism: The Place of Medicine in Later Victorian Protestant Missionary Thinking," in *The Church and Healing,* p. 271.
39. Ibid., p. 277.
40. Raymond W. Albright, *A History of the Protestant Episcopal Church* (New York, 1964), p. 361.
41. Protestant Episcopal Church, Standing Liturgical Commission, *Prayer Book Studies* (New York, 1950–), vol. 24: Pastoral Offices, p. 11.
42. *The Book of Common Prayer* [1979] (New York, 1977), p. 459. The book was first approved by General Convention in 1976 and published in 1977, but did not become official until approved a second time by General Convention in 1979.
43. See Stuart Mews, "The Revival of Spiritual Healing in the Church of England, 1920–1926," in *The Church and Healing,* pp. 299–331; and Charles W. Gusmer, "Anointing of the Sick in the Church of England," *Worship* 45(5):262–272.
44. Albright, *History,* p. 361.
45. "Report of the Joint Commission on the Ministry of Healing," Protestant Episcopal Church in the U.S.A., *Journals,* 1964, p. 564. See also *The Ministry of Healing: Report of the Committee appointed in accordance with Resolution 63 of the Lambeth Conference, 1920* (London, 1924).
46. *The Report of the 1920, 1930, and 1948 Conferences* (London, 1948), p. 182, from the 1930 report.
47. *Exorcism: The Findings of a Commission Convened by the Bishop of Exeter,* ed. Dom. Robert Petitpierre, O.S.B. (London, 1972), p. 16.
48. Ibid., pp. 9–10.
49. *Prayer Book Studies,* vol. 24: Pastoral Offices, p. 4.
50. *Lambeth Conference, 1958,* sec. 2, p. 143.
51. Ibid., sec. 2, pp. 146–151.
52. *Book of Common Prayer* [1979], p. 423.
53. *General Convention: Journals,* 1979, AA-125.
54. Ibid., AA-136.
55. James B. Simpson and Edward M. Story, *The Long Shadows of Lambeth X* (New York, 1969), p. 289. See also *General Convention: Journals,* 1964, p. 294.
56. *Prayer Book Studies,* vol. 24: Pastoral Offices, p. 19.
57. *Book of Common Prayer* [1979], p. 493.
58. *Lambeth Conference, 1958,* sec. 2, pp. 169–170.
59. *General Convention: Journals,* 1967, Appendix 22.9.
60. Ibid., 22.10.
61. *General Convention: Journals,* 1970, p. 466.
62. William Temple, *Christus Veritas: An Essay* (London, 1949), p. 218.
63. Ibid., p. 219.
64. *General Convention: Journals,* 1973, p. 595.

65. *Blue Book,* 1982, p. 133.
66. *General Convention, Journals,* 1973, p. 595.
67. Ibid., 1976, sec. C.1.
68. *Blue Book,* p. 131; *The Episcopalian* 149 (November 1984):1, 7.
69. *General Convention: Journals,* 1973, p. 596.
70. Ibid., pp. 596–597.
71. Ibid., 1967, pp. 492–493.
72. Ibid., 1976, C.108.
73. Ibid., 1976, AA.121–122. See entire report, AA.123–147.
74. Ibid., 1973, p. 594.
75. *Lambeth Conference,* 1948, Pt. II, pp. 3–4.
76. Ibid., p. 5.
77. *General Convention: Journals,* 1973, p. 590.
78. Ibid., pp. 590–591.
79. Ibid., p. 591.

CHAPTER 9

The Anabaptist

Tradition

WALTER KLAASSEN

The Anabaptist movement arose in the third and fourth decades of the sixteenth century in Switzerland, Germany, and the Netherlands. Its founder, Konrad Grebel (ca. 1498–1526), was a disciple of Huldreich Zwingli of Zurich, leader of the Protestant Reformation in Switzerland. Because Grebel and his followers insisted on rebaptizing persons who had been baptized in infancy, Zwingli in 1525 dubbed them Anabaptists, meaning persons who have been rebaptized.

After a period of initial uncertainty about the proper relationship between church and state, and a failed attempt to establish the end-time kingdom of saints at Münster in Westphalia in 1534, Anabaptists united on the following principles: a congregational church separate from the state and the world at large, a strong emphasis on following Christ in daily obedience and on being ready to suffer and even endure martyrdom, and a personal responsibility for religious decisions expressed in the baptism of adult believers only and a rigorous church discipline. The Anabaptists lived in small, self-governing congregations, whose elected leaders exercised firm control over beliefs and behavior. Members devoted much time to group Bible study and celebrated their unity and commitment to Christ by baptism and the Lord's Supper.

Because of their opposition to the union of church and state and their refusal to bear arms, swear oaths, hold public office, or even accept government protection for their church, Anabaptists suffered persecution

271

at the hands of both Roman Catholic and Protestant authorities. As a result, thousands joined "the noble army of martyrs." Except in the Netherlands, the survivors fled their urban homes for sanctuary in the country, where they developed a reputation for honesty, hard work, and agricultural expertise—traits that made them desirable settlers on many noble estates in Europe. Their rural lifestyle, together with the loss of the early educated leaders, who sacrificed their lives for the cause, gave rise to a confirmed social and religious conservatism that lasted for three centuries.

The nonconformity of the Anabaptists led to successive migrations: from Tyrol to Moravia and from the Netherlands to the Kingdom of Poland beginning in the 1530s; from Switzerland and the Palatinate to Pennsylvania beginning in 1683; from Prussia to Russia in 1789; from Russia to Canada, the United States, and Paraguay in 1874, 1923, and 1945; and from Canada to Mexico, Brazil, Bolivia, and Belize since 1919. In the sixteenth century they moved because of persecution; later, because of pacifism, separation from the world, and economic considerations. Except in Tyrol and Moravia, where the Catholic Inquisition totally exterminated Anabaptists, the migrations always left behind a remnant.

Because of the prominence of Menno Simons (ca. 1496–1561), a former Dutch priest who emerged as the movement's best-known leader in the late 1530s, most Anabaptists came to be called Mennonites. However, two groups—the Hutterites and the Amish—have maintained a separate identity. The Hutterites, named after their leader Jacob Hutter (d. 1536), fled from Tyrol and other parts of Europe to Moravia, where in 1533 they began establishing communities modeled after the early Christian church. They differed from other Anabaptists chiefly in their adherence to an absolute "community of goods," which meant holding property in common and giving up private income. With one brief interruption of their communitarian life in the nineteenth century, when they nearly disappeared, they have remained faithful to the basic form of community life given them by Hutter, working large communal farms called Bruderhofs. Today most of them live in North America, where they number some 25,000 members.

The Amish derive their name from Jacob Amman (b. 1644), a preacher among the Swiss Anabaptists. In 1693 he began censuring his Mennonite brethren for having become too worldly, especially in matters of church discipline. A true Christian, he argued, should avoid all contact with a member—even a spouse—who had been put under the ban, a practice called "shunning." His intransigence on this point led to a schism that has persisted until the present. Over the years some Amish have rejoined the Mennonites, but about 75,000 continue to live in self-sufficient communities in Canada and the United States, where they began to settle in the early eighteenth century. The most visible mark of Amish separation from the world is their wearing of very conservative antique clothing.

Today there are just short of one million Mennonites in the world, concentrated mostly in Europe and North America, but also sprinkled in roughly equal numbers throughout Latin America, Africa, and Asia. North American Mennonites are divided into twelve main groups, the largest being the (Old) Mennonite Church, the General Conference Mennonite Church, and the Mennonite Brethren Church. Over the years these three groups have become extensively acculturated—so much so that in their attitudes toward technology and in their church practices they are now barely distinguishable from non-Mennonites. A fourth group, the Old Order Mennonites, so named because they maintained the "old order" of church and worship customs and rejected modern technology, separated from the Mennonite Church in North America following 1872.

Spiritual life in Mennonite churches everywhere is relatively vigorous, expressing itself in worldwide mission work, education at all levels, medical service, and the relief of suffering through the Mennonite Central Committee. This reflects the traditional Anabaptist view that deeds legitimize creeds. Emphasis on family and community remains strong. Today, more than at any other time since the sixteenth century, Mennonites are conscious of being a "peace church," seeking to address violence in the world with a variety of programs that go far beyond simple pacifism.

From the beginning Anabaptists have accepted the major doctrines of the historic Christian creeds. However, two distinctive emphases have shaped their attitudes toward health and healing: their view of the church as a congregation, the visible demonstration of the presence of God's kingdom; and their conviction that deeds are necessary to salvation.

While congregationalism formed a part of Reformation theology, it constituted the essence of the Anabaptist tradition, defining God's visible church. Unless one could see the covenanted and disciplined congregation in a given place, there was no assurance of the presence of the church—word, sacrament, and hierarchy notwithstanding.[1] Anabaptists never talked of "the mystical body" or "the invisible church." Their church was a visible, concrete certainty, in which members became sisters and brothers in the family of God, welded together in obedience and in faithfulness with their elder brother, Jesus. For Anabaptists, the congregation provided the actual borders that separated the church from the world. Although they avoided slipping into exclusivism, they always assigned first priority to caring for "those of the household of faith."[2]

Membership in this caring family of God brought with it the gift of well-being—insofar as that was attainable in a world in which the Antichrist was attempting to destroy God's "little flock."[3] The chief characteristic of well-being was *gelassenheit,* the ancient mystical non-resistant surrender to the will of God, the abandonment of all self-will, all struggling for security, and all attempts to save one's soul and body. True *gelassenheit* promised the cessation of inner conflict and disharmony over all the "ills that flesh is heir to," including physical ailments.[4]

The Anabaptist emphasis on deeds rather than creeds stemmed from a fervent biblicism. Like other Christians through the centuries, members of the Anabaptist family laid "that flattering unction to their souls" that they were more biblical than anyone else. But unlike their Lutheran and Calvinist contemporaries, they tended to excise all authorities other than the Bible from their lives, a trait symbolized by the burning of all books except the Bible in Münster in 1534.[5] They believed that "the times of restitution" spoken of in *Acts* 3:21 had come. Hence they deliberately modeled themselves in a literal way on the New Testament teachings regarding personal behavior, separation from the world, and the details of worship and church organization. They even emulated Paul's epistles in their letters of edification to one another.[6] On the basis of the world view found in the New Testament, they believed not only that God worked through his chosen few in a visible manner, but that the Adversary went about alternately as a roaring lion, a wolf in sheep's clothing, or an angel of light, afflicting the just and seeking in every way to trick them into apostasy.

Anabaptists would brook no "interpretation" of Scripture (that is, the use of anything beyond the text), which they regarded as the devil's way of muddying the clear fountain of truth. Such uncompromising biblicism stood in the way of developing a systematic presentation of doctrine. Besides, during their first fifty years they suffered virtually unremitting persecution that provided no settled existence and no leisure for scholarly activity. The writings on doctrine that have survived were produced during periods of involuntary retirement in prison or dashed off in response to the attacks of opponents.[7] The first Anabaptist confession, drawn up at Schleitheim in Switzerland in 1527, focused on the radical separation of church and world, details of church order, and specific ethical imperatives. It emphasized obedience and purity of life rather than purity of doctrine. Belief in Jesus as Son of God, Anabaptists said repeatedly, was of no consequence unless one did what he commanded. Because good deeds—"works of faith"—provided irrefutable evidence of faith, Anabaptists saw them as necessary to salvation. Unlike other Protestants, they did not separate faith from works; thus, they could at the same time speak of justification by faith alone and of the necessity of works for salvation.[8]

In a lengthy passage in his major work, Bernhard Rothmann, the sixteenth-century theologian of Anabaptist Münster, explained the relationship between faith and works: "The sum of it is this: God desires obedience and performance of his will. These two therefore mark the true Christian: genuine faith in Christ, and holy behavior according to all his commandments."[9] The view Rothmann expressed characterized Anabaptism during its formative period and shaped the tradition throughout its history. Anabaptists experienced none of the exuberant liberation felt by Martin Luther when he discovered that his compromised holy works had nothing whatever to do with God's acceptance of him. Instead they deliberately and joyfully assumed the yoke and burden of divine command. Hence they invested enormously in right action and cared greatly about the details of ethical correctness. This accounts for the importance the Amish, Hutterites, and Old Order Mennonites have attached to "separated" clothing.

The activism characteristic of the Anabaptist tradition since its beginnings stemmed from the view that people are free to choose their own course and are responsible for the course they choose. While in Reformed Protestantism the spring of action was often the need to provide evidence of election, among Anabaptists it was the need to justify one's chosenness. Thus in times of sickness one's attitude of resignation, which could be personally chosen, assumed greater importance than healing.

The Early Tradition

Anabaptists in the sixteenth century rarely addressed questions of health and illness. However, like many other Christians, they acknowledged health to be a gift of God and looked upon illness as one of his methods for training and chastising his children. Their belief in the restoration of New Testament conditions might have led them to expect miraculous healings from illness as a sign of the coming Kingdom, but early records report no such miracles.

Two factors may account for this. First, New Testament writers, especially Paul, said little about illness. When Paul did refer to his own affliction in 2 *Corinthians* 12:7–9, a favorite Anabaptist text, he identified it as a means of divine chastening, illustrating God's strength being made perfect in weakness. The single reference in Anabaptist writings to *James* 5:14–15, the classic New Testament text that called for the elders to anoint the sick with oil, noted simply that the oil was "not the Pope's,"—a response not unlike John Calvin's in *The Institutes*.[10]

The second reason for their silence stemmed from their identification of miraculous healings with such "popish" practices as pilgrimages to healing shrines and appeals to the curative power of relics. Because such customs seemed "unbiblical," Anabaptists rejected them—along with other forms of miraculous healing. This suspicion of divine healing remained characteristic of Mennonite attitudes into the twentieth century, when the influence of the holiness movement and a new reading of Scripture, which emphasized the role of faith in many New Testament healings, produced some exceptions.[11]

Because of their strong emphasis on human volition, Anabaptists often assumed a direct causal connection between sin and sickness. If one granted this assumption, it seemed presumptuous to expect God to heal miraculously. If one denied it, as some Anabaptists did, there still remained the possibility that God used sickness to teach humility and patience. And if he did, sickness was a blessing, not something to be eliminated.

Regardless of their position on these matters, Anabaptists presumably found no greater joy in physical pain and infirmity than anyone else. We know that their afflictions sometimes severely strained the prized state of *gelassenheit,* frequently leaving it in tatters. Even Menno Simons could not resist complaining about his physical ailments.[12] Paul Glock, a sixteenth-century Hutterite missionary who became ill while serving a nineteen-year imprisonment for his faith, railed against his jailers and interrogating clerics for suggesting that his illness was punishment for his heresy.[13] Like most other Christians, Anabaptists attempted to cure their physical ailments and prayed for healing.[14] They inquired about each other's health and on occasion gave medical advice to fellow believers.[15] Above all, they reminded one another that life in the "great village of this bleak world's wilderness" was short and that they would soon be in the great and glorious mansions of their Lord, where pain and suffering were unknown.[16]

Although the early Anabaptists wrote little about health and healing, they frequently engaged in caring and curing activities. Whenever they enjoyed relative toleration and stable community life, they developed the office of deaconess, particularly during the sixteenth and seventeenth centuries and primarily in the Netherlands and in the communities of the Vistula delta. Deaconesses were usually widows who, being chosen by the congregations, devoted themselves to the care of other widows, orphans, the poor, the elderly, and the sick. Of a deaconess in Amsterdam it was said that "she visited the sick and feeble, especially the women, and . . . she was obeyed as a mother in Israel and a servant of Jesus Christ."[17] Anabaptists found the precedent for this practice in the New Testament church and incorporated it as a formal office in the Dordrecht Confession of 1632, the single most important Mennonite confession of faith.[18]

A number of Mennonite preachers in the Netherlands were trained physicians who ministered to both body and soul, and the Hutterites were famous for their skilled barber-surgeons, who traveled from community to community, carrying their drugs and medicines in wagons. The great enemy of the Moravian Hutterites, the Jesuit Christoph Andreas Fischer, implied that these apprentice-trained healers had no rivals for excellence because "the Christians" (that is, Catholics), and especially the Moravian nobility, preferred their services to those of non-Hutterites.[19] Although the Hutterite surgeons charged outsiders for their services—an important source of community revenue—they provided free care to fellow believers.

In addition to their itinerant practices, these surgeons administered the mineral baths found in Hutterite communities. The Regulation of Medicinal Baths *(Bader-Ordnung)* of 1654 provides a fascinating glimpse into seventeenth-century medicine.[20] It admonishes surgeons to look to their profession, their soul's salvation, and the common good. They are to be ornaments of their profession and confession wherever they work. They are to read extensively in the Scriptures and in pharmaceutical books and gather herbs and roots for their medicines. They are to be especially careful in prescribing drugs lest they become responsible for a patient's death. They are to keep their instruments clean and in repair so as to avoid causing pain and discomfort. They are to be on call always and pay special attention to the needs of the infirm and aged. Thus God will hear their faithful prayers for the prospering of their work.

The Hutterites paid particular attention to preventive measures, especially with respect to children. Sixteenth-century schoolmasters were instructed to care for their students with gentleness and love, to plan and supervise their diet, and to keep them clean in order to reduce the danger of contagion. Sick children were to have separate washing and toilet facilities, and their clothing, bed-linen, and dishes were to be cleaned separately. The hands of adults were to be thoroughly washed after examining the mouths of sick children. Children with scalp and skin lesions (for example, eczema) were to receive special combs and brushes.[21]

Deeds

Rejection and persecution drove Anabaptists into quietism in the late 1500s, and for four hundred years they remained relatively passive. In the late nineteenth century, however, the main group of Mennonites broke out of their cultural and religious isolation and discovered the biblical command to give all sufferers a cup of water "in the name of Christ." Mennonites in Russia, Germany, and the United States revived the old Anabaptist deaconess service, which by this time had become popular among other Protestants (in part because of Anabaptist influences). Like their Protestant sisters, the new Mennonite deaconesses emphasized nursing, and by 1908 they were running hospitals in Kansas and Nebraska. The deaconesses in charge of these hospitals were formally ordained to this service and were required to wear a special habit, but they did not take a vow of chastity (though many remained celibate).[22] By the mid–twentieth century, however, deaconesses were beginning to disappear. The ministers' manual of the General Conference Mennonite Church published in 1950 omitted any reference to ordination of deaconesses and instead assigned deacons the task of caring for the sick.

Whereas the Amish, Hutterites, and Old Order Mennonites continued into the twentieth century to care for their aged parents and the chronically ill at home, the more acculturated Mennonites established nursing homes and homes for the aged in virtually every Mennonite community around the world. These institutions were funded by fees and government grants as well as by personal contributions of money and labor from members of the Mennonite community. Although trained nurses were in attendance, medical care in these institutions remained minimal. Instead, they emphasized a homelike and caring atmosphere that allowed the aged and the ill to derive strength and support from the communities in which they had lived.

The tradition of mutual aid remained strong among twentieth-century Anabaptists. For example, the Amish and Old Order Mennonites, who avoided medical insurance because of its tendency to diminish community responsibility, cared for farmers who fell ill and assisted them with their field work and daily chores. Acculturated Mennonites also provided for one another in times of illness, but they increasingly resorted to more formal means. In 1888 the Franconia Conference (Pennsylvania) of the Mennonite Church led the way by creating a Beneficial Society to insure members and their families against illness. During and after the Great Depression a number of other Mennonite groups in the United States and Canada established associations for easing the burdens of medical costs. Typical of these arrangements was the Mennonite Health Society of Coaldale, Alberta, begun in 1928, which contracted with a local physician, usually a Mennonite, to render professional services to subscribers and their families for a monthly fee of one dollar per family. The Coaldale Society, like some others, also established its own hospital and nursing service.[23] Such experiments exemplified the fusion of traditional mutual-aid practices with modern risk-sharing plans.

In 1908, thriving Mennonite communities in the United States and Canada began establishing general hospitals, occasionally in conjunction with schools of nursing, as expressions of care for those in the "household of faith." Eventually there were over twenty of these institutions, including the previously created deaconess hospitals.[24] Because these hospitals functioned as extensions of the normal home and church community, they were staffed mostly by Mennonites who could empathize with older members and care for them in an intimate, homey, friendly atmosphere. These hospitals also admitted as many non-Mennonites as they could accommodate, thus fulfilling Christ's mandate to care for the sick. At first these facilities were supported solely by voluntary contributions from Mennonites and the communities in which they were located. More recently, as many have evolved into general hospitals for the wider community, they have accepted financial support from government and philanthropic agencies.

When acculturated Mennonites joined in the great missionary movement in the late nineteenth century, they immediately instituted medical work in India, China, Africa, and the East Indies. The newly acquired wealth of North American Mennonites allowed the missionaries to build clinics, hospitals, and leprosaria and to train medical personnel.[25] In undertaking mission work, the Mennonites were probably influenced more by the example of other Protestant bodies than by antecedents within their own tradition; yet in some ways they were merely extending to outsiders the care they had always provided to members of their own communities.

Although the various branches of the Anabaptist family have doggedly pursued their separate identities based on ethnic and theological differences, nearly all of them have worked together at the task of relieving human suffering through the Mennonite Central Committee, an inter-Mennonite service agency. Founded in 1919 to relieve the human suffering caused by World War I, this expression of "holy behavior according to His commandments" rapidly expanded its activities after World War II.[26] Financed by contributions from North America, it built hospitals in Paraguay to serve not only the rapidly growing Mennonite communities, but also the indigenous population.

The Committee's major involvement in health and healing began in 1947 with the establishment of mental health centers in the United States. During World War II, Mennonite young men, along with many others who refused to take up arms, worked in state mental hospitals as a form of alternative national service. A number of these men found the experience so rewarding that they continued to serve as regular staff after the war. Strongly motivated by the conviction that the way of Christ was the way of love, patience, and nonviolence, they objected to the careless and sometimes brutal treatment of mentally afflicted people in these public institutions. The prison-like atmosphere, cheerless accommodations, unsympathetic ward attendants, and custodial approach to care so appalled these Mennonites they began to talk about the need for centers where the mentally ill would be treated in a Christlike way.

The first of eight Mennonite Mental Health Service centers opened its doors in 1947 in Hagerstown, Maryland. Based on the belief that it was possible to combine psychiatry with the Christian values of caring, community, and respect for human dignity, these centers attempted to provide "a loving, home-like, and rural environment where work and activities would be natural components." In addition to trained professional psychiatrists, the staff included nonmedical personnel and volunteers who stressed the "importance of the interpersonal approach to the care and treatment of the mentally ill." Instead of locking patients up in their rooms, the centers encouraged them to become involved with the local Mennonite community. Although funded by community gifts, government grants, and patient fees as well as church contributions, the centers have maintained a vital relationship to the Mennonite church and have upheld the ideal of service "in the name of Christ." Elmer Ediger, for many years administrator of Prairie View, one of the centers near Newton, Kansas, wrote: "the Mennonite experience of suffering and isolation provided a subsoil of experience which helped the mental health movement to take root and flourish. . . . Religious motivation guided them toward this type of constructive reaction to hurts that threatened their self-image."[27]

In Germany, Switzerland, and the Netherlands, where Mennonites were often culturally integrated with their respective societies, they generally availed themselves of public medical institutions rather than creating their own. However, in Russia, particularly in the Mennonite communities of the Ukraine, where secular facilities were often not available, they engaged in a broad spectrum of medical activities. Ukrainian Mennonites became involved in health care during the Crimean War of 1854–1855, when they were called upon to care for a large number of wounded soldiers. After the war, some of these Mennonites continued to practice medicine as civilian *feldschers,* a military term designating an army surgeon's assistant. Eventually short training programs for *feldschers* were offered, often at community expense. These programs, along with similar ones for training midwives, brought institutionalized medical care to Mennonite communities for the first time in modern history.

With the appearance about 1880 of a fully qualified medical doctor, Ukrainian Mennonites expanded their medical services to include clinics, hospitals, and pharmacies, all of which provided free drugs and medical care at community expense.[28] In addition to general hospitals, they established industrial hospitals to care for workers in Mennonite factories. In 1911 they opened their first mental hospital, Bethania, and three years later they built a sanatorium to aid people suffering from tuberculosis. These medical institutions flourished in Russia until the Stalin era, when many Mennonites were deported to Soviet Central Asia and their communities destroyed. Today, Mennonites in the Soviet

Union, like all other citizens, receive state medical care. They have no institutions of their own.

Beliefs and Practices

In spite of their centuries-long separatism, Anabaptists adopted many of the health practices of the societies in which they lived. From the beginning they frequently relied on popular folk medicines, using, for example, herbal remedies prescribed by neighbors or local healers. Mennonites in France in the eighteenth and nineteenth centuries acquired a reputation for being skilled herbalists and for being adept at curing both humans and animals with folk medicines.[29] Some Anabaptist immigrants to America brought with them a quasi-religious form of folk healing called *braucherei* or powwowing (an Algonkian word for the work of a medicine man). Practitioners of this art, both professional and domestic, used incantations and rituals to remove warts, extract pain, counteract the "evil eye," or cure sick animals.[30] One twentieth-century Mennonite grandmother described her practice as follows:

> You want me to tell you about Divine Healing. I am not anxious to say. As so many people don't believe in it. I do, as I know what it done for two of my boys. . . . A neighbor taught me. You measure patient with a Thread, from the crown on back of head to end of spine, then on the limb to heel, on to big toe. If you are in health you are exactly 7 times as long as your foot. If decay of flesh is present, you are too short.
> Then we stroke patient from crown to toe 3 times with a slow hand and Ask in *His* name a prayer, repeat in a week for 3 wks, then rest 3 wks, measure again. They are often all rite [*sic*] by then. It's very simple. But Scripture says, If we ask anything in His name He will give it. There's no witchery about it. But a skinny person can't do it. Must be vigorous and healthy. . . . There are other ways too. But this is all I know about. . . . I forgot to say we never accept money for powwowing. Then it would not help. 'Tis love for your neighbor.[31]

Like other forms of folk healing, powwowing, which persists to this day among certain Amish and Mennonite groups, has tended to supplement rather than supplant scientific medicine. Although the Amish and the Hutterites have sometimes preferred chiropractors and naturopaths to physicians (because they seemed to offer more personalized service), most Mennonites have warmly—even uncritically—embraced modern medicine.[32] As long as medical practices seemed compatible with the values of the tradition, they were given a Christian rationale and incorporated into the life of the community.[33] This process facilitated acculturation, but it may also have compromised the witness of Mennonites, who have rarely raised their voices against medical abuses.

On most issues relating to life's passages, Anabaptists have shared the beliefs of other Christians, trusting that the beginning and end of human life rested in the hands of God. Although they regarded any child who survived the hazards of birth and infancy as a miracle, a special gift from God, they rejected infant baptism. Only after a child came to a knowledge of good and evil and passed from blamelessness to culpability, from innocence to responsibility, could he or she make a deliberate choice for or against the salvation God offered to all. Baptism thus represented the most important passage of human existence. In the early years of the movement, when church membership brought with it the threat of suffering and perhaps martyrdom, baptism was delayed until the late teens or early twenties. And among the Amish, Hutterites, and Old Order Mennonites, for whom baptism still represents the acceptance of accountability, the ancient practice holds.[34] Among other Mennonites, the absence of persecution removed the prime reason for delaying baptism; thus parental concern about "a decision for Christ" and other factors have lowered the baptismal age to early adolescence.

Until the present century, Mennonites paid little attention to the problems of aging. They sometimes commented in a melancholy way about the inevitability of growing old or expressed a desire to "depart and be with the Lord" and their loved ones, but little more. In the twentieth century, however, most acculturated Mennonites in Europe and North America began to share in the general perceptions regarding aging in industrial societies. Mennonites improved the lot of the aged by providing group homes, but even community-centered care did little to ease the deep trauma suffered by a farmer or a businessman suddenly torn from his daily routine and rendered dependent. Mennonite women seemed to have weathered this transition much more easily because they had never been independent and even in old age they could often continue their accustomed domestic duties.

Mennonites have characteristically displayed a profound ambivalence toward death. With Protestants they shared the joyful liberation of salvation by faith alone, which in theory freed them from worries about dying without having fulfilled the demands of God. But at the same time they shared with Catholics an emphasis on works as an essential part of the process of justification, which gave rise to gnawing fears that they had not achieved the required purity of life. This antinomy has continued to influence Mennonite life into the present, prompting, on the one hand, an outpouring of sacrificial service on behalf of others as a way of fulfilling the law of Christ while creating, on the other, a heavy burden of guilt for ethical failures. Thus Mennonites have at the same time joyfully anticipated death as liberation from present suffering while experiencing deep anxiety about the judgment to follow. In view of this situation, it is not surprising that manic–depressive states, often directly related to guilt, account for most of the mental illness among the Amish and the Hutterites, who, perhaps because of their powerful community ethos, seem less prone to mental illness than the general population.[35]

Martyrdom played a prominent role in the early history of Anabaptism. The sixteenth-century martyrs, who fully expected to pass from earthly rejection to heavenly exaltation with Christ, looked upon their experience as the crowning fulfillment of the law. For them, martyrdom removed the ambivalence about death and the fear of judgment precisely because it represented the complete fulfillment of the demands of God. The absence of martyrdom in recent centuries has given rise to a sense of guilt among some Anabaptists, particularly prosperous Mennonites. Hutterites, Amish, and Old Order Mennonites have replaced martyrdom with an ascetic separation and discipline, much as monastic renunciation became the new martyrdom for Christians after Constantine.

Death in Mennonite communities has always been an occasion for the rallying of community support for the bereaved.[36] Burial associations relieved the burden of funeral expenses, while neighbors, especially in rural communities, volunteered their services. In recent years many Mennonite pastors have received special clinical training in counseling the dying and comforting the bereaved.

During the formative years of the Anabaptist tradition, women played a visible role in the life of the church, sometimes serving as evangelists or dying as martyrs. Their prominence may have resulted from the radical revolt against clericalism and a celibate clergy by Anabaptists, who went further than other Protestant reformers in dismantling traditional church structures. Nevertheless, Anabaptist women rarely occupied leadership positions in the church, and within the family they remained subordinate to their husbands, who from time to time admonished them to resist the temptation to rise above their biblically defined position.[37]

The pattern of subordination continued unchanged until the present century. Although Mennonite women regularly taught in Sunday schools and served as ordained missionaries abroad, until only a few decades ago in many rural communities in Canada they were not allowed to participate in church business meetings or to share in making church decisions. Today women function as pastors in North American Mennonite churches, though they often struggle to overcome entrenched traditional attitudes. In the Netherlands there have been women pastors since the beginning of this century.

Sixteenth-century Anabaptists, influenced by their literal reading of the New Testament, viewed marriage as a penultimate commitment, entered upon solely for purposes of procreation. If loyalty to spouse conflicted with loyalty to Christ, Christ won. Thus divorce and separation occurred with relative frequency.[38] Later, as women became increasingly subordinate, divorce virtually disappeared from Anabaptist communities, owing perhaps to the increasingly important role played by the family in a community that grew only by biological propagation. Today, divorce remains an anathema among the socially conservative groups of the tradition, although it has become relatively common among acculturated Mennonites, especially the educated and professional class.

On most questions of sexuality, Mennonite opinion in recent years has increasingly reflected the norms and fashions of contemporary society.[39] On the one hand, Mennonites still consider premarital and extramarital sex to be among the most serious sins; on the other, growing numbers of them have come to share the permissive views on sexual morality generated by the sexual revolution. Officially, they continue to reject homosexuality as a legitimate form of sexual behavior, but a vocal organization of Mennonite homosexuals now exists. Although therapeutic abortions are condoned, virtually all Mennonites, who stress the sanctity of life, oppose abortion on demand.

In recent years Mennonites have displayed extensive concern for disabled persons suffering from mental retardation, learning disabilities, and physical handicaps. A special Mennonite Disabilities Committee under the Mennonite Central Committee has led out in this movement by providing a congregational study guide. As a result, new churches are now built on only one level to accommodate wheelchairs. In Kitchener, Ontario, a special task force headed by handicapped people has established a program for "independent living" for the physically handicapped.

Mennonites, like other Christians, have begun paying increasing attention to the ethical issues raised by such developments as test-tube babies, artifical insemination, recombinant DNA research, and euthanasia, but no clear pattern of response has yet emerged. Because of their biblicism, their continuing preoccupation with ethical minutiae, and their concern for purity, Mennonites find these issues, like divorce and homosexuality, extraordinarily difficult to deal with. Hence they are tempted to ignore them.

In 1960 Paul M. Miller, a Mennonite pastor, summed up contemporary Anabaptist views of sickness and health in a book titled *How God Heals.* God's highest will for people is Christ-likeness, not necessarily physical health, he wrote. God uses suffering as a method of discipline and growth to liberate his people from their slavery to material and physical things and to promote Christ-likeness. Thus suffering can be redemptive both for the sufferer and others. The apostolic gift of healing has been given to the church, the obedient and praying body of believers, not to individuals. The expectation of miraculous healing should not lead people to neglect medical services, for these are God's gifts of love to be used together with prayer. The prayers of a believing congregation express Christian compassion in a way medical science cannot. Illnesses brought on by hostility, tension, or suppressed guilt require the healing of love and acceptance.[40] From this statement we can see that, despite centuries of change, especially during the last hundred years, the Anabaptist tradition has remained remarkably consistent in its basic attitudes toward health and healing.

Notes

1. W. Klassen and W. Klaassen, eds., *The Writings of Pilgram Marpeck* (Scottdale, PA, 1978), pp. 455–456; R. Stupperich, ed., *Die Schriften Bernhard Rothmanns* (Münster, 1970), p. 241.
2. J. C. Wenger, ed., *The Complete Writings of Menno Simons* (Scottdale, PA, 1956), p. 842, records caring for adversaries.
3. W. Klaassen, ed., *Sixteenth Century Anabaptism: Defences, Confessions, Refutations,* trans. F. Friesen (Waterloo, Ontario, 1982), p. 160; Klassen and Klaassen, *Writings of Pilgram Marpeck,* p. 416.
4. G. H. Williams and A. M. Mergal, eds., *Spiritual and Anabaptist Writers* (Philadelphia, 1947), pp. 279–84; Stupperich, *Schriften Bernhard Rothmanns,* p. 321.
5. Richard von Dulmen, ed., *Das Tauferreich zu Münster 1534–1535* (München, 1974), p. 100.
6. See the letters of Pilgram Marpeck in Klassen and Klaassen, *Writings of Pilgram Marpeck,* pp. 303–554, and of Paul Glock in Klaassen, *Sixteenth Century Anabaptism,* pp. 120–174.
7. See Peter Rideman, *Account of our Religion, Doctrine and Faith* (London, 1950); and "Reply to Martin Micron" and "Epistle to Martin Micron" in Wenger, *Writings of Menno Simons,* pp. 835–943.
8. Stupperich, *Schriften Bernard Rothmanns,* p. 244–245.
9. Ibid., p. 247.
10. John Calvin, *The Institutes* (Philadelphia, 1960), book IV, chap. 18, sec. 21, pp. 1468–1469.
11. *Divine Healing: A Symposium,* Paul Erb, ed. (Scottdale, PA, 1952).
12. Wenger, *Writings of Menno Simons,* p. 674.
13. Klaassen, *Sixteenth Century Anabaptism,* pp. 154–157, 160.
14. Wenger, *Writings of Menno Simons,* pp. 1057ff.
15. Klaassen, *Sixteenth Century Anabaptism,* p. 167; Klassen and Klaassen, *Writings of Pilgram Marpeck,* p. 515.
16. Wenger, *Writings of Menno Simons,* pp. 1052–1054.
17. Quoted in "Deaconess," *The Mennonite Encyclopedia,* eds. H. S. Bender and C. Krahn, 4 vols. (Scottdale, PA, 1955–1959), 2:22.
18. John H. Leith, ed., *Creeds of the Churches* (Richmond, VA, 1973), p. 301.

19. Robert Friedman, "Hutterite Physicians and Barber-Surgeons," *Mennonite Quarterly Review* 20 (1953):128–136. On Mennonite preacher-physicians, see *Mennonite Encyclopedia,* 3:553.

20. The translated text is appended to John L. Sommer, "Hutterite Medicine and Physicians in Moravia in the Sixteenth Century and After," *Mennonite Quarterly Review* 20 (1953):125–127.

21. H. S. Bender, "A Hutterite School Discipline of 1578 and Peter Scherer's Address of 1568 to the Schoolmasters," *Mennonite Quarterly Review* 5 (1931):232–241.

22. "Deaconess," 2:24.

23. "Coaldale Hospital," *Mennonite Encyclopedia,* 1:630–631.

24. *Mennonite Encyclopedia,* 3:551; 2:817–818.

25. Ibid. 3:551; Lena Graber, "Nursing Service at Dhamtari Christian Hospital," *Gospel Herald* 47 (August 17, 1954): 784–785.

26. C.J. Dyck, ed., *The Mennonite Central Committee Story,* vol. 1: *Documents* (Scottdale, PA, 1980). The *Mennonite Quarterly Review* devoted the entire July 1970 issue of vol. 44 to the work of the Mennonite Central Committee.

27. Elmer Ediger, "Influences on the Origin and Development of Mennonite Mental Health Agencies," *Mennonite Quarterly Review* 56 (1982):33, 39.

28. "Medicine and the Mennonites in Russia," *Mennonite Encyclopedia,* 3:555; "Medicine," ibid., 3:551.

29. Jean Seguy, "Religion and Agricultural Success: The Vocational Life of the French Anabaptists from the Seventeenth to the Nineteenth Centuries," *Mennonite Quarterly Review* 47 (1973): 209–217.

30. Gerald C. Studer, "Powwowing: Folk Medicine or White Magic?" *Pennsylvania Mennonite Heritage* 3 (July 1980): 17–23; Levi Miller, "The Role of a Braucher-Chiropractor in an Amish Community," *Mennonite Quarterly Review* 55 (1981): 157–171. See also John A. Hostetler, "Healing Arts and Cures," *Christian Living* 1 (August 1954):7; Hostetler, "Folk and Scientific Medicine in Amish Society," *Human Organization* 22 (1963–1964): 269–275; and Hostetler, *Amish Society* (Baltimore, 1963), pp. 330–331.

31. Quoted in Studer, "Powwowing," p. 18.

32. John A. Hostetler, *Hutterite Society* (Baltimore, 1974), p. 267; Hostetler, *Amish Society,* p. 316.

33. For an example, see S. Grubb, "Church Hospitals," *The Mennonite* 40 (July 9, 1925): 1–2.

34. Hostetler, *Hutterite Society,* pp. 220, 235–243; Hostetler, *Amish Society,* pp. 79–81.

35. Hostetler, *Hutterite Society,* pp. 262–263; Hostetler, *Amish Society,* p. 322. See also Joseph W. Eaton, "Adolescence in a Communal Society," *Mental Hygiene* 48 (January 1964):66–73; Eaton, "Folk Psychiatry," *New Society,* August 29, 1963, pp. 9–11; J.W. Eaton, R.J. Weil, and B. Kaplan, "The Hutterite Mental Health Study," *Mennonite Quarterly Review* 25 (1951): 47–65; and John W. Bennett, "Social Theory and the Social Order of the Hutterian Communities," ibid. 51 (1977):305.

36. Hostetler, *Amish Society,* p. 199.

37. Klaassen, *Sixteenth Century Anabaptism,* p. 128.

38. Hostetler, *Hutterite Society,* p. 238; Klaassen, *Sixteenth Century Anabaptism,* pp. 55–58.
39. J. Howard Kauffman and Leland Harder, *Anabaptists Four Centuries Later* (Scottdale, PA, 1975), pp. 179–180, 261–274.
40. Paul M. Miller, *How God Heals* (Scottdale, PA, 1960).

CHAPTER 10

The Baptist

Tradition

Timothy P. Weber

Most Baptists find their roots in seventeenth-century English Puritanism, from which they derived their most distinctive view: belief in a "gathered" church made up of converted and baptized believers and organized along congregational or democratic lines. The earliest Baptists were Puritans who withdrew from the Church of England to form new congregations of "convinced believers." John Smyth (ca. 1554–1612), a former Anglican priest who pastored a Separatist congregation from 1606 to 1608, led a group of about eighty exiles to Amsterdam. There, probably under the influence of Dutch Mennonites, Smyth rejected infant baptism and in 1609 convinced most of his followers that only believing persons should be baptized. Smyth then baptized himself and about forty others by affusion (pouring) and soon suggested that they join the Mennonites. Some of Smyth's congregation refused to accept this realignment and, under the leadership of Thomas Helwys (ca. 1550–1616), returned to London in 1612 to establish the first Baptist church on English soil.

From the beginning, English Baptists remained fiercely independent, often disagreeing over doctrine. For example, they argued over whether Christ had died for everyone or just the elect (General vs. Particular Baptists). But they all shared a number of basic commitments. They believed in the priesthood of all believers, rejected notions of clerical hierarchy, practiced baptism by immersion (a mode widely adopted by 1640), and called for religious freedom. Although they occasionally drew up creeds or confessions of faith, Baptists avoided a binding creedalism, taking care to preserve freedom of conscience on doctrinal matters ("soul liberty") and to allow for the possibility that new light and truth might come from the Bible, which they made their only rule for faith and life. Because such notions were not widely accepted in seventeenth-century England, Baptists suffered occasional persecution until the Act of Toleration (1689) provided some relief. They grew substantially during the evangelical awakenings of the mid-eighteenth century and in the 1790s organized for more effective missionary expansion.

The Baptist movement's greatest success, however, occurred in the United States. Roger Williams founded the first Baptist church in the New World in 1639 at Providence, Rhode Island; but Baptist membership remained small until the First Great Awakening in the 1740s. By the American Revolution, Baptists, who played a significant role in the coming of religious liberty, could be found in all the colonies. The Second Great Awakening, in the early nineteenth century, brought the movement unprecedented growth. Given their new influence, Baptists began to form cooperative societies to promote home and foreign missions and religious publishing.

In large part because of the independent spirit and theological diversity of American Baptists, their history has been marked by division and controversy. In 1845 they divided over the slavery issue, giving rise to the Southern Baptist Convention. In 1880 Black Baptists organized their own convention, which soon split over a property dispute (1916) into the National Baptist Convention of the U.S.A. and the National Baptist Convention of America. In the twentieth century, Baptists in the North have parted company a number of times over doctrinal, financial, and organizational issues.

By the early 1980s there were over thirty Baptist denominations in the United States, of which only six had memberships of over a million: Southern Baptist Convention (13 million); National Baptist Convention of the U.S.A. (6.5 million); National Baptist Convention of America (3.5 million); American Baptist Churches of the U.S.A. (2.1 million); National Primitive Baptist Convention (2 million); and Baptist Bible Fellowship (1.2 million). Of the thirty-five million Baptists in the world, nearly thirty million live in America. The remainder can be found on every continent, thanks to a foreign-missions emphasis among most Baptists.

Like many other Christians, Baptists have concerned themselves with matters of health and medicine without making them central to their practice or theology. While they have concentrated their efforts more on saving souls than curing bodies or preserving health, they have often found ways of ministering to both body and soul at the same time. Most Baptists have been favorably disposed to medicine, but they have never adopted any particular approach to medical treatment nor developed any special health regimen, such as a distinctive diet. On the whole, they have been rather ambivalent about human suffering, seeing it both as a curse for sin and a gift of grace to produce spiritual stamina.

The Place of Suffering in the Christian Life

Throughout their history there is remarkable consistency in the way Baptists have viewed suffering: On the one hand, it is a result of sin and a fearful reminder of the Fall; on the other hand, it is often used by God to bring about spiritual growth in the Christian.

The typical Baptist perspective was held by John Gill (1697–1771), an English Particular Baptist pastor and professor of divinity, who believed that all human suffering stemmed from Adam's sin, which he called "the *pandora* from whence have sprung all spiritual maladies and bodily diseases; all the disasters, distresses, mischiefs and calamities that are, or have been in the world."[1] Human suffering is therefore inevitable. Because the Fall made the human race mortal, "it is liable . . . to various diseases."[2] Sickness, pain, the agonies of childbirth, and death are certain in this life. Even redemption in Jesus Christ does not eliminate the physical effects of sin. In salvation, the historic Baptist confessions declare, people of faith are redeemed and forgiven, but the residues of sin remain.[3] According to the Second London Confession of 1677, when the elect are "effectually called" to repentance and faith, they are regenerated and have a "new Spirit created in them." The Spirit then starts the sanctification process by which the "whole body of sin is destroyed, and the several lusts thereof, are more and more weakened, and mortified." "This Sanctification is throughout, in the whole man, yet imperfect in this life; there abideth still some remnants of *corruption* in every part."[4] This means that while the Christian's soul is making spiritual progress, there is still considerable spiritual and physical imperfection. The "old nature" fights with the "new nature" in "a continual and irreconcilable war."[5] Only at the resurrection of the body will the process be complete, with all of the effects of the Fall reversed.[6] Virtually all of the major Baptist confessions say the same thing, whether they are early or late, British or American, Calvinist or Arminian.[7]

Nevertheless, while Baptists believed that suffering would come in this life, they also expected, by God's grace, to be able to profit from it. In his providence God uses pain in a variety of ways. Sometimes suffering expresses God's anger at human sin and is intended to produce reflection and repentance. At other times God allows it to promote spiritual maturity. Often God's purposes are hidden from the sufferer.

Thus "diseases, disasters, and distresses" both reveal and conceal the divine will.

It is easy to document such beliefs among Baptists. Roger Williams (1603–1683), one of the founders of the Baptist movement in America, wrote *Experiments of Spiritual Life and Health* (1652) for his wife during her recovery from a severe illness which left her depressed. Williams reminded her that one of the signs of spiritual health was a "humble, a patient, and thankful submission to the afflicting and chastening hand of God."[8] Suffering softened the heart and made it susceptible to divine guidance. He compared the effects of suffering on the human spirit to "the ground mollified upon a thaw, fit to be broken up, or like the ground moistened with storms and showers from heaven, ready in some hopeful turn for the Lord's most gracious seed and heavenly planting."[9] Williams believed that there was a close connection between physical and spiritual suffering.

> As it is in the restoring of the body to health or in the preserving of it in a healthful condition, it is often necessary to use the help of sharp and bitter things—bitter pills, bitter potions, bitter medicines, sweating, purging, vomitings, bloodlettings, etc.—so it is with our souls and spirits and preservation of the health and cheerfulness of the spiritual and the inner man.[10]

Similarly, other Baptists of the seventeenth and eighteenth centuries saw suffering as a normal part of the Christian life through which God worked for human benefit. It was the Christian's duty to make sure that these "checks of conscience" made one better, not bitter.[11]

Sometimes, then, suffering was more than a punishment for sin. It could be a gift of grace. That is the way Charles Haddon Spurgeon (1834–1892), no stranger to suffering himself, looked at it. Spurgeon was the pastor of the Metropolitan Tabernacle in London and the most influential English Baptist in the nineteenth century. For the last twenty years of his life, he suffered from a variety of ailments which forced him to curtail his pastoral ministry at various times. Through his experience, he developed the conviction that ill health was God's gift.

> I venture to say that the greatest earthly blessing that God can give to any of us is health, *with the exception of sickness*. Sickness has frequently been of more use to the saints of God than health has. . . . A sick wife, a newly made grave, poverty, slander, sinking of spirit, might teach us lessons nowhere else to be learned so well. Trials drive us to the realities of religion.[12]

He firmly believed that his bouts with rheumatism, gout, and neuralgia made him a better pastor, preacher, and person.

In short, Baptists have understood human suffering in different ways. It may be punishment for sin or part of God's plan to make better people. According to Baptist evangelist Billy Graham (b. 1918), "The fire of chastening purifies our lives and deepens our spirit."[13] But sometimes God's purposes remain hidden. "When God allows these things to happen, there is a reason which will eventually be known to the individual—most likely not until we get to heaven."[14] In the meantime, the Christian must be patient and trust God.[15]

Positive Views Toward Prayer and Medicine

The attitudes of Baptists toward suffering did not create hostility toward healing ministries or antipathy toward physicians and the healing arts. Baptists did not refrain from trying to alleviate suffering through prayer and medicine just because God used human suffering to punish sinners and sanctify the saints. In fact, medical doctors have played significant roles in Baptist history. Peter Chamberlen (1601–1683), one of the earliest converts to sabbatarian views among English Baptists and a pioneer in the development of obstetrical forceps, pastored the Mill Yard Seventh Day Baptist Church in London while maintaining a medical practice that included serving as a personal physician to English monarchs.[16] John Clarke (1609–1676), one of the founders of Rhode Island and an early American Baptist leader, was a trained physican. After practicing medicine in London, he immigrated to Boston in 1637, where he resumed his profession and eventually became a Baptist. During the 1640s he pastored Baptist churches and practiced medicine in Rhode Island; and during his long diplomatic assignment in England to secure a new charter for the colony, he supported himself by practicing medicine.[17] Similarly, a number of trained physicians played prominent roles in the early days of the National Baptist Convention, the largest black denomination in the United States. In the 1880s and 1890s, men like H.C. Lewis in San Antonio, Jacob J. Durham in South Carolina, T.H. Ewing and T. Edward Perry in Kansas City combined the two most highly respected professsions in the black community, physician and minister.[18] Such examples demonstrate that Baptists historically have seen no essential conflict in combining spiritual and health-oriented ministries.

From the beginning, then, Baptists found ways to combine faith and medicine. God used physicians to heal the sick, they reasoned; but he also used other means. Probably the most important was prayer. Baptists believed that when people got sick, they should pray to be healed. Although God allowed his people to suffer, he was not unmoved by their pain and often intervened on their behalf.

Sometimes prayer was accompanied by the anointing of the sick with oil, as described in *James* 5. Evidently this ritual was quite common among English Baptists in the mid-seventeenth century. In the 1640s, for example, it was widely reported that numerous healings had occurred after the sick had been anointed by elders.[19] Some English Baptists classified anointing the sick as a regular ordinance (sacrament) of the church; others practiced it irregularly. Vavasor Powell (1617–1670), an early Welsh Baptist leader, declared that "visiting the sick and . . . [anointing] them in the name of the Lord is a gospel ordinance and not repealed."[20] Baptist elders who anointed with oil did not urge the sick to shun physicians. Calling a doctor and being anointed with oil were part of the same healing process.[21]

Early American Baptists practiced similar rites. Morgan Edwards, a collector of Baptist historical sources in the late eighteenth century, found numerous reports of miraculous healings after anointing with oil. Yet he had to admit that the practice seemed to be dying out in his day. "The present generation of Baptists in Pennsylvania and the several other colonies (German Baptists excepted) have somehow reasoned themselves out of the practice of anointing the sick for recovery."[22]

It is difficult to determine how widespread this healing rite was among early Baptists. None of the major Baptist confessions in the seventeenth, eighteenth, or nineteenth centuries refers to it as a regular ordinance of the church. Standard Baptist manuals on church procedures ignore the practice.[23] But anointing may have been done in an informal and *ad hoc* fashion. The Free Baptists of New England, for example, anointed with oil well into the twentieth century, although they made no mention of it in their church manuals.[24]

One thing does seem clear. By the end of the nineteenth century, many Baptists appeared to have more confidence in modern medicine than they had in prayer and healing rituals. To a large extent this reticence stemmed from a reaction against the so-called faith-cure movement. Many Baptists, theological conservatives among them, believed that faith healing involved too much emphasis on divine intervention and not enough on the ordinary means of grace. Augustus Strong (1836–1912), president of Rochester Theological Seminary at the turn of the century, criticized this aspect of the faith cure:

> We would grant that nature is plastic in God's hand; that he can work miracles when and where it pleases him; and that he has given promises which, with certain Scriptural and rational limitations, encourage believing prayer for healing in cases of sickness. But we incline to the belief that in these later ages God answers such prayer, not by miracle, but by special providence, and by gifts of courage, faith and will, thus acting by his Spirit directly upon the soul and only indirectly on the body. . . . The Scripture

promise to faith is always expressly or impliedly conditioned by our use of means. . . . It is vain for the drowning man to pray, so long as he refuses to lay hold of the rope thrown to him. Medicines and physicians are the rope thrown to us by God; we cannot expect miraculous help while we neglect the help God has already given us. . . . The atonement has purchased complete salvation, and someday salvation shall be ours. But death and depravity still remain, not as penalty, but as chastisement. So disease remains also. Hospitals for incurables and the deaths even of advocates of faith-cure show that they too are compelled to recognize some limit to the application of the New Testament promise.[25]

A large number of Baptists by the end of the nineteenth century shared Strong's views. Even those who believed in prayer for healing did not want to be identified with Christian Scientists and other advocates of "mind-cure." They believed in divine healing but rejected the kind of hyper-supernaturalism that constantly expected, and even demanded, "signs and wonders." In Britain, Charles Spurgeon made his regular pastoral rounds during an outbreak of cholera and obtained what he described as an embarrassing reputation for healing sick folks through his bedside prayers. Spurgeon believed in and practiced prayer for the sick, but he did not want to be known as a "faith-healer."[26]

Some Baptists refused to let the confusion over faith healing deter them. A.J. Gordon (1836–1895), prominent Baptist minister from Boston, believed that God was still in the healing business. In 1882 he published *The Ministry of Healing*, in which he argued that though "grace is vastly more important than miracles . . . miracles have their place as shadows of greater things."[27] The reasons for the decline in the healing ministry, Gordon claimed, were the church's lack of faith, the fear of deception, and the corroding effects of rationalistic and liberal theology. Departing from the standard "baptistic" view, Gordon alleged that in Christ's death, he became the "sickness-bearer as well as the sin-bearer."[28] Because the atonement provided for physical healing, Christians should expect it and pray for it, though Gordon was quick to add that sometimes God chose not to answer the prayer of faith because suffering and even death better served his inscrutable purposes.[29] Gordon believed that anointing the sick with oil was an ordinance of the church, along with baptism and the Lord's Supper, and suggested that it be reinstituted as a normal part of church life.[30]

Some Baptists were attracted to this teaching, especially those partial to "holiness" or "perfectionist" doctrine. Gordon himself was involved in the Keswick movement, which taught that through a total surrender of the will to Christ, one could overcome the old sinful nature and live the "victorious Christian life."[31] A few Baptists who accepted Keswick teaching joined the Pentecostal movement in the early twentieth century, where faith healing was a major emphasis. In a 1979 Gallup Poll, twenty percent of the Baptists in the sample identified themselves with the pentecostal–charismatic movement.[32]

Most Baptists, however, did not adopt this view of divine healing. In fact, by the middle of the twentieth century, it was often difficult to tell the difference between Baptist conservatives and liberals on this issue. Many conservatives who believed in the possibility of supernatural healing nevertheless maintained that the age of miracles was all but over and that people who sought divine healing might be deluding themselves into fanaticism. Some even denied the applicability of anointing the sick with oil, a rather intriguing position for people who believed in the inerrancy of the Bible.[33]

Baptists, therefore, have maintained a diverse approach to matters of faith and medicine. They have recognized that suffering is a normal part of the human condition, due, theologically speaking, to the sinfulness of the race. Yet, they have also believed that suffering can have positive side effects, that God may use it to bring sinners to repentance and to help saints in their spiritual development. Baptists have generally maintained a positive view toward medicine and have often joined it to the practice of prayer and rites of healing. But in comparison to some other faith traditions, Baptists have never made health or medical concerns central. They have, however, occasionally isolated a few health-related practices and addressed them with evangelical fervor.

Alcohol and Tobacco

Few health issues have agitated Baptists more than the consumption of alcohol. Nevertheless, even here Baptists have had difficulty speaking with one voice. Because of their democratic and decentralized polity, Baptists have not had the official mechanism for deciding issues for everyone. Each congregation makes and enforces its own rules. Denominational conventions and associations can only offer advice or, when that fails, use unofficial coercion. No matter how strong the pressure from denominational bodies, Baptists have insisted that believers on the local level still retain the right to come to their own conclusions.

On the early American frontier, where Baptists experienced their most significant growth, the use of alcohol was widespread. It was viewed as a preventative of disease and a necessary accompaniment to everything from house-raisings to harvests. Making, selling, and consuming hard liquor were all acceptable practices among frontier Baptists, who often paid their preacher's salary partly in whiskey. This tolerant view of drinking, however, did not mean that Baptists took drunkenness

lightly. Records of early nineteenth-century frontier Baptist congregations show that men and women who could not hold their liquor were
expelled from membership.[34]

When the temperance movement gained national recognition in the
1820s, Baptists responded to it in different ways. Early on, Baptists in
New England opposed temperance as often as they supported it, especially when the movement changed its emphasis from moderate
drinking to total abstinence.[35] Free Will Baptists, however, were an
exception. In 1828 they advised that no member use ardent spirits,
except for medicinal purposes; and by 1832 they refused to ordain
drinkers to the ministry and threatened to expel liquor dealers from
membership.[36]

Such a response, however, was not universal. In the West and South,
pre–Civil War Baptists showed little enthusiasm for the national temperance movement. The Primitive Baptists, for example, rejected any
religious or reform society outside the local church because they could
find no biblical precedent for such action. Many other antebellum
Baptists believed that churches as churches should not take a position
on such matters: They were called to preach the gospel, not reform
society. Still others were put off by the relationship of northern temperance advocates to other radical causes such as abolitionism and early
feminism.[37] But opposition to nationally organized temperance societies
did not mean that Southern Baptists were uninvolved on the local level.
Many individual Baptists were ardent adversaries of the liquor traffic.
In the late 1820s, Abner Clopton, a physician turned pastor, organized
Baptists into the Virginia Society for the Promotion of Temperance
(1826), which led anti-alcohol forces in the state.[38]

It was not until the 1870s that Southern Baptists began to make
official (but nonbinding) pronouncements on alcohol. All Baptist state
conventions in the South, with the exception of North Carolina, passed
resolutions against the users and sellers of alcohol.[39] By the 1880s, total
prohibition was the Baptist position in the South, and many Baptists
were willing to organize politically to achieve it. For example, the
Baptist state convention of Tennessee supported a prohibition amendment to the state constitution in 1887, and Baptist leaders used every
rhetorical device at their disposal in its behalf. The editor of the *Baptist*
suggested that anyone who refused to vote in favor of prohibition was
"neither fit for the land nor the dung hill." Let him be consigned to
hell, "where his stench of a decayed and rotten manhood may be
consumed day and night forever and ever."[40] Another Baptist author
blamed the liquor traffic for virtually every social ill and predicted that,
if left unchecked, it would "destroy virtue and immolate the fair daughters of Tennessee on the altar of lust."[41]

When reformers founded the Anti-Saloon League (1895) to work for a national prohibition amendment, Southern Baptists endorsed it, often taking up collections to aid the League's political program. This marked a significant turning point in the approach of Southern Baptists on this issue. Heretofore, they had avoided overt political action at the national level and any cooperation with northerners in reform causes. But they finally made an exception.[42] In 1896, after years of debate, the Southern Baptist Convention (SBC) adopted a resolution that condemned anyone who manufactured, sold, or drank alcohol and recommended that such people be excluded from church membership.[43] Although the Convention never officially endorsed the Prohibition Party, many of its constituents supported it, a few of them running for office on the party's ticket.[44] By the 1920s, the SBC had a Committee on Temperance and Social Service, which carefully monitored local and national elections and recommended that "wet" candidates be driven from office.[45]

Even when such political measures failed, Baptists maintained their antipathy toward alcohol. Baptists made an elaborate religious case against intoxicants, even when consumed in moderate amounts. The Bible taught that wine was a mocker and deceiver (*Prv.* 20:1) and that it led to spiritual ruin.[46] But there was another side to the biblical argument. Did not Jesus turn water into wine (*Jn.* 2:1–11), and did not Paul advise Timothy to "use a little wine for thy stomach's sake" (1 *Tm.* 5:23)? Such textual obstacles were not insurmountable, even for teetotalers. Using a circular argument, some Baptists reasoned that because Jesus never did anything sinful and the use of intoxicating liquor is sinful, the wine he made at the wedding feast of Cana could not have been real wine.[47] Furthermore, Paul's recommendation to Timothy concerned only the medicinal use of wine; because science had produced nonalcoholic medicines, the use of wine was no longer warranted.[48]

In addition to the biblical rationale, Baptists also amassed medical and social arguments. Alcohol was bad for health, injurious to society, disastrous to family life, and psychologically detrimental to the individual.[49] No matter which kinds of arguments were used, the ultimate solution to the problem was always spiritual: Only the grace of Jesus Christ could save people from the ravages of drink. Politics and social programs may fail to achieve their ends, but conversion to Jesus Christ never does.[50]

Despite such a strong anti-alcohol tradition, there is some evidence that Southern Baptist practice is changing. In 1984 Ronald Sisk of the Southern Baptist Christian Life Commission complained that Southern Baptists were drinking just like everybody else. According to a recent survey, forty-eight percent of Southern Baptists drink and sixteen percent of those become alcoholics. Twenty-five percent of Southern Baptist young people reported using alcohol during the previous year. Sisk concluded that "somewhere along the way, a lot of Baptists stopped listening to our annual sermons on abstinence."[51]

Baptists in the North also joined the prohibition movement and discouraged the private manufacture, sale, and use of liquor. Walter Rauschenbusch (1861–1918), leader of the social–gospel movement and a Baptist seminary professor of church history, made temperance an important part of his program to realize the Kingdom of God. He called the use of intoxicants one of the "marks of barbarism" and urged Baptist churches to do everything in their power to end not only the liquor traffic, but the social sentiment that made drinking acceptable.[52]

Most English and Canadian Baptists felt the same way about temperance. As early as the 1840s, English Baptist ministers were organizing temperance societies in their local congregations; and eventually a few Baptists—Isaac Doxsey, Dawson Burns, John Clifford, and Charles H. Spurgeon—became temperance leaders at the national level.[53] In Canada, Baptists and Methodists led the strong temperance movement which reached its zenith in the late nineteenth century.[54]

Baptists have been much more ambivalent about tobacco, another personal habit with health consequences, than alcohol. Nowhere has this been more evident than among Southern Baptists in America. In the nineteenth century some Baptists condemned tobacco use as a sin second only to drunkenness; others considered it helpful in soothing the nerves, promoting digestion, and preventing "local scurvy."[55] The chief reason for such diversity is not hard to find. Large numbers of Baptists in the American South not only smoked, chewed, and dipped tobacco, but made their livings from it. Southern Baptist clergy in tobacco-growing areas understood clearly that the financial well-being of their congregations depended on the size of the year's tobacco crop and the price that it brought at market. During the nineteenth century, many Baptists in the South never thought twice about tobacco use. At best, tobacco was one of life's great pleasures; at worst, it was one of life's tolerable vices. Thus when Edgar Young Mullins (1860–1928), a pastor who later became president of the Southern Baptist Theological Seminary in Louisville, gave up his tobacco habit in 1887, it was noteworthy—and uncalled for. According to his wife, "There was no prejudice against a preacher's smoking in the South at that time, and nothing to coerce him." Mullins himself seemed bemused by his decision and was unable or unwilling to cite any reason for it.[56]

Nevertheless, some Baptists had strong convictions on the subject. They vehemently attacked tobacco and called on fellow believers to forsake it. Because they were biblicists, they occasionally found themselves in a difficult position. How could they be so dogmatic about the sinfulness of tobacco use when the Bible was silent on the subject? Although they could not cite chapter and verse against the "evil weed," they did take their stand on the Bible. They claimed that certain general commands, if taken seriously, prohibited tobacco use. For instance, Paul ordered the Thessalonians to "abstain from all appearance of evil" (1 *Thes.* 5:22) and reminded the Colossians that "whatsoever ye do in word or deed, do all in the name of the Lord Jesus, giving thanks to God and the Father by him" (*Col.* 3:17). Furthermore, Paul inquired, "What? Know ye not that your body is the temple of the Holy Ghost which is in you, which ye have of God, and ye are not your own? For ye are bought with a price: therefore glorify God in your body, and in your spirit, which are God's" (1 *Cor.* 6:19–20). In light of such passages, one Baptist asked, "Do you 'glorify God in your body and spirit, which are his,' by the use of tobacco? If you do not, then you are solemnly bound by your Christian profession to give it up."[57]

When biblical arguments failed to persuade, scientific ones were used. Opponents of tobacco cited the testimony of medical experts who blamed tobacco for a long list of ailments, including heart trouble, insomnia, lung disease, nervousness, and imbecility. One editor claimed that there was a close connection between tobacco and alcohol abuse: "The way that leads down to a drunkard's grave and to a drunkard's hell is strewn thick with tobacco leaves."[58]

Most Baptists, however, remained unconvinced. Baptist periodicals carried advertisements for tobacco products, and some church newspapers regularly featured articles on tobacco-farming methods and market conditions. In one extreme case of ambivalence, the editor of the *Religious Herald* in Richmond, Virginia, urged his readers, on biblical and medical grounds, to abstain from tobacco, but added that if they chose to do otherwise, they should at least buy from the tobacco companies that advertised in his newspaper.[59]

Even Baptists who defended or at least tolerated tobacco use occasionally had to admit that it created problems. Denominational gatherings, clergy get-togethers, and annual meetings of the Southern Baptist Convention were often thick with smoke; and tobacco chewers had to be reminded not to spit on the carpets. Sunday morning churchgoers complained about people chewing tobacco during services. One obviously disgusted Baptist wondered what Christ thought of those who turned His house into a "tobacco chewer's spitbox."[60] Churches that failed to keep people from chewing during worship were forced to provide them with spittoons, which, according to opponents, only served to encourage the practice.[61]

By the end of the nineteenth century, there was some evidence that tobacco use was on the decline among Baptists in the South; but for the most part, church leaders consistently refused to condemn it. According to Rufus Spain, by 1900 "Baptist ministers and laymen alike continued to smoke, chew, and dip, though perhaps with a slightly uneasy conscience."[62]

During the twentieth century, medical evidence has steadily increased concerning the harmful effects of tobacco, yet Southern Baptists have remained deeply divided over the issue. In 1984, for the first time ever, the Southern Baptist Convention took a stand against tobacco. The "messengers" who met in Kansas City pondered whether it was Christian, in light of tobacco's documented ill effects, to traffic in its trade. Consequently, they passed a resolution that called on tobacco farmers to switch to another crop and urged the federal government to cease its subsidies to them. Because such resolutions are not binding on local churches, rank-and-file Southern Baptists are free to dissent, and they have. Opposition has centered in North Carolina, the South's premier tobacco-growing state. The North Carolina State Baptist Convention repudiated the SBC's action and threw its support behind the state's tobacco farmers. Although the convention recognized tobacco's health risks, it also cited the severe moral and ethical questions that would be created by the decline of tobacco production. As one North Carolina Baptist pastor put it, "I don't look on tobacco as being a moral issue. I look at it as being a respectable product. It provides an economy for North Carolina farmers and, quite frankly, without it my church couldn't survive."[63] In such cases, some Baptists are moved more by economic issues than by moral or medical ones. Obviously, for those directly tied to the tobacco economy, the dilemma is a real one.

Medical Missions: Organizing for Medical Care

Although Baptists had long been concerned about issues of health and medicine, they did not organize to provide medical care until the middle of the nineteenth century. To a large extent the impetus for building hospitals and other medical facilities came from foreign missions. Once Baptists became convinced that medical care was a legitimate form of evangelical ministry, they strongly supported organized health care, both at home and abroad.

The Baptist foreign missionary movement began in the late eighteenth century. In 1792 William Carey (1761–1834), an English Baptist minister and shoemaker, published An Enquiry into the Obligation of Christians to Use Means for the Conversion of the Heathens, in which he rejected the "hyper-Calvinism" that had stifled evangelistic work by Particular Baptists.[64] Thanks in large part to Carey's pamphlet, the Baptist Missionary Society (BMS) was organized in 1792.[65] Three months later, the society appointed its first missionaries: John Thomas

(1757–1801), a trained physician who had practiced medicine for the Royal Navy and the East India Company, and William Carey. Because Dr. Thomas already could speak Bengali and some Sanskrit, the society decided to send the pair to India. The new mission originally settled in Calcutta, but because of strong opposition from the British East India Company, Carey and Thomas in 1800 moved to Serampore, in Dutch territory. There the work prospered, despite Thomas's quick demise. Building on the foundation laid by Carey and Thomas in India, by 1875 British Baptists expanded their missionary work to Jamaica, West Africa, and China.[66]

American Baptists commissioned their first foreign missionary in 1814. Adoniram Judson (1788–1850), appointed in 1812 as a missionary to Burma by the American Board of Commissioners for Foreign Missions (Congregationalist), changed his views on baptism and became a Baptist during his passage to the Orient. When Judson informed the American Board of his new convictions, it terminated support. The American Baptist Trienniel Convention, organized in 1814 to encourage missions, quickly stepped in, making Judson its first appointee. By the 1850s, American Baptists had missionary work in France, Germany, Greece, Siam, Haiti, and southern India;[67] and by the turn of the century, they were established in China, Assam, Spain, the Congo, and the Philippines.[68] Not even the division of American Baptist churches over the slavery issue dampened missionary enthusiasm. One of the first acts of the new Southern Baptist Convention (1845) was to form the Foreign Mission Board, which eventually sent missionaries to Hong Kong and South China, Liberia, Nigeria, northern China, Italy, Mexico, Brazil, and Japan. In the early twentieth century, Southern Baptists opened additional missions in South America, Europe, and Palestine.[69] From 1850 to 1950 other Baptist missionary societies proliferated. Although many of these organizations grew out of institutional and theological disputes, they produced an unprecedented advance in Baptist missionary activity.[70]

Physicians were involved from the beginning of the missions movement. Dr. John Thomas, Carey's colleague in India, used his medical skill to win the mission's first convert: Krishna Pal became a Christian after Dr. Thomas set his broken arm.[71] However, most early Baptist missionary physicians saw themselves as evangelists first and medical experts second. Initially, they practiced most of their medicine on fellow missionaries and their families, attending to the health needs of native peoples only as time and energy allowed. Many of these physicians preferred preaching to doctoring. Dr. George Washington Burton, for example, who was sent by the Southern Baptists to Shanghai in 1851, spent more time doing evangelism than healing the sick, although he did manage to establish several dispensaries and maintain a private medical practice on the side.[72]

In the beginning, at least, most Baptist missionary societies wanted it that way. Their main emphases were on evangelism and education. From their standpoint, missionaries—even medical personnel—were sent and supported to save souls. While few members objected to missionaries responding to the desperate physical needs around them, Baptists as a whole expected them to concentrate on spreading the gospel. Baptists believed that medicine was an effective tool for evangelism and that healing the body was often the first step to healing the soul. For that reason, many agencies in the nineteenth century insisted that missionary doctors be theologically trained and properly ordained Baptist ministers before sending them out. It was not until after 1850 that Baptist mission agencies started to give medicine the same support that they had given evangelism and education.[73]

To a large extent, this change in attitude resulted from the growing involvement of Baptist women in foreign missions. In the 1870s Northern Baptist women organized a number of missionary societies, including the Free Baptist Woman's Missionary Society in 1873.[74] Southern Baptist women organized their Woman's Missionary Union in 1888.[75]

These societies, which raised funds and recruited and supported women missionaries, were often more successful than their male counterparts at arousing and sustaining interest in the missionary cause. These women's societies also stressed healing ministries more than the male-controlled societies did. They aggressively recruited women physicians and nurses, convinced that they had a unique role to play overseas. Many native women would not allow male doctors to examine them. This reticence was especially evident in places like India and the Moslem countries, where women were sequestered. Consequently, local custom often placed half the population beyond the reach of medical missions—until women physicians arrived.

Baptists commissioned their first women missionary doctors in 1879, ten years after the Methodist Episcopal Woman's Foreign Missionary Society sent out the first woman physician ever appointed to any field by any society. These pioneering Baptists were Eleanor Mitchell, a fifty-year-old doctor from Wisconsin who had served as a nurse in the Civil War before going to Burma, and Dr. Carolina H. Daniels, who went to Swatow, China. Over the next few decades, Baptist women doctors and nurses entered missionary service by the score, often finding that there were more opportunities overseas than on the home front.[76]

Thanks to the increased attention to the healing ministry, Baptists began to establish dispensaries and hospitals as a normal part of their missionary work. By the end of the 1870s, most foreign fields had at least one medical dispensary where basic medicines were distributed and the simplest medical procedures were performed; in many places, hospitals provided more substantive medical care, sometimes offering the best treatment available for hundreds of miles. In China and India, Baptists established nurses' training schools and medical colleges for the preparation of native physicians. In addition, they set up leprosy and tuberculosis sanatoriums, maternity hospitals, and mobile medical clinics.[77]

Once Baptists caught the vision for building hospitals, they did so with great enthusiasm. In some cases, individual congregations or state associations back home assumed responsibility for a particular medical facility, raising building funds and keeping the hospital well-supplied once it was built.[78] Northern Baptists, who were renamed American Baptist Churches of the U.S.A. in the 1970s, started building medical facilities and training schools in the 1860s; by 1983 they operated eighty-nine clinics, six nursing schools and a medical college, fourteen dispensaries, and twenty-one hospitals in Zaire, India, the Philippines, Thailand, Haiti, and Nicaragua.[79] Between 1900 and 1923, Southern Baptists built eleven hospitals and dispensaries in China alone and assisted Chinese Christians in establishing and maintaining their own.[80] Seventh Day Baptists founded their first medical mission at Liuho, outside Shanghai, in 1902 and constructed a major hospital there in 1912.[81] In the 1920s, National Baptists built a hospital in Monrovia, Liberia, that became the leading medical center for the country.[82] Not long after its founding in the 1940s, the Conservative Baptist Foreign Mission Society began medical work overseas.[83]

British Baptists did not lag far behind. In 1894 Dr. Vincent Thomas applied to the Baptist Missionary Society as a medical missionary. Up to that time, the BMS had never considered the few physicians whom it had appointed as full-fledged missionaries. But Dr. Thomas's appeal led the Society to rethink its position. By 1901 the BMS concluded that "the medical man or the nursing sister, no less than the evangelist or the teacher, could claim to have a *missionary vocation*" and founded the Medical Mission Auxiliary to support its new emphasis.[84]

In addition to building medical institutions and designating medical work as a legitimate missionary task, most agencies encouraged—and sometimes required—missionary candidates to acquire a basic knowledge of medical procedures, which often amounted to little more than a crash course in first aid. Many missionaries found that even such a meager investment of time and effort paid large spiritual dividends later on. For example, on one occasion in the late nineteenth century, E.C. Smyth, a British Baptist missionary in China's Shantung province, was asked to see a boy who had swallowed his mother's brass ring. Chinese doctors had tried their folk remedies (such as piercing his neck with needles, shaving his head, blistering his skin with hot coals), but to no avail. Although he had little medical training, Smyth administered an emetic; and in a few minutes "sickness accomplished what the needles and blistering had failed to do." As a result, Smyth was able to convert the boy and his family and soon established a Baptist church in their village.[85]

Despite its new status in missions, medicine was still closely tied to the work of witness. Medical service remained "pre-evangelism," and doctors were expected to convert their patients as well as heal them. Therefore, in Baptist dispensaries and hospitals, the gospel was as freely dispensed as medication. In India, for example, "Bible women" (trained women evangelists) conducted services for people in hospital waiting rooms. Evangelistic meetings were held in the wards. Hospital chaplains and tract-society colporteurs made rounds in order to discuss spiritual issues with patients as well as their visiting friends and relatives. Physicians openly evangelized their patients and prayed with them about their physical and spiritual problems.[86] In Baptist medical facilities, then, Bibles were as common as bedpans. As a result, no one who used Baptist medical facilities could have avoided being presented with a clear and sometimes aggressive gospel appeal.

Baptists believed that such tactics were appropriate and needful. After all, Baptist missionaries were there to confront people with the claims of Christ and win them for the kingdom of God. Acts of compassion and verbal witness were inseparable. Baptist doctors and nurses performed their duties in Jesus' name, and few medical missionaries saw any reason to keep quiet about spiritual matters or tone down the message that they were sent to proclaim. Healthy bodies without saved souls were not enough.

Despite the alliance between medical and evangelistic missions, in the twentieth century many Baptists began to question the relationship. There were two main reasons for this reevaluation. The first was financial. A considerable decline in donations to mission boards during the 1920s curtailed the ability of Baptists to maintain expensive medical programs and personnel overseas.[87] A second reason was theological. Like many Protestants in the late nineteenth and early twentieth centuries, Baptists, especially in the North, were torn apart by theological conflict between liberals and conservatives.[88] Changing theological perspectives affected the missionary enterprise as much as they did the peace of Baptist schools and churches. Many liberals no longer accepted the traditional motive for foreign missions: the saving of the lost so that they could escape the wrath of God. William Newton Clarke (1840–1912), the Baptist seminary professor who wrote evangelical liberalism's most influential textbook,[89] rejected the belief that people who did not accept Jesus Christ as Saviour were headed for an eternity in hell.[90] This view not only called into question the traditional rationale for Baptist missions, it also weakened the historical relationship between evangelism and medicine. The liberal perspective, many traditionalists feared, might lead to doing medicine for its own sake, rather than as an aid to winning lost souls to Christ.

By 1930 the breakdown of consensus had created a crisis. A group of Northern Baptist businessmen called for a study of the current state of foreign missions. Representatives from seven Protestant denominations were organized into a commission, and, with money supplied by Baptist John D. Rockefeller, Jr., they travelled to China, Burma, India, and Japan in order to analyze the situation. Their observations and recommendations were published in *Re-Thinking Missions: A Laymen's Inquiry After 100 Years.*[91]

While the report did not recommend the abandonment of mission work, it called for a radical transformation: for missionaries to be more open-minded in their dealings with non-Christian religions and more humanitarian, rather than evangelistic, in their approach. The report also addressed the traditional relationship between medicine and evangelism, observing that while

> the spoken word may have its appropriate place in the hospital . . . the use of medical or other professional service as a direct means of making converts, or public services in wards and dispensaries from which patients cannot escape, is subtly coercive, and improper. . . . Enlightened non-Christians frequently express their scorn of institutions which proselytize the sick and helpless, who are least able to resist.

The authors of the report urged that medicine be practiced along more "professional" lines, without the disturbing pressures to evangelize.[92]

Furthermore, the *Inquiry* went on, agencies should strive for higher standards of professionalism in their medical programs. Well into the twentieth century, many mission hospitals were primitive by western standards. As late as 1926, for example, the Etta Waterbury Memorial Hospital in Udayagiri, India, which was considered one of the best Baptist missionary hospitals in the world, had no electricity, gas, or running water. Water had to be transported by hand, and operations were performed by the light of an oil lamp.[93] For a variety of reasons, in many places simple sanitation and hygiene were hard to come by, and doctors had to perform surgery on the floor of mud huts or turn old doors and packing crates into operating tables.[94] Understandably, physicians who practiced in remote areas had very little opportunity to "keep up." The *Inquiry* noted such lapses of professionalism and suggested that it would be better to have fewer hospitals, more specialists, and higher standards than to maintain many mediocre institutions.

To say the least, the *Laymen's Inquiry* provoked considerable discussion, especially in the Northern Baptist Convention. For the most part, however, Northern Baptists rejected the report's suggestion that missionary doctors downplay evangelism in their medical work.[95] Baptists in the South, where theological liberalism had made few inroads, paid scant attention to the *Inquiry*. In 1982, for example, Southern Baptists were still insisting that they built mission hospitals "for the dual purpose of expressing Christian compassion and as a means of witness through which persons may acknowledge Christ as Lord."[96]

Organizing for Health Care at Home

Once Baptists established the role of medicine in the work of the gospel, they also applied their principles at home. In the United States, the first Baptist hospital grew out of the efforts of a St. Louis layman, Dr. W.G. Mayfield, who in 1884 took a patient into his home to administer spiritual and medical care. That act of charity grew into the Missouri Baptist Sanitarium in 1890 and the Missouri Baptist Hospital a short time later.[97] Likewise, in 1903 the Tabernacle Baptist Church of Atlanta, under Pastor Len G. Broughton (who had been a practicing physician before entering the ministry), opened a small infirmary next to the church in order to serve people who could not afford regular medical care. That modest work eventually turned into the Georgia Baptist Hospital. By World War I, Baptists all over the South were building hospitals. In 1923 the Southern Baptist Convention created a Hospital Commission to oversee the construction of hospitals in New Orleans, Louisiana, and Jacksonville, Florida; but for the most part, Baptists kept their hospitals under the control of local associations or state conventions.[98] In 1981, of the thirty-four Southern Baptist state conventions, eleven owned and operated approximately fifty medical facilities of one kind or another.[99]

Baptists believed that such institutions, like their hospitals overseas, served a spiritual as well as a medical purpose. In 1960 the Southwide Baptist Hospital Commission declared that "a Baptist hospital exists to bring men into a saving relationship with God through faith in Jesus Christ by means of direct personal witness as occasion presents, and by a positive Christian interpretation of the experience of disease, disability, and death."[100]

Southern Baptists also founded medical and nursing schools. In conjunction with Wake Forest College in North Carolina, they founded the Bowman Gray School of Medicine in 1902;[101] and Baylor University in Texas established a medical school (1903), school of nursing (1917), and school of dentistry (1918).[102]

Although not nearly as aggressively as Southern Baptists, Baptists in the North also built hospitals. Russell Conwell, who turned a struggling Baptist church in Philadelphia into the Baptist Temple (and Temple University), started the Samaritan Hospital in 1892 "in the hope that it would do Christ's work . . . to so do those charitable acts as to enforce the truth Jesus taught."[103] In time, Conwell's Temple University opened a medical school to train the city's poor for medical careers. Similarly, the Ruggles Street Baptist Church in Boston started the New England Baptist Hospital in 1893, an institution that subsequently grew into a leading medical center in the Northeast. The Northern Baptist Convention (American Baptist Churches) created an Association of Baptist Homes and Hospitals in 1933, which by 1965 supervised eight hospitals, sixty-eight homes for the aged, and fourteen children's homes.[104]

Baptists never developed a distinctive approach to medical care, but, as their contributions to organized medical care illustrate, they did find ways to combine a deep concern for spiritual life with an active interest in health and well-being. Although Baptists occasionally treated medicine and health care as means to a greater end (evangelism), the fact remains that they expended enormous time, energy, and money to heal the sick, whenever and wherever they found them.

Caring for the Person

Despite their proven ability to build institutions, Baptists have cared most about people. This can be clearly seen in their emphasis on pastoral care. Frontier Baptists, for example, believed that personal behavior was "church business." Fighting spouses, the sexually perverse or promiscuous, drunkards, crooked business dealers, and gossips were all liable for church discipline. The goal, however, was restoration, not exclusion. Therefore, Baptist elders and deacons acted as pastoral counselors who exhorted, instructed from the Bible, and prayed with erring ones.[105]

Until the twentieth century, pastoral care consisted of heavy doses of moralistic and biblical advice. But with the rise of psychology and psychotherapy, Baptists adjusted their approach.[106] The University of Chicago Divinity School was the first Baptist seminary to offer a course in the psychology of religion (1904). Chicago pioneered in "functionalism," the belief that religion's main role is to help people adjust to their environment. In 1906, Chicago theologian Edward Scribner Ames, a follower of William James, suggested that theology and "functional psychology" join forces and that theological truth be judged by its ability to help people adjust to life.[107] Not everyone followed Ames's radical approach, but soon Baptist seminaries were integrating psychology into their programs.[108] In 1920, Gaines Dobbins of the Southern Baptist Seminary in Louisville announced his intention to "capture psychology for Christ." He believed that second to the Bible, psychology was the most important subject for pastors to master.[109] During the 1920s and 1930s, then, Baptist seminaries added courses, and even departments, in pastoral care and counseling. By 1944, all Southern Baptist seminaries had such programs, and by the 1980s, the same could be said about virtually all other Baptist seminaries. A few even offered degree programs in those areas. Furthermore, when the need for the clinical training of pastors led to the development of clinical pastoral education, a program of supervised training for theological students and pastors, most Baptists lent their enthusiastic support.[110]

Most Baptists have seen psychology and psychotherapy as allies of religion. Harry Emerson Fosdick (1878–1969), a prominent liberal Baptist minister from New York who put pastoral counseling at the center of his ministry, believed that good preaching was "personal counseling on a group scale."[111] More recently, Wayne Oates (b. 1917), of the Southern Baptist Seminary and the University of Louisville, introduced many Baptists to psychologically informed pastoral care through the discipline of psychology of religion.[112] Consequently, most Baptist ministers subscribed to a "team approach" to pastoral care and willingly referred their "clients" to other more qualified professionals.[113] Naturally, Baptists have disagreed about how psychological theories and techniques of psychotherapy should be used in pastoral work. But most have recognized that there is a psychological as well as a spiritual dimension to human life and that not all personal problems have easy religious solutions. Most Baptist pastoral counselors have employed psychological categories and techniques within their own theological and biblical framework, fully aware that, if they are not careful, they can manipulate people through the improper use of Scripture and prayer.

It is not altogether clear the extent to which these sentiments filtered down to the pew. Just because seminaries maintained psychologically sophisticated programs in pastoral care did not necessarily mean that pastors, who in many Baptist denominations were not seminary graduates, and laypeople went along. There remained in the rank and file a largely unspoken prejudice against psychotherapy. Many Baptists who might talk to a minister would refuse to see a psychotherapist because they thought that real Christians did not have psychological problems.

A big part of the pastoral counseling that went on in Baptist churches has had to do with personal behavior that has health consequences. For the most part, Baptists have been concerned about health-related behavior only when there is a moral or religious dimension to it. Thus Baptists opposed alcohol because it breaks up families, lowers natural inhibitions, and ruins one's relationship to God, not just because excessive use destroys liver function.

Consequently, Baptists have always cared deeply about human sexuality because of its moral implications. Most Baptists have had a positive view of sex, within certain limits. Traditionally, they believed that sexual intercourse belongs only in marriage, which rules out any homosexual, premarital, or extramarital sexual activity. Sex between married persons has been considered much more than a reproductive act; it is an experience of pleasure, joy, and intimacy. But the biblical rules are clear: "Chastity before and after marriage is the norm of sexual relations. . . . Adultery is the violation of 'one flesh' unity, the ontological aspect of marriage."[114]

When expressed outside the limits laid down by Scripture, most Baptists have believed, sex is sinful and destructive. Illicit sex has disastrous personal and social consequences. In the early twentieth century, Walter Rauschenbusch condemned a number of sexual sins, including masturbation, promiscuity, and lust. "An evening out; a broken girl; a shamed family; a syphilitic baby; scrophulous [sic] bodies for several generations. Show us the last results at the beginning and we should sober up."[115] Sexual immorality led to prostitution, venereal disease, and loss of self-respect and self-control.[116] Thus, breaking God's sexual standards often produced its own punishment, as fundamentalist Baptists especially liked to point out. For example, the outbreak of AIDS in the homosexual community during the 1980s was commonly called "Jerry Falwell's revenge" because of the Baptist fundamentalist leader's condemnation of all homosexual practice.[117]

In order to uphold sexual standards, Baptists traditionally monitored social and personal behavior. Many more conservative Baptists, for example, have condemned dancing, dressing immodestly, "mixed bathing" (which refers to males and females swimming together), moviegoing, and novel-reading because they may arouse sexual passions and lower inhibitions. Baptists warned their young people about the dangers of sexual stimulation, often referred to as necking, petting, or "making out."[118]

Recently, many Baptists have shown increasing interest in sex, thanks to its rediscovery by American evangelicals at large. American evangelicalism, which historically has been rather ambivalent toward sexuality—sometimes even in marriage—experienced a sexual renaissance in the 1970s. Marabel Morgan's *The Total Woman* was a runaway bestseller in evangelical circles.[119] It celebrated "Christian" sexuality and suggested that Christian wives should spice up their sex lives by dressing enticingly in baby-doll nighties and leather boots and having intercourse with their husbands in unusual places around the house, such as in the kitchen or under the dining room table. Many Baptists eagerly embraced this rather liberated approach to married sex; and a few of them actually contributed to the genre: Tim and Beverly LaHaye, leaders in Baptist fundamentalism and the Moral Majority, produced their own sex manual, *The Act of Marriage: The Beauty of Sexual Love*.[120]

Such a profound shift in attitudes proves that Baptists have not been immune to social change in the twentieth century. As traditional mores have shifted, so have many Baptist practices, although it is difficult to determine the degree or the extent of such change. With the exception of some conservatives, most Baptists are no longer as concerned about mixed bathing, dancing, and moviegoing as they used to be. Large numbers have evidently lost their sexual shyness. Other issues concerning human sexuality get more attention.

Birth control has never been seen as a major problem by most Baptists. Southern Baptists have criticized the papal ban on birth control and have endorsed for married couples "methods of planned parenthood and the dissemination of planned parenthood information."[121] Most Baptists prefer to leave such matters to personal discretion.[122]

The practice of abortion has been much more controversial among Baptists, who have lined up on both sides of the issue. In 1971, the Southern Baptist Convention voted to support legislation that allowed "abortion in cases of rape, incest, clear evidence of severe fetal deformity, and carefully ascertained evidence of the likelihood of damage to the emotional, mental, and physical health of the mother."[123] Supporters of the resolution claimed that it steered a middle course between the extremes of abortion on demand and the view that all abortion was murder. Many Southern Baptists, however, were not satisfied with that position and organized to reverse it. In 1974, they failed to pass a resolution that called for a constitutional amendment against abortion.[124] In 1976, they failed again but did manage to amend the 1971 resolution so that it could not be seen as promoting "permissive legislation."[125] After turning down resolutions in favor of a constitutional amendment in 1977, 1978, and 1979, the SBC of 1980 finally voted to endorse "legislation and/or a constitutional amendment prohibiting abortion except to save the life of the mother."[126] Subsequent conventions have reaffirmed and even strengthened the 1980 resolution.[127] In contrast to the Southern Baptist stance on abortion, in 1983 pro-life advocates in the American Baptist Churches in the United States failed to get an anti-abortion resolution passed at their convention.[128] In short, it is impossible to generalize about the Baptist view on abortion: Some allow abortion under certain circumstances, while others call it murder under any conditions.[129]

In addition, many Baptists have become aware of the enormous bioethical issues facing people in and out of the health-care professions.

Although nothing like consensus has emerged, Baptists have begun to grapple with issues of euthanasia, infertility, genetic engineering, and the like. Paul D. Simmons of the Southern Baptist Theological Seminary, for example, has done much to awaken Baptists as well as others to some of the life and death issues confronting modern society.[130]

Conclusion

From one perspective, Baptist people have never made health issues a primary concern. They have never had a distinctive diet or endorsed a particular approach to medical care. They have been more interested in evangelizing and building churches. But because of their stress on the importance of the individual, they have occasionally become interested in various health-related matters. Their concern for souls led them to oppose alcohol and to build health-care institutions. Their concern for morality led them to follow, at least until recently, traditional views of sexual morality. As people who care about people, Baptists have been willing to consult (and become) physicians and psychologists in order to alleviate human suffering. Whereas their theology tells them that pain is inevitable in this life, few Baptists have been willing to leave it at that.

Notes

1. John Gill, *The Body of Divinity* (London [1769] 1839), p. 324. See also Augustus H. Strong, *Systematic Theology* (Old Tappan, NJ, 1907), pp. 869–881; and Dale Moody, *The Word of Truth* (Grand Rapids, MI, 1981), pp. 322–325.
2. Ibid., p. 342.
3. For a collection of Baptist creeds, see William L. Lumpkin, *Baptist Confessions of Faith* (Philadelphia, 1959).
4. *The Second London Confession,* ch. XIII, ibid., pp. 267–268.
5. Ibid., p. 268.
6. Ibid., p. 293.
7. Compare, for example, *The Second London Confession* (1677), the Orthodox Creed of the General Baptists (1678), and the New Hampshire Confession (rev. 1853), ibid., pp. 268, 316, 365.
8. Roger Williams, *Experiments of Spiritual Life and Health,* ed. Winthrop Hudson (Philadelphia, 1951), p. 69.
9. Ibid., pp. 90–91.
10. Ibid., pp. 94–95.
11. See also Edwin S. Gaustad, ed., *Baptist Piety: The Last Will and Testimony of Obadiah Holmes* (Grand Rapids, MI, 1978), p. 117.
12. C.H. Spurgeon, *Autobiography,* 2 vols. (Edinburgh, 1973), 2:414.
13. Billy Graham, *Till Armageddon: Perspectives on Suffering* (Waco, TX, 1981), p. 85.

14. Ibid., p. 87.
15. See also B.W. Woods, *Understanding Suffering* (Grand Rapids, MI, 1974); Jerry Falwell, *When It Hurts Too Much to Cry* (Wheaton, IL, 1984).
16. Russel J. Thomsen, *Seventh-Day Baptists: Their Legacy to Adventists* (Mountain View, CA, 1971), pp. 18–21.
17. *Encyclopedia of Southern Baptists*, 4 vols. (Nashville, 1958), 1:292–293; Thomas Armitage, *History of the Baptists*, 2 vols. (New York, 1887), 2:669–673.
18. Samuel William Bacote, *Who's Who Among the Colored Baptists of the United States* (Kansas City, 1912), pp. 98–110, 112–113, 114–117, 270–272.
19. Armitage, *History of the Baptists*, 2:518–519.
20. Quoted in A.J. Gordon, *The Ministry of Healing* (Houston, 1882), pp. 79–80.
21. Armitage, *History of the Baptists*, 2:568.
22. Morgan Edwards, *Materials Towards a History of American Baptists*, quoted in Gordon, *The Ministry of Healing*, pp. 243–244.
23. For example, *A Treatise on the Faith and Practice of the Free Baptists* (Boston, 1848); Edward T. Hiscox, *The Baptist Church Directory* (New York, 1859); F.M. McConnell, *McConnell's Manual for Baptist Churches* (Philadelphia, 1926); Wayne R. Rood, ed., *A Manual of Procedures for Seventh-Day Baptist Churches* (Plainfield, NJ, 1972); Howard B. Foshee, *Broadman Church Manual* (Nashville, 1973); William Roy McNutt, *Polity and Practice in Baptist Churches* (Philadelphia, 1935); Norman Maring and Winthrop Hudson, *A Short Baptist Manual* (Valley Forge, PA, 1965).
24. M. Phelan, *New Handbook of All Denominations* (Nashville, 1930), p. 57.
25. Strong, *Systematic Theology*, pp. 132–133.
26. John T. McNeill, *History of the Cure of Souls* (New York, 1951), p. 271.
27. Gordon, *The Ministry of Healing*, p. 207.
28. Ibid., pp. 16–17.
29. Ibid., pp. 198–205.
30. Ibid., pp. 29–38.
31. John C. Pollock, *The Keswick Story* (Chicago, 1964).
32. Robert Mapes Anderson, *Vision of the Disinherited: The Making of American Pentecostalism* (New York, 1979), p. 64; Vinson Synan, *The Holiness-Pentecostal Movement in the United States* (Grand Rapids, MI, 1971), pp. 147–148; Richard Quebedeaux, *The New Charismatics II* (San Francisco, 1983), p. 221; Sidlow Baxter, *Divine Healing of the Body* (Grand Rapids, MI, 1979), passim.
33. See, for example, Samuel Fisk, *Divine Healing Under the Searchlight* (Schaumburg, IL, 1978).
34. Alice Felt Tyler, *Freedom's Ferment* (Minneapolis, 1944), pp. 311–312; William Warren Sweet, *Religion on the American Frontier: The Baptists, 1783–1830* (New York, 1964), pp. 37, 52.
35. Ian R. Tyrrell, *Sobering Up: From Temperance to Prohibition in Antebellum America, 1800–1860* (Westport, CT, 1979), pp. 56–57, 146–147.
36. Norman A. Baxter, *History of the Free Will Baptists* (Rochester, NY, 1957), pp. 109–113.

37. C.C. Pearson and J. Edwin Hendricks, *Liquor and Anti-Liquor in Virginia, 1619–1919* (Durham, NC, 1967), pp. 105–107; Rufus Spain, *At Ease in Zion: A Social History of Southern Baptists, 1865–1900* (Nashville, 1961), pp. 174–175.

38. Pearson and Hendricks, *Liquor and Anti-Liquor in Virginia,* pp. 88–89.

39. Spain, *At Ease in Zion,* p. 185.

40. *Baptist* 1 (September 17, 1887):6; Paul Isaac, *Prohibition and Politics: Turbulent Decades in Tennessee, 1885–1920* (Knoxville, 1965), p. 39.

41. *Tennessee Baptist* 20 (June 25, 1887):3.

42. Robert T. Handy, *A History of the Churches in the United States and Canada* (New York, 1976), p. 285.

43. Southern Baptist Convention, *Proceedings, 1896* (Nashville, 1896), p. 45; Spain, *At Ease in Zion,* p. 185.

44. Ibid., p. 195.

45. George Kelsey, *Social Ethics Among Southern Baptists, 1917–1969* (Metuchen, NJ, 1973), pp. 131–151.

46. Wyatt R. Hunter, "The Liquor Problem as Seen from the Bible," *The Baptist Record* 85 (January 16, 1964):3.

47. Joe T. Odle, "The Bible and Legalized Wine," *The Baptist Record* 84 (May 17, 1962):4.

48. W.R. White, "Public Enemy Number One," *Christian Faith in Action,* ed. Foy Valentine (Nashville, 1956), p. 69; Spain, *At Ease in Zion,* p. 186.

49. For a sampling of such arguments, see Henry Tiffany, "The Liquor Traffic: Biological Enemy No. 1," *Religious Herald* 114 (May 15, 1941):4–5; Henry Tiffany, "The Liquor Traffic: Economic Enemy No. 1," ibid., 114 (May 22, 1941):4; Henry Tiffany, "The Liquor Traffic: Moral Enemy No. 1," ibid., 114 (May 29, 1941):4; Wayne E. Oates, *Alcohol In and Out of the Church* (Nashville, 1966).

50. Spain, *At Ease in Zion,* p. 186; Louis Bristow, *Healing Humanity's Hurts* (Nashville, 1927).

51. *The Denver Post* (August 3, 1984).

52. Walter Rauschenbusch, *A Theology for the Social Gospel* (Nashville [1917] 1978), pp. 63–64; Walter Rauschenbusch, *Prayers of the Social Awakening* (Boston, 1909), pp. 111–112.

53. J.C. Carlile, *The Story of English Baptists* (London, 1905), pp. 261–262; Brian Harrison, *Drink and the Victorians: The Temperance Quest in England, 1815–1872* (Pittsburgh, 1971), pp. 179–181.

54. Handy, *A History of the Churches in the United States and Canada,* p. 351.

55. *Religious Herald* (May 9, 1878):1; Spain, *At Ease in Zion,* p. 202.

56. Isla May Mullins, *Edgar Young Mullins* (Nashville, 1929), p. 44.

57. *Religious Herald* (April 7, 1870):1.

58. Ibid. (December 17, 1896):1.

59. Ibid. (June 27, 1869):3; Spain, *At Ease in Zion,* p. 203.

60. *Biblical Recorder* (June 28, 1876):1.

61. Spain, *At Ease in Zion,* p. 204.

62. Ibid., p. 205.

63. Rev. Hoyt M. Lock, quoted in *The Christian Century* 101 (August 15–22, 1984):768. See also ibid. 101 (September 26, 1984):866; *Newsweek* (June 25, 1984):59–60; Peter J. Boyer, "Study Linking Tobacco,

Morality Dilemma for Farmers, Churches," *The Denver Post* (April 29, 1984):6C.

64. For a facsimile version of the original, see William Carey, *An Enquiry into the Obligations of Christians to Use Means for the Conversion of the Heathens,* with an introduction by Ernest A. Payne (London, 1961).

65. Fred T. Lord, *Achievement: A Short History of the Baptist Missionary Society* (London, 1942).

66. Carlile, *The Story of English Baptists.*

67. Henry C. Vedder, *A Short History of Baptist Missions* (Philadelphia, 1927).

68. Edmund F. Merriam, *A History of American Baptist Missions* (Philadelphia, 1900); Robert G. Torbet, *A History of the Baptists,* 3rd ed. (Valley Forge, PA, 1980), pp. 331–355.

69. Baker J. Cauthen et al., *Advance: A History of Southern Baptist Foreign Missions* (Nashville, 1970).

70. Albert W. Wardin, Jr., *Baptist Atlas* (Nashville, 1980), p. 49; William J. Hopewell, Jr., *The Missionary Emphasis of the General Association of Regular Baptists* (Chicago, 1963).

71. Carlile, *The Story of English Baptists,* p. 181.

72. Franklin T. Fowler, "The History of Southern Baptist Medical Missions," *Baptist History and Heritage* 10 (1975):194–203.

73. R. Pierce Beaver, *American Protestant Women in World Mission* (Grand Rapids, MI, 1968), p. 131.

74. Mary Davis, *History of the Free Baptist Woman's Missionary Society* (Boston, 1900).

75. Fannie E. S. Heck, *In Royal Service: The Mission Work of Southern Baptist Women* (Richmond, VA, 1927).

76. Beaver, *American Protestant Women,* pp. 131–139, 174–177.

77. John Spencer Carman, *Rats, Plague, and Religion: Stories of Medical Mission Work in India* (Philadelphia, 1936); Dana M. Albaugh, *Between Two Centuries: A Study of Four Baptist Mission Fields, Assam, South India, Bengal-Orissa, South China* (Philadelphia, 1935); Henry Raymond Williamson, *British Baptists in China, 1845–1952* (London, 1957).

78. Nellie G. Prescott, *The Baptist Family in Foreign Mission Fields* (Philadelphia, 1926).

79. *Yearbook of the American Baptist Churches of the U.S.A. 1983* (Valley Forge, PA, 1983), pp. 70–153.

80. *Encyclopedia of Southern Baptists,* 2:844–845.

81. Thomsen, *Seventh-Day Baptists,* pp. 85–86.

82. Owen D. Pelt and Ralph Lee Smith, *The Story of the National Baptists* (New York, 1960), pp. 155–157.

83. Conservative Baptist Foreign Mission Society, *Founded on the Word and Focused on the World: The Story of the Conservative Baptist Foreign Mission Society* (Wheaton, IL, 1978).

84. Lord, *Achievement,* pp. 88–89.

85. Ibid., p. 86.

86. For example, see Gordon S. Seagrave, *The Life of a Burma Surgeon* (New York, 1960); and Gordon S. Seagrave, *Waste-Basket Surgery* (Philadelphia, 1930).

87. Winthrop Hudson, *Religion in America,* 3rd ed. (New York, 1981), p. 375.

88. William R. Hutchison, *The Modernist Impulse in American Protestantism* (Cambridge, MA, 1976); George Marsden, *Fundamentalism and American Culture* (New York, 1980).
89. William Newton Clarke, *An Outline of Christian Theology,* 10th ed. (New York, 1901).
90. William Newton Clarke, *A Study of Christian Missions,* 2nd ed. (New York, 1901).
91. William Ernest Hocking, ed., *Re-Thinking Missions: A Laymen's Inquiry After 100 Years* (New York, 1932).
92. Ibid., pp. 200–201.
93. Prescott, *The Baptist Family,* p. 41.
94. Ibid., pp. 46–47.
95. P.H.L. Lerrigo, *Northern Baptists Rethink Missions* (New York, n.d.), pp. 87–108.
96. *Annual of the Southern Baptist Convention, 1982* (Nashville, 1982), p. 99.
97. O.K. Armstrong and Marjorie Armstrong, *The Baptists in America* (Garden City, NY, 1979), p. 369.
98. William Wright Barnes, *The Southern Baptist Convention, 1845–1953* (Nashville, 1954), p. 218; *Encyclopedia of Southern Baptists,* 1:651–653.
99. *Annual of the Southern Baptist Convention,* 1982, p. 89.
100. Davis C. Woolley, ed., *Baptist Advance* (Nashville, 1964), p. 340.
101. *Encyclopedia of Southern Baptists,* 2:1472–1473.
102. Ibid. 1:150–153; Walter H. Moursund, *A History of Baylor University* (Houston, TX, 1956).
103. Agnes R. Burr, *Russell H. Conwell and His Work* (Philadelphia, 1926), p. 290.
104. Armstrong and Armstrong, *Baptists in America,* pp. 370–372.
105. Sweet, *Religion on the American Frontier,* passim.
106. See E. Brooks Holifield, *A History of Pastoral Care in America* (Nashville, 1983), for an excellent overview of this subject.
107. Edward Scribner Ames, "Theology from the Standpoint of Functional Psychology," *American Journal of Theology* 10 (1906):219–232.
108. Albert L. Meiburg, "The Heritage of the Pastoral Counselor," in *Introduction to Pastoral Counseling,* ed. Wayne Oates (Nashville, 1959), pp. 3–18.
109. Gaines Dobbins, "Capturing Psychology for Christ," *Review and Expositor* (1936):436. See also his "Theological Education in a Changing Social Order," ibid. (1935):193–194.
110. *Encyclopedia of Southern Baptists,* 3:1905–1906.
111. Holifield, *History of Pastoral Care,* p. 220. See also Harry Emerson Fosdick, *On Being a Real Person* (New York, 1943).
112. See especially the work of Wayne Oates: *Religious Factors in Mental Illness* (New York, 1955); *Pastoral Counseling in Social Problems: Extremism, Race, Sex, Divorce* (Philadelphia, 1966); *New Dimensions in Pastoral Care* (Philadelphia, 1970); *The Bible in Pastoral Care* (Philadelphia, 1953); *Protestant Pastoral Counseling* (Philadelphia, 1962); *The Psychology of Religion* (Waco, TX, 1973).
113. A. Donald Bell, "Calling in the Help of Other Counselors," in *Introduction to Pastoral Counseling,* pp. 170–184; Richard K. Young, "The Process of Multiple Interview Counseling," ibid., pp. 117–129.

114. Henlee H. Barnette, *The New Theology and Morality* (Philadelphia, 1967), p. 65.
115. Rauschenbusch, *Theology for the Social Gospel,* p. 268. See also Dores Sharpe, *Walter Rauschenbusch* (New York, 1942), pp. 396–397.
116. J. M. Price, *Christianity and Social Problems* (Nashville, 1928), pp. 169–182.
117. Jerry Falwell, *Listen, America!* (Garden City, NY, 1980), pp. 180–186. See also *Annual of the Southern Baptist Convention,* 1976, p. 58; ibid., 1977, p. 50.
118. Price, *Christianity and Social Problems,* pp. 161–163, 173–176; Spain, *At Ease in Zion,* p. 207; Kelsey, *Social Ethics Among Southern Baptists,* pp. 171–175.
119. Marabel Morgan, *The Total Woman* (Old Tappan, NJ, 1973).
120. Tim and Beverly LaHaye, *The Act of Marriage: The Beauty of Sexual Love* (Grand Rapids, MI, 1976).
121. Dale Cowling, "The Pope is Wrong," *Arkansas Baptist* 67 (August 8, 1968):5; James A. Lester, "The Papal Ban on Birth Control," *Baptist and Reflector* 135 (February 6, 1969):6; *Annual of the Southern Baptist Convention,* 1967, pp. 74–75.
122. William B. Lippard and Frank A. Sharp, "What is a Baptist?" in *Religions in America,* ed. Leo Rosten (New York, 1975), pp. 32–33.
123. *Annual of the Southern Baptist Convention,* 1971, p. 72.
124. Ibid., 1974, p. 76.
125. Ibid., 1976, p. 58.
126. Ibid., 1977, p. 53; ibid., 1978, p. 65; ibid., 1979, pp. 50–51; ibid., 1980, pp. 48–49.
127. Ibid., 1982, pp. 64–65.
128. *Yearbook of the American Baptist Churches of the U.S.A. 1983,* pp. 251–252.
129. Falwell, *Listen, America!,* pp. 165–180.
130. Paul D. Simmons, *Birth and Death: Bioethical Decision Making* (Philadelphia, 1983); Paul D. Simmons, ed., *Issues in Christian Ethics* (Nashville, 1980).

CHAPTER 11

The Wesleyan-

Methodist

Tradition

HAROLD Y. VANDERPOOL

Methodist origins reach back to the late 1720s in Oxford University when John (1703–1791) and Charles (1707–1788) Wesley and other kindred-minded students organized a Holy Club, through which they sought to recapture the piety and power of the Apostolic Church. Because of their strict, disciplined methods of study, fasting, prayer, communion, spiritual introspection, and good works among prisoners and others, they were soon labeled reproachfully as "Methodists." By the 1740s, when the early Methodist societies were expanding rapidly within the Anglican church, John Wesley counseled society members that the new name *Methodist* was but a mark of the newness and power of their Christian commitment.[1]

The primary impetus of early Methodism lay not in literalistic rule-keeping or other-worldly piety, but in its burning determination to recover the life and thought of the early Church as depicted in the Bible and the classical writings from the first centuries of the Christian era. For many years, Methodists remained a fervent minority within the

317

greater Church of England, a minority that considered itself loyal to the parent church's traditions and institutions, yet eager to stir and empower it to live by the ideals that initially brought it into being.

The passions and actions of John Wesley and others nevertheless led to the emergence of a new Protestant denomination. Although the activities of the early Methodist societies were designed so as to compliment rather than interfere with the policies and regular worship services of the Anglican Church, gradually Methodism separated itself from the parent body. Independence was achieved in America before Wesley's death in 1791 and shortly after his death in England.

As a dynamic, closely knit, evangelical tradition, Methodism grew rapidly in England, America, Canada, South Africa, and elsewhere. In America, for example, Methodism expanded from 1,160 members in 1773 to 8,500 in 1780; 57,630 in 1790; 511,150 in 1830; 5.5 million in 1900; and some 14 million in 1982. In 1982 the total world membership of all Methodist denominations included about 20 million official members in more than 100 nations. The largest of these denominations, the United Methodist Church in the United States, contained approximately 10 million members, while the largest branch of the parent Methodist Church in Britain had a membership of about 800,000. Other national figures included 1.4 million Methodists in India; 760,000 in South Africa; 400,000 in Korea; and 200,000 in Mexico and the Caribbean.[2]

Racial, economic, political, and ideological influences caused Methodism to divide into several separate denominations in the nineteenth century and then to overcome internal divisions and unite ecumenically in the twentieth century. In response to racial biases, the African Methodist Episcopal (AME) Church under Richard Allen and others emerged as an independent denomination beginning in Philadelphia in 1816. For similar reasons, in New York, the African Methodist Episcopal Zion (AMEZ) Church was formed in 1820. In 1982 the AME Church had some 2,210,000 members, and the AMEZ Church approximately 1,134,000 members. Desires for greater democratization, more participation by the laity, and more active roles for women lay behind the emergence of the Primitive Methodist connection in England in 1811 and the Methodist Protestant Church in America in 1830. Questions of slavery and sectionalism split the main body of American Methodists into the Methodist Episcopal Church (North) and South in 1844. Several Holiness and Nazarene denominations separated from mainline Methodism after 1894, prompted by desires to recapture personal holiness, experience spiritual gifts, and resist theological liberalism. The Methodist Protestant Church and the Methodist Churches (North) and South reunited in 1939. This body then joined with the Evangelical United Brethren in 1968 to form the United Methodist Church.

In spite of considerable diversity, Methodists have shared certain common traditions. These include a reliance on the Bible as Scripture, an indebtedness to the articles of faith of the Anglican or Episcopal churches, an honoring of many of the teachings and principles of John Wesley, including his *General Rules for Methodist Societies* (1743) and his numerous sermons, an accenting of a life of Christian holiness, and a sharing of the many hymns of Charles Wesley. Like Lutherans and Calvinists, Methodists believe in the sufficiency of Scripture, human spiritual depravity, and salvation by grace through faith. Methodists, however, traditionally accent certain distinctive theological themes, notably, that through grace God creates all humans so as to be sufficiently free to resist or accept salvation (universal prevenient grace, as opposed to irresistable grace for those predestined or elected by God), that through the active power of the Holy Spirit all may know that they are saved through the experience of an inner transformation and of a continuing trust in the love of God (as opposed to intellectual assent to Christian doctrine), and that all may be empowered through the Spirit to love God with all their being and their neighbors as themselves (Christian perfection).[3] Furthermore, because Methodist theology was shaped by several legacies, including Continental Protestantism and Anglicanism, the classical thinkers of the first centuries of the Christian era (the Fathers of the ancient church), and German Pietism, Methodists have played active and influential roles in efforts to unite diverse branches of Christianity (the Ecumenical Movement).

Methodism was and is highly organized. The early movement was almost totally controlled by John Wesley, who divided each local society into small, homogeneous bands and larger, mixed classes directed by handpicked men and women leaders. From Methodist ranks, Wesley also appointed lay preachers, many of whom made itinerant rounds or circuits to respective societies. After 1744, an advisory conference of preachers met annually, out of which activity Annual Conferences became the basic organizational unit for Methodist churches throughout the world. In England, ministers were elected as superintendents of geographical Conference areas, while in America a threefold order of ministry developed: deacons (ordained ministers), elders, and bishops, the last of whom, unlike Anglican bishops, are elected rather than appointed. Conferences are subdivided into districts, which are supervised by elders appointed by bishops. In turn, bishops and lay representatives meet in General Conferences from which stem the highest legislative enactments of each national Methodist body. The specific policies of the General Conferences are carried out by a network of boards and agencies including Boards of Publication, Church and Society, Global Ministry, and Higher Education for America's United Methodist Church. After 1881, Methodists began gathering in multinational ecumenical conferences, from which emerged the World Methodist Conference, a conclave that gathers each decade to investigate common and worldwide problems and challenges.[4]

Methodists have established numerous colleges, universities, and theological seminaries. In America, these include Boston University and Theological Seminary; Drew University and Theological Seminary (Madison, New Jersey); Duke University and Divinity School (Durham, North Carolina); Emory University and the Candler School of Theology (Atlanta, Georgia); Southern Methodist University and the Perkins School

of Theology (Dallas, Texas); as well as the Iliff School of Theology
(Denver, Colorado) and the University of Southern California School of
Religion (Los Angeles). The Methodist Publishing House, the oldest
(1789) and largest religious publishing concern in the world, was circulating fifty-five different periodicals by 1984.[5]

------------- ··⟨∞⟩·· -------------

Past and present, directly and indirectly, Methodists have viewed John
Wesley (1703–1791) as a central source of insight and inspiration. The
sources of Methodist faith and life are, of course, much older than
Wesley, yet he became the lens through which the Bible and Christian
tradition were interpreted. Individuals like John's brother Charles and
the great Calvinist evangelist George Whitefield (1714–1770) also contributed greatly to the dynamics and expansion of Methodism, yet
Wesley's influence was immeasurably greater and more enduring than
theirs or that of any other individual.[6] An understanding of the meaning
and significance of medicine and health within the Methodist tradition
must therefore begin with the life and thought of this fervent, fascinating
reformer.

John Wesley

More than any other major figure in Christendom, John Wesley actively
involved himself with the theory and practice of medicine and with
the specific principles and practices of ideal physical and mental health.
On a lesser scale, he also advocated and relied upon the supernatural
power of God for the healing of human infirmities. This chapter surveys
Wesley's historic medicine–health legacy, whereby medical and religious
healing, as well as a variety of rules regarding human health, were set
forth as necessary addenda to Christian living. The chapter focuses on
the details and dynamics of this by and large uncharted story of medical
and health concerns and deals secondarily with some of the complex
ways these concerns were informed by respective theological, medical,
scientific, philosophical, and national traditions. It also charts how
Methodists over time dealt with life's final passage, human death.

John Wesley first began to read books on "anatomy and physic
[medicine]" shortly after entering Christ's Church College in Oxford
University in 1721 at the age of seventeen.[7] He continued to read such
works in his leisure hours until 1731, when he studied medicine more
seriously for several months in preparation for his and his brother
Charles' (1707–1788) missionary expedition to the New World colony
of Georgia. He did this in order to "be of some service to those who

had no regular physician among them."[8] Such preparation was in keeping with an ecclesiastical tradition shared alike by Anglican and Puritan clergy, who believed that a knowledge of the theory and practice of medicine would enable ministers to contribute to the physical and spiritual well-being of their parishioners in the absence of trained physicians.[9] While serving in America, Wesley continued to study books on anatomy and surgery. He also witnessed at least one autopsy and experimented with a vegetarian diet in hopes that self-denial would increase his effectiveness.[10]

Between 1741 and 1746, Wesley grew increasingly unorthodox in his medical activities. This period precisely paralleled the most creative and formative period of Methodist history and followed the deeply troubling time when Wesley was suspended from his chaplaincy in Georgia over a scandalous love affair, returned to England (1738), searched mightily for a way to find rest for his soul, experienced conversion, and began forming Methodist societies.[11] In April 1741, Wesley chose eight or ten society members to visit sick persons regularly. Within a month, others were chosen to visit the sick every other day, provide for their needs, and meet every Tuesday to review what had been accomplished.[12] Having renewed his study of medicine with the counsel of an apothecary and surgeon, Wesley in 1745 published his first medical tract, an alphabetical list of sixty-three "distempers" from "ague" (fevers) to "wounds." With each listing, Wesley attached several cheap, safe, and easily concocted remedies, each of which was to be tried one after another until treatment was secured.[13] About this time he adopted the "desperate expedient" of administering medicines himself to persons unable to afford hospitals, physicians, apothecaries, and surgeons.[14]

In 1747, Wesley published the first edition of *Primitive Physick,* which listed remedies for some 250 maladies and contained a carefully constructed introduction about the history and theory of medicine, including a list of rules for maintaining health.[15] The popularity of *Primitive Physick* surprised even Wesley. Within five years of its release, nine editions were required, and it had been widely dispersed throughout the British Empire and in "neighboring nations." At least thirty-eight English and twenty-four American editions appeared by 1880.[16] Satirists and critics soon branded Wesley as a quack in medicine, religion, and politics, claiming that

> Starv'd *Bodies* with apt *Nostrums* he controuls,
> and with worse Physic stupefies their Souls.[17]

Yet Wesley remained generally unfazed by such criticisms. To one physician–critic who argued that *Primitive Physick* was a "quack pamphlet" filled with injudicious, ignorant, and injurious remedies, Wesley replied that because the doctor's critique had increased the demand for his book, would he not "please publish a few further remarks" on it.[18]

Although the therapies in *Primitive Physick*—the use of cold baths, lemonade, tar-water, toad pills, and warm puppies on the belly—are a world removed from contemporary medicine, they either reflected or were compatible with popular opinion at the time.[19] For example, Thomas Dover, a well-known disciple of the famous physician Thomas Sydenham, prescribed pills made from dried and powdered toads for asthma; and Wesley's suggestions that the powder of mushroom puff-balls would stop the bleeding of open wounds and that the yeast of beer would remove corns from the feet echoed advice given by Sir Robert Boyle, one of the founders of the Royal Society.[20] Wesley's recommendation of sheep's milk for bloody urine was identical to that proposed by the apothecary Nicholas Culpepper.[21] Wesley, however, utilized current opinion creatively. Compared to others, he wrote more plainly, generally prescribed less harsh, less complicated, and more readily available remedies, and simplified the organization of his book.

Although *Primitive Physick* represented John Wesley's most important and popular contribution to medicine, it was far from his last writing on the subject. In 1748 he wrote a letter-pamphlet opposing the drinking of imported tea, primarily because tea "gives rise to numerous disorders, particularly those of the nervous kind," and because the money it consumed could be used to aid the poor and sick.[22] After conducting numerous experiments and witnessing its effectiveness, Wesley in 1759 composed a treatise on the curative effects of electricity, which he titled *The Desideratum; or, Electricity Made Plain and Useful*. At least five editions of this book were published. Drawing from the ideas of Benjamin Franklin and others, he first discussed the properties of electricity, then gave descriptions about its ability to cure cramps, deafness, back pains, toothaches, and so on.[23]

Wesley's summary of the terrible physical and mental effects of masturbation appeared in 1767 under the title *Thoughts on the Sin of Onan*, which was republished as *A Word to Whom it May Concern* in 1779. Written for both sexes and largely bowdlerized from a treatise by the Swiss physician Simon A.D. Tissot, Wesley's pamphlet was designed for modest persons who he said could not bear to read the gross, indelicate, even beastly discussions of the subject by Tissot and others. Wesley first indicated how "self-pollution" produces dullness, effeminancy, loss of appetite, paralytic disorders, and even madness, blindness, and the gout. He then discussed both the prevention and cure of the bodily disorders caused by the sin of masturbation.[24]

In 1769 and 1774, Wesley published edited abbreviations of Dr. Tissot's *Avis au Peuple* (1762) and Dr. William Cadogan's *A Dissertation on the Gout* (1771). He edited the first because he admired Tissot's tender concern for his fellow creatures, his descriptions of diseases (which *Primitive Physick* notably lacked), and his use of generally inexpensive and safe remedies.[25] Cadogan's *Dissertation*—the thesis of which credited the cause of gout to intemperate living—was controversial and widely read. Having registered his belief that Cadogan oversold his ideas, Wesley praised his general understanding of disease etiology, as well as many of his specific recommendations.[26]

Toward the end of his life, Wesley wrote pamphlets entitled *Thoughts on Nervous Disorders* (1784) and *The Duty and Advantage of Early Rising* (1789). In the former, he asserted that although many nervous disorders were caused by lack of faith and piety, other "purely natural" causes included drinking distilled liquors and tea, not exercising sufficiently, and sleeping too much. He credited Dr. Cadogan for identifying several of these causes, but noted that Cadogan had not identified the unhealthful effects of "sleeping longer than nature requires."[27] In *The Duty and Advantage of Early Rising,* Wesley expanded on the thesis that oversleeping caused "all nervous disease."[28]

Each of Wesley's medical writings was designed for practical use and priced for popular consumption. Some, like *Primitive Physick,* were largely composed by Wesley himself, while others, like *The Desideratum* and *Advices with Respect to Health* were edited and abbreviated in a *Reader's Digest* fashion from the works of those with whom he basically agreed. Yet Wesley's activities did not end with the written word. In the early 1740s he appointed several Methodist society members as regular visitors of sick persons. Viewing these male and female visitors as similar to the deacons and deaconesses of "the primitive church," upon which the Methodist movement was patterned, Wesley regarded the care of the sick as a standard feature of Methodism—and a service especially suited for women, whose "vile bondage" he eloquently resisted.[29] By 1746, convinced that sick persons were not being cared for effectively by regular physicians, hospitals, or even Methodist visitors, he decided to set up dispensaries in which he and others would examine and treat those who came for help.[30] The several rooms that he later set aside for electrical therapy extended these efforts to distribute inexpensive medical care to a broad spectrum of English citizens.[31]

Similar to his passionate concern to restore primitive or apostolic Christianity, Wesley praised the virtues of *primitive* physick. He sought to rescue both medicine and the church from those who had corrupted them, to purify and revitalize them by returning them to their ancient, plain, practical, and efficacious beginnings. He wanted "to reduce Physick to its ancient Standards . . . to make it a plain intelligible Thing, as it was in the Beginning."[32] By *beginning* he meant the long tradition after the Fall of Adam and Eve in which humans gradually discovered effective remedies through trial and error, then passed these traditions along to later generations. Wesley observed that American Indians suffered little because they employed quick and "generally infallible" cures.[33] Like the ancient Greeks and Romans, these primitive Americans relied on the healing powers of nature, the author of which is God.[34]

Ancient or primitive medical remedies have certain basic characteristics, Wesley asserted. They are efficacious and useful because they are founded upon trial-and-error experiments and experience.[35] They are plain, simple, safe, and inexpensive, because they are readily found in ordinary plants, animals, and inorganic substances.[36] These qualities paralleled the "plain and simple" Gospel proclaimed by Wesley, a Gospel unfettered by theological abstractions, available to all humans irrespective of wealth or station in life, curative for body and soul, and readily found in the churches, squares, and fields of England.[37] Wesley displayed his conscious awareness of the interconnections among nature, God, and medical healing in several of his writings, including his book on electricity. In that book, he asserted that electricity was the fundamental cause of attraction and repulsion in nature—like gravity in the cosmos. As a powerful, universal, secondary cause of motion, electricity, like gravity, points to God. Wesley regarded electricity as "pure" and "elementary" fire from which vulgar, culinary fire is kindled. It enters the body primarily through breathed air and enlivens the body by coursing through blood and nerves so as to make each human and animal "a kind of fire machine."[38] Wesley thus viewed restoration of the power and flow of electricity as a superbly effective, simple, and inexpensive medical therapy.

In keeping with his times, Wesley emphasized that poor health habits often caused disease and that good ones could be medically efficacious. Specifically, he believed that a lack of exercise; intemperance in eating, drinking, and sleeping; strong displays of emotion (or the passions); and unhealthful habits in clothing, housing, bathing, and breathing caused numerous ailments, so he set forth guidelines for the control of each of these.[39] He edited the medical works of writers who laid "much stress upon regimen," even as had "the ancient [Greek and Roman] physicians," and he borrowed the list of health rules found in the preface of *Primitive Physick* from a popular book by Dr. George Cheyne, whose work had made a lifelong impression on Wesley as a student in Oxford.[40] Like the remedies Wesley recommended, these rules of regimen represented plain, easy, and inexpensive ways to regain and maintain health.

Wesley used these theories of medicine and disease as the cutting edge for a moral critique of the medical profession of his time. He accused most apothecaries and physicians of practicing medicine out of greed and personal aggrandizement. Prompted by these motives, they made medicine mysterious and unintelligible rather than plain; they compounded medical ingredients to make it impossible for most common persons to effect their own cures; they mixed exotic, expensive, and harmful chemicals to render their services necessary; they used technical terms to disguise, rather than reveal, what they were doing; they bled, blistered, and purged the sick without proof of medical efficacy; and they branded those (like Wesley) who advocated simple and workable remedies with the pejorative name *empirik*.[41] Wesley thought it very unlikely that "the gentlemen of the faculty [of medicine]" would use safe and inexpensive therapies like electricity, for that would demonstrate their greater concern for sick persons than for themselves and their cohorts, the apothecaries.[42]

These criticisms explain some of Wesley's motives for breaking with tradition and practicing medicine himself. He personally knew too many poor persons pining away in sickness with no means to pay medical professionals for medicines that would do them little good anyway. He could not in good conscience wait for wealthy doctors like the prominent Richard Meade to arrive in their carriages, then treat their patients with medicines more likely to kill than cure.[43] He decided to practice and write about medicine without incurring personal debts to medical professionals. Yet he continued to praise those "great and good" doctors who displayed "a tender sense of the sufferings of . . . [their] fellow creatures," and he continued to recommend "a Physician that fears God" for those struck with uncommon, complicated, or life-threatening illnesses.[44] In these matters he weighed both himself and medical professionals in the scales of Christian benevolence and justice.

Throughout his life John Wesley also displayed great concern for the preservation of physical and mental health, which he linked to the same principles of regimen that were useful in curing disease. He regarded physical health as being highly dependent upon exercise, diet, sleep, and cleanliness. Informed by contemporary writers and personal experience, he set forth specific recommendations concerning each of these.

In both eating and drinking he urged temperance, a careful monitoring of one's personal responses to various types of food, and control over what was consumed. He believed in the long-standing adage: Christians should not live to eat, but rather eat to live.[45] For Wesley, temperance in eating meant consuming only the kind and quantity of food that would impart maximum strength and energy. Persons seeking health should, for example, curtail their consumption of salty, greasy, pickled, and highly seasoned foods. They should also fast occasionally; eat plenty of bread, eggs, and vegetables; and, if weak in digestion, avoid foods like rich pies and unripe fruit. He regarded fresh well-water as the best drink, milk as nourishing, and limited amounts of wine and ale as acceptable; but he described distilled liquors as "a certain though slow poison."[46] For reasons of health and Christian benevolence, he thought that persons of all ages should drink herbal and mint teas or cocoa rather than the stronger and expensive imported teas from the Far East.[47]

Like George Cheyne and William Cadogan, John Wesley valued the healthful effects of exercise and cleanliness. He recommended at least two hours of walking or, for less vigorous persons, horseback riding per day. House-bound persons should ride on wooden rock-horses or knead their flesh with brushes or rollers. Body and clothes should be washed regularly, the former especially in cold water, which Wesley considered exceedingly healthful. Wesley's health advice also included ridding oneself of lice and itches; burying human excrement; and avoiding the unclean, unwholesome, and self-indulging habit of smoking tobacco or dipping snuff.[48]

Wesley recommended seven or, at most, eight hours of sleep as conducive to healthy vigor, warning that if people stayed in bed longer than that, their flesh would become soaked and "parboiled," then soft and flabby. At the same time, the nerves would become weak and "quite unstrung," making slothful persons susceptible to nervous disorders and sinful indulgence, notably masturbation.[49]

Viewing physical and mental health as inextricably intertwined, Wesley believed that drinking tea or distilled liquor, sleeping too long, or failing to exercise could lead to mental disorders such as nervousness, faintness, or "lowness of spirits." Persons suffering from lowness of spirits—depression in today's language—typically felt "a kind of faintness, weariness, and listlessness," lost their relish for daily activities, and often looked upon life itself as a burden.[50] In Wesley's opinion, violent or irregular passions—including great joy followed by despair, piercing emotional desires that remained unsatisfied, anger, and tormenting fear—indicated mental disorders. As such, they were to be treated by both physical regimen and disciplined emotional control.

How, then, could human passions be controlled and channeled so as to enable persons to be active, tranquil, and full of purpose and joy? Wesley believed that "the sovereign remedy" for all emotional miseries lay in a love of God, through which the mind could achieve "unspeakable Joy and perfect Calm."[51] He said:

Grief, Desire, Hope deferred, make the heart sick, with a sickness that drugs cannot cure. What can cure it, but the peace of God? No other medicine under heaven. What but the love of God, that sovereign balm for the body as well as the mind?[52]

Wesley's assertion that the love of God affects body and mind is a crucial point of departure for exploring his understanding of human nature, his underlying theology, and his fundamental reasons for practicing medicine and setting forth guidelines for physical and mental health. Regarding human nature, he viewed the human body as a fearfully and wonderfully created "machine," the anatomy, composition, sustaining, and weakening of which excited his continued study and curiosity.[53] Lodged in and inextricably linked to this body was an "inward principle" or "soul" capable of sensing, judging, reasoning, willing, and expressing passions or affections like love, hatred, sorrow, and hope. Wesley considered the soul as the spiritual "image of God" in humans, and viewed it as so vitally united with the imperfect human body that the apprehensions, judgments, and decisions of the soul were inevitably confused, disordered, and unrighteous. Although he considered body and soul as "widely different natures"—the former material, the latter immaterial—Wesley regarded them as unalterably symbiotic with each other. The "corrupted body" presses down upon and afflicts the thoughts, moods, and morals of the soul, while the afflicted soul can "weaken a strong constitution, and lay the foundation of such bodily disorders as are not easily removed."[54] Given this distinctly psychosomatic perspective, Wesley deeply committed himself both to a restoration of the love, peace, and goodness of the soul and to the alleviation of bodily infirmities—including ordinary, acute, and chronic sickness, as well as hunger, poverty, and all conditions responsible for human suffering. He believed that suffering was inevitable, that it could ultimately strengthen faith and would forever counter human pride, but he felt commissioned by God to alleviate anguish and sickness wherever possible.[55]

John Wesley primarily regarded himself neither as a physician nor as a social reformer, but as a minister and ambassador of true religion for the salvation of humankind—spiritual, physical, and social. His practice of medicine and advocacy of health were thus ultimately rooted in his theological understanding of salvation, through which he proclaimed that all humans are spiritually depraved, that by grace all are empowered to choose whom they will serve, that through faith all may be justified or forgiven of sin, that all may then know assuredly that they are saved because they love God with all their soul (mind, affections, and spiritual endowment) and manifest their faith and love through holiness of life and through continual good works (sanctification or holiness to the point of Christian perfection), and that all may know, love, and serve God throughout eternity.[56] Wesley's medical activities were embedded in two aspects of this theology of salvation: First, medical care was essential for partially restoring the body so that the soul in its totality might be relieved, reached, and possibly rescued;

and second, medical activities manifested fruits of sanctification, namely, acts of goodness and mercy for God and humans. Wesley's health advocacy was an essential element in his understanding of sanctification and Christian perfection, a theme that led him to give great attention to the nature of the Christian life.[57] Many of his health-related principles directly pertained to the holiness and purity of the body—notably regulations regarding diet, sleep, and cleanliness. It is thus not surprising that in the middle of his treatise on Christian perfection, Wesley summarized his ideas on food, drink, exercise, and sleeping,[58] and that strictures against self-indulgence and the drinking of distilled liquors were thus included in the *General Rules of the United Societies* (1743).[59] Other principles addressed mental health, the essense of which lay in loving God with one's heart (affections), mind (thinking and reasoning), and soul.[60] Wesley viewed this love as antithetical to self-pride, self-willfulness, and self-love, which led to anger, jealousy, and unhappiness. Drawing upon New Testament Scripture, he called for a "crucifixion of the heart" and a complete love of God, whereby Christians would be freed from anger, jealousy, fear, doubt, and despair and empowered through grace to live joyously, meekly, peacefully, purposefully, and altruistically.[61] He thus equated holy desires and emotions with healthy mental states and posited a connection between unholy spiritual expressions and unhealthy emotional conditions. Wesley made regulations regarding healing and health essential features of evangelical Protestantism. By so doing, he became a far more influential figure in ecclesiastical history than has yet been realized.

In several of his most important medical writings, John Wesley said that sick persons should "use that medicine of medicines, prayer" in addition to remedies and regimen.[62] Although he believed that prayer instilled inner peace and strength, he had more than emotional consequences in mind when he encouraged sick persons to pray. In fact, he believed that God could and sometimes would directly intervene to cure both physical and mental illness. Such cures were rightly called "miraculous," said Wesley, because they could not be credited to "natural or ordinary causes," but must be viewed as works "of omnipotence wrought by the supernatural power of God."[63]

Behind this belief in supernatural cures lay Wesley's acceptance of the accuracy and veracity of the world according to the New Testament, including the existence and malicious influence of the devil, demons, and witches. He knew that many English citizens dismissed reports of witches and apparitions as "old wives' tales" and that infidels had "hooted witchcraft out of the world." Yet he believed that witches existed and apparitions occurred because the Bible spoke of them and because such manifestations had been regarded as true by so many credible witnesses for so many ages of human history.[64] He nevertheless believed that these phenomena and supernatural cures should be accepted only after diligently researching all "the facts" and striving first to account for them "in a natural way." He thus consciously sought to steer a "middle way" between what he called "well-attested accounts" and those that were unconvincing.[65]

Wesley's middle way between natural and supernatural curing can be summarized as follows: He regularly relied upon natural methods of curing, but remained open to unaccountable supernatural interventions. For example, he constantly attended to his own medical needs and expected to be healed by "the ordinary use of outward means." Nevertheless, believing that God could and would interpose into nature according to "His own sovereign will," he prayed to God and, on one occasion, claimed to have been mysteriously relieved from incapacitating pain.[66] Wesley also published accounts of miraculous cures of Methodists and others suffering from leprosy, paralytic disorders, infectious diseases, fits of madness, and sicknesses considered terminal by physicians; and he claimed to know of many more instances than those he reported.[67] He emphasized that the greatest miracles he had witnessed were the wholly transformed lives of persons led to trust and love God completely.[68]

The miraculous healings recounted by Wesley were described as occurring after prayer, as sometimes being accompanied by visions or apparitions, and, in keeping with standard eighteenth-century defenses of biblical prophesy and miracles, as being validated by credible witnesses. Wesley did not view himself as a divine healer endowed with special gifts of the Holy Spirit, and he expelled one George Bell from the Methodist societies for claiming miraculous powers, including the ability to cure with spittle and biblical formulas.[69] For Wesley, supernatural healing was possible for all persons who called upon God in prayer. He warned, however, that such healings should not be expected as answers to prayer, because they were not merited and because humans could not presume to know or control the will of God. It is in this light that the brief recommendations of prayer in Wesley's medical works should be understood: as a "medicine of medicines," prayer instills trust and peace, but it is also an "unfashionable" source of ancient power universally and freely available to those who seek and ask.[70]

Even as Wesley believed that Methodists should live according to biblical standards of purity and piety in life, so also he believed that their deaths should attest to the truth of their faith and the fullness of their sanctification. In his *Plain Account of Christian Perfection,* for example, he described in detail the death of Jane Cooper, whom he called a "witness of Christian perfection" in life and death. Cooper contracted smallpox and experienced convulsions and extreme suffering.

Yet the more she weakened and suffered, the more she displayed a strengthening of faith, "smiles of triumph," a commitment to the strict doctrine of Methodism, and a love for God and Christ.[71]

Dying saints like Jane Cooper exemplified the virtues of a fully sanctified life marked by assurance, a complete resignation to the will of God, and a joyful hope that they would soon be united with departed Christians and the heavenly hosts. Such persons would be able to face God, Christ, and the angels at that great and awful Day of Judgment, which Wesley said would likely last for several thousands of human years as each person gave an account of every action, idle word, thought, and intention of the heart. They would then avoid the agonizing, sleepless, never-ending torments of Hell, in the midst of which condemned sinners would *"gnaw their tongues* for anguish and pain."[72]

The passage from life to death presented a critical time for the dying individual, for family and friends, and for the Methodist community. This passage could either be terrifying or expressive of hope and joy. It could also serve either to validate or undermine the spirit and truth of Methodism. Wesley believed that the key to a good and exemplary death lay in a long life of love for God, accompanied by a surrendering of willfulness and fleshly appetites. One of the signs of the truth of Christianity generally and Methodism specifically was that upon facing death, even in the midst of a plague, Christians would display peace, resignation, and joyful expectations rather than anxiety and fear.[73]

The Evangelical Era, 1790–1880

For some ninety years after Wesley's death in 1791, Methodism perpetuated many of his traditions regarding theology, a life of piety, maintaining and enhancing health, and the use of prayer for supernatural healing. Methodism upheld these traditions during this period for at least three reasons. First, its ranks had been tightly organized and controlled for half a century by Wesley, who continually pruned away those who disagreed with him or failed to live by the rules of scriptural holiness summarized by himself and Charles in 1743. Each society was divided into classes of twelve under the supervision of handpicked leaders, who were to visit each member at least once a week to make sure that required duties were being carried out. Negative duties included no buying or selling of distilled liquor, no wearing of gold or costly clothing, and no "softness, and needless self-indulgence"; positive duties included "visiting or helping those that are sick or in prison," self-denial, regular church attendance, a life of prayer and biblical study, and periodic fasting.[74] Second, by separating from American Episcopalianism in 1784 and from the Church of England shortly after Wesley's death, Methodism was able to sustain much of its distinctive character and orientation under the leadership of persons intensely loyal to its original polity, piety, and theology.[75] Third, the most fundamental challenges to the biblical world view of Wesley and early Methodism— notably modern biblical criticism, Darwinian evolution, and secular psychology—did not emerge until after 1850 and thus did not begin to transform Methodist thought and piety until the last decades of its evangelical era.[76]

In spite of maintaining fundamental continuity with its beginnings, however, Methodism during its evangelical era began to alter several emphases and ideas of its founder. Most significantly, Wesley's concern for medical theory and therapy was largely preempted by Methodism's evangelical outreach, by the intense controversies engendered by slavery, and by a rising campaign against the drinking of alcoholic beverages. Methodists also expended great energy in missionary activity and building churches, colleges, and seminaries. They joined forces with other evangelical Protestants to oppose slavery and support temperance. Such engagements led to theological as well as medical changes. During this era it became increasingly difficult to distinguish Methodist beliefs and patterns of living from those of other evangelicals.

Even though over forty-five English and American editions of *Primitive Physick* appeared between 1791 and 1881, it cannot be assumed that Methodists adhered to Wesley's specific theories and therapies after his death.[77] In fact, although *Primitive Physick* was regularly published in America under official church auspices,[78] alterations began as early as 1793, when Francis Asbury (1745–1816), one of the superintendents of the Methodist church in America, asked Henry Wilkins to revise Wesley's medical handbook and to append to it one by Wilkins. This Wilkins–Wesley publication was widely sold through the Methodist Publishing House.

Bishops Francis Asbury and Thomas Coke (1747–1814), two of the most influential figures in American Methodism during its first fifty years, wrote a letter–preface to the Wilkins–Wesley volume. In the spirit of Wesley, they expressed interest in both the souls and bodies of their readers and earnestly recommended the book because physicians were few and often unskilled, and money for doctors was limited. Although the bishops preferred "simple remedies," they noted that Wesley's *Primitive Physick* had been revised to suit American physicians, the American climate, and the constitutions of American citizens.[79]

In particular, Wilkins modified Wesley's understanding of medical theory and therapy to accommodate the practice of regular physicians who were using remedies Wesley had opposed. Wilkins had received his M.D. in 1793 from the Medical College of the University of Pennsylvania, where the famous Benjamin Rush (1745–1813) was teaching.

Rush profoundly influenced medical theory and practice in America during the late eighteenth and early nineteenth centuries by advocating "heroic" levels of therapeutic bloodletting, purging with calomel (mercurous chloride), and dosing with tartar emetic (a toxic compound for removing so-called stomach poisons).[80]

Wilkins placed his own publication, *The Family Advisor; or, A Plain and Modern Practice of Physic,* at the front of the combined book, where chapters were arranged according to different diseases. Wilkins defined each disease, described its causes and symptoms, and discussed how patients should be managed and cured. While his recommendations for "management" used many of the principles of diet, rest, and exercise found in Wesley's writings, a number of Wilkins' "cures" were precisely those Wesley had opposed. In contrast to Wesley, who had decried "dangerous" chemicals, large doses of quinine, and bloodletting, Wilkins regularly recommended bleeding (often repetitively), "puking," purging the bowels, blistering, or a combination of therapies.[81] And whereas Wesley had said that flesh bitten by a mad dog should be plunged into cold water for twenty days or (as Galen recommended) treated by taking two spoonfuls of crawfish ashes for forty days, Wilkins believed that the wound should be cut out or, if that were impossible, "filled with gun powder, and this burned." In lieu of these treatments, Wilkins urged that patients be rubbed with mercurial ointment for six hours until they salivated freely.[82]

Wilkins' revisions of *Primitive Physick* reflected a thorough-going fusion—perhaps confusion—of Wesley's simple remedies with heroic therapy. While many of Wesley's remedies were kept, others were deleted, and new ones were added. For ague (intermittent fever), Wilkins kept Wesley's sixth (yarrow herbs boiled in new milk), tenth (spirits of hartshorn in water), and eleventh (eating a small lemon, rind and all) recommendations, but he added strong doses of laudanum. For apoplexy (a stroke involving loss of sense and voluntary motion), he retained Wesley's use of cold baths and water-drinking, but added induced vomiting, copious bleedings, and sending for "a good physician immediately."[83]

This tendency to adjust Wesley's medical views to prevailing opinion appears to have occurred both in England and America. Wesley may have encouraged this by his own revisions of *Primitive Physick* and by remaining somewhat open to physicians' criticisms. Furthermore, a number of physicians, surgeons, and apothecaries, both in England and America, became Methodists, one of whom in England preached Wesley's funeral sermon.[84] At any rate, no Methodist minister after Wesley sought to write comprehensively and voluminously on medical curing, and none sought to return medical theory and therapy to pre-modern or primitive modalities.

Wesley's accent on workable, efficacious remedies and his over-arching concern for body and soul nevertheless continued to be visible, particularly in the regular "Health and Disease" columns in Methodist periodicals. The most widely read of these periodicals in America was *The Christian Advocate*, probably the most popular magazine in the United States in the middle decades of the nineteenth century.[85] The editors of this journal scoured books, articles, and farm almanacs for practical recommendations regarding everything from anesthesia to smallpox. An article on smallpox spoke of its causes, cure, and pre-vention, suggesting exercise, bathing, a regular diet, and vaccination for the last of these. It carefully described home-administered vaccination and urged the care of "a skillful physician" for those contracting the disease.[86] Articles on such topics as anesthesia and blood transfusions enthusiastically reported new medical developments available to doctors, while notes on saving drowned persons or curing ulcerations on the feet gave do-it-yourself procedures.[87]

It is difficult to determine precisely when Methodist ministers ceased prescribing and administering medicines. In England and America many others besides Wesley filled the dual roles of minister and physician. In America, for example, Francis Asbury, Thomas Coke, and numerous circuit riders viewed it as a duty to prescribe medical remedies for the sick.[88] By 1830, however, several factors, including developments within medicine and the inclusion of an increasing number of physicians and surgeons in the Methodist fellowship, appear to have brought this minister-physician tradition to an end. In 1817 an American Methodist was found guilty of acting contrary to the standards of a minister of the Gospel by practicing medicine against the counsel of his presiding elder. After 1820, Methodists generally decided either to preach or practice medicine, not do both.[89] By the 1860s, clear lines of demarcation existed between these "once united" professions, and Methodists rou-tinely praised the medical profession. Indeed, they increasingly asso-ciated medical science with human progress, against which ministers would commit a "breach of courtesy" should they even recommend untested medicines to laypersons.[90] Behind these positions lay a con-troversy over ministerial endorsements of patent medicines and the advertising of these medicines in Methodist periodicals. By the early 1860s, the editors of *The Christian Advocate* had taken a stand against such endorsements and advertisements as "unwarrantable interference with an honorable profession."[91]

The medical dispensaries established by Wesley apparently never survived his death, but there is evidence that societies inspired by, but independent from, Methodism sought to attend to the needs of the sick poor from the 1780s through the 1860s.[92] The tradition of visiting the sick continued after Wesley, but in modified ways. Class leaders were expected to comfort, encourage, and pray for the sick. Many Methodist women found a special calling as visitors of the sick, through which they were able to display theological knowledge and rhetorical gifts.[93]

The autobiographies and biographies of Methodists reveal how the converting of nonbelievers took precedence over all other concerns in this intensely evangelical era. Female and male visitors entered the homes of the sick to explore the conditions of their souls and to warn them of "the wrath to come" should they die unconverted.[94] Certain that the world had never witnessed such a mighty harvesting of souls since the apostolic era, some Methodist preachers became virtually oblivious to sickness. One itinerent, for example, recounted how he "hasted away" from his "exceedingly ill" wife and infant son, only to find that his firstborn had died in his absence. He took "consolation," however, from the fact that he had not been absent on his "own account" but had been "in the cause of my heavenly Father."[95]

Enthusiastic evangelism also led many Methodists to view disease as a divine punishment upon those who, although free and able to turn to God, persisted in their worldly ways. Some Methodists claimed that all pain and sickness should be viewed as God's "punishments and correctives for our sins and follies." Others said that individual afflictions were not clear indications of divine displeasure, but that plagues and national calamities were.[96] Yellow fever, typhus, and cholera epidemics were regularly viewed as the judgments of an all-wise and all-powerful God upon dissolute, intemperate, and sometimes filthy human communities. During epidemics ministers sought—often with success—to convert the fearful and unchurched.[97]

While Methodism during its evangelical era significantly altered the medical theories, therapies, and patterns of organized care set forth by John Wesley, it by and large perpetuated his ideas regarding physical and mental health. Rank-and-file Methodists generally abided by Wesley's rules of eating, drinking, sleeping, exercising, and clean living. Indeed, these rules appear to have become all the more important for Methodist evangelicals because they served to distinguish the saved from the lost, those who lived according to patterns of primitive Christianity from those who did not. Members who drank distilled liquor, took opium, smoked tobacco, dipped snuff, or stirred up sensual passions by dancing were viewed as indulging in un-Christian, worldly, sinful activities, as both corrupting their bodies—the "temples of the Holy Spirit"—and endangering their immortal souls.[98] Those who showed concern for their health and displayed lives of temperance and chastity were praised as models of the purity and simplicity of the gospel.[99] Principles of good health continued to be equated with essential aspects of scriptural holiness.

Like Wesley, Methodists in this period also supported their views of health with recent scientific and medical opinion. Columns on "Health and Disease" in *The Christian Advocate,* for example, summarized medical reports on the harmful physiological effects of smoking, on the beneficial effects of hard work, and on the value of eight hours of sound sleep. Articles by medical doctors also discussed at length the structure and care of eyes and ears and recommended regular exercise, bathing, and a proper diet.[100] Such medical information, however, continued to be linked to Scripture and tradition, which in the case of distilled liquors led to a moderate stand. Many of the leaders of the temperance movement that began in England and America in the 1820s were espousing total abstinence from all alcoholic beverages by the late 1830s. Methodists in both England and America, bolstered by medical and scientific opinion, opposed this radical stand—by appealing to the Bible and Christian tradition, including Wesley.[101] As liquor, beer, and wine became identified with numerous social and physical ills and as national prohibition became equated with social reform, however, this moderate stance declined among Methodists in England (in the 1880s) and America (in the 1890s).[102]

Drunkenness was nevertheless condemned wholesale. Like evangelical sermons on divine chastisement through epidemic diseases, Methodist sermons often used intoxication to illustrate the wages of sin. One minister who credited drunkenness with "every conceivable thing terrible or revolting . . . [and] all the crimes, of every form and every hue," described graphically the suicides and pitiful deaths of those enslaved to liquor. Others recounted the punishments of inebriated actors, or wedding parties, or, worst of all, backsliders.[103]

Methodists also preached against the sinfulness of dancing by describing "numerous" examples of beautiful young women struck with fatal fevers after having stirred up their passions and over-exerted themselves on the dance floor.[104] Dancing was equated with un-Christian lust, unhealthy and possibly destructive emotions, and was condemned as expensive, a waste of time, antithetical to the domestic roles of women, and opposed to biblical standards of sexuality and family unity.[105]

On the whole, Methodist evangelicals reiterated the views of mental health and holiness set forth by Wesley. Adam Clarke (1762–1832), a prominent British Methodist whose prolific theological works and biblical commentaries circulated widely in America, summarized the interplay between holiness and mental happiness in bold strokes:

> Misery was never known until sin entered the world; and happiness can never be known by any man, till sin be expelled from his soul. No holiness,

no happiness . . . no plenary and permanent happiness, without plenary and permanent holiness.[106]

Clarke, however, dichotomized body and soul, describing the former as deriving gratification and health from "natural things" and the latter as being an altogether "different nature" and requiring saving grace and divine goodness before it could experience peace and joy. When separated from God by sin, humans experienced mental turmoil, misery, and depression. By loving God and living according to scriptural precepts, they would enjoy peace, cheerfulness, zeal, and the absence of malice or ill will toward others. Like Wesley, Methodist evangelicals viewed love for God and holy living as essential for mental health, but unlike him, they no longer accented the interplay between body and soul by which the soul expressed itself through the constitution and conditions of the body, and the body shared in the grace of creation.[107]

Although it is impossible to determine how many ministers and Methodist laypersons believed in, attempted, or witnessed supernatural cures, reports of such activity continued to appear in England and America in popular stories and in official Methodist publications throughout the evangelical era. Like Wesley, his evangelical heirs viewed these healings as divine answers to prayer, not as the work of healers endowed with special gifts of the Holy Spirit. On the popular level, the remarkable deliverances from maladies such as cancer, fevers, crippling rheumatism, and sore throats were viewed as no less amazing than the numerous stories about remarkable judgments upon drunkards, revelers, and reprobates. Nor were supernatural healings through prayer regarded as being different in kind from miracles attributed to prayers requesting the rescue of imperiled individuals, the salvation of families from starvation or misfortune, or the control of rain and storm.[108] Methodist publications carried accounts of miraculous cures from the time of Wesley's death through the late nineteenth century, and books on the qualifications and responsibilities of class leaders continued to urge visitors of the sick to "pray for them that they may be healed."[109]

Methodist responses to the challenge of the notorious prayer test in 1872 illuminate Methodist attitudes toward the healing power of prayer at the time. This challenge, issued by the British physicist and natural philosopher John Tyndall (1820–1883), sought to counter religious superstition with scientific method and theory. Tyndall proposed that a single ward in a hospital be singled out in order to see whether prayer had any appreciable influence on healing the sick. The proposal quickly made the news.[110] Although Methodists labeled it as being little more than the dissembled sarcasm of a "materialistic sceptic," the test called forth serious replies. Methodists talked about the impossibility of measuring faith or love, about amazing cures wrought by God beginning with John Wesley, and about recent incidents of healing. One Methodist told of the remarkable healing of a child who had been deemed incurable by her physician. The writer said he could describe "many such instances" and claimed that the life of every minister "abounded" with such stories. Others asserted that although Methodists "condemned" those who failed to use medical skill, they nevertheless regarded any slighting of the healing power of God through prayer as "impiety."[111] In spite of an increasing chasm between scientific validation and traditional religious belief, Methodist confidence in divine healing in response to prayer had not yet been surrendered.[112]

The tradition of displaying the power and consolation of faith at the time of death blossomed full force during Methodism's evangelical era. In fact, deathbed scenes became a literary genre representing one of the supporting "evidences of Christianity" in this generation that was thoroughly enamored of defenses of the faith based on "evidence."[113] In keeping with evangelical styles of argumentation, Methodists and other Protestants vividly contrasted the deaths of saints and sinners. Numerous stories, tracts, and sermons described how believers spent their last hours in confidence and joyful hope because they trusted in God and were resigned to his will. Dying Christians followed biblical examples by comforting and inspiring relatives and leaving them with special words and commissions. Dying saints were credited with unique religious insight and were viewed as possible subjects of supernatural manifestations.[114] Methodists thus continued to nurture the art of dying. Regardless of age, sex, or circumstance, life's final passage became a veritable pulpit for every believer. More particularly, Methodist deathbed rites reflected the testimonials, exchanges, and emotional dynamics of Methodist class meetings.[115]

For the wicked, it was not so. A young woman struck with a fatal illness after a dancing party died in utter despair upon losing her soul for a night of pleasure. A young man fatally injured during a horse-riding accident cried repeatedly "how hard it is to die without religion!" A powerfully strong, but pleasure-seeking reprobate suddenly seized with a dangerous malady died in such agony and pain that he bit off, then tried to swallow, his lower lip.[116] Methodist writers described nonbelievers as passing from this world hopelessly, regretfully, angrily, and insensitively, and dying infidels as facing anguish, dread, and prolonged agony—none more than Voltaire or Thomas Paine.[117] Such stories illustrate both how death and dying were interpreted through evangelical lenses and how piety and positive emotional states, as well as impiety and negative emotional responses, were viewed as interrelated.

Modern Methodism Since 1880

In the last decades of the nineteenth century, Methodism faced a new cultural world. Rural life, small towns, and partially industrialized cities characterized the social world of John Wesley and evangelical Methodism, while urbanization, labor unions, mass communication, public amusements, and a reliance on science and technology typified Western societies after 1880. Wesley and Methodist evangelicals had opposed "worldly" fashions, books, and entertainment in the name of scriptural and practical holiness. Like a spartan phalanx, each Methodist church was relatively hard to enter, tightly disciplined by ministers and class leaders, and ever ready to exclude those not subject to its control. By 1880, however, Methodist traditionalists were lamenting the spiritual decline and lax discipline of the church—specifically, the degree to which "the day of elegant written pulpit essays, quartette choirs, and frigid gentility had come, and that of the class-meeting was past."[118] Church trials and expulsions became less and less common and finally ceased occurring almost entirely.[119] Increasingly, Methodists lost touch with the lower social classes and participated more in the high culture of the times. To the chagrin of traditionalists, the change underway in the 1850s had become a social revolution by the 1900s.[120] Toward the end of this period, Nazarene and Holiness splinter groups left mainline Methodism for greater scriptural piety. These groups retained strict prohibitions against dancing and consuming any form of alcoholic beverage, generally accommodated themselves less to modern medical care, and accented the healing power of prayer. The several Holiness Pentecostal groups that Methodism helped spawn made miraculous healing a central tenet of faith and practice.

Intellectual changes during these same decades were also revolutionary. Whereas a literal belief in the Bible and its miracles sustained the thought of Wesley and evangelical Methodists, a natural, scientific perspective predicated upon radically different assumptions about the age, origins, laws, and limits of nature and cosmos shaped the thinking of modern Methodists. Momentously, a new understanding of the Bible emerged from the hands of linguistic and historical critics, whose work undermined the Mosaic authorship of the first five books of the Old Testament, showed that the *Book of Isaiah* was written by at least two authors, pointed out the differences and inconsistencies among the four Gospel accounts, and demonstrated how Christians in the apostolic era mistakenly expected the return of Christ in their generation.[121] Out of this matrix, Protestant liberalism—which after the 1890s included large segments of Methodism—developed as a movement determined to uphold belief in God and the power and relevance of the teachings of

Jesus and the Old Testament prophets in the social and intellectual context of its time.[122]

By 1880, Methodism had effectively severed most of its ties with John Wesley's medical theories and therapies. Methodist publishing houses no longer printed *Primitive Physick;* ministers and physicians practiced in distinct professions; and the profession of medicine received official praise rather than criticism. Although some Methodist publications continued educating their readers about developments in medicine—like bone replacements, skin grafts, and public health—their distance from Wesley's legacy grew increasingly great.[123] This distance was symbolized by an article in *The Christian Advocate* entitled "Wesley and Physic," which praised Methodism's primary founder for his concern for body and soul, but added that his remedies had been "singularly speculative" and had been harvested from "old wives and old valetudinarians."[124]

At the same time that Methodists were dismissing and misinterpreting Wesley's therapies, a new era was dawning with respect to medical-care organizations. Aware of Methodism's historical charitable concerns for the sick and the poor, modern Methodists found a new cause in the building of hospitals, the first of which, the Seney Methodist Episcopal Hospital in Brooklyn, was dedicated in 1882. By 1923, seventy-five Methodist hospitals and clinics had opened to persons of any faith. Many included dispensaries where medicines and supplies could be purchased under cost; all were overseen by a standing Board of Hospitals and Homes.[125] By 1960, some seventy-six general hospitals were being operated under Methodist auspices—a number second only to Lutheranism among Protestant denominations in America. This dynamic movement drew its inspiration from John Wesley's benevolent concerns, as well as from the determination of liberal Protestants to transform society according to the principles of Jesus and the Hebrew prophets (the so-called Social Gospel). Methodism's Social Gospel activities included programs dealing with health, crime, labor relations, poverty, and racism.[126]

In association with the church's new social services, especially hospitals and dispensaries, Methodists revived the office of deaconesses after 1888. This office for women, which appears to have faded away after Wesley's death, owed its revival to European Anabaptist influences. The deaconess movement grew rapidly within Methodism in the first decades of the twentieth century, but thereafter nurses increasingly replaced deaconesses in Methodist hospitals.[127]

The roles of Methodist women were not limited to homemaking, serving as deaconess, nursing, and teaching. In fact, by 1880 Methodist authors were asserting that women "should have fully as good an education in medicine as men," and hence should be trained as phy-

sicians. Their intellectual capacities, sympathy, and acuteness of observation were praised as ideal qualities for modern physicians.[128] In
contrast, women were not allowed to become ministers in the mainline
American Methodist churches until 1956, when only one-third of the
Methodists in the United States believed that men and women "should
have equal and identical rights" professionally. By the 1980s, women
were increasingly occupying Methodist pulpits, and some married clergy
couples were working together.[129]

After World War II, Methodists responded to heightened demands
for training ministers as chaplains in prisons, mental institutions, the
Veterans Administration, and general hospitals. Clinical training for
chaplains was closely aligned with interdenominational agencies in this
ecumenical era.[130] The work and training of chaplains built on several
decades of interdisciplinary reflection about theology and psychology.
Beginning in the 1920s—and expanding into a steady stream of books,
journals, and articles in the 1930s—pastoral psychology had developed
as a discipline exploring the roles of ministers for the physically sick,
mentally ill, or troubled. In spite of the creative work of chaplains in
hospital settings; of many studies and pronouncements regarding the
interconnectedness of body, mind, and spirit; and of numerous summons
for doctors and ministers to work together; very little cooperative
interaction seems to have occurred between doctors and parish ministers.[131]

During the first decades of the modern era, Methodists continued
to advocate long-standing positions regarding physical health—positions
confirmed by numerous scientific studies of diet, exercise, and hygiene.
In fact, John Wesley's rules on eating, drinking, cleanliness, and exercise
are reflected virtually wholesale in secular health manuals that accent
moderate amounts of low-salt, low-cholesterol foods, supplemented by
regular exercise.[132]

During its modern era, Methodism focused particularly on the unhealthful effects of tobacco and alcoholic beverages. After 1892, for
example, a "solemn judgment" against cigarette smoking and any other
habitual use of tobacco was added to the "special advices" section of
the official Doctrines and Discipline of the Methodist church.[133] No
health-related issue addressed by modern Methodists compared to its
intense opposition to the consumption of liquor. As noted previously,
the defenders of moderate drinking who appealed to Scripture and to
Wesleyan tradition lost ground in England and America in the 1880s
and 1890s. During their first world conference in 1881, Methodists in
both nations and in foreign fields gave great attention to the evils of
intemperance. By the end of the century, an overwhelming majority of
ministers, and apparently a majority of laypersons, had become teetotalers.[134] Between 1875 and the 1940s in England, Methodism threw

its weight behind parliamentary restrictions of drinking and the liquor trade, but its highly active temperance campaign had to settle for moral persuasion through voluntary organizations. In America, Methodists in the North and South united in a common cause against alcohol in any consumable form. As ardent prohibitionists, Methodists helped secure the passage of constitutional amendments against the sale or transportation of alcoholic beverages, first on a state, then (in 1919) on a national level.[135]

By 1933, when the prohibition amendment was repealed in America, Methodists worldwide had begun to view social drinking and drunkenness as one of a number of interconnected social problems and evils—including political corruption, economic exploitation, broken marriages, and mental illness.[136] By the mid-1940s, the Methodist Board of Temperance was working with the Yale Center of Alcohol Studies, Alcoholics Anonymous, and similar organizations. Like others in American society, Methodists came to conclude that "alcoholism" was a disease, a physical addiction symbiotic with social and psychological factors such as loneliness and insecurity, and to view alcoholics as needing care and rehabilitation. Significant contributions regarding the care and counseling of alcoholics were made by the Methodist pastoral theologian Howard J. Clinebell, Jr., whose work was informed by the Yale Center and who became exceedingly influential in Methodist seminaries. Clinebell explored the manifold interconnections between alcoholism and psychospiritual needs and analyzed various psychodynamic and theological approaches to the problem, including the pros and cons of its being considered a sickness.[137] Methodism's legacy of opposing the consumption of alcohol remained strong as late as 1959, when the results of a national survey indicated that sixty-three percent of Methodists believed in total voluntary abstinence and national prohibition—as opposed to a national average of thirty-eight percent. This legacy was also reflected in the 1972 *Book of Discipline* of the United Methodist Church, which asserted that abstinence from alcohol and marijuana constituted "a faithful witness to God's liberating and redeeming love."[138]

The complex changes in Methodist views of mental health merit much more extensive investigation than they have received.[139] From the time of Wesley through the evangelical era, Methodists fused notions of mental health with scriptural holiness. This tradition continued among the Holiness Christians who separated from the mainline Methodist denominations in the last decade of the nineteenth century.[140]

The emerging disciplines of psychology and pastoral care in the modern era introduced new understandings of the inner workings of the human psyche. Notions of the unconscious, the instincts of sexuality and aggression, concepts of repression and sublimation, and contrasts between inferiority and superiority or introvertedness and extrovertedness all became analytical categories for educated westerners, as well as common notions in popular culture. These concepts influenced traditional Methodist views of mental health and religious holiness in several respects, leading ministers to realize the depths to which "the entire membership of the church" was subject to periods of anxiety, depression, anger, jealousy, and drug-dependency in various forms.[141] This realization made it impossible to assume that Methodists or any other Christians could live according to any superficial interpretation of the standards of scriptural perfection advocated by John Wesley— standards requiring that the inner self be totally motivated by self-denying love. In fact, by 1959 a national survey of Methodist opinion in America indicated that only 11.9% of laypersons and clergy still believed that "Christians could expect through the power of God to attain perfect love in this life."[142] In contrast to Adam Clarke in the evangelical era, modern Methodists no longer regarded a person's spirit as the pure creation of God residing in a natural body, but rather viewed the soul as both natural and God-given. These altered views of the inner self accompanied changing patterns of external living, namely increased participation in and acceptance of "worldly" activities and amusements. By the 1950s, Methodist leaders were publicly asserting that their members were "about as broad and liberal in their codes of behavior as . . . other leading Protestants."[143]

Owing to these changes, Methodist theologians and counselors balanced their theological heritage with psychological insight for the purpose of defining and securing mental health. Given both the diversity of psychological theory and the theological pluralism within Methodism, this balance predictably assumed various forms. In the 1920s, James Albert Beebe, professor of pastoral theology in Boston University's School of Theology, spoke of mental peace and happiness as resulting from the "healing personality" of pastors; from counseling techniques for relieving repression, depression, and other mental afflictions; and from prayer and daily meditation.[144] In an exceedingly popular book in the late 1930s, Henry C. Link, a Methodist psychologist, used Carl Jung's distinction between introverts and extroverts in proposing that true happiness was to be found in turning away from the selfishness and introversion of childhood to a life molded and inspired by Jesus Christ, "the great exponent of the unselfish life" and an "extrovert to a degree which few can hope to achieve."[145] On a far more profound level, after the second World War, pastoral theologians like Howard Clinebell, Jr., Carroll A. Wise, and Paul E. Johnson explored interrelationships between modern psychology and theology, including the ways religion and moralistic preaching can be used destructively. Wise's investigation of the psychological insights and depths of Wesley's thought pointed to the latter's realistic awareness of human freedom and dependency, of human impotence and growth, and of the degrees to which healing and grace were mediated through experience and relationships.[146] The thought of Wise and others broke beyond Social Gospel liberalism by drawing upon the perspectives of Protestant Reformers, Wesley, and crisis theologians like Karl Barth and Paul Tillich. Finding deep interconnections between the dark picture of the inner self as drawn by psychotherapy and the views of human nature in Reformation and Wesleyan theology, Albert Outler (b. 1908), a dominant Methodist figure in recent decades, argued that humans are fundamentally disposed toward misery and self-destruction, even though they possess sadly disfigured inner righteousness. They could find psychological well-being and goodness only "by God . . . in communication with God, in and through the God-Man," Jesus Christ.[147]

Modern Methodists have furthermore regarded human sexuality as an integral aspect of human wholeness. The views of human sexuality set forth in the *Book of Discipline* of 1972 illustrate several of the important changes that occurred after the evangelical era. Here sex is recognized as "a good gift of God," which must be "acknowledged and affirmed" personally and socially in order for persons "to be fully human." This dimension of humanness can be understood only through a combination of insights from the disciplines of medicine, theology, and the humanities. Although the *Book of Discipline* describes homosexuality as being "incompatible with Christian teaching," it affirms that "homosexuals, no less than heterosexuals, are persons of sacred worth," whose civil rights must be protected.[148] The 1980s have witnessed extensive debates about homosexuality. In contrast, masturbation is rarely discussed in Methodist circles—probably because many pastors do not oppose it unless it undermines a person's self-esteem and mental health.[149]

It is impossible to determine how many Methodist ministers and laypersons have ceased relying on divine healing through prayer. Clearly, by the 1920s such a reliance received no emphasis among molders of Methodist thought. In his 1923 guidelines for visiting the sick, for example, Beebe made no mention of divine intervention through prayer. Instead, he viewed prayer and the minister's presence as easing and composing the "restless" minds of the sick, thereby inducing moods "favorable" to recovery.[150] Nevertheless, a minority of Methodists retained confidence in the possibility of divine healing: Twenty-nine percent of Methodist ministers surveyed in 1954 responded "yes" when asked if they had "attempted to perform a spiritual healing."[151]

It is possible that the number of Methodist ministers who had attempted spiritual healing in the mid-1950s had increased from earlier decades, because by the 1950s a resurgence of divine healing was underway in both England and America. This resurgence was encouraged by the positive mind-cure work of Norman Vincent Peale (b. 1898), a Methodist by birth and education, and by the post–World War II television healing services of Oral Roberts (b. 1918), a Pentecostal who joined the Methodist church in 1968. Notable proponents of divine healing within Methodism include Leslie D. Weatherhead (1893–1976), at one time the president of the Methodist Church in England and, in America, Albert E. Day, who founded the New Life Clinic in which Olga Worrell (b. 1906) received her early training. Worrell has for many years actively promoted healing through "paraelectricity," a fringe perspective in America's holistic health campaign.[152]

Advocates of divine healing within Methodism during the last thirty years make limited claims about its frequency, and they regularly emphasize that such healing is supplementary to natural and scientific medical interventions. Weatherhead and Worrell attribute divine healings to auras or emanations—forces viewed as mediated to sick persons through the laying on of hands—that they believe will eventually be identified and measured.[153] Others express embarrassment about faith healers who try to imitate methods of curing described in the New Testament, recognize that one century of scientific therapy has been more effective than many centuries of religious healing, and oppose the guilt and psychological harm resulting from viewing sickness as punishment from God. They nevertheless maintain that on occasion God directly intervenes from outside the realm of ordinary experience and heals those who seek blessing through prayer.[154]

By the beginning of Methodism's modern era, the tradition of saints dying in bliss and sinners dying in terror was being overtly questioned. One Methodist critic of this tradition, for example, said in 1882 that dying persons probably were unconscious of what they or others said, that alleged deathbed visions were "doubtless subjective," and that the terrors of sinners were due to the widespread fear of eternal punishment that pervaded communities at the time.[155] Although no clear story of changing Methodist beliefs and practices about dying exists, it appears that Methodists, like their neighbors, die in increasing numbers in hospitals according to the unostentatious dynamics of hospital routines. They may welcome visitations and prayer, but they have ceased believing that death is particularly noteworthy or memorable.[156] One of the reasons for this change lay in the fact that the majority of modern Methodists became "emancipated from the prescientific view of a physical heaven 'up there' and a physical hell 'down there.' "[157] Methodists had also abandoned the practice of fervent evangelical witnessing, which had been sustained by the dynamics and symbolic significance of traditional class meetings. Instead, they affirm "dying with dignity," namely dying in the midst of loving personal care and free from useless life-prolonging medical technology.[158]

Beginning in the nineteenth century, Methodist ethics focused on social reform in the name of Christian benevolence, justice, and holiness. With these principles, Wesley had both criticized the medical profession of his time and established a variety of institutions for needy, neglected, and dispossessed persons. The first two of these principles inspired modern Methodists to build and maintain numerous hospitals and clinics throughout the world.

The Methodist church never developed an institutional tradition of reflection on the rightness or wrongness of specific medical interventions. Individual Methodists, however, occasionally set forth views about the transcience and tragedies of life by reflecting upon the limits of medicine and the meaning of sickness and deformity; and contemporary Methodists like Harmon L. Smith at Duke University and J. Robert Nelson at Boston University's School of Theology and the Institute of Religion in Houston's Texas Medical Center have been exploring issues in medical ethics, as well as fundamental philosophical and religious perspectives on bioethics and life's nature and meaning.[159] These matters will likely become an increasing concern in the future and give rise to churchwide investigation and judgments. The early indications of this trend appeared in the brief references to abortion (justifiable in instances of "tragic conflicts of life") and dying with dignity in the 1972 *Book of Discipline*.[160] When such work leads to clear and forceful positions and criticisms regarding modern medicine, Methodism will have recaptured yet another of its historic traditions from John Wesley.

Notes

1. John Wesley, *Advice to the People Called Methodists* (Bristol, 1745); V.H.H. Green, *John Wesley* (London, 1964), pp. 24–37.
2. Frank Baker, "Methodism," *The Encyclopedia Americana*, 30 vols. (Danbury, CT, 1983), 18:793–796; Edwin Scott Gausted, *Historical Atlas of Religion in America* (New York, 1976), pp. 75–83.
3. Green, *John Wesley*, pp. 109–122; Baker, "Methodism," pp. 793–794; Colin W. Williams, *John Wesley's Theology Today* (New York, 1960), pp. 39–206; Albert C. Outler, ed., *John Wesley* (New York, 1954), pp. 25–33; Umphrey Lee, *John Wesley and Modern Religion* (Nashville, 1936), pp. 110–272.
4. Baker, "Methodism," pp. 794–796; Edwin H. Maynard, "Methodists," *Collier's Encyclopedia*, 24 vols. (New York, 1984), 16:66–69; *The Book of Discipline of the United Methodist Church 1972* (Nashville, 1972); Frank S. Mead, *Handbook of Denominations in America* (New York, 1961), pp. 151–163.
5. Maynard, "Methodists," p. 67; Mead, *Handbook of Denominations*, p. 156; John O. Gross, "The Field of Education, 1865–1939," in *The History of Methodism*, ed. Emory Stevens Burke, 3 vols. (New York, 1964), 3:243–249.

6. Green, *John Wesley,* pp. 67–76.
7. John Wesley, *The Letters of the Reverend John Wesley,* ed. John Telford, 8 vols. (London, 1931), 2:307.
8. Wesley, *Letters,* 1:11, 2:307; and John Wesley, *The Journal of the Reverend John Wesley, A.M.,* ed. Nehemiah Curnock, 8 vols. (London, 1938), 2:534, 3:161.
9. George Herbert, *A Priest to the Temple, or, The Country Parson* (London, 1652), pp. 274–278; Ronald L. Numbers and Ronald C. Sawyer, "Medicine and Christianity in the Modern World," in *Health/ Medicine and the Faith Traditions,* eds. Martin E. Marty and Kenneth L. Vaux (Philadelphia, 1982), pp. 140–144.
10. Wesley, *Journal,* 1:111, 180, 185, 188, 217.
11. Green, *John Wesley,* pp. 45–66; John Lawson, "The People Called Methodists—2. Our Discipline," in *A History of the Methodist Church in Great Britain,* eds. Rupert Davies and Gordon Rupp, 3 vols. (London, 1965), 1:190–199.
12. Wesley, *Journal,* 2:448, 453–454.
13. Wesley, *Letters,* 2:307; John Wesley, *A Collection of Receipts for the Use of the Poor* (Newcastle, 1745).
14. Wesley, *Letters,* 2:307.
15. John Wesley, *Primitive Physick; or, An Easy and Natural Method of Curing Most Diseases,* 12th ed. (Philadelphia, 1764), p. xvii.
16. G.S. Rousseau, "John Wesley's *Primitive Physick* (1747)," *Harvard Library Bulletin* 16 (1968):242–256.
17. Albert M. Lyles, *Methodism Mocked* (London, 1960), p. 119.
18. Wesley, *Letters,* 6:225–226; William Hawes, *Examination of the Reverend Mr. John Wesley's Primitive Physick,* 2nd ed. (London, 1780); and Richard P. Heitzenrater, *The Elusive Mr. Wesley,* 2 vols. (Nashville, 1984), 1:134–144, 2:128–138.
19. Rousseau, "John Wesley's *Primitive Physick,*" pp. 242–256; and Eunice Bonow Bardell, "Primitive Physick: John Wesley's Receipts," in *Pharmacy in History* 21 (1979):111–121.
20. Kenneth Dewhurst, *The Quicksilver Doctor: The Life and Times of Thomas Dover* (Bristol, 1957), p. 148; Wesley, *Primitive Physick,* 12, 24, 32; and Robert Boyle, *Medicinal Experiments; or, A Collection of Choice and Safe Remedies,* 4th ed. (London, 1703), pp. 9, 70.
21. Wesley, *Primitive Physick,* pp. 23, 72; and Nicholas Culpepper, *The English Physician* (Boston, 1708), pp. 12, 27.
22. John Wesley, "A Letter to a Friend Concerning Tea," in *The Works of the Rev. John Wesley, M.A.,* 27 vols. (Bristol, 1771–1774), 24:264–283.
23. John Wesley, *The Desideratum; or, Electricity Made Plain and Useful,* in *The Works of the Rev. John Wesley,* 24:284–369; and A. Wesley Hill, *John Wesley Among the Physicians* (London, 1958), pp. 83–110.
24. John Wesley, *A Word to Whom it May Concern* (Bristol, 1779), pp. 2–16.
25. John Wesley, *Advices with Respect to Health Extracted from a Late Author* in *The Works of the Rev. John Wesley* (Bristol, 1773) 25:150–156; and Hill, *John Wesley,* pp. 54–82.
26. John Wesley, *An Extract from Dr. Cadogan's Dissertation on the Gout* in *The Works of the Rev. John Wesley,* (Bristol, 1774) 26:3–52; and John Rendle-Short, "William Cadogan, 18th Century Physician," *Medical History* 4 (1960):288–309.

27. John Wesley, "Thoughts on Nervous Disorders," *Arminian Magazine* 9 (1786):52–54, 94–97.
28. John Wesley, *The Duty and Advantage of Early Rising* (London, 1789), pp. 3–10.
29. Wesley, *Letters,* 2:306; Wesley, *Journal,* 2:447, 454; and John Wesley, "On Visiting the Sick," in *The Works of the Rev. John Wesley, M.A.,* 7 vols. (New York, 1856), 2:335–336.
30. Wesley, *Letters,* 2:95, 307; and Wesley, *Journal,* 2:273.
31. Wesley, *Journal,* 4:190–191.
32. Wesley, *Primitive Physick,* pp. viii–ix.
33. Ibid., pp. iii–v.
34. Ibid., pp. v–ix; and Wesley, *A Survey of the Wisdom of God in the Creation,* 3 vols. (Bristol, 1770).
35. Wesley, *Primitive Physick,* pp. vi–vii, xi; Wesley, *Desideratum,* pp. 367–368; Wesley, *An Extract from Dr. Cadogan's Dissertation,* pp. 5–7; and Wesley, *Advices With Respect to Health,* p. 156.
36. Wesley, *Primitive Physick,* pp. vi–x; Wesley, *Desideratum,* pp. 285–288; and Wesley, *Advices With Respect to Health,* pp. 151–156.
37. John Wesley, *An Extract from Dr. Cadogan's Dissertation,* p. 10; Wesley, *A Plain Account of Christian Perfection,* 14 vols. (London, 1752); and Wesley, "The Scriptural Way of Salvation," in *The Works of the Rev. John Wesley, M.A.* (Bristol, 1771), 3:252–270.
38. Wesley, *Desideratum,* pp. 284–293; Wesley, *A Survey of the Wisdom of God in the Creation,* 2:101–107; and Wesley, "What is Man?" in *The Works of the Rev. John Wesley, M.A.* (London, 1831), 7:225–226.
39. Wesley, *Primitive Physick,* pp. iv–v, xiii–xvi; Wesley, *A Word to Whom it May Concern,* pp. 9–12; and Wesley, *The Duty and Advantage of Early Rising,* pp. 4–8.
40. Wesley, *Advices With Respect to Health,* p. 151; Wesley, *An Extract from Dr. Cadogan's Dissertation,* pp. 8–10; Chester R. Burns, "The Nonnaturals: A Paradox in the Western Concept of Health," *Journal of Medicine and Philosophy* 1 (1976):202–211; Wesley, *Letters,* 1:11; Wesley, *Primitive Physick,* pp. xiii–xvi; and George Cheyne, *An Essay on Health and Long Life,* 4th ed. (Dublin, 1725).
41. Wesley, *Primitive Physick,* pp. viii–ix; Wesley, *Advices with Respect to Health,* pp. 151–156; Wesley, *Letters,* 4:195, 5:325.
42. Wesley, *Desideratum,* pp. 287–288.
43. Wesley, *Letters,* 2:95, 307.
44. Wesley, *Primitive Physick,* pp. ix–x, xviii; and Wesley, *Advices with Respect to Health,* pp. 150, 156.
45. John Wesley, *The Manners of the Ancient Christians,* 4th ed. (Bristol, 1771), p. 14.
46. Wesley, *Primitive Physick,* pp. xiv–xvi; Wesley, *A Word to Whom It May Concern,* pp. 11–12; Wesley, *An Extract from Dr. Cadogan's Dissertation,* pp. 4–7; Wesley, *Letters,* 3:78, 6:18, 185–186; and Wesley, *Advices with Respect to Health,* p. 151.
47. Wesley, *A Letter to a Friend,* pp. 265–273; Wesley, *A Word to Whom It May Concern,* p. 10; and Wesley, *Letters,* 4:14.
48. Wesley, *Primitive Physick,* p. xv; Wesley, *An Extract from Dr. Cadogan's Dissertation,* pp. 8–9; Wesley, *Letters,* 4:213, 5:42, 132–133, 6:59.

49. Wesley, *The Duty and Advantage of Early Rising,* pp. 3–6; Wesley, *Letters,* 4:278–279, 7:75; Wesley, *A Word to Whom it May Concern,* p. 10; and Wesley, "Thoughts on Nervous Disorders," pp. 94–97.
50. Wesley, "Thoughts on Nervous Disorders," pp. 52–54, 94–97.
51. Wesley, *Primitive Physick,* p. xvi.
52. Wesley, *An Extract from Dr. Cadogan's Dissertation,* p. 10.
53. Wesley, *A Survey of the Wisdom of God in the Creation,* 1:8–87; Wesley, "What is Man?," pp. 225–226; and J. Robert Nelson, *Human Life* (Philadelphia, 1984), p. 43.
54. John Wesley, "Heaviness Through Manifold Temptations," in *The Works of The Rev. John Wesley, M.A.* (London, 1831), 6:94–95; Wesley, "The Heavenly Treasure in Earthen Vessels," *The Works of the Rev. John Wesley, A.M.* (London, 1831), 7:346–348; Wesley, *A Survey of the Wisdom of God in the Creation,* 1:92–93.
55. Wesley, "Heaviness Through Manifold Temptations," pp. 95–103; Wesley, "What is Man?," pp. 229–230.
56. Wesley, "The Scriptural Way of Salvation," in *The Works of the Rev. John Wesley, M.A.,* pp. 254–270; Wesley, "The New Birth," in *The Works of the Rev. John Wesley, M.A.,* (Bristol, 1771), 3:290–310; Wesley, "Scriptural Christianity," in *The Works of the Rev. John Wesley, M.A.,* (Bristol, 1771), 1:67–91; Wesley, "What is Man?," pp. 228–230; Williams, *John Wesley's Theology,* pp. 57–73, 98–140.
57. Albert Outler, "The Place of Wesley in the Christian Tradition," in *The Place of Wesley in the Christian Tradition,* ed. Kenneth Rowe (Metuchen, NJ, 1976), pp. 14–32.
58. John Wesley, *A Plain Account of Christian Perfection* (London, 1952 [1765]), p. 84.
59. John and Charles Wesley, *The Nature, Design, and General Rules of the United Societies,* 8th ed. (London, 1761 [1743]).
60. Wesley, *A Plain Account of Christian Perfection,* pp. 11, 19–20, 80; and Wesley, "The Scriptural Way of Salvation," pp. 255–256.
61. Wesley, *A Plain Account of Christian Perfection,* pp. 80–84; Wesley, "Heaviness Through Manifold Temptations," pp. 101–103.
62. Wesley, *Advices with Respect to Health,* p. 156; see also *Primitive Physick,* p. xiii; and Wesley, *An Extract from Dr. Cadogan's Dissertation,* pp. 10–11.
63. Wesley, *Letters,* 2:135, 210.
64. Wesley, *Journals,* 4:212–213; 5:178, 265–271, 375; 6:212–213; Wesley, *Letters,* 2:251–253.
65. Wesley, *Journals,* 5:103.
66. Wesley, *Letters,* 2:257.
67. Ibid. 2:210, 253–258; Wesley, *Journals,* 2:283–298; 3:56; "The Narrative of an Extraordinary Cure," *Arminian Magazine* 5 (1782):251–255; "A Narrative of the Cure of Susannah Arch," ibid. 5 (1782):312–317; "The Miraculous Cure of a Dutch Woman," ibid. 9 (1786):43–44; and Henry D. Rack, "Doctors, Demons, and Early Methodist Healing," in *The Church and Healing,* ed. W.J. Sheils, vol. 19 of *Studies in Church History* (Oxford, 1982), pp. 137–152.
68. Wesley, *Letters,* 2:105, 262–263.
69. Rack, "Doctors, Demons," pp. 149–150; Wesley, *Letters,* 2:258, 5:317.
70. Wesley, *Primitive Physick,* p. xiii; Wesley, *An Extract from Dr. Cadogan's Dissertation,* pp. 10–11; Wesley, *Advices with Respect to*

Health, p. 156; and Wesley, *A Word To Whom it May Concern,* p. 17.

71. Wesley, *A Plain Account of Christian Perfection,* pp. 62–69; Outler, *John Wesley,* p. 32.

72. Wesley, *Letters,* 6:213, 222; Wesley, "The Great Assize," in *The Works of the Rev. John Wesley, M.A.* (Bristol, 1771), 1:298–321; John Wesley, "Of Hell," in *The Works of the Rev. John Wesley, M.A.* (New York, 1856), 2:147–154.

73. John Wesley, ed., "An Extract from Mr. Vincent's Account of the Plague in London," *Arminian Magazine* 5 (1782):203–206.

74. John and Charles Wesley, *General Rules of the United Societies,* pp. 4–9; also found in *The Book of Discipline of the United Methodist Church* 1972, pp. 66–68.

75. John Lawson, "The People Called Methodists," pp. 183–210; John Walsh, "Methodism at the End of the 18th Century," in *A History of the Methodist Church in Great Britain,* 1:277–315; and Richard M. Cameron, "The New Church Takes Root," in *The History of American Methodism* 1:241–290.

76. Sidney E. Ahlstrom, *A Religious History of the American People* (New Haven, 1974), pp. 763–784; and James Hastings Nichols, *History of Christianity* (New York, 1956), pp. 255–282.

77. Rousseau, "John Wesley's *Primitive Physick,*" pp. 254–255.

78. James Penn Pilkington, *The Methodist Publishing House,* 2 vols. (Nashville, 1968), 1:89.

79. Thomas Coke and Francis Asbury, "To the Members of the Methodist Episcopal Church," in *The Family Advisor To Which is Annexed Mr. Wesley's Primitive Physick,* ed. Henry Wilkins, M.D., 6th ed. (New York, 1818), pp. 9–10.

80. Fielding H. Garrison, *An Introduction to the History of Medicine,* 4th ed. (Philadelphia, 1929), pp. 378–380; and Charles E. Rosenberg, "The Therapeutic Revolution: Medicine, Meaning, and Social Change in Nineteenth-Century America," in *The Therapeutic Revolution,* eds. Morris J. Vogel and Charles E. Rosenberg (Philadelphia, 1979), pp. 3–25.

81. Wesley, *Primitive Physick,* pp. viii–xiii; Wesley, *Advices with Respect to Health,* pp. 151–156; Wilkins, *Family Advisor,* pp. 8–135.

82. Wilkins, *Family Advisor,* pp. 52–53, 134.

83. Wilkins, *Family Advisor,* pp. 12–14, 17–18.

84. J. Robertson, "Concerning Systems of National Philosophy," *Arminian Magazine* 2 (1779):89–91; Leslie F. Church, *More About the Early Methodist People* (London, 1949), pp. 35–42, 202; and James B. Finley, *Sketches of Western Methodism* (New York, 1969 [1854]), pp. 260–282.

85. William R. Cannon, "Education, Publication, Benevolent Work, and Missions," in *The History of American Methodism,* 1:577–578.

86. "Small Pox," *Christian Advocate* 47 (January 25, 1872):31.

87. B.A. Brooks, "Anesthesia," ibid. 48 (June 19, 1873):193; "Blood Transfusion," ibid. 51 (March 23, 1876):89; "Saving Human Life," ibid. 48 (April 21, 1873):271; "The Earth Cure for Ulcers," ibid. 47 (February 15, 1872):55.

88. Church, *More About the Early Methodist People,* p. 42; James Asbury, *The Journal and Letters of Francis Asbury,* ed. J. Manning Pitts (London,

1958), 3:500; and Wade Crawford Barclay, *Early American Methodism* (New York, 1950), 2:12–13.

89. Barclay, *Early American Methodism,* p. 13.

90. "The Medical Profession," *Methodist Quarterly Review* 47 (1865):100–115, quotations from pp. 114–115.

91. Pilkington, *Methodist Publishing House,* pp. 457–458.

92. Maldwyn Edwards, *After Wesley* (London, 1935), pp. 117–118; Erik McCoy North, *Early Methodist Philanthropy* (New York, 1914), pp. 45–52; and Abel Stevens, *The History of the Religious Movement of the 18th Century Called Methodism* (New York, 1864), pp. 472–474.

93. Henry Fish, *The Class-Leader's Manual* (London, 1849), pp. 91–93.

94. Joseph H. James, *The Life of Mrs. Mary D. James* (New York, 1886), pp. 42–74; William Myles, *Advice to the Afflicted* (London, 1804), p. 12; and William Carvosso, *A Memoir of Mrs. William Carvosso* (Nashville, 1874), pp. 154–156.

95. Thomas Ware, *Sketches of the Life and Times of Rev. Thomas Ware* (New York, 1840), pp. 235–236; and Stevens, *The History of the Religious Movement,* pp. 467–471.

96. Myles, *Advice to the Afflicted,* p. 5; and "Yellow Fever," *Methodist Magazine* 5 (1822):387–390.

97. "Progress in the Indian Cholera," *Methodist Magazine and Quarterly Review* 16 (1832):450–474; and William Wyatt, *The Life and Sermons of Rev. William Wyatt* (New York, 1879), pp. 78–79.

98. Leslie F. Church, *The Early Methodist People* (New York, 1949), pp. 188–217; "The Christian Care of the Body," *Christian Advocate* 50 (April 15, 1875):15; Maxwell Pierson Gaddis, *Footprints of an Itinerant* (Cincinnati, 1856), pp. 154–155, 372–376; "Tobacco," *Methodist Magazine and Quarterly Review* 13 (1831):273–292; R. Tabraham, *An Earnest Address to Christians . . . in the Common Use of Tobacco and Snuff* (London, 1844), pp. 4–12; J. Townly Crane, *An Essay on Dancing* (New York, 1851), pp. 105–115; and Thomas Olivers, *An Answer to Mr. Mark Davis' Thoughts on Dancing* (London, 1792), pp. 3–88.

99. William Ross, "A Short Account of the Life and Death of Dr. Loredon," *Methodist Magazine* 3 (1820):252–255, 290–295.

100. "The Effects of Tobacco on Man and Animals," *Christian Examiner* 47 (October 3, 1872):319; B. Nash, "Tobacco," ibid. 49 (February 5, 1874):42; "The True Remedy for Trouble," ibid. 47 (October 10, 1872):324; and "Take Enough Sleep," ibid. 47 (March 14, 1872):87; S. Henry Clark, M.D., "The Use and Abuse of Eyesight," *Methodist Quarterly Review* 43 (1861):104–126; and Clark, "The Hearing Ear," ibid. 45 (1863):106–128.

101. Maldwyn Edwards, *Methodism and England* (London, 1943), pp. 100–105; and "The Temperance Movement," *Christian Advocate* 49 (April 23, 1874):132.

102. Edwards, *Methodism and England,* pp. 105–118; and Richard M. Cameron, *Methodism and Society in Historical Perspective* (New York, 1961), pp. 244–248.

103. Gaddis, *Foot-Prints,* pp. 151–155, 372–373, 377 (quotations); Donald E. Byrne, *No Foot of Land* (Metuchen, NJ, 1975), p. 90; and Carvosso, *A Memoir,* pp. 137–138.

104. "Evil Effects of Dancing," *Methodist Magazine* 2 (1819):348–349; Crane, *An Essay on Dancing,* pp. 109–110; and Gaddis, *Foot-Prints,* p. 136.
105. Crane, *An Essay on Dancing,* pp. 105–115; Adam Clarke, *Christian Theology,* ed. Samuel Dunn (New York, 1842), pp. 400–401; Cameron, *Methodism and Society,* pp. 222–223; Edwards, *Methodism and England,* pp. 220–221.
106. Clark, *Christian Theology,* p. 392.
107. Clark, *Christian Theology,* pp. 390–393; Fish, *Class-Leader's Manual,* pp. 43–55; and George C. Robinson, "Spiritual Depression," "Christian Perfection," "Rejoicing in God," and "Self-Will," in *Seed-Thought: A Handbook of Doctrine and Devotion* (New York, 1863), pp. 37–38, 111–114, 124–126, 138–139.
108. Byrne, *No Foot of Land,* pp. 17, 134–142, 156–165.
109. T. Hanby, "A Short Account of the Life and Death of Ann Brooks," *Arminian Magazine* 16 (1793):144–147; and R.H. Howard, "A Novel Test of the Efficacy of Prayer," *Christian Advocate* 47 (August 29, 1872):273; Fish, *Class-Leader's Manual,* p. 94.
110. Stephen G. Brush, "The Prayer Test," *American Scientist* 62 (September–October, 1974), 561–563.
111. Howard, "A Novel Test," p. 273; W.C. Conant, "Bible Therapeutics," *Christian Advocate* 47 (October 17, 1872):329.
112. "Remarkable Prayer Cure," *Christian Advocate* 48 (August 28, 1873):278.
113. Davis W. Clark, ed., *Death-Bed Scenes* (New York, 1852) p. 22; and "Short Reviews," *Methodist Quarterly Review* 34 (1852):156.
114. Clark, *Death-Bed Scenes,* pp. 15–20, 133–443; Robinson, *Seed-Thought,* pp. 34–35; William Ross, "A Short Account . . . of Dr. Louden," *Methodist Magazine* 3 (1820):252–255, 290–294; and "The Death of John Davis," ibid. 2 (1819):77–80; and Harold Y. Vanderpool, "The Responsibilities of Physicians Toward Dying Patients," in *Medical Complications in Cancer Patients,* eds. J. Klastersky and M.J. Staquet (New York, 1981), pp. 118–120.
115. A. Gregory Schneider, "Sentimental Community: The Ritual Drama of Happy Dying Among Nineteenth-Century American Evangelicals," unpublished paper, 1981, pp. 7–35.
116. Gaddis, *Foot-Prints,* pp. 135–138, 140–143.
117. Clark, *Death-Bed Scenes,* pp. 469–555; and Byrne, *No Foot of Land,* pp. 84–90.
118. O.P. Fitzgerald, *The Class-Meeting* (Nashville, 1880), p. 48.
119. Cameron, *Methodism and Society in Historical Perspective,* pp. 265–266.
120. Henry Brown, *The Impeding Peril* (New York, 1904), pp. 7–60; Cameron, *Methodism and Society in Historical Perspective,* pp. 266–292.
121. William Newton Clark, *Sixty Years with the Bible* (New York, 1912); Ahlstrom, *Religious History,* pp. 763–784; and William Strawson, "Methodist Theology, 1850–1950," in *A History of the Methodist Church in Great Britain,* 3:197–210, 222.
122. Edwards, *Methodism and England,* pp. 207–227; Strawson, "Methodist Theology," pp. 182–231; William J. McCutcheon, "American Methodist Thought and Theology, 1919–1960," in *The History of American Methodism,* 3:261–327.
123. "Change of Treatment in Disease," *Christian Advocate* 55 (June 1880):382; "A Remarkable Operation," ibid. 56 (September 15, 1881):587;

and "The Public Influence of the Medical Profession," ibid. 57 (March 23, 1882):190.

124. "Wesley and Physic," *Christian Advocate* 57 (January 26, 1882):62; and A.B. Prescott, "Nostrums: Their Demonstrative Composition and Real Power," ibid. 56 (May 26, 1881):335.

125. Ralph Diffendorfer, ed., *The World Service of the Methodist Episcopal Church* (Chicago, 1923), pp. 602–613.

126. Diffendorfer, *World Service,* pp. 602–603; "The Dedication of a Hospital," in *Doctrines and Discipline of the Methodist Episcopal Church* (New York, 1936), pp. 632–639; and Walter G. Muelder, *Methodism and Society in the Twentieth Century* (New York, 1961), pp. 308–311; Cameron, *Methodism and Society in Historical Perspective,* pp. 299–325.

127. C. Golder, *History of the Deaconess Movement* (Cincinnati, 1903), pp. 33–45, 316–335; Diffendorfer, *World Service,* pp. 593–599, 613–614.

128. "Women Physicians," *Christian Advocate* 55 (May 6, 1880):302; and "Carlyle on Female Physicians," ibid. 56 (April 28, 1881):270.

129. S. Paul Shilling, *Methodism and Society in Theological Perspective* (New York, 1960), pp. 295, 302; Baker, "Methodism," p. 795.

130. McCutchen, "American Methodist Thought," pp. 326–327; and Charles F. Kemp, *Physicians of the Soul* (New York, 1947), pp. 243–261, 274–276.

131. Kemp, *Physicians of the Soul,* pp. 94–107, 213–225, 236–237; and Lewis H. Allison and R. Paxton Graham, "Co-operation of Minister and Doctor," in *Religion and Medicine,* ed. John Crowlesmith (London, 1962), pp. 169–179.

132. E.g., M.R. Drury, *At Hand* (Dayton, OH, 1895), pp. 9–10, 51–52, 113–114; Donald B. Ardell, *High Level Wellness* (Emmans, PA, 1977).

133. *Doctrines and Discipline of the Methodist Episcopal Church* (New York, 1936), p. 81.

134. Edwards, *Methodism in England,* pp. 106–107; and Cameron, *Methodism and Society in Historical Perspective,* p. 248.

135. Edwards, *Methodism in England,* pp. 108–118; and Cameron, *Methodism and Society in Historical Perspective,* pp. 248–262.

136. *Doctrines and Discipline,* p. 80.

137. Howard J. Clinebell, Jr., *Understanding and Counseling the Alcoholic Through Religion and Psychology* (Nashville, 1968 [1956]); Muelder, *Methodism and Society in the Twentieth Century,* pp. 299–300, 342–343.

138. Schilling, *Methodism and Society in Theological Perspective,* p. 151; and *The Book of Discipline* (1972), p. 89.

139. William A. Clebsch, "American Religion and the Cure of Souls," in *Religion in America,* eds. William C. McLoughlin and Robert N. Bellah (Boston, 1966), pp. 249–265; and Edwin S. Gausted, Darline Miller, and G. Allison Stokes, "Religion in America," *American Quarterly* 31 (Bibliography Issue, 1979):250–283.

140. Strawson, "Methodist Theology," pp. 225–229.

141. James Albert Beebe, *The Pastoral Office* (New York, 1923), pp. 287–289.

142. Schilling, *Methodism and Society in Theological Perspective,* pp. 150, 283.

143. Ralph W. Sockman and Paul A. Washburn, "What is a Methodist?" in *Religion in America,* ed. Leo Rosten (New York, 1975 [1952]), p. 176.

144. Beebe, *The Pastoral Office,* pp. 287–289.

145. Henry C. Link, *The Return to Religion* (New York, 1937), pp. 45–51.
146. Clinebell, *Understanding and Counseling the Alcoholic;* Paul E. Johnson, *Psychology of Pastoral Care* (New York, 1953); and Carroll A. Wise, *The Meaning of Pastoral Care* (New York, 1966).
147. Albert C. Outler, *Psychotherapy and the Christian Message* (New York, 1954), pp. 53–54, 68–69; also David E. Roberts, *Psychotherapy and a Christian View of Man* (New York, 1950), pp. 104–117, 129–143.
148. *Book of Discipline* (1972), p. 86.
149. Leslie D. Weatherhead, "Present-Day Non-Medical Methods of Healing," in *Religion and Medicine,* ed. John Crowlesmith (London, 1962), pp. 62–63.
150. Beebe, *The Pastoral Office,* pp. 284–285.
151. Don H. Gross, *The Case for Spiritual Healing* (New York, 1958), p. 9.
152. Walter W. Dwyer, *The Churches' Handbook for Spiritual Healing* (New York, 1958), pp. 15–58, 66–68; Olga Worrell, "Experiencing the Role of Spiritual Faith Healing in Holistic Health," *Journal of Holistic Health* 3 (1978):37–41; Worrell, "Unconventional Healing," in *Wholistic Dimensions in Healing,* ed. Leslie J. Kaslof (New York, 1978), pp. 180–181; and Harold Y. Vanderpool, "The Holistic Hodgepodge: A Critical Analysis of Holistic Medicine in America Today," *Journal of Family Practice* 19 (December 1984):773–781.
153. Weatherhead, "Present-Day Non-Medical Methods of Healing," pp. 41–57.
154. Erastus Evans, "The Significance of the New Testament Healing Miracles for the Modern Healer," in *Religion and Medicine,* ed. John Crowlesmith (London, 1962), pp. 80–88; and William Strawson, "The Theology of Healing," ibid., pp. 110–111.
155. "Last Words of the Dying," *Christian Advocate* 57 (August 24, 1882):29.
156. Harold Y. Vanderpool, "Responsibilities of Physicians Toward Dying Patients," pp. 117–133; and August M. Kasper, "The Doctor and Death," in *The Meaning of Death,* ed. Herman Feifel (New York, 1959), pp. 259–270.
157. Sockman and Washburn, "What is a Methodist?" p. 174; and Schilling, *Methodism and Society,* p. 289.
158. *The Book of Discipline* (1972), p. 87.
159. Harmon L. Smith, *Ethics and the New Medicine* (Nashville, 1970); and J. Robert Nelson, *Human Life: A Biblical Perspective for Bioethics* (Philadelphia, 1984).
160. *The Book of Discipline* (1972), pp. 86–87.

CHAPTER 12

The Unitarian

and Universalist

Traditions

SPENCER LAVAN

GEORGE HUNTSTON WILLIAMS

The Unitarian and Universalist churches of North America arose from differing origins, but both were essentially American religious movements. Unitarianism represented a progressive liberalization of the Puritan Calvinist congregationalism found in New England, although outside the region, especially in Pennsylvania, it also derived inspiration from old England, notably through the ministry of Joseph Priestley. Universalism originated in Great Britain, but from a Methodist background; by the end of the eighteenth century it had appeared in varying versions in America and was spreading rapidly.

The name *Unitarian* refers specifically to belief in the unity of the godhead and disavowal of the Trinity. It was applied originally to the Arian theology that Christ was of "like substance" but not of the "same substance" as God; this is the identifying theological concept of the movement. Unitarians in Boston and other towns of eastern New England at the end of the eighteenth century thought of themselves as liberal or catholic Christians. Their espousal of free will and their conviction about the goodness of the heavenly Father carried the movement into many of the historic parishes and other institutions of Puritan New England including its first college, Harvard.

The name *Universalist* refers to those who rejected the Calvinist position that only "the elect" would be saved in favor of the view that all could be saved by God's grace through the Lord Jesus Christ. While the concepts behind both the Universalist and Unitarian faiths have their origins in heresies of early Christianity, there is no direct link between the modern movements originating in America and England and the ancient theological views. Both churches emerged indirectly from the Continental and English Radical Reformations of the sixteenth century, but particularly from liberalizing trends in English Presbyterian and Scottish nonconformist religious communities. Both churches were organized around congregational polity, according to which each congregation was responsible for calling its own minister and functioned without control by bishops or national organizations.

Unitarians in New England first described their theology as "liberal Christianity" at the start of the nineteenth century. Universalists date their origins to the arrival in New Jersey of John Murray in 1770. Murray, a Trinitarian, became pastor of the first organized Universalist congregation, in Gloucester, Massachusetts. American Universalism, focusing on a unitarian theology with emphasis on new social and ethical concerns, more truly emerged under the leadership of Hosea Ballou. The theological perspective of early Universalism is stated most explicitly in the 1803 Winchester, New Hampshire, Profession, which emphasized the scriptural character of Universalism, a God of love revealed in Jesus Christ, and a doctrine of happiness and holiness aimed at maintaining the social order and practicing "good works" in order to determine the status of a Universalist in the afterlife. This determination was not left to God alone, but rather derived from the way a person's morality was played out in life.

Unitarian Christianity, standing against both Calvinist theology and the evangelical fervor of the Great Awakening, was shaped by men as important in American history as Thomas Jefferson, Benjamin Franklin, and Thomas Paine, all of whom were attracted to deism, which limited God's activity to the creation of the universe. Deism, however, was not the position of the Reverend William Ellery Channing (1780–1842), the nineteenth-century Unitarian leader from Boston's Federal Street Church. His theology was that of "supernatural rationalism" which accepted the validity of the Scriptures, but examined them and other religious phenomena in the light of reason. Channing set the ideological tone for American Unitarianism on a national level with his sermon "Unitarian Christianity," delivered in Baltimore in 1819; nevertheless, he, himself, eschewed involvement in the organization of the American Unitarian Association, established in Boston in 1825 on exactly the same day a sister association of Unitarian churches was founded in London. During

his thirty-seven-year ministry in Boston, Channing became the outstanding theological and social–ethical spokesperson for the movement.

During the nineteenth century, both movements were predominantly
situated in New England. Unitarians not only engaged in domestic
missionary outreach to the poor and unchurched, but also led in the
development of cultural institutions, including Harvard College. Universalists took hold especially in the more rural areas spreading from
Maine and Vermont across upstate New York and on to the Midwest.
By 1850, the Universalists claimed 529 congregations, of which 285
were in New England, plus a number of colleges and theological schools.
State conventions existed even in the South and Midwest, where churches
were few. At the end of the century, there were 1,000 congregations
serving about 50,000 members, but by 1950 the number of churches
had dwindled to 300. The Unitarians had 246 churches in 1850, 455
in 1900, but only 357 in 1950. Throughout the first half of the twentieth
century membership remained in the low 70,000s; however, rapid development in the South and West in the 1950s swelled ranks to 100,000
by 1958. Since the merger of the two denominations in 1961, members
have taken a more active role in spreading the message of the faith.
Current membership of more than 1,000 congregations of the Unitarian
Universalist Association is 150,000. Small Unitarian movements exist in
the United Kingdom and on the continent, including in Hungary and
Romania, all affiliated (like the North American denomination) with the
International Association for Religious Freedom founded in 1900.

In the context of American social and cultural development, the two
denominations were known in the nineteenth century for their contributions to social reform. Their theology was much influenced by Transcendentalism, the New England echo of German Romantic idealism
exemplified by the Transcendentalist minister-turned-lecturer Ralph Waldo
Emerson and activist pastor and Old Testament scholar Theodore Parker.
Idealistic Transcendentalism led, in the late nineteenth century, to the
Free Religious Association, which sought to develop a liberal faith beyond
the bounds of Christianity. In the first half of the twentieth century,
Unitarians and to a lesser extent Universalists were involved in controversies among liberal Christians, world-religion theists, and explicit hu-
manists.

A major problem in analyzing each tradition is that of authority. While
other traditions can cite religious laws or the teachings of their founder
as the source of authority by which members should act, Unitarians
and Universalists have never possessed any voice of authority. Neither
the President of the American Unitarian Association nor the General
Superintendent of the Universalist Church of America was ever authorized to speak for the whole denomination. Individual ministers have
freely expressed their views, while local churches or designated denominational meetings, whose jurisdiction was limited to those they represented, could vote to urge specific social policies.

A representative statement of faith, written by James Freeman Clarke
(1810–1888), enjoyed popularity throughout the denomination. While

never accepted as a creed, this statement was frequently affirmed at Sunday worship for many decades and was summarized in five points: (1) the Fatherhood of God; (2) the brotherhood of man; (3) the leadership of Jesus; (4) salvation by character; and (5) the progress of mankind onwards and upwards forever.

Since the merger in 1961, the Unitarian Universalist Association of North America has focused on social activism, service, and outreach (rather than traditional missionary work) and on the development of new forms of worship. The increased role of women in leadership is reflected in the fact that women now represent fifteen percent of settled ministers throughout the United States and Canada.

The Principles and Purposes reflecting the current perspective of the denomination were agreed to by a vote of the 1984 General Assembly.

> We, the member congregations of the Unitarian Universalist Association, covenant to affirm and promote
> The inherent worth and dignity of every person;
> Justice, equity and compassion in human relations;
> Acceptance of one another and encouragement to spiritual growth in our congregations;
> A free and responsible search for truth and meaning;
> The rights of conscience and the use of the democratic process within our congregations and in society at large;
> The goal of world community with peace, liberty and justice for all;
> Respect for the interdependent web of all existence of which we are a part.

A second section of the statement traces the roots of the tradition to the mystical and prophetic traditions of Judaism and Christianity as well as to the perspectives of humanism, reason, science, and the world's great religious faiths.

The Unitarian theological theme "unity of the godhead" and the Universalist theme "salvation for all" had no direct immediate consequences for health or medicine. But the two traditions that developed such distinctive traits in North America after 1800 entered into a new understanding of death and dying that differed from that of antecedent Puritan Calvinism. Both traditions subscribed to a belief in free will leading to salvation and repudiated their inherited Calvinist–Pauline teachings about predestination. The newly emerging churches, as creedless institutions, encouraged individualism, free will, and personal and social responsibility. Both stressed a hopeful view of life and life after death in sharp contrast to the pessimism and fear of death sometimes engendered by Calvinist theology.

Neither denomination directed its members to adhere to specific positions on matters relating to health, wellness, disease, or medical treatment. As churches originating in Puritan congregational Christianity, they traditionally celebrated life's passages: birth through baptism or dedication, coming of age through confirmation and membership into a congregation, marriage through conventional and unconventional marriage ceremonies, and death by funeral service and burial or, more recently, by cremation and memorial service.

Resistance to Puritan Calvinism in New England led, at the start of the eighteenth century, to a modified religious position known as Arminianism. While accepting the Puritan Commonwealth or Zion established during the seventeenth century, the Arminians recoiled against the determinism of Calvinist theology as well as against the revivalism of Jonathan Edwards and the Great Awakening of the 1740s. The view that God looks benevolently over his universe and allows either "salvation by character" (Unitarian) or "universal salvation" (Universalist) emerged from the post-Revolutionary Enlightenment in America. Three philosophies in particular helped to shape these two religious visions and their views of life and death: John Locke's philosophy of rights stated in the Declaration of Independence; the deism articulated by Thomas Paine and Benjamin Franklin, postulating a creator God no longer directly active in human affairs; and Scottish "Common Sense" Realism, according to which religious truths are received through sensations and reflections as well as from Scriptural revelation.

Arminian ministers such as Charles Chauncey and Jonathan Mayhew, serving Boston congregationalist pulpits in the mid–eighteenth century, accepted and developed the psychological views of John Locke that knowledge comes through sensation and reflection. The Harvard Unitarian moral philosophers of the early nineteenth century also added the teachings of the Scottish Realists about reason, prudence, and self-love as they articulated what one historian has called "the Unitarian conscience."[1] Both deism and the philosophy of the American Republic reflected contemporary ideas that were very much a part of the background shaping both religious movements.

Unitarianism and Universalism were, in the nineteenth century, two distinct yet parallel religious traditions serving the needs of different socioeconomic groups. Unitarianism in Boston and many eastern seaboard towns and rural areas was a religion of the old elite. Universalism in urban areas reflected the interests of the newly prosperous, while in rural areas it attracted small farmers and tradespersons. With each offering a new stress on individual freedom of thought and responsibility of action based on an affirmative view of life, there emerged a vigorous ethic of social service to meet the health and welfare needs of persons both within and outside the immediate religious communities. The roots of this ethic lay clearly in the Puritan cultural background.

Each tradition, as well as the merged denomination, has spoken clearly on issues of health and medicine at various national gatherings and through denominational publications. The roles of articulate members in setting new standards and breaking new ground in areas from temperance to sex education are at least half the history to be reported here. Although the individuals cited had no authority comparable to that of a bishop, their persuasive voices resonated through both church and world. Their work has been as important in developing the identity of these churches over the past 185 years as general pronouncements have been.

One of the first such exemplars was the prominent Philadelphia physician Benjamin Rush (1745–1813), coming from a Presbyterian background, who expressed sympathy with Universalists by joining their 1790 Philadelphia convention and aiding in polishing their first statement of faith. Rush developed the Philadelphia Dispensary for the Medical Relief of the Poor, which during its first five years (1786–1791) served nearly eight thousand patients. Although his medical practice was not related to his religion, Rush clearly demonstrated a transition from the Reformed view of illness as God's punishment for sin toward the hope of Universalism. "A belief in God's universal love to all his creatures," Rush stated, "and that he will finally restore all those of them that are miserable to happiness is *polar* truth. It leads to truths upon all subjects. . . . It establishes the *equality* of mankind. . . ."[2]

Rush's remarks on the progress of intellectual, moral, and political truth in post-Revolutionary America closely resembled those of his Universalist contemporary, the theologian Hosea Ballou (1772–1852), who wrote in his 1805 *Treatise on the Atonement* that:

> Man's main object, in all he does, is happiness; and were it not for that, he never could have any other particular object. What would induce men to form societies; to be at the expense of supporting government; to acquire knowledge; to learn sciences, or till the earth, if they believed they could be as happy without as with?[3]

This view provided the foundation for his doctrines of "disinterested benevolence" (akin to that in New England theology) and universal salvation through the grace of God and Jesus Christ. The implications of his theology for an involvement in caring and curing, a positive attitude toward life, and concern for death and dying were profound: When a religion teaches its adherents to find fulfillment and to feel adjusted to the world, they develop a natural approach to living.

Health and Religious Reform

William Ellery Channing (1780–1842), minister and civic leader for thirty-seven years in Boston, stood out as the public voice for Unitarianism before 1860 who demonstrated a strong strain of individualism coupled with moral responsibility. Among the many themes addressed in Channing's persuasive preaching were those of personal health and well-being, conditions far easier to achieve for wealthy Boston Unitarians of his Federal Street congregation than for the socially and culturally separated, less well-educated urban populations around him. Channing articulated his doctrine of health in his lecture on "the Elevation of the Laboring Classes" (1840), in which he wrote: "Health is the working man's fortune and he ought to watch over it more than the capitalist over his largest investments. Health lightens the efforts of the body and mind."[4] Channing also supported the movement in the popular press to discuss issues in health and physiology. Although known best for his dynamic liberal and social activist preaching, he was a shy man, uncomfortable in social situations, who rarely visited the sick and distressed.

Octavius Brooks Frothingham (1822–1895) described how the vestiges of Calvinism were softened but still part of the ministry of his father at Boston's First Church (Unitarian). The senior Frothingham's life

> was consumed in services to individual souls, rendered in public and private. [His] diary has in it nothing but records of prayers with the sick, visits of consolation to the afflicted, ministrations of hope to the dying, benedictions over the dead, words of admonition or cheer for those entering upon the duties of existence. . . . The religion was essentially the old one, softened by thought, knowledge, experience, feeling; a faith rather than a creed, a sentiment more than a dogma . . . a religion of the heart.[5]

Frothingham's description documents specifically the daily tasks of caring and curing in a typical Unitarian parish ministry in the 1830s where Channing's most significant preaching, published in six volumes, documents the expressed ideas of the new faith.

Horace Mann (1786–1859), a devoted member of Channing's church who helped to reform the American education system, also expressed deep concern about issues of health and well-being. His essay on "The Laws of Physical Life," included in one of his annual reports as Massachusetts Secretary of Education, prompted the physician Edward Jarvis (1803–1884), himself a Unitarian, to review the essay for the Unitarian journal, the *Christian Examiner,* in an article that explored the relation of science to religion. In discussing each person's responsibility to care for the body, Jarvis wrote that "our health and comfort, our fulness and power of life depend on our faithful discharge of that responsibility, on our fulfillment of the conditions of our earthly existence, and that from our unfaithfulness . . . from the laws of our being, come our pains, our ailments and our early death."[6]

Jarvis explicitly rejected a still prevailing Calvinist view that because life is a mystery and diseases are God's chastening, "all attempts to increase our strength or protract our life will be but an ineffectual struggle against the Almighty."[7] Although he recognized God as the source of our being, he believed that "God has put our lives, partially at least, into our own hands." Believing that nothing in life was left to chance and that God's laws were fixed, Jarvis attributed the causes of premature death to the breaking of the physical laws of health, by overexertion, for example. In a marvelous passage he argued that "A multitude, crowded into a church to hear the gospel preached, suffer as surely from the corrupted and carbonized air as a crowd at the theater, listening to profaneness or looking upon sin."[8] Through the efforts of persons such as Mann and Jarvis, by 1840 the focus of issues of health and well-being had shifted to environment and personal responsibility outside of any specifically religious context.

The Unitarian minister Charles Follen, a German immigrant professor at Harvard, introduced athletics and gymnastics into the curriculum after 1825. One of his students described how physical fitness entered the curriculum:

> The Delta, where Memorial Hall now stands, was furnished with masts, parallel bars and the then usual variety of apparatus for athletic training and exercise. . . . We exercised under Dr. Follen's instruction and supervision. He taught us to run with a minimum of fatigue, with body thrown slightly forward, the arms akimbo, and breathing only through the nose.

Follen's ideas on physical fitness and exercise seemed deeply to influence the early generations of ministers and were further developed by ministers such as Theodore Parker and Thomas Wentworth Higginson. The latter's *Outdoor Papers*, published in 1863, included chapters on "Physical Courage," "The Health of Our Girls," "Gymnastics," and "Letters to a Dyspeptic."[9] The notion of exercise and fitness was naturally a part of taking responsibility for health.

Channing's sermon on the occasion of the death of Follen (killed accidently in January 1840) set out a Unitarian position on suffering attributing it in part to human ignorance and guilt. Life, he declared,

> has a heavy burden . . . deep wounds for each; and I state that we may . . . understand that suffering is not accidental, but designed for us, that

it enters into God's purpose . . . God intends that we shall suffer (because) . . . every organ of the body in consequence of the delicacy of its structure, and its susceptability of influences from abroad becomes an inlet of acute pain. . . . There are still deeper pains, those of conscience . . . when startled by new revelations of slighted duties, of irreparable wrongs to man, of base unfaithfulness to God. . . . Thus suffering comes from and through our whole nature.[10]

Decades before the advent of modern psychology, Channing demonstrated here a remarkably sophisticated understanding of the inner workings of the human body and spirit, explaining pain or evil as resulting from a falling away of God's standards.

Channing addressed the meaning of death in his 1834 Easter sermon, "The Future Life," using as a text, *Ephesians* 1:20, "he raised him from the dead, and set him at his right hand in heavenly places." The text itself gives an indication of the seriousness with which Channing and his contemporaries took such scriptural passages. In this case, we have not only the sermon itself, but also the reaction of Horace Mann, who was sitting in the pews that Sunday grieving over the death of his first wife. When the virtuous die, Channing explained, they join Christ to experience unutterable happiness. While death severs a deceased person's ties to the world, it does not obliterate that person, for a new channel of love is opened to the survivor. Describing a state of being after death in which the best conditions of life on earth would be continued, Channing taught that the deceased would find bliss both in Christ and in God. Channing's scribe, Elizabeth Peabody (1804–1894), reported that Mann was "lost in exaultation" and that the sermon "gave laws to the imagination and landmarks to the affections" he had never known before—thus providing evidence of the effectiveness of Channing's message on the meaning of death and immortality for a parishioner personally struggling with the issue.[11]

The widely read *Christian Examiner,* a major Unitarian publication, covered a broad range of religiously related issues. Published between 1824 and the 1860s, it frequently carried articles on health and medicine. Universalist journals such as *The Ladies' Repository* and the *Universalist Quarterly* regularly addressed theological issues from a more popular viewpoint than that found in the *Christian Examiner.* One piece from *The Repository,* "Reflections Upon Death" (1839), stated that it was natural to fear death, but that the gloom associated with the Calvinist attitude toward death should no longer concern Universalists. Another article appearing in the same year, "Unavoidable Evils," described old age and death as inevitable: "The good and the wise will not call them evils, they belong to our present state of existence and we take them as an inheritance." However, the author argued that sickness and bodily pain are not inevitable, for no calamity is certain "until we have taken every effort to remove it."[12] In one sermon published by the American Unitarian Association in 1833, the Reverend Orville Dewey observed that "mistaken and exaggerated ideas of the evil of death tend evidently to prevent the calm and settled expectation of dying, and rational and just views of the preparation for it."[13]

Unitarianism and the Medical World of Boston

Unitarianism achieved its greatest strength among the business and professional leaders of Boston. In fact, one historian has referred to Unitarianism as "the Boston religion."[14] Although the establishment of such institutions as Harvard Medical School (1782) and the Massachusetts General Hospital (1821) predated the impact of organized Unitarianism or Universalism in Boston, it is of significance that the liberal Reverend John Bartlett (1784–1849), chaplain of the city's only almshouse, led the campaign for a major hospital, which became Massachusetts General, and was responsible, in 1818, for organizing the McLean Asylum for the Insane.[15] There is no question that the physicians promoting these new medical institutions—the same men who founded the antecedent of the *New England Journal of Medicine*—were personally shaped by the post-Puritan ethic preached from liberal Christian pulpits throughout the area. This ethic was derived from a sense of "noblesse oblige," a conviction that the well-to-do had a responsibility to support social and cultural institutions.[16]

According to one scholar, the medical and cultural institutions of Boston were linked "by structure, operations and personnel."[17] The evidence suggests that the dominant medical group centered on Massachusetts General Hospital, just as the Unitarian cultural group centered on the Boston Atheneum (library) and Lowell Institute (lecture center). The city's medical and cultural circles intersected significantly: some forty-six percent of the boards of trustees of these Unitarian-founded institutions served both the library and hospital between 1820 and 1850, and forty-three percent of the Boston Dispensary trustees from 1800 to 1860 were also members or relatives of members of the Massachusetts Historical Society. Because of the links between Unitarianism and the city's emerging institutions, the spiritual message that influenced liberal Christians in the pew cannot be separated from the apparently secular medical institutions of their central community.

Medical and Social Reform

Unitarian and Universalist attitudes toward life and death and the institutions that grew from the active presence of the new liberal faith required a specific program of outreach. Involvement in domestic missionary work was best exemplified in the ministry of Joseph Tuckerman (1778–1840) to the poor and immigrant peoples in Boston, a work begun in 1825 that still functions under its original name, the Benevolent Fraternity of Unitarian and Universalist churches. The effectiveness of Tuckerman's inner-city mission in Boston was clearly evident from the spread of such ministries to Portsmouth, Baltimore, and other cities. Tuckerman's visit to British Unitarians in 1833–1834 led to the creation of similar domestic missions to the poor and unchurched in ten major English cities.[18]

With fellow Unitarians such as Horace Mann, Dorothea Dix (1802–1887), and physician Samuel Gridley Howe (1801–1876), Channing built bridges between the medical and pastoral professions, attempting as a liberal Christian to reach beyond the parish to the fields of education and care for the mentally ill, the blind, and the retarded. Howe, who with his wife Julia Ward Howe attended James Freeman Clarke's Church of the Disciples, had served as a physician to the Greeks in their war against the Turks. On returning to Boston he was encouraged to apply his skills to working with the blind. The establishment of the New England Institute for the Blind in 1831 was the direct result of his work and demonstrates the application of moral principles preached from Unitarian and Universalist pulpits addressing societal needs. Physician Samuel Woodward, first superintendent of the Worcester State Hospital in Massachusetts, though a Connecticut congregationalist, "accepted the prevailing faith in the perfectability of man" and was both influenced and supported in his work by Channing and Mann.[19] Woodward advocated "moral treatment" for the insane, emphasizing the importance of environmental influences in treating the mentally ill. Edward Jarvis also promoted moral therapy, and helped to develop a public health program in Massachusetts. A founder of the American Statistical Association, Jarvis worked to define diseases clearly and precisely. His biographer described his work as embodying "many of the intellectual, social and religious currents of his age . . . unifying knowledge with morality and reason."[20]

About 1840 a new movement, Transcendentalism, based on idealism rather than the philosophy of reason and sensation, arose within Unitarianism, offering a strong criticism of the perceived sterile life of the churches. Although Transcendentalism is more often identified as a literary movement led by Bronson Alcott, Ralph Waldo Emerson, Henry David Thoreau, and Margaret Fuller, the movement also emerged as a left wing of Unitarianism. The Reverend Theodore Parker (1810–1859), a leading proponent of Transcendentalism, combined his theological views with radical social action. In his *Lessons from the World of Matter and Man,* an anthology of essays, he asserted that "no Hebrew or Christian revelation shall make me doubt the infinite loving-kindness of God to saint and to sinner, too."[21] In the same essay, Parker criticized St. Paul for his "false estimate of the body." To Paul's statement "I know there is no good thing in my flesh," Parker responded vigorously: "He knew nothing like it. . . . God put no bad thing there; it is full of good things. . . . Do you think God in making man gave him a body that was fit to be trod only under foot, with no good thing in it?"[22] Reiterating the common Unitarian and Universalist belief that "old age is the only natural death, the only one that is unavoidable and must remain so," Parker concluded that "as virtue is the ideal life of man, so is old age the ideal death."[23]

Parker and Ralph Waldo Emerson (1803–1882), the Transcendentalist and former Unitarian minister, were highly critical of the views and practices held by a majority of Unitarians, who only twenty years earlier had been looked upon by Calvinists as radical. Many Transcendentalists, as well as others among the laity and clergy not necessarily identified with Transcendentalism, drew upon their strong reliance on individualism and reason as well as on their search for ideals to approach caring and curing in new and controversial ways.

Strong undercurrents associated with phrenology, spiritualism, and homeopathy emerged in both denominations. During her travels in America in 1834–1835, Harriet Martineau (1802–1876), a noted and controversial English Unitarian, called the attention of American liberal Christians to phrenology.[24] Johann Spurzheim, a German physician who helped develop phrenology, sufficiently impressed leaders of the liberal Christian community in New England that the membership of the Boston Phrenological Society read like a "Who's Who" of Unitarianism. Phrenology also found a sympathetic response among Unitarian psychiatrists and hopeful Universalists, for it provided a means of connecting mind and matter, teaching that mind was not a unit but composed of independent and identifiable faculties, located in different regions of the brain. This new science also taught that persons could cultivate different faculties by following the natural laws that governed physical development and human behavior. For phrenologically inclined psychiatrists, it offered a physical explanation for normal and abnormal functions of the brain. One historian of Universalism quotes a contemporary source: "One could hardly enter a Universalist minister's study but there hung a chart, or stood a bust like the guardian angel of the place, with the 'organs' all marked out and numbers on the cranium."

Spiritual healing became a major interest of a cross section of Universalists at mid-century. Three Universalist ministers became advocates and supporters of the first great American spiritualist, Andrew Jackson Davis (1826–1910), author of publications such as *The Great Harmonia, Concerning the Seven Mental States* (1852) and *The Principles of Nature: Her Revelations and a Voice to Mankind* (1847). In these works, Davis claimed to have received revelations in a mesmerized state, reflecting his skill as a medical clairvoyant. His journal, *The Univercoelumm,* numbered among its contributors mostly "ex-Universalist ministers or Swedenborgians." Although it may seem odd, the connection between Universalism and spiritualism emerged from four principles utilized to make spirit communication credible: "a rejection of supernaturalism, a firm belief in the inviolability of natural law, a reliance on external facts rather than on an inward state of mind, and a faith in the progressive development of knowledge."[25] That Davis's spiritualist teachings had a major impact is suggested by the fact that his volume *The Physician* went through ten editions by 1880.

Homeopathy, a popular mid-century medical sect, strongly influenced Universalists and Unitarians. Developed in Germany, homeopathy taught that a principle of vitalism pervaded and animated the body. Homeopathy utilized two approaches to healing: "like cures like" and the administration of diluted doses of medicines. Disease was not considered a separate entity affecting one specific organ, but a derangement of the "immaterial vital principle." The natural approach to healing found great appeal among Transcendentalists, who stood an ideological pole apart from the rational scientific approach of the great Boston and Harvard physicians. Homeopathy became a religious cause for some ministers, one of whom stated, "Religion itself has undergone a spiritual revolution since the date of [its] discovery." Another wrote that if homeopathy became the only medical method, "then, for the first time, will the Gospel of the Kingdom of Grace be preached, and received as God ordered it to be received."[26]

Among the patients of the homeopathic physician William Wesselhoeft were Theodore Parker, Bronson Alcott, Elizabeth Palmer Peabody, Julia Ward Howe, and Thomas Wentworth Higginson. Like the Unitarian Transcendentalists he served, Wesselhoeft was an optimist who stressed that "health and longevity were the normal state and natural right of the human race; that the healthy body would resist external causes of disease to an incalculable extent." He joined Universalists and Unitarians in espousing temperance, gymnastics, and hydropathy as well as homeopathy. One might well ask why such an outstanding group of New England leaders would turn to an alternative form of medicine hardly known today, when other members of their religious community remained in the forefront of scientific medicine in Boston. The answer would seem to lie in the very issues that separated the Transcendentalists from the Boston Unitarian establishment and interested them in the mystical teachings of Emmanuel Swedenborg about which Emerson had written. The emphasis here lay in "impatience with a mechanistic approach to the universe, a conviction that nature was an emanation of spirit, [and] a desire to unify experience." Going beyond the "common-sense" philosophy of reason and experience to a more meaningful idealism, they applied such principles to their lives by creating utopian communities such as Brook Farm and Fruitlands. In this context, it seems natural that homeopathy would appeal to them as a medical alternative.[27]

Oliver Wendell Holmes, Sr. (1809–1894), physician, author, lyceum lecturer, and sometime dean of Harvard Medical School, was an active Unitarian layman and friend to many of the Transcendentalists. When it came to the practice of medicine, Holmes stood clearly with the orthodox tradition and not with homeopathy. In a work entitled, "Homeopathy and its Kindred Delusions" (1842), he described homeopathy as a "mingled mass of perverse ingenuity, of tinsel erudition, of imbecile credulity, and of artful misrepresentation." Holmes's adamant opposition reflects his belief that the public was being seduced by many forms of medical quackery.[28]

Women and Health

Women in both liberal Christian movements played a significant role in the discussion of health and medical concerns. Elizabeth Blackwell (1821–1910), the first woman in America to receive an M.D. degree, was a close friend of the Reverend William Henry Channing (William Ellery Channing's nephew) and a member of his Cincinnati church. In 1871, she lectured on "The Religion of Health," which reflected both the religious concerns of liberal Christianity and the statistical approach to public health problems advocated by Jarvis and others in England and America. Stressing how health issues affected not only the poor but everyone, she wrote:

> Health depends upon the observance of all the laws of our complex nature; it applies to the mind as well as the body. . . . Hygiene is based upon the physical and moral perfectability of man, of which it furnishes the proof. Health may be described in two words—morality, competence.[29]

Blackwell also addressed issues pertaining to women's health care, including the hygienic advantages of sexual morality and the abuses of sex. In her book *Counsel to Parents on the Moral Education of their*

Children (1883), Blackwell advocated a direct and positive role for the church in sexual education. The church that allows such discussion "is bound to rouse every young man and woman of its congregation to the perception that respect for the ennobling principle of sex, with fidelity to purity, is a fundamental condition of religious life."[30]

Her sister-in-law, the Reverend Antoinette Brown Blackwell (1825–1921), one of the first women ministers, wrote extensively in her later career on issues concerning women's health and well-being. In *The Sexes Throughout Nature* (1875), she argued forcefully against the view that girls could not compete with boys and therefore did not deserve the same level of education.[31] Throughout her writings, Blackwell sought to reconcile her theological and feminist views with the teachings of Charles Darwin on biological evolution and Herbert Spencer on social evolution, views that caught the spirit of progressivist thinking in both denominations toward the end of the century.

Both the Unitarian and Universalist churches were alive with women in the cause of women's rights and health reform. Mary Livermore, Louisa May Alcott, and Clara Barton were among those most involved in hospital care during the Civil War.[32] The writings of these women and those of Susan B. Anthony, Julia Ward Howe, and Elizabeth Palmer Peabody, though not accepted by everyone in both churches, were widely known and appreciated. Mary Ellen Richmond (1861–1928), a Unitarian from Baltimore who developed her skills in a church-based social service organization, later developed the case-work method, spelled out in her book *Friendly Visiting Among the Poor,* for systematically dealing with the needs of the poor. Included are chapters on health, recreation, and the role of the church in contributing positively to organized charitable work.[33]

New Approaches

By the end of the nineteenth century, both Unitarianism and Universalism were so diverse one could argue that attitudes toward health, disease, and medicine among the membership were dictated more by general cultural forces than by influences within the churches themselves. On the controversial issues of birth control and contraception, differing views emerged. At the end of the 1870s, the Society for the Suppression of Vice in Boston actively supported the Comstock laws prohibiting distribution of contraceptives or educational materials on sexual matters. Although the Society was not itself Unitarian, it attracted the Reverend Edward Everett Hale and several Unitarian laymen who joined numerous religious conservatives in this cause. In Connecticut, Universalist layman and legislator Phineas T. Barnum (best known for his establishment of the circus) lobbied for a bill to prohibit the sale or distribution of contraceptive devices. The Free Religious Association, a radical progressive offshoot from Transcendentalism which invited the participation of all religious liberals, whether Christian or not, vigorously opposed the Comstock laws. The Reverend Francis Ellingwood Abbott (1836–1903), editor of the association's periodical, *The Index,* boldly defended Ezra Heywood and D.M. Bennett, who had been arrested for advocating birth control and marriage reform in the 1870s. Clearly there was no consensus about contraception and freedom of the press within the two denominations a century ago.[34] By the 1930s and 1940s, however, birth control advocate Margaret Sanger was preaching from Unitarian pulpits, and ministers and members were helping to found local chapters of Planned Parenthood. Some church buildings were even used for birth control clinics.

If there was a major medical outreach from Unitarianism, it was in the establishment of the U.S. Sanitary Commission, "Lincoln's Fifth Wheel," during the Civil War. Henry Whitney Bellows (1814–1882), minister of All Souls Unitarian Church in New York, responded to needs evident at the start of the war by working zealously with women's organizations to establish the Commission, a precursor of the American Red Cross, founded some years later by Universalist-born Clara Barton. The Sanitary Commission, when federally funded, was significantly over-represented by Unitarians. Because the Commission intended to be interdenominational rather than evangelical, it represented a liberal Christian approach in its national effort to care for the war wounded. A self-proclaimed Evangelical Sanitary Commission attacked the offical aid organization because of its strong Unitarian, Catholic, and Jewish participation.[35]

The development in the 1880s of a chair of Christian Social Ethics at Harvard Divinity School, to which Francis Greenwood Peabody (1847–1936) was appointed the first professor, was of true significance to the history of health care in the two denominations. Peabody, one of the first liberal Christian ministers and professors to systematically apply Christian principles to social problems, examined such questions as charity, temperance, labor, prisons, and divorce. Although he rarely addressed medical issues directly in his numerous writings,[36] Peabody influenced his successor at the Divinity School, the Unitarian physician Richard Clark Cabot (1868–1939), a member of Kings Chapel. While holding his professorship at the Divinity School from 1920–1933, Cabot also served on the faculty of Harvard Medical School and on the staff of the Massachusetts General Hospital, where he originated the patient-care conference as early as 1913. Between them, Cabot and Peabody taught several generations of Unitarian graduates at the Divinity School.[37]

In contrast to the Christian emphasis predominant at Harvard, a new religious humanism emerged within both traditions at the turn of the century, which attempted to speak to the world without reference to God, the scriptures of the past, traditional worship, or church structures. In 1933, thirty-four persons, thirteen of whom were Unitarian or Universalist ministers, signed a Humanist Manifesto which included at least three affirmations relating to health and well-being. One, rejecting the body–mind dualism, insisted "on an organic view of life." Another urged humanists to find religious emotion expressed in "a heightened sense of personal life and in a cooperative effort to promote social well-being." A third stressed "reasonable and manly attitudes" in pursuit of a "path of social and mental hygiene" while discouraging "sentimental hopes and wishful thinking."[38] Humanist Manifesto II, published in 1973, also included a number of Unitarian Universalist ministers, several of whom had signed the first document. One section, on "Ethics," focused on human autonomy and situational ethics, positions advocated by some liberal Christians in the health care field, but certainly not agreed upon by more conservative Unitarians and Universalists, who wanted their ethical standards to be more theologically grounded. One paragraph stressed the value and dignity of the individual, while another asserted unequivocally that the rights to sexual behavior in any form between consenting adults performed in the context of "intimacy, sensitivity, respect and honesty in interpersonal relations are encouraged." This broke ground for the later denominational support for the rights of gays and lesbians both as laypersons and clergy.

Principles and Programs in the Twentieth Century

Both Unitarian and Universalist denominations issued "declarations" at various times addressing the social and, by implication, the medical ills of society. For example, a 1917 Universalist Declaration called for "universal brotherhood" and an end to "the evils of unjust social and economic conditions which condemn one to be born in filth and squalor of the slums" while others were born amidst undeserved luxury. Included in this working program were safeguards to marriage so that every child "shall be born with sound physical, mental and moral heritage; to guarantee to every child the best conditions of housing, food, recreation and education; to create a maximum standard of living where limits are only set by capacity." In some ways these statements seem to reflect the eugenics movement with its concern for improved human development through heredity. In other ways, it reflected the continuing concern in the churches to improve social and environmental conditions in which everyone lived. This latter point was evident because the declaration also supported equal economic, social, and political rights for women; drew attention to the danger of drugs and tobacco in undermining the health and character of American youth; and called for a national prohibition on the manufacture and sale of liquor and severe restrictions on tobacco production. One section included a demand for some form of social insurance to replace individualistic and inadequate methods of charity.[39]

Throughout their histories, neither denomination actively developed programs in foreign missions. Although each began with considerable enthusiasm and attracted numerous adherents, American and English religious liberals generally believed that active evangelism was inappropriate. They did support missions in India, Japan, and the Sandwich Islands—but with the aim of educating, not converting. Perhaps the closest to a mission program were the two service committees set up to aid refugees from the Spanish Civil War in France as well as others during the Second World War, but now merged and operated almost entirely on a professional basis. More recently, medical missions have been part of the service committee's work in Africa, the Caribbean, Europe, and among native Americans. Using a style of operation developed prior to the Peace Corps, the committee sent teams to specific villages to provide nutritional, public health, and medical training. Recently, a large grant has provided special services to women and children in India. The motivation behind these activities was the Unitarian Universalist commitment to helping people help themselves.[40]

Since 1945, the denominationally supported yet independent Beacon Press has regularly published controversial books in fields related to health care, medicine, and women's issues as well as in theology, politics, and sociology. Although many of these publications have been neither by nor specifically for church members, they have been sold at church bookstores and have come to the attention of church members through denominational publications. Because such books as *Morals and Medicine* (1954) by Episcopalian minister Joseph Fletcher, *Human Guinea Pigs* (1968) by British physician Maurice Pappworth, and *Explaining Death to Children* (1967), edited by Reform Rabbi Earl Grollman, have addressed religious and medical issues from a liberal religious viewpoint, they seem to have precluded the need for Unitarian Universalists to write such books for themselves. This is not to say that the denomination has not developed religious education materials and pamphlets on these subjects. However, because it has derived so much religious sustenance on biomedical issues from Reform Judaism, Ethical Culture, and various secular sources, it has not actively encouraged the exploration of such topics within its own ranks.[41]

Concern for the affective life of church members has developed significantly during the past two decades. Many ministers have received accreditation as pastoral counsellors; and the criticism of social ethicist James Luther Adams that the strong emphasis on reason throughout Unitarian Universalist history inhibited many members from coming to terms with the emotional side of their being has become increasingly less valid.[42]

Both denominations have taken progressive positions on such issues as mental health, gay rights, abortion, and death and dying well ahead of other groups affiliated with the National Council of Churches. The Reverend Stephen Fritchman, for example, received national attention in 1963 because of his campaign for reform of funeral practices instigated by Jessica Mitford's best-seller, *The American Way of Death.* The Reverend Donald McKinney serves as president of Concern for Dying and was appointed in 1984 to Governor Mario Cuomo's task force studying life support and the terminally ill in New York State. The Legislative Conference of Unitarians and Universalists in Maryland (LEGICUUM), which meets annually, devoted its 1984 meeting to the discussion of medical ethical issues with legislators and scholars.

In the years immediately following the merger in 1961, general resolutions passed at General Assemblies frequently dealt with such pressing issues as civil rights and the Vietnam War, but in 1964, the General Assembly also called for Congress to vote for Medicare. The meetings in 1971 and 1979 focused on the need for a national health plan. Many resolutions in the 1970s addressed environmental problems, urging stricter enforcement of existing clean air acts and proposing a system for universal education on the world ecological crisis.

Resolutions favoring the legalization of abortion, an issue tied closely to women's rights, have passed General Assembly numerous times; a 1963 resolution, ten years before the Supreme Court legalized abortion in the *Roe v. Wade* decision allowing control over abortion to rest with a woman and her physician, called for enactment of a uniform statute making abortion legal except when performed by someone unqualified. The creation in the early 1980s of an Abortion Task Force by the First Unitarian Society of Madison, Wisconsin, demonstrated that a thoughtful and democratic study of the issue could involve many members of the church. The congregation stood at neither extreme on the issue, but preferred to see abortion used only when truly necessary and without undue restrictive discrimination against those unable to pay for needed abortions.[43]

Although Unitarian Universalists have often discussed biomedical issues in denominational pamphlets and ministerial sermons—and perhaps more so now than in the past, because women fill fifteen percent of all pulpits—there are few clearcut positions to which all members subscribe. Individual freedom and commensurate responsibility still remain at the core of theological understanding and hence at the core of ethical action as well.

Notes

The authors wish to offer their gratitude to the following persons for their assistance in various aspects of the research of this project: The Reverend Alan Seaburg, archivist of the Unitarian Universalist collection at Harvard Divinity School's Andover Harvard Library; Dr. Conrad Wright, Professor of American Church History at Harvard; Eugene Taylor; Sanbourne Bockhoven, M.D.; Anne Rose, Ph.D.; Catherine Albanese, Ph.D.; Gerald Grob, Ph.D.; Robert Webb, Ph.D.; Russell Miller, Ph.D.; and the Reverend William C. Saunders.

1. Daniel Howe, *The Unitarian Conscience: Harvard Moral Philosophy, 1805–1861* (Cambridge, MA, 1970).
2. For Rush's views, see Carl Binger, *Revolutionary Doctor: Benjamin Rush 1746–1813* (New York, 1966), pp. 182 and 194. Rush's statement quoted in *Universalism in America: A Documentary History of a Liberal Faith,* ed. Ernest Cassara (Boston, 1971), p. 92.
3. Hosea Ballou, *Treatise on the Atonement,* quoted in *Universalism in America,* ed. Cassara, p. 98.
4. William Ellery Channing, "On the Elevation of the Laboring Classes," in *The Works of William E. Channing, D.D.* (Boston, 1885), pp. 59–60.
5. O.B. Frothingham, *Boston Unitarianism: 1820–1859* (New York, 1890), p. 37.
6. Edward Jarvis, "Law of Physical Life," *Christian Examiner* 17 (September 1843):1–31.
7. Ibid., p. 2.
8. Ibid., p. 21.
9. Andrew Preston Peabody, *Harvard Reminiscences* (Boston, 1888); Thomas Wentworth Higginson, *Outdoor Papers* (Boston, 1863).
10. William Ellery Channing, "A Discourse Occasioned by the Death of the Reverend Dr. Follen," in *The Works of William Ellery Channing,* pp. 608–609.
11. William Ellery Channing, "The Future Life," in *The Works of William Ellery Channing,* pp. 359–366. For Mann's reaction to the sermon, see Jonathan Messerli, *Horace Mann: A Biography* (New York, 1972), pp. 178–179.
12. "Reflections Upon Death," *Ladies Repository* 8 (July, 1839):214; "Unavoidable Evils," ibid., p. 214.
13. Orville Dewey, *On Erroneous Views of Death* (Boston, 1833), p. 6.
14. E. Digby Baltzell, *Puritan Boston and Quaker Philadelphia* (New York, 1979), p. 199.
15. A brief biography of Bartlett appears in Samuel A. Eliot, *Heralds of a Liberal Faith: The Pioneers* (Boston, 1910), pp. 179–184.
16. See Baltzell's chapter on "The Learned Professions," *Puritan Boston,* pp. 355–356 for a discussion of Boston's Unitarian physicians.
17. Ronald Story, *The Forging of an Aristocracy* (Middletown, CT) p. 18; see also pp. 162, 172–173.

18. See Daniel T. McColgan, *Joseph Tuckerman: Pioneer in American Social Work* (Washington, DC, 1940); and Channing's tribute to Tuckerman in *The Works of William E. Channing,* pp. 578–599. Tuckerman's annual reports exist in pamphlet form. On the domestic ministry in Liverpool, see Ann Holt, *A Ministry to The Poor* (Liverpool, 1936).

19. On the liberal Christian role in moral treatment, see J. Sanbourne Bockhoven, "The Unitarian Contribution to the Early History of American Psychiatry," *Proceedings of the Unitarian Historical Society,* XII, 2, (1959), 1–7. On the connections between Woodward, Channing and Mann, see Gerald Grob, *The State and the Mentally Ill* (Chapel Hill, NC, 1966), p. 44.

20. See Gerald Grob, *Edward Jarvis and the Medical World of the Nineteenth Century* (Knoxville,TN, 1978), p. 69.

21. Theodore Parker, "The Nature of Man," in *The World of Matter and Man* (Boston, 1910), p. 47. Emerson's essays on "Old Age" and "Immortality" will be of interest as well. See *The Complete Works of Ralph Waldo Emerson,* Centenary Edition, ed. Edward Waldo Emerson, 12 vols. (Boston and New York, 1903–1904).

22. Parker, *The World of Matter and Man,* p. 64.

23. Ibid., p. 65.

24. Harriet Martineau, *Society in America,* 2 vols., (London, 1837).

25. Critical discussion of phrenology appeared twice in *The Christian Examiner* in 1834: The first essay was a review article by psychiatrist Isaac Ray of George Combe's *A System of Phrenology* (May 1834), pp. 221–248, and the second a review of Spurzheim's *Phrenology or the Doctrine of Mental Phenomena* (November 1834). For the role of Universalists in phrenology and spiritualism, see Russell Miller, *The Larger Hope,* vol. 1 (Boston, 1979), pp. 222–225. See also J. William Broadway, "Universalist Participation in the Spiritualist Movement of the Nineteenth Century," *Proceedings of the Unitarian Universalist Historical Society,* XIX, Part 1 (1980–1981), pp. 1–15.

26. Joseph Kett, *The Formation of the American Medical Profession: The Role of Institutions, 1780–1860* (New Haven, CT, 1968), p. 139.

27. Ibid., pp. 135, 153–154.

28. See E.M. Tilton, *Amiable Autocrat: A Biography of Dr. Oliver Wendell Holmes* (New York, 1947); and Oliver Wendell Holmes, "Homeopathy and Its Kindred Delusions," in *Medical Essays: 1842–1882* (Boston, 1891). For a fascinating discussion of life in the Boston Unitarian and reforming community in this period, see also Julia Ward Howe, *Reminiscences* (Boston, 1899).

29. Elizabeth Blackwell, "The Religion of Health," in *Essays in Medical Sociology* (London, 1902), pp. 228–229.

30. Elizabeth Blackwell, *Counsel to Parents on the Moral Education of their Children* (New York, 1883), p. 153.

31. Antoinette Brown Blackwell, *The Sexes Throughout Nature* (New York, 1875), p. 153.

32. See Mary A. Livermore, *My Story of the War: A Woman's Narrative of Four Year's Personal Experience* (Hartford, CT, 1890); and Louisa May Alcott, *Hospital Sketches* (1863).

33. Mary Ellen Richmond, *Friendly Visiting Among the Poor* (New York, 1906).

34. The best description of these events is in Carol Flora Brooks, "The Early History of Anti-Contraceptive Law in Massachusetts and Connecticut," *American Quarterly* 18 (1966):3–23. For the history of the Free Religious Association, see Stow Persons, *Free Religion* (New Haven, CT, 1947).

35. W.Q. Maxwell, *Lincoln's Fifth Wheel: The Political History of the United States Sanitary Commission* (New York, 1956). For a perspective from within the tradition, see Walter Donald Kring, *Henry Whitney Bellows* (Boston, 1979).

36. Among F.G. Peabody's works relevant to this study are *Jesus Christ and the Social Question* (New York, 1906) and *Reminiscences of Present Day Saints* (Boston, 1927), containing short biographies of James Freeman Clarke, Edward Everett Hale, Charles Follen, and others.

37. Among the more relevant writings of Richard C. Cabot are *Social Service and the Art of Healing* (New York, 1909), *Social Work* (Boston, 1919), *The Art of Ministering to the Sick* (New York, 1936), and *Christianity and Sex* (New York, 1937).

38. For a recent study of the three most significant early humanist ministers, see Mason Olds, *Religious Humanism in America: Dietrich, Reese and Potter* (Washington, DC, 1978). The texts of *Humanist Manifestos I and II* have been republished by Prometheus Books (Buffalo, 1973) in pamphlet form.

39. "A Declaration of Social Principles," *The Universalist Leader* 99 (November 3, 1917):6. See also Hugh Emerson Lalone, *And Thy Neighbor as Thyself* (Boston, 1939), for a discussion of social outreach in Universalist history.

40. For a detailed history of the missions in India, see Spencer Lavan, *Unitarianism and India: A Study in Encounter and Response* (Boston, 1977).

41. A survey of press publications since 1945 indicates an increasingly high number of books on health and medicine. Two recent exceptions to the generalization that Unitarian Universalists are not publishing in this field are the books by ministers on marriage and sexuality, Ronald Mazur, *Common Sense Sex* (Boston, 1973) and David Sammons, *The Marriage Option* (Boston, 1977).

42. See James Luther Adams, *On Being Human Religiously* (Boston, 1976), p. 42. See also Carl Wennerstrom's essays in *Pastoral Care in the Liberal Churches,* eds. James Luther Adams and Seward Hiltner (Nashville, 1970).

43. The texts of all resolutions passed by the General Assembly since merger are in the Unitarian Universalist Association Directory for the following year. For a Unitarian defense of a right-to-life position, see George Huntston Williams "The Social, Theological, and Biological Context of Abortion," *Linacre Quarterly* 50, (1983):335–354. Williams develops the ethical model he calls "the sacred condominium" in another article, "Safer Footing than Blind Reason, Stumbling Without Fear: Reflections on Bioethics in our Civic, Religious, Historical, Professional Context," in Leonard J. Nelson, ed., *The Death Decision* (Ann Arbor, MI, 1984), pp. 127–179.

CHAPTER 13

The Disciples of Christ-Church of Christ Tradition

DAVID EDWIN HARRELL, JR.

The Disciples of Christ is an American-born religious group formed in 1832 by the merging of the Christian movement led by Barton Stone (1772–1844) and the Reforming Baptists led by Thomas Campbell (1763–1854) and his son, Alexander Campbell (1788–1866). Most of the early leaders of the movement, including Stone and the Campbells, had been Presbyterians. Stone was one of the promoters of the Great Revival in the West in the early nineteenth century. Distressed by Presbyterian opposition to the revival, in 1804 Stone and five other Kentucky ministers left the church, announcing in a statement called "The Last Will and Testament of the Springfield Presbytery" their intention to be "Christians only."

Thomas Campbell came to America in 1807, having been a minister in Northern Ireland. Disturbed by the sectarian spirit of American Presbyterians, Campbell clashed with the Synod, and in 1809 he was suspended from the ministry. Campbell and a few of his friends then formed the Christian Association of Washington (Pennsylvania), and he wrote a fifty-six–page explanation of his views entitled *The Declaration and Address* (1809). Alexander Campbell arrived in America shortly after the publication of his father's views. Twenty-one years old at the time, Alexander Campbell had been influenced by the reforming ideas of Scottish evangelist Robert Haldane while studying for a year in Glasgow, and he immediately embraced his father's independent position. Within a few years he became the unquestioned leader of the movement. The Campbells associated with the Baptist church from 1815 to 1830; during that time their followers were generally called Reformers.

Preaching similar pleas for Christian union and in frequent contact with one another in Kentucky, the Stone and Campbell movements sealed a remarkably successful union in 1832. Alexander Campbell favored the name Disciples of Christ, while the Stone churches generally called themselves the Christian Church. Many local congregations were known as Churches of Christ. All three names have been used throughout the movement's history. The new church spread rapidly with the westward migration of population; at the time of the union in 1832 it had an estimated 22,000 members, and by 1860 that figure had grown to about 200,000.

Two ideas undergirded Disciples' thought, both of them highly marketable amid the optimism on the American frontier in the 1830s. First was an emphasis on Christian union. Second was a call for the "restoration of the ancient order of things," a plea to return to New Testament Christianity. The Disciples were New Testament primitivists, believing that they could find there a pattern for all Christian behavior. The watchword of the movement, stated in 1809 by Thomas Campbell, was "where the Scriptures speak, we speak; and where the Scriptures are silent, we are silent." From the "Last Will and Testament of the Springfield Presbytery," which urged all men to take "the Bible as the only sure guide to heaven," to the statement in the *Declaration and Address,* which defined the aim of the Christian Association of Washington as "promoting a pure evangelical reformation, by the simple preaching of the everlasting gospel, and the administration of its ordinances in an exact conformity to the Divine Standard," Disciples worked to discover the apostolic patterns that would bring a millennium of Christian unity.[1]

While conceiving of themselves as protesters against sectarian division, the Disciples quickly became a part of the denominational competition in the American Midwest and South. Alexander Campbell's influence was particularly strong among the Baptists, and in some areas of the West the new movement devastated Baptist associations. The church spread rapidly westward from Ohio and Kentucky and as far south as Tennessee and Texas.

The years after the Civil War form a second epoch in Disciples' history. The religious census of 1906 revealed that the church had grown to about 1,150,000 members, but it also reported the completion of a schism that separated perhaps fifteen percent of the membership from the main body. The dissenting churches (which generally used the name Churches of Christ) were predominantly southern, rural, and poor.

While the tensions of the late nineteenth century had clear sectional and social underpinnings, the dividing of the movement also had a doctrinal focus. Conservative Disciples increasingly lost interest in Christian union as an impractical ideal; liberal Disciples discarded legalistic restorationism as an impractical and divisive strategy. The most visible issues that divided churches were support for the missionary society which had been founded in 1849 and the scripturality of the use of instrumental music in worship.

In the absence of authoritative denominational organizations, editors of religious papers played important roles as leaders of the Disciples of Christ. The most powerful journal during the late nineteenth century was the *Christian Standard* (1866–present), established in 1866 in Cincinnati by Isaac Errett (1820–1888). The most influential journal among the conservatives of the South was the *Gospel Advocate* (1855–present), edited for over half a century by David Lipscomb (1831–1917) in Nashville, Tennessee. By the end of the century, however, leadership of the movement had fallen into the hands of James H. Garrison (1842–1931), who in 1874 became editor of the *Christian–Evangelist* (1863–present), which was published in St. Louis. Garrison was grounded in the nuances of Disciples theology, but he was irenic in spirit and encouraged a new generation of Disciples leaders (including his son, Winfred Ernest) to reestablish contact with the mainstream of American Protestantism.

In the early twentieth century, the Disciples suffered a second major division and a slowing growth rate. As a new generation of Disciples liberals (particularly a group associated with the University of Chicago) pushed for a more ecumenical view of the church's mission and a more liberal understanding of the Scriptures, conservative opposition solidified around the *Christian Standard.* In the 1920s the conservatives began withdrawing support from Disciples organizations and in 1927 established a rival North American Christian Convention. The conservative congregations, loosely affiliated in the Undenominational Fellowship of Christian Churches and Churches of Christ, in 1979 had an estimated membership of about 1,050,000. By that date the membership of the noninstrumental music Churches of Christ had reached an estimated 1,600,000.

The more liberal wing of the movement, which used the name the Christian Church (Disciples of Christ), had a membership of 1,231,061 in 1979. That church had developed a full body of boards and commissions in the twentieth century, headquartered mostly in Indianapolis and St. Louis. In 1968 the church restructured into a representative and more centrally controlled organization, losing perhaps one-third of its listed congregations in the move and completing the second schism, which had been in progress since the 1920s. Liberal Disciples have been important leaders in modern ecumenical activities. The *Christian Century* began as a Disciples journal (founded as the *Christian Oracle* in 1884), and its editorial corps was long dominated by Disciples.

First generation leaders of the Disciples of Christ were almost entirely preoccupied with the doctrinal questions implicit in the restoration of the ancient order of things. One historian wrote,

> Disciples in the earlier period had special reasons for aloofness from social problems, and even for hesitating to make positive pronouncements on disputable questions of personal conduct. The primary reason was their concentration on restoring the unity and the apostolic order of the church and on the conversion of individuals according to the spiritual "plan of salvation."[2]

In perhaps the most important statement of his beliefs, *The Christian System,* published in 1839, Alexander Campbell only passingly alluded to the moral and ethical content of Christian thought.[3]

If Disciples leaders said little specifically about the relationship of Christianity to one's health and well-being, they shared many orthodox Christian understandings with other American evangelical Protestants, which flavored their views about life and death. All of the church's early leaders acknowledged that much of the Christian message was practical and personal; some feared that the movement had been too singularly devoted to doctrinal reform. In 1833 Barton Stone warned of the "danger of dwelling too long upon doctrinal disquisitions, to the neglect of practical piety" and challenged his readers to "labor to have our own hearts and lives reformed."[4] In *The Christian System,* Campbell confirmed the importance of moral principles: "If I were to classify in *three* chapters the whole Christian institution, after the fashion of the modern schools, . . . I would designate them Christian *faith,* Christian *worship,* and Christian *morality.*"[5]

Influenced by the Scottish Common Sense philosophy of the nineteenth century, most early Disciples leaders were convinced that all nature, including humans, was governed by God's natural law and that revelation and experience taught men how to relate harmoniously with that law. Alexander Campbell developed a full-blown philosophy that called for educating the "whole man": "True science affirms that all that is in man, and only what is in him, is to be educated; that every organ and sense and power, whether animal, intellectual, moral or religious, can be improved, and ought to be improved by education."[6] The preservation of physical health, while rarely discussed at any length, was the assumed responsibility of Christians. While the "animal" nature of humanity was the lowest of God-given attributes, it was important in God's scheme of things: "The human soul incarnate operates only through organs, and through organs only can it be operated on."[7] Respect for God's moral law was crucially important to one's physical well-being:

If this be apparent to the philosopher, who sees the bearings of physical nature upon the physical and moral constitution of man, much more evident is it to the student of the Bible, that the violation of moral principle, not only in consequence of the constitution of the realms of nature, but also and more especially in pursuance of every divine law and institution, must be accompanied with pain.[8]

The rationalistic, natural-law orientation of early Disciples leaders guarded the movement against the pseudo-scientific health movements of the nineteenth century. In an 1852 lecture, Campbell lionized inductive science and denounced as fraudulent "phrenology, animal magnetism, clairvoyance, spiritual rappings, etc."[9] While a few early Disciples preachers (most notably Barton Stone) believed that miraculous healing could be restored to the church, most Disciples accept a dispensational interpretation of the Bible that connected miracles with revelation and discounted all claims of present divine intervention with natural law.[10] Campbell believed that the rise of modern science was inseparably connected with the rise of Protestantism. He regarded Roman Catholicism as a haven of superstition and irrational thought; in 1837 he debated Bishop John Purcell of Cincinnati in one of the most famous Protestant–Catholic confrontations of the nineteenth century.[11] The light of reason applied to natural law and to revelation, Campbell believed, would lead to personal and social happiness.

One other idea important in the thought of first-generation Disciples leaders was an optimistic postmillennialism, which they shared with many other evangelical Christians of their day. Disciples have always held disparate views of the millennium, and after the Civil War millennial ideas had little effect on the movement. A few early Disciples leaders flirted with the fervent premillennial enthusiasm connected with William Miller's prediction that Christ would return to earth in the 1840s, but for the most part they embraced the optimistic hope that the United States would lead the world into a period of political, religious, and moral enlightenment which would introduce the desired reign of Christ on earth. While Campbell vacillated in his views of the millennium, and with the approach of the Civil War despaired of any hope for an early reign of justice and peace, he nonetheless believed that it was God's will to relieve human suffering and establish social peace. When his magazine, the *Millennial Harbinger* (1830–1866), was launched in 1830, included among its objectives was "to develop the powers of the human mind, and to prepare man for rational and social happiness."[12]

Employing these general assumptions, Disciples leaders wrote occasionally on subjects relating to health and well-being, though often their beliefs appeared only as hidden assumptions encased in doctrinal pronouncements. In an address on "Life and Death" Campbell labored mostly to destroy the theories of "soul-sleeping" and "purgatory" before finally concluding that the "sublime, awful and tremendous" meaning of death was summed up in the contemplation of "salvation and damnation."[13] The subject of marriage was discussed frequently in Disciples papers (and was even more frequently a matter of concern in the records of the local churches), but almost invariably the discussions were doctrinal, treating such questions as the validity of marriage between Disciples and non-Disciples and the scriptural grounds for divorce.[14]

Early Disciples assumed that violations of God's moral law would inevitably result in "pain"; they often argued from that conviction to support other beliefs. For instance, in the midst of early nineteenth-century agitation for the government to stop the delivery of the mail on Sunday, Campbell opposed the restrictive legislation on the grounds that it discriminated against such minorities as Jews and constituted the establishment of religion.[15] On the other hand, most early Disciples agreed that Sunday laws, understood strictly as "human institutions," were reasonable and useful: "It gives necessary rest to men and beasts that labor, and tends to the adoption of regular habits."[16] Novel reading was condemned because it "dissipates and weakens the mind, and renders it unfit to investigate truth"; such "frivolities" as dancing were also judged to be dangerous to one's health.[17]

Early Disciples leaders commonly proscribed the use of tobacco—largely because they judged it to be unhealthful. One early preacher summarized his objections: "The injurious effects of tobacco are seen in its causing vomiting, purging, universal trembling, staggering, convulsions, languor, feebleness, relaxation of the muscles, great anxiety of mind and a tendency to faint, and blindness."[18] He also composed a quatrain about tobacco:

Tobacco is an Indian weed:
It was the Devil sowed the seed:
It drains your pocket, stains your clothes,
And makes a chimney of your nose.[19]

The moral issue that most clearly implicated the issue of health in the minds of most Disciples, and the issue that increasingly came to dominate the attention of church leaders, was drinking. Like most American Protestants in the nineteenth century, the Disciples at first showed only a mild interest in temperance reform, but by the 1850s they were actively supporting legal prohibition. There were many reasons for the growing support for the prohibition movement, including a burgeoning body of theological argument in its behalf and the increasing Protestant fear of Catholic immigration. But whatever the other reasons, Disciples vigorously supported their case with health arguments. While some of the older generation continued to demand "more cogent reasons and authoritative arguments than have as yet been given . . . to satisfy my mind that a *temperate* use of what is provided by an indulgent Providence is sinful," the dominant view came to be that alcohol was a "deadly poison."[20] In 1843, a Tennessee editor put the question in a millennial setting:

> *Christians,* is it not part of almost every prayer you offer, that God will soon open upon the world the millennial day? Are you acting in accordance with your prayers, by lending your influence to help forward this glorious cause of moral improvement [prohibition], which must prevail ere the millennium shall fully come? . . . Do you make the poison, or do you use it, or do you sell it? Never open your lips, then, to pray for the millennium.[21]

Probably the most important way in which Disciples' teaching effected the well-being of the church's early nineteenth-century members had to do with the structuring of local congregations. Throughout most of the nineteenth century, local churches were by far the most important organizational units in the movement, although a weak network of denominational institutions did begin to emerge in the middle of the century. Disciples leaders believed that a strong local congregation was at the heart of restoring New Testament Christianity. Early Disciples leaders argued that each local church was autonomous under the rule of its elders and should appoint deacons (and perhaps deaconesses) to care for the physical needs of its members. In an early article on New Testament church organization, Alexander Campbell wrote: "Christian congregations, in primitive times, had need of money or earthly things, as well as we. . . . A deacon or deacons had the charge of the treasury, and were ex-officio treasurers. . . . They were not only to take care of the contributions, but to dispense or appropriate them according to the directions of the brethren."[22]

The church record books of the early nineteenth century confirm that the elders in most local congregations not only scrutinized the moral condition of their members but their physical condition as well.[23] Frequently the women of a church met to "sew and make garments for the poor and needy" of the congregation.[24] Jessie B. Ferguson, minister of the strong Nashville, Tennessee, Disciples church, reported that his congregation had appointed "brethren and sisters in each ward [of the city], whose duty it is to visit once every week, every member of the church in their several wards, and report their temporal and spiritual condition upon every Lord's day. We may thus have a full report every week, so that no one suffers in our midst."[25] A visitor to the Disciples church in Walnut Grove, Illinois, described the benevolent program of that congregation:

> These same brethren have reared up two poor houses within the bounds of the congregation, where the old and the maimed who love and obey the Lord, find comfortable homes with a good supply of the good things of this world.—This looks like old-fashioned Christianity, and very unlike that cold hearted . . . policy so prevalent with many churches.[26]

The strong emphasis of the Disciples on the local congregation frequently flared into an outspoken anti-institutionalism. While a majority of the early leaders of the church were not opposed to religious societies and cooperation on doctrinal grounds, nearly all were highly suspicious of denominational organization. Most imbibed of the spirit expressed by Alexander Campbell in an early issue of the *Christian Baptist* (1823–1830):

> The early Christian churches were not fractured into missionary societies, Bible societies, education societies; nor did they dream of organizing such in the world. The head of a believing household was not in those days a president or manager of a board of foreign missions; his wife, the president of some female education society; his eldest son, the recording secretary of some domestic Bible society; his eldest daughter, the corresponding secretary of a mite society; his servant maid, the vice-president of a rag society. . . . They knew nothing of the hobbies of modern times. In their church capacity alone they moved.[27]

This anti-institutional bias, combined with the doctrinal preoccupation of the early years of Disciples history, seriously retarded the growth of benevolent and eleemosynary institutions in the movement.

These anti-institutional prejudices diminished somewhat in the 1840s; in 1849 a missionary society was formed with the tacit approval of Alexander Campbell. In 1846, Lewis L. Pinkerton, one of the most liberal thinkers among the first-generation Disciples leaders, established the Kentucky Female Orphan School in Midway, Kentucky, with the design of "clothing, feeding, and educating orphan girls."[28] Campbell commended the enterprise as "humane and Christian"; he believed it "would seem to merit the kind consideration of the philanthropic and wealthy portion of the Christian community."[29] The Kentucky school was the only benevolent institution successfully launched in the loosely knit movement in the years before the Civil War.

The Middle Period, 1865–1920

While still extremely interested in doctrinal questions, the second-generation leaders of the Disciples of Christ ranged wider in their theological and social probings than had the church's founders. Much of the earlier theological base remained clear—the emphasis on New Testament example, the appeal to reason and science—although the Civil War destroyed the optimistic postmillennialism of the early nineteenth century. But the most inauspicious development of the second generation was the growing diversity within the church. Doctrinal differences led to two schisms that left three distinct churches. It is not surprising that Disciples also came to speak more disparately about humans and their environment.

All Disciples continued to agree that health was a proper Christian concern. Most still believed that the principles of natural law governed physical health:

> If we did not violate the laws of nature, humanity would be largely free from the pains and aches, the debility and suffering, that now renders the existence of so many miserable. . . . It is not right to charge our afflications of body or mind, to the Lord. He does not willingly afflict any one; . . . it is as wrong for us, in the sight of God, to violate the physical, as it is the moral law.[30]

In some ways, Disciples' confidence in science reduced the importance of religion in human healing; the church increasingly looked upon physicians as God's healing instruments. "The Christian physician is as truly a messenger of God as the minister," wrote one editor. "The division of labor in divine things is recognized in the New Testament."[31]

Prohibition overshadowed all other social issues in late nineteenth- and early twentieth-century Disciples thought. In every wing of the dividing movement, the church's papers were flooded with articles urging support for the prohibition movement. In 1879 James H. Garrison, soon to be recognized as the foremost leader of the liberal element in the church, declared that "the question of American slavery was never anything but a baby by the side" of the prohibition of alcohol.[32] While the prohibition hysteria remained a complicated social phenomenon, it provided a platform for Disciples' most vocal proclamations on the sanctity of the human body. Almost uniformly, late nineteenth-century Disciples accepted the diagnosis that alcohol was a "violent poison."[33] D.R. Dungan, an Iowa preacher and probably the leading prohibition advocate of the late nineteenth century, warned that drinking was directly responsible for a long list of diseases and that it induced "insanity" and "mental disability and idiocy." While other arguments for the prohibition of alcohol abounded, every attack began with a listing of the deadly results of the habit.[34]

Second-generation Disciples also fortified a wide range of other moral teachings on the ground that they involved the principles of good health. As in the early nineteenth century, the arguments against the use of tobacco most closely paralleled the case against alcohol. "Christianity holds up to us a high type of manhood and womanhood that ought to make us turn away with loathing from all unclean practices," wrote the editor of a Disciples journal in 1897. "The highest moral and intellectual efficiency forbids the use of this injurious narcotic."[35]

There was not always total agreement about what contributed to good health. As liberal church leaders began to relax the restraints on such recreations as dancing, they appealed to the need for healthful recreation. "Whether we need amusements or not, is not primarily a religious, but a physiological question," wrote Isaac Errett in 1866.[36] On the other hand, conservative Disciples writers regaled their readers with both religious and health warnings against the dangers of "popular amusements." While dancing was generally condemned as sexually promiscuous, a Tennessee preacher believed that it was also unhealthful; participating in such "violent exercise" in "the close and vapid air of the ball-room," he warned, was "likely to bring on disease that will carry one to a premature grave, examples of which I have in mind at this time."[37] Countless other "frivolities" were judged by the same health standards. For example, in warning against roller skating, James H. Garrison argued that: "Physicians testify that it is highly injurious to health."[38] Even women's dress, a constant source of concern to many conservative preachers, was expected to pass a health test. After reading of a Chinese mother who disfigured the feet of her little girl, an Alabama preacher wrote:

> I know a clever, good girl, who has driven the color from her face, is sickly and cannot walk straight. Oh, but she has the beautiful figure of a wasp.
> . . . These Christian mothers destroy the breast bones and ribs of their daughters with an eye-letted vice, and then turn them deformed upon society to drag out a miserable life filled with groans, and sighs—a perfect cheat upon a husband and the human family.[39]

Disciples views on marriage, divorce, and sex change little in the late nineteenth and early twentieth centuries, although those topics were more frequently discussed. Generally, church leaders decried what they perceived as a loosening moral standard in American society, particularly the passage of laws that allowed divorce for causes other than adultery. All agreed that "teaching and training the young people in the principles of Christianity must not be overlooked."[40] On the other hand, it became increasingly clear that Disciples remained divided in their views on marriage and divorce. In 1891 one preacher publicly complained about the "loose manner in which the marriage relation is treated by some of our preachers."[41] On all such moral issues, Disciples continued to believe there was a Christian path to happiness and morality, but they by no means agreed about the details.

Perhaps nothing illustrated the diverging mind of the Disciples of Christ better than their disparate views on human suffering and its relation to the Christian message. Conservative Disciples continued to view suffering largely as a product of God's providence, often imposed as a "punishment for our sins."[42] One writer advised: "Adversity is God's rod by which he chastises the people for their sins, and seeks to turn them again into the right way."[43] Suffering was God's corrective. "The Christian view of trial," wrote a Tennessee Disciple in 1881, "makes it a benign necessity, a boon rather than a bane."[44]

While this view of human suffering blunted any general interest in social reform, it did not produce a simple disregard for suffering. Suffering existed by the providential will of God, but it was the responsibility of the church to do its best to relieve it. Over and over conservative church leaders urged Disciples to care for the poor and sick, noting, for example, that "the winter is upon us, and there are many poor . . . to be looked after."[45] Often these exhortations were directed to individuals. Again and again in the late nineteenth century the *Gospel Advocate* called attention to suffering in Nashville and the South and urged the able to help those less fortunate than themselves. Drought, the cold winter, the advent of "hard times," an epidemic of yellow fever, or some other catastrophe would set off a series of pleas for benevolence. Typical was an appeal made by David Lipscomb in 1875:

> We daily see numbers of people, especially Negroes in and around the highways of this city whose countenances but too plainly tell of the cold and starvation they are enduring. The death rate in Nashville has averaged about twenty a week during the winter. Public charity does something but there are numbers whom it never reaches. . . . The only way . . . to prevent further suffering, is for each one to do what he can for the poor of his immediate neighborhood.[46]

Conservative Disciples preserved, and perhaps expanded, the earlier emphasis on congregational benevolence. The most widely accepted benevolent precept among them was: "It is the duty of every congregation to provide for its own poor."[47] "The provisions for the poor under Christianity," wrote Elisha G. Sewell, "are such that if the churches . . . do their duty, there will be no necessity for the poor to borrow."[48] "Let each church be provided with competent deacons," wrote another preacher, "and let these deacons take the oversight of temporal matters, seeing that none suffer for food, for such is their duty."[49]

Most conservative Disciples leaders retained an anti-institutional bias and objected to the rise of "human institutions to see to the wants of the poor."[50] Most insisted that each congregation should take care of its own suffering members. J.T. Walsh of North Carolina wrote: "The Church of God keeps the Lord's treasury filled. She takes care of her own poor. She feeds her own hungry, and clothes her own naked. She feeds and clothes her own Widows and Orphans."[51]

There is no way to measure how adequately the local churches lived up to this model of a succoring community. Some apparently did. A Kentucky minister wrote to a friend in 1869: "I have succeeded in getting the congregations at Gamaliel, and Free Will, monroe co *[sic]* . . . to put their Deacons to hunting up the *poor widows* and other *poor* of the congregations and feeding and clothing them. Is this in apostolic taste and order?"[52] A California preacher reported in 1878: "No matter how industrious or temperate a Christian may be, sickness or old age, or some unexpected casualty, may make him dependent on charity. All our churches provide funds in such cases. All our ministers, elders and deacons consider it a part of their duty to visit and relieve the poor of Christ's flock."[53] No doubt many local churches did provide both support and aid to the sick and suffering in their midst.

While conservative Disciples continued to stress the importance of local churches, the growth of denominational organization and a more sophisticated leadership pushed a majority of the churches in other directions. Liberal Disciples became increasingly concerned about the causes of suffering, seeing social injustice as a proper Christian concern. At the same time, they also turned to political and institutional means to find solutions to the problems of suffering. Beginning in the 1870s, many Disciples leaders became outspoken advocates of social reform, and the church became deeply involved in building benevolent and humanitarian institutions.

In 1894, in an article entitled "The State of the Cause," James H. Garrison summarized the changes that he had observed in his lifetime as a Disciple:

> In the past the church has been all too neglectful of . . . the welfare of human society. A marked change for the better, however, is evidenced by many signs. Never before has the ministry taken so deep an interest in the great social problems which affect the well being of man here in the world as they do today. . . . Without departing in the least from the spirit and

aim of the gospel, but with a fuller and truer apprehension of its aim and spirit, we would urge upon our ministers and members the importance of extending practical sympathy and aid to all wise movements, looking to the purification of our political life, the removal of unjust burdens from the shoulders of the oppressed, the enactment of laws for the better protection of the life and the health of the toiling masses, . . . in a word, to lend their influence and assistance to whatever will help to lessen crime, diminish the burdens of the weak, protect the home, purify our public life and make the world a more desirable place in which to live. The church that neglects this side of its Christian duty on the plea of separation of church and state, or for fear of soiling its heavenly robes, will find itself in the rear of the procession as the army of the Lord passes through the opening gates of the Twentieth Century.[54]

One important result of this heightened social conscience was the building of a network of institutions. In 1903 the secretary of the Disciples Home Missionary Society wrote:

There can be no restoration of apostolic Christianity to the world until we restore apostolic benevolence to the Church of Christ. We can submit no better evidence of our being the Church of Christ than our care for the poor whom Christ has made his ambassadors to the church. This should not be wholly committed to Catholics and lodges.[55]

The orphan school in Midway continued to flourish in the years after the Civil War and was joined by a number of similar institutions in the late nineteenth century. A second home for orphans was established in 1884 in Louisville; widows were admitted to the home beginning in 1912. In 1886 a number of women members from the First Christian Church in St. Louis took the lead in beginning the National Benevolent Association to coordinate charity work among the Disciples. The group opened a home for widows and orphans in St. Louis in 1889, and ten years later, with the backing of the leaders of the denomination, the group became the coordinating agency for the church's benevolent work. In 1920, when the National Benevolent Association, along with several other independent church agencies, transferred legal control of its work to the newly formed United Christian Missionary Society, the association was operating twelve homes for children and the aging.[56]

As individuals, Disciples made several efforts to build hospitals in the late nineteenth century, largely as humanitarian ventures. The most successful was the Axtell Christian Hospital founded in 1887 in Newton, Kansas, by Dr. and Mrs. J.T. Axtell; in 1925 it became a formal work of the Kansas Christian Missionary Society.[57] Several other efforts to build hospitals were less successful because of the limited size of the denomination and the competition for funds from the growing number of social and missionary organizations related to the Disciples.[58]

As the Disciples expanded their foreign missions in the late nineteenth and early twentieth centuries, they depended heavily on medical institutions to support their efforts. By 1927, the United Christian Missionary Society was sponsoring four hospitals in the Belgian Congo; four in China; four hospitals, one tuberculosis sanatorium, one leper asylum, and two orphanages in India; three hospitals in the Philippines; and one hospital and one orphanage in Tibet.[59]

Diverging Paths, 1920–1985

By 1920 the Disciples of Christ movement had come to span virtually the whole spectrum of Protestant theology and social thought. Leaders of the Churches of Christ, recognized as a separate church in the religious census of 1906, remained fervent New Testament literalists, intent on restoring the ancient order of things in the twentieth century. Both their doctrinal teaching and their social thought seemed a re-creation of the concerns of the first generation of Disciples leaders. Tennessee and Texas farmer–preachers continued to exhort their congregations to use their God-given reason to interpret the revealed law of God, to honor their bodies as part of God's natural order, and to care for their neighbors through individual and congregational charity. At the other end of the spectrum, national leaders of the Disciples of Christ surfaced in the forefront of the ecumenical movement. The church produced more than its share of eminent scholars, and Disciples leaders contributed to many of the avant-garde social movements of the twentieth century.

In between these two extremes lay thousands of Disciples local churches filled with such incongruous mixtures of members they frequently had difficulty defining their own placement within the movement. In 1940, the pastor of the Central Christian Church in Fayetteville, Arkansas, tried to explain the nuances within her religious movement to the Historical Records Survey office in Little Rock:

> I can understand your perplexity as to how Central Christian Church should be classified. . . . In the course of a century and a half, a rather complete denominational setup has developed, repudiated by the great middle-class rank and file, but fostered by a very skillful minority which controlled the conventions and gave out misleading publicity to the press. It by no means represents the principles underlying the movement. . . . The lines I have indicated are not sharply defined. Many churches whose names appear in the Disciples of Christ yearbook have their fingers crossed about the whole

setup, and believe in local autonomy, just as we do. Often both groups are represented in the same congregation.[60]

The glue that held most of the churches together was the historical Disciples' belief that agreement was necessary only on matters of "faith" that were set forth "in express terms or by approved precedent" in the New Testament. All else was considered "opinion." In the mind of Alexander Campbell, wrote historian Harold Lunger, "social ethics . . . remained largely a matter of individual interpretation and judgement."[61]

Within the context of diversity, most Disciples continued to view the relationship of religion and health in ways similar to their forebears, expounding more fully ideas that could be found earlier in the movement. They continued to view prayer for the sick as a proper Christian responsibility of the local church. "It would seem that the best approach to the matter of healing by the Church," wrote the editor of the *Christian Evangelist* in 1957, "would be to acknowledge freely the basic place of prayer as integral in maintaining or regaining health. . . . Certainly, the Church must play a vital part in the healing processes and health needs of the congregations."[62] Increasing numbers of Disciples explored the meaning of death and suffering in the Christian context, but they generally treated the subjects in the same conventional ways as had earlier Disciples.[63]

Most of the more liberal Christian churches continued to support a program of institutional benevolence both at home and abroad. In 1981 the National Benevolent Association was supervising twelve facilities for "older adults" as well as caring for about 1,500 "children and mentally retarded" in eight centers. Most overseas work supported by the church was done through ecumenical missions programs that were strongly medically oriented. The Disciples retained control of their mission program in Zaire, which had been launched in 1899 and which by the 1980s included the operation of five hospitals and clinics and fifteen dispensaries, staffed by a total of fifty-six persons.[64] The non-cooperating, more conservative Christian churches also supported several overseas medical missions.[65]

Three questions involving Christian healing seemed to some twentieth-century Disciples to demand reconciliation with their historical beliefs. First was the rise of Pentecostalism, particularly as represented in the healing evangelists who crisscrossed the nation in the aftermath of World War II. For liberal Disciples, the Pentecostal message posed no major threat. They condemned the "bizarre practices and unjustified claims" of the revivalists, but like most mainstream Protestants, had no theological objections to a renewed emphasis on the miraculous.[66] But to the conservatives in the Churches of Christ, Pentecostalism seemed to be a resurrection of the superstition and irrationality which

Alexander Campbell had denounced in the Roman Catholicism of his day.

Since the 1920s, the Churches of Christ and the rapidly growing Pentecostal denominations have competed keenly for the loyalty of the common people of the South and Midwest. They conducted scores of debates beginning in the 1930s and came to know one another's doctrines almost as well as their own.[67] The Churches of Christ based their opposition on a simple explication of Alexander Campbell's dispensationalism: miracles served the divine purpose of confirming the New Testament revelation and then ceased.[68] While God might answer prayers in some inscrutable way, he would not perform miracles that violated his natural laws. Christians should look to medical treatment for healing—faith healing was an illusion or a fraud.

In the 1950s and 1960s, the Churches of Christ became the most outspoken and vitriolic critics of the independent healing revivalists such as Oral Roberts. The beginning of a healing crusade would likely elicit a series of newspaper advertisements by a local Church of Christ challenging the evangelist to debate and offering a one thousand dollar reward for documentary evidence that a miracle had occurred. A typical article in the Sacramento *Union* in 1955 read:

> We will give $1,000.00 reward, which is on deposit in a North Highlands bank, for acceptable evidence of one case of instantaneous and miraculous divine healing of cancer that has been pronounced in a state of malignancy by competent medical authority, active tuberculosis, withered limbs, or paralysis. Testimony of three reputable Sacramento County physicians upon whom we are mutually agreed, will be accepted as sufficient evidence. We stand ready to deny in public discussion that such power is given to men today.[69]

Sometimes the messages continued after the campaigns closed. In 1955, the following advertisement appeared in a Jacksonville, Florida newspaper after the close of a Roberts campaign:

> In view of the fact that a revival campaign has just concluded, in which claims were made both over the radio and through the mails that many had been healed, . . . the Churches of Christ felt compelled to take this means of bringing out the fact that NOT ONE SINGLE CASE OF MIRACULOUS DIVINE HEALING CAN BE PRODUCED.[70]

Churches of Christ ministers openly labeled the crusades a "sham and a hoax" and charged that the Pentecostal revivalists were "fake healers."[71] In the 1980s, probably no other religious group in the nation stood in more adamant opposition to any expectation of divine intervention in human affairs.

A second twentieth-century health issue that caused considerable discussion about the historical beliefs of Disciples was the reappearance of debate in the Churches of Christ over institutional benevolence. In the 1950s and 1960s, the Churches of Christ experienced a division much like the one that had separated the conservative churches from the mainstream of the Disciples movement a half century earlier. The division had much of the same sociological underpinning that the earlier one had: the Churches of Christ had grown dramatically since 1900 and had come to include many middle-class, college-trained members. As a new and more sophisticated leadership emerged in the churches, so did a variety of institutions dependent on the independent congregations for their livelihood. Particularly important were a number of orphan homes which had grown from a new impetus to support "practical Christianity" in a movement that continued to be preoccupied with doctrinal correctness. By the 1950s, the Churches of Christ were embroiled in a new battle between anti-institutional prejudices rooted in the continued insistence on the exact replication of the New Testament church and a concern for a more visible benevolent witness. The result was a schism which separated perhaps fifteen percent of the most conservative Churches of Christ from the remainder of the group. At least in theory, these arch-conservative churches were also the most scrupulous promoters of the local church as a community of succor and benevolence.[72]

While the most conservative Disciples in the twentieth century struggled to preserve the historical message they had inherited from the past, the liberal wing of the movement searched for ways to accommodate the rapidly changing ideas of the post–World War II era. Challenged by a wave of nontraditional ideas about such subjects as homosexuality and abortion in the 1960s, most conservative Disciples reacted with predictable abhorrence and shock.[73] But liberal Disciples entertained the new ideas seriously and found a way to place them in the church's historical tradition.

By the postwar years, it was clear that the liberal church had abandoned many of the older moral absolutes accepted by past generations of Disciples. Condemnation of the "drink disease" and advocacy of prohibiton had changed to explorations of methods for treating "alcoholism."[74] By the 1970s, the restructured Christian Church (Disciples of Christ) began passing formal resolutions on moral and ethical issues in its representative General Assemblies. One student of those resolutions summarized the "discernable trends": (1) clear protection of the individual right of decision, (2) a liberal tone in the positions adopted on questions related to the governance of the whole society, and (3) "the absence of rigid pronouncements designed to govern individual life-styles."[75] Disciples liberals used the movement's historical defense of liberty of conscience in nonessential beliefs to protect the defenders of abortion and homosexual rights. "If you ask about the moral correctness of having an abortion, the appropriate expression of human sexuality, seeking a divorce, consuming drugs or participating in any number of other activities which raise questions of an ethical or moral nature," advised a *Handbook* published in 1980, "the Christian Church (Disciples of Christ) will *not* provide a systematic blueprint for your personal behavior."[76] The reason for such flexibility, explained the author, was the Disciples heritage of liberty:

> While Disciples as a body may disapprove of the general practice of abortion, they recognize a greater danger of legislating a single moral opinion for all persons, thereby abridging the freedom of individual choice. On moral–ethical questions related to personal behavior, Disciples tend to affirm and reaffirm this position which is a cherished part of their heritage.[77]

The tolerance of liberal Disciples was an ultimate expression of the old Disciples slogan: "In essentials unity, in opinions liberty, in all things charity."

Conclusion

At first glance, the Disciples of Christ movement appears to be almost devoid of a healing tradition. Nineteenth-century Disciples leaders were totally preoccupied with doctrinal questions, and Disciples thought on such questions as death, suffering, and health largely reflected the intellectual baggage Disciples brought with them out of the Presbyterian and Baptist churches. Nor has subsequent Disciples history been far different from that of those mother churches. Being theologically orthodox, the Disciples easily made the same social and intellectual transitions that affected other evangelical groups in America. By the 1980s, the movement's heirs were scattered from the most conservative to the most liberal fringes of the American religious spectrum.

A few distinctive Disciples beliefs did, however, seem to play some role in determining how the churches reacted to human needs. Particularly important in the nineteenth century (and among conservatives in the twentieth) was the Disciples emphasis on the local congregation. In the Churches of Christ, local elders still frequently oversee both the moral and physical well-being of their flock—providing prayer for the sick and assistance for the needy as well as remonstrances to the wayward.

Modern Disciples also remain the heirs to a rationalistic mindset and a dispensational theology which questions the miraculous intervention of God in the day-to-day affairs of humans. Those theological assumptions are much clearer in the conservative wing of the movement, but even among liberal Disciples the espousal of causes is likely to be supported by producing New Testament proof texts.

Finally, the Disciples' belief in liberty of conscience allows almost complete freedom in the area of personal beliefs. Even in conservative Churches of Christ a member would be allowed the private right to support abortion (though probably not homosexuality), and every wing of the movement would allow contradictory opinions about marriage and divorce and on such issues as birth control. While the Disciples tradition of liberty has been immensely useful in preserving the oft-divided movement from falling into total anarchy, it has also precluded the development of any distinctive healing message by the church.

Notes

1. Charles Alexander Young, *Historical Documents Advocating Christian Union* (Chicago, 1904), pp. 2, 78.
2. Winfred Ernest Garrison and Alfred T. De Groot, *The Disciples of Christ* (St. Louis, 1948), p. 421.
3. Alexander Campbell, *The Christian System* (Bethany, VA, 1839).
4. "Editor's Address," *Christian Messenger* 7 (January 1833):3.
5. Campbell, *The Christian System*, p. 129.
6. Alexander Campbell, *Popular Lectures and Addresses* (St. Louis, n.d.), p. 460.
7. Ibid., p. 461.
8. Ibid., p. 465.
9. Ibid., pp. 186–212.
10. "Laying on of Hands," *Christian Messenger* 5 (December 1831):273–274; Campbell, *Popular Lectures and Addresses*, pp. 157–162.
11. *A Debate on the Roman Catholic Religion: Held in Sycamore Street Meeting House, Cincinnati, from the 13th to the 21st of January, 1837, Taken Down by Reporters, and Revised by the Parties* (Cincinnati, 1837).
12. "Prospectus," *Millennial Harbinger* 1 (January 4, 1830):1.
13. Campbell, *Popular Lectures and Addresses*, pp. 403–452, esp. p. 449.
14. See David Edwin Harrell, Jr., *Quest for a Christian America* (Nashville, 1966), pp. 196–198.
15. See "Reply to Mr. Watterman," *Millennial Harbinger* 5 (May 1834): 213–217.
16. Bradford Clark, "The Christian Sabbath," *Primitive Christian and Investigator* 2 (December 1836):193; see also Robert Richardson, *Memoirs of Alexander Campbell*, 2 vols. (Philadelphia, 1868), 1:515–537.
17. "Popular Literature—No. VI," *Millennial Harbinger*, Third Series, 1 (December 1844):599; see also Harrell, *Quest for a Christian America*, pp. 185–190.
18. Jacob Creath, *A Tract on the Use and Abuse of Tobacco* (n.p., 1871), p. 6.
19. Jacob Creath, "Tobacco," *Christian Pioneer* 8 (March 5, 1868):64.

20. "To the Editor of the Christian Index," *Millennial Harbinger* 2 (September 1831):429–430; see also David Edwin Harrell, Jr., *The Social Sources of Division in the Disciples of Christ* (Athens, GA, 1973), pp. 208–210.
21. "The Temperance Reformation a Harbinger of the Millennium," *Christian Journal* 2 (October 7, 1843):110.
22. "A Restoration of the Ancient Order of Things. No. XIX," *Christian Baptist* 4 (May 1827):211.
23. For instance, see Church Register and Record of the South Elkhorn Church, 1817–1897; and Walter Scott Notebook, unpublished manuscripts, Bosworth Memorial Library, College of the Bible, Lexington, Kentucky.
24. See Walter Scott [untitled notice], *Evangelist* 8 (March 1840):72.
25. "Every City Ought to Have Its Sunday School," *Millennial Harbinger,* Third Series, 4 (April 1847):203.
26. T.J. Matlock, "State Meeting in Illinois," *Western Evangelist* 2 (October 1851):314–416.
27. "The Christian Religion," *Christian Baptist* 1 (August 1823):6–7.
28. Harry Giovannoli, *Kentucky Female Orphan School* (Midway, KY, 1930), p. 29.
29. "Contemplated Female Orphan School," *Millennial Harbinger,* Third Series, 3 (July 1846):419.
30. Mrs. Augusta Smith, "A Word in Season," *Gospel Advocate* 24 (June 15, 1882):374.
31. "The Healing Ministry of the Church," *Christian-Evangelist* 61 (January 31, 1924):143.
32. "Brevities," *Christian* 17 (February 27, 1879):1.
33. Geo. E. Flower, "What They Say, Number II," *Christian Standard* 13 (July 15, 1876):226.
34. See David Roberts Dungan, *Rum and Ruin; the Remedy Found* (Oskaloosa, IA, 1879), pp. 11–60.
35. "Our Easy Chair," *Christian-Evangelist* 34 (January 14, 1897):19.
36. "Theaters and Gaming," *Christian Standard* 1 (August 11, 1866):140.
37. "Dancing," *Gospel Advocate* 23 (September 8, 1881):568.
38. "Boston Miscellany," *Christian Evangelist* 22 (March 26, 1885):195.
39. "None Are So Blind as Those Who Will Not See," *Gospel Advocate* 20 (January 3, 1878):6–7.
40. "Divorce," *Christian Companion* 24 (June 1885):218.
41. G.W. Warner, "False Marriage," *Christian Oracle* 8 (November 12, 1891):725.
42. "Query," *Gospel Advocate* 16 (December 2, 1875):1141.
43. Hugh Tucker, "The Indifference of Christians and the Benefits of Hard Times," *Christian Oracle* 13 (November 5, 1896):709.
44. J.M. Trible, "The Christian Theory of Trial," *Gospel Advocate* 23 (May 19, 1881):307.
45. "Editorial Jottings," *American Christian Review* 28 (December 24, 1885):412.
46. "Destitution, Its Cause," *Gospel Advocate* 17 (March 4, 1875):227.
47. "A Wrong Practice," *Gospel Echo* 6 (October, 1868):390.
48. "Queries," *Gospel Advocate* 27 (May 20, 1885):306.
49. "Kansas Echoes," *American Christian Review* 28 (March 5, 1885):73.
50. J.S. Durst, "Christian Duties," *Gospel Advocate* 20 (January 3, 1878):3.
51. "The Law of Love," *Watch Tower* 4 (September, 1876):107.

52. Isaac Tipton Reneau to John Mulkey, January 11, 1869, Isaac Tipton Reneau Papers, Lexington Theological Seminary, Lexington, Kentucky.
53. "California Letter," *American Christian Review* 21 (April 9, 1878):115.
54. *Christian-Evangelist* 31 (December 6, 1894):774.
55. Benjamin Lyon Smith and George B. Ranshaw, "Yearbook," *The American Home Missionary* 10 (December, 1903):399.
56. See J. Edward Moseley, *The Concern for Benevolence Among Disciples of Christ* (St. Louis, n.d.); and Harrell, *Social Sources of Division*, pp. 62–69.
57. Moseley, *The Concern for Benevolence*, p. 37.
58. See Harrell, *Social Sources of Division*, p. 37.
59. *1927 Yearbook* (St. Louis, 1927), pp. 201–202.
60. Historical Records Survey, Arkansas, Records Inventory Files, 1936–1942, Box 415, Special Collections, University of Arkansas.
61. Harold Lunger, *The Political Ethics of Alexander Campbell* (St. Louis, 1954), p. 27.
62. "What is Faith Healing?" *Christian-Evangelist* 95 (March 20, 1957):650.
63. See *The Christian-Evangelist Index, 1863–1958,* 3 vols. (St. Louis, 1962), 1:2714–2719; Batsell Barrett Baxter, *The Problem of Human Suffering* (Nashville, n.d.); Homer Hailey, *The Problem of Suffering* (Athens, AL, n.d.).
64. Shirley L. Cox, ed., *Yearbook & Directory, 1981* (Indianapolis, 1981), pp. 183–236.
65. See "Teacher to Go to Mashoka," *Christian Standard* 93 (October 31, 1959):612; *Christian Standard Index, 1866–1966,* 6 vols. (Nashville, 1972) 4:2151.
66. "What is Faith Healing?" p. 650; also see "Prayer and Medicine," *Christian-Evangelist* 91 (January 21, 1953):52; Jacques Zimmerman, "Gifts of Healing," *The Christian* 111 (January 21, 1973):66.
67. See Gus Nichols and C.J. Weaver, *Nichols-Weaver Debate* (Nashville, 1944); B. Sunday Meyers and W. Curtis Porter, *The Porter-Meyers Debate* (Monette, AR, 1956); Ray Vaughn and G.K. Wallace, *Wallace-Vaughn Debate* (Shreveport, LA, 1952).
68. See A.G. Hobbs, *Have Miracles Ceased?* (Ft. Worth, TX, 1953); James M. Tolle, *Have Miracles Ceased?* (Beaumont, TX, n.d.).
69. *Sacramento Union,* October 7, 1955, p. 13.
70. *Florida Times-Union,* April 15, 1955, p. 3.
71. V.E. Howard, *Fake Healers Exposed,* 6th printing, rev. (West Monroe, LA, 1970), pp. 3, 29; see also "The Truth About Faith Healers," *The Odessa (Texas) American,* February 20, 1957, p. 7.
72. See David Edwin Harrell, Jr., *The Emergence of the "Church of Christ Denomination"* (Lufkin, TX, n.d.); Cecil Willis, *The Taproot of Digression: "No Pattern-ism"* (Marion, IN, n.d.).
73. See "The Atrocious Sin of Abortion," and "Seeking Homosexual Vote," *The Sower* 29 (September–October 1984):4; George T. Jones, *Reverence for Human Life* (Louisville, n.d.).
74. See *The Christian-Evangelist Index, 1863–1958,* 1:13.
75. D. Duane Cummins, *A Handbook for Today's Disciples* (St. Louis, 1981), p. 46.
76. Ibid., pp. 46–47.
77. Ibid., p. 45; see also General Office of the Christian Church (Disciples of Christ), *Yearbook & Directory, 1979* (Indianapolis, 1979), pp. 86–88.

CHAPTER 14

The Mormon

Tradition

Lester E. Bush, Jr.

The Church of Jesus Christ of Latter-day Saints was organized in 1830 in the "burned-over district" of upstate New York by a 25-year-old farmer and onetime seeker of treasure named Joseph Smith (1805–1844). Smith preached a restoration of primitive Christianity and divinely bestowed authority, and offered as evidence of his prophetic call *The Book of Mormon,* a theological narrative set against the backdrop of ancient America, and translated, he said, from a set of inscribed "golden plates" revealed to him in a vision.

Guided by an ongoing series of revelations, Smith led his growing band of primitivist seekers on a complex odyssey which, over a period of nearly two decades, eventually led to the Great Salt Lake Valley. From New York, the group first moved simultaneously to the Western Reserve of Ohio (temporary headquarters of the church) and western Missouri (the site designated by Smith as Zion, the New Jerusalem to which Christ would shortly come to usher in the millennium), and thence to Illinois on the Mississippi, where Smith was killed in 1844. It was from Illinois that Smith's successor, Brigham Young (1801–1877), led the Mormon pioneers of 1847 to their safe haven in the West.

Not long after announcing the Restoration, Joseph Smith began to depart from his initial primitivist notions—to the alienation of many of his followers—and soon developed a hierarchical style of leadership that combined the New Testament ideals of communitarianism, apostolic

witness, and guidance by the Holy Spirit at both individual and institutional levels; the Old Testament models of a gathering, prophets, and
polygyny; and Smith's own innovations, including an increasingly stratified priesthood of all adult male believers and a theocratic government
with himself as the undisputed leader and sole spokesman for God.

At a time when doctrinal innovations were moving the new church
away from American religious and social norms, gathering converts
swelled the Mormon community to the point of dominance over other
local institutions. This led to a series of confrontations between the early
Mormons and their neighbors, and ultimately to an 1838 "extermination
order" by the Missouri governor which drove the Mormons from that
state.

Reestablished in a sparsely settled area of Illinois, the Mormons
enjoyed several years of relative peace, and constructed the city-state
of Nauvoo, to which some 16,000 saints gathered. This was the period
of Smith's most expansive theological innovation, as he elaborated on
earlier texts and tenets and introduced some of Mormonism's most
distinctive doctrines: the plurality of Gods, man's potential Godhood,
exaltation (salvation) of the dead through vicarious ordinances, secret
(though not uncommon) temple ceremonies with a promise of eternal
family relationships, and the practice of "celestial" or plural marriage.
It was this latter practice, more than any other factor, that led to schism
within the Nauvoo community and ultimately to Smith's murder in
1844.

Within three years of the prophet's martyrdom, the Mormon vanguard
(now under the firm leadership of Brigham Young) came to the end of
their odyssey, in the Great Basin of the mountain West. Perhaps half
the Nauvoo-area Mormon community followed this vanguard; many
who remained behind affiliated with various groups, some still extant
today, which accepted the earlier Restorationist claims of Joseph Smith
but rejected the theology of the Nauvoo period. By far the largest of
these is the Reorganized (in 1860) Church of Jesus Christ of Latter Day
Saints, now headquartered in Independence, Missouri, and numbering
some 200,000 members worldwide.

Shored up by literally thousands of immigrating British and Scandinavian converts, Mormons in Utah for the remaining five decades of
the nineteenth century waged a holy struggle on two fronts: against a
hostile natural environment as pioneers further colonized the Great
Basin, and against a United States government determined to abolish
Mormon theocracy and polygamy. The first struggle was won, but the
second was lost. Plural marriage (as a practice) was abandoned in 1890,
and thereby Utah achieved independent statehood; polygamy as a principle as well as Mormon theocracy was discarded about 1904, in response
to Senate hearings on the seating of newly elected United States Senator
(and Mormon Apostle) Reed Smoot.

The twentieth century has seen Mormonism evolve from an innovative
"peculiar people" to an increasingly programmed, quintessential American religion. Although now devoid of many of its more colorful (or

radical) aspects, it maintains as central tenets ideals that arose during its earliest days: prophetic leadership, an open canon, humankind's potential Godhood and the plurality of Gods, the potential exaltation of all humankind through vicarious ordinances, and continuity of family association past mortal life. While the church has survived the abandonment of plural marriage and, recently, the reversal of its exclusionary policy toward blacks, it continues to face serious challenges in the form of a groundswell of feminism, a growing body of Third World converts (to about twenty percent of current membership), an elderly and increasingly fundamentalistic hierarchy, a cumbersome bureaucracy ill-prepared for an exponential membership growth (to a total now exceeding five million) and a challenge to its doctrinal and social integrity from an increasingly pluralistic society. Responses to such challenges, as in the past, will undoubtedly emerge from a tension between reliance on revelatory enlightenment of an authoritative hierarchy on the one hand and accommodation to the demands of social, economic, and political realities on the other.

————··◁∞▷··————

Most Morman social and intellectual traditions have been distinctly evolutionary in nature. While themes viewed within the faith, sometimes retrospectively, as "fundamental" often persist over time, a marked progression in both perspective and practice is also usually identifiable. The history of the Mormon interaction with health and medicine is no exception to this general pattern.

The Formative Years, 1830–1844

To judge by their initial revelations and commentary, the early Mormons viewed health and disease in the same heterogeneous light as many of their countrymen. While a Christian primitivist perspective was often evident in the King James Bible context invoked in these sources, everyday perspectives of Jacksonian America were equally evident.[1]

By and large, these earliest comments were brief and incidental to other concerns. A notable exception is found in an important revelation on health announced by Joseph Smith in February 1833. Termed the *Word of Wisdom* after a phrase included in an introduction to the published version, this revelation guaranteed to those who led righteous and dietetically appropriate lives

> health in their navel, and marrow to their bones and [they] shall find wisdom, and great treasures of knowledge, even hidden treasures; and shall run and not be weary, and shall walk and not faint; and I the Lord give

unto them a promise, that the destroying angel shall pass by them, as the children of Israel, and not slay them.[2]

As specified in this Word of Wisdom, righteous and healthful living involved both proscriptions and prescriptions. The former, in general accord with botanic and orthodox medical condemnations of "stimulants" as then defined (but short of the extremes of Sylvester Graham's then popular vegetarian health crusade), advised that

> wine or strong drink . . . is not good. . . . [S]trong drinks are not for the belly, but for the washing of your bodies. . . . [T]obacco is not for the body, neither for the belly, and is not good for man, but is an herb for bruises. . . . [H]ot drinks [soon interpreted to mean coffee and tea] are not for the body or belly. . . . [F]lesh . . . of beasts and of the fowls . . . are to be used sparingly; and . . . only in times of winter, or of cold, or famine.

The prescriptions, by contrast, were more sweeping, and advised that "all wholesome herbs [are] for the constitution, nature, and use of man—Every herb in the season thereof, and every fruit in the season thereof. . . . [F]lesh also of beasts and of the fowls. . . ." Such recommendations were reinforced through passing references in other revelations, one of which, for example, pointedly noted that "whoso forbiddeth to abstain from meats, that man should not eat the same, is not ordained of God; for behold the beasts of the field, and the fowls of the air, and that which cometh of the earth, is ordained for the use of man, for food, and for raiment." Additional prescriptive guidance was limited to the passing word of counsel in another revelation that the faithful should "retire to thy bed early, that ye may not be weary; arise early, that your bodies and minds may be invigorated."

Although the prophetic authority with which these ideas were advanced was certainly new to recent converts, the recommendations themselves clearly were not—representing as they did the dominant view among authorities on health reform. Perhaps sensitive to the strongly held, but divergent views then current—as well as feeling some discomfort with anything that might be thought a creed—Smith carefully labeled the Word of Wisdom at the time of publication "not by commandment or constraint." Nonetheless, violation of this code quickly became contributory, if not sufficient, grounds for expelling recreants from some early congregations. Within a very few years, however, changed circumstances, including the geographic and administrative concentration of the church community directly under Joseph Smith, led to a much more tolerant attitude. Smith himself occasionally disregarded some of the divine counsel, and his view that some stimulants had an appropriate "medicinal" role (for example, in cases of fatigue and melancholy) further undermined an inflexible application of the health code. Although a firm doctrinal commitment to the dietary guideline remained, it was not viewed as the panacea one might have anticipated at the time of its introduction in 1833.

Even in theory, safeguarding one's health was never truly viewed as merely a matter of adhering to a divine health code. While no comprehensive Mormon treatise on the nature of disease was penned, a variety of supplemental perspectives on the question is evident in early writings and commentaries. These no doubt derived from many sources, both within and without the church.

To begin with, there obviously were circumstances—which must have been viewed as commonplace, given the death rates then current, especially among young children—when, in the words of another revelation, an individual simply had been "appointed unto death" by the Lord.[3] In this case, apparently nothing would avail.

Similarly, death and disease were at times viewed, or at least described, as instruments in the divine hand. They could be the vehicle (for example, in the case of the cholera pandemic of 1832–1833) whereby divine chastisement was meted out to wicked nations or individuals. With many others, Mormons saw divine plagues as heralding the last days, warning readers of their journals that "all flesh is grass, but, that amidst all the judgements of the Lord, the righteous have never been forsaken."[4] Even when the faithful themselves later were seized by cholera—as happened to a third of a small Mormon expeditionary force organized in hopes of reclaiming Missouri properties—it was immediately pronounced a "consequence of the fractious and unruly spirits that had appeared among them." Any type of intervention under such circumstances was futile, if not dangerous, as Joseph Smith made clear:

> At the commence [of the attack of cholera], I attempted to lay on hands for their recovery, but I quickly learned by painful experience, that when the great Jehovah decrees destruction upon any people, and makes known this determination, man must not attempt to stay his hand. The moment I attempted to rebuke the disease I was attacked, and had I not desisted in my attempt to save the life of a brother, I would have sacrificed my own.[5]

Conversely, however, illness was sometimes described as providing the opportunity whereby the presence of God's healing power within the church could be displayed. In fact, the "gift of healing" among the membership was very soon identified (along with the gifts of tongues, prophecy, revelation, and visions) as both an "article of faith" and a confirmation of the church's divine mandate.

Illness, and even death, was also variously characterized as a divine test—of both the faith and determination of the Saints. This was particularly so during the difficult early pioneer years, during which time the Latter-day Saints were particularly wont to compare themselves to saints tested in biblical times.

Finally, again following the biblical model, some illnesses were said to be the manifestation of demonic possession. Indeed what was termed by Joseph Smith "the first miracle in the church" occurred when he was called to the home of an early convert who was "suffering very much in his mind, and his body acted upon in a very strange manner; his visage and limbs distorted and twisted in every shape and appearance possible to imagine; and finally he was caught up off the floor of the apartment and tossed about most fearfully." Taking the man by the hand, Smith "rebuked the devil," and immediately the victim "spoke out and said that he saw the devil leave him and vanish from his sight."[6]

Theologically, death itself, and particularly the troublesome death of infants, was dealt with very early in the Mormon experience. The *Book of Mormon* stated clearly that "all little children [who die] are alive in Christ, and also all they that [die who] are without the law."[7] Like many of their Christian contemporaries, the early Mormons thus turned in the face of death to a vision of eternal rewards in the life hereafter. As developed by Joseph Smith over the next decade, however, this vision had some distinctive aspects. In time, Smith characterized death as a necessary and proper rite of passage, as was birth, in a larger (as later termed) "plan of salvation." Every mortal being, he eventually taught, existed as an individual spirit prior to being born into mortality. These spirits elected to undertake the moral test inherent in living in "the world," and also thereby took on a physical body requisite to their progression through the eternities. Human life was the union of a spirit with its earthly body to form a "soul." At death the spirit and body again separated, but were permanently reunited at the time of resurrection. Resurrected souls accounted before God for their conduct on earth, and those worthy of ultimate exaltation eventually become as God themselves, parenting their own "spirit children" who continued the unending cycle by in turn taking on mortal bodies and undergoing a similar "test." God, himself, according to Smith, was one who had passed through mortal experiences analagous to those of the nineteenth-century saints, who could find hope and solace in the face of earthly tragedies through the knowledge that if they kept the faith "to the end" they would achieve a comparable station. In the words of a popular couplet penned by a later church president, "As man is now, God once was; as God is now man may be."[8]

The problem of the tangible suffering experienced by many enroute to this eventual reward was not the subject of much formal, systematic reflection, either in these early years or thereafter. Those who addressed the subject usually viewed suffering both as an experience implicit in mortality ("inherited" in a completely naturalistic sense, as was death, from Adam), and as a necessary part of the earthly experience which prepared the righteous eventually to become as God.[9]

When actually dealing with those who were ill, Smith and his primitivist followers turned for guidance first to the counsel of St. James (5:14–15) that, if there were "any sick among you? Let him call for the elders of the church; and let them pray over him, anointing him with oil in the name of the Lord: And the prayer of faith shall save the sick, and the Lord shall raise him up." A revelation reported just months after the organization of the church counseled that "whoso shall ask it in my name, in faith, they shall cast out devils; they shall heal the sick; they shall cause the blind to receive their sight, and the deaf to hear, and the dumb to speak, and the lame to walk."[10] Several later revelations specifically commanded church elders to exercise this gift of healing.

Also very early came another revelation which dealt with those who were sick but spiritually weak:

> And whosoever among you are sick, and have not faith to be healed, but believe, shall be nourished with all tenderness with herbs and mild food, and that not by the hand of an enemy. And the elders of the church, two or more, shall pray for and lay their hands upon them in my name, and if they die shall die unto me, and if they live they shall live unto me.[11]

The implicit endorsement of botanic remedies ("herbs and mild food") was consistent not only with biblical examples, but as well with the use of herbal remedies in the narratives contained in the *Book of Mormon*. Moreover, herbalism was the predominant orientation of most early converts, not a few of whom were themselves Thomsonian practitioners, who rejected the bleedings and calomel dosing of regular physicians in favor of indigenous botanical remedies.

In practice, the early Mormons drew on both their doctrinal legacy and their diverse backgrounds. The sick were administered to and blessed by elders who generally anointed the affected part, or head, or both, with specially consecrated olive oil. Given the considerable incidence of disease on the nineteenth-century American frontier, this healing ritual was very common in early Mormon communities. Diarist Wilford Woodruff, early Mormon apostle and in 1890 church president,[12] catalogued well over a thousand administrations to the sick during his lengthy career, noting that "many were healed by the power of God. Devils were Cast out, the Dumb spake, the Deaf heard, The blind saw, the lame walked, The sick were raised up and in one instance the dead were raised in the Case of my own wife After the spirit left her body."[13]

By the early 1840s women, although not ordained to the priesthood, were performing the same ordinances. Additionally, a practice developed, without clear antecedent, in which "rebaptism" was performed as a healing ritual. The results of all these efforts, to the eye of contemporaries such as Woodruff, were very often miraculous.

Most actual medical treatment was either through self-help (including patent medicines) or at the hands of one of the many botanic or Thomsonian physicians who gathered to Mormonism. (There were very few orthodox M.D.s among the converts, and they—along with the Thomsonians—were often chosen as Smith's personal secretaries or close advisers.) In his youth, Joseph had been spared the loss of a osteomyelitic leg through the brilliant efforts of the distinguished and orthodox Dr. Nathan Smith, using pioneering surgical procedures. Unfortunately the family's negative recollection of the event centered more on the initial (and accepted) orthodox recommendation of amputation. The death of Joseph's beloved older brother, Alvin, with a lump of orthodox calomel lodged in his bowels, and several other untoward experiences further supported a family inclination against the so-called heroic therapy of regular physicians. Not surprisingly, Joseph as Mormon prophet chose a botanic practitioner as his personal physician.

In the early 1840s, botanic healers and midwives began to be "called" and "set apart" by church leaders to perform their work in the community, and a botanic board of health was established in Mormon-controlled Nauvoo. Smith, meanwhile, condemned the notion—held by some converts—that the use of medicine ("roots and herbs") was "of the devil," recommending instead that "if you send for a Dr at all send in the first stages" and on occasion commending some of his own preferred remedies.[14]

A few public-health measures, principally drainage of sloughs, were undertaken around Nauvoo to combat the "miasma" which blew over the community from the adjacent Mississippi. While this may have helped somewhat, malaria continued to decimate the Saints throughout their stay in the area. An equally serious problem, contaminated water, remained completely unrecognized, as it did nationally; thus water-borne disease also took a major toll, especially among the young. Smith's recommendation that immigrating converts locate in the lower parts of the city (nearer the river), that water from shallow wells be used in preference to river water, and that both were "more healthful to drink than spring water," in hindsight could hardly have been more medically off-target.[15] At the time, however, this would not have been apparent. Moreover, there was the overriding issue that Smith's principal detractors were concentrated in the higher parts of town.

Although not strictly public-health issues, there were other aspects of community life that might be said to have fostered the general health of early Mormons. From the earliest days, Mormon social life was characterized by a very positive attitude toward recreation. This probably reflected Smith's general physical prowess, gregarious personality, and perhaps some compensatory competitiveness on his part following a sickly childhood. Sports, especially wrestling, were a common pastime. Dancing, too, despite an initial rejection as too much of "the world," soon became a prominent Mormon diversion, and has continued so to the present day. An active program of home visits to all members by assigned "teachers" who assumed spiritual and often temporal responsibility for their "families" was begun very early, and also continues to the present, as does the practice of occasional congregation-wide fasting on behalf of the sick. During the nineteenth century the effectiveness of such activities was probably enhanced by the fact that the Mormons were a geographically concentrated community, as well as a gathering of believers.

Despite all of Nauvoo's acknowledged health problems, cemetery sexton reports do not show the community to have fared any worse overall than other frontier communities of the day. Much obviously remained to be learned everywhere. And in the final analysis, notwithstanding the theological, even apocalyptic, overtones often associated with death and disease, on the day-to-day level Mormons viewed such events with much the same pragmatism as they did other natural occurrences. One church leader was probably entirely representative when he matter-of-factly wrote from the vicinity of the promised New Jerusalem (in Missouri), "Here sickness comes, and where does it not? The ague and fever; the chill fever, a kind of cold plague, and other diseases, prey upon emigrants till they are thoroughly seasoned to the climate. Here death puts an end to life, and so it does all over the globe."[16] Similarly, disciple Woodruff, finding himself, like many others, still afflicted with malaria following one of the most heralded community-wide faith healings in Mormon history—and despite three botanic emetics and fifteen minutes of steaming—sought relief with no erosion of his faith in the "highly recommended" quinine-containing "Sapington's Anti fever pills." "[B]lessed be the Lord," he reported, "they have entirely broaken [sic] the ague entirely to all appearance."[17]

The Pioneer Years, 1846–1869

The pioneer years saw no major changes in Mormon teachings on health and disease. Righteous living continued, at least rhetorically, to be the key to good health. The context of the discussion, however, was expanded well beyond the Word of Wisdom to include, most notably, participation in divinely mandated plural marriage. The good health of Mormon children was cited by church leaders as a natural consequence of parental compliance with God's decrees, the "physiologic side of the question" being "one, if not the strongest, source of argument in favor" of the practice of polygamy.

Non-Mormons held to a similar moral physiology, but used the *poor* health of these same children as proof of the "gross" and "sensual" nature of the Mormon religion. In descriptions published in medical journals throughout America, the astonishingly rapid emergence of a "new race" was described, manifesting the degenerate characteristics acquired over many ages by the inhabitants of densely populated Old World cities. In the words of a widely reprinted medical correspondent, "the yellow, cadaverous visage; the greenish-colored eyes; the thick, protuberant lips; the low forehead; the light, yellowish hair; and the lank, angular person, constitute an appearance so characteristic of the new race, the production of polygamy, as to distinguish them at a glance."[18] Beauty being in the eyes of the beholder, the Mormons, in turn, saw the "generally sickly and shortlived" children of New England as a direct manifestation of the vices of the non-Mormon East.[19]

If anything, the early Utah years saw a further relaxation in the general attitude toward the proscriptions of the Word of Wisdom. Those setting out on the overland trek west were officially advised to include coffee, tea, and alcohol—which had acquired the status of mini-panacea in orthodox medicine—among their supplies. And the typical Mormon family (including that of Brigham Young) continued to use one or more of these items on a regular basis. Periodic suggestions that the divine health code be made a "commandment" were rebuffed by Young, who nonetheless continually urged compliance with its recommendations. At the same time, he often preached words of practical nutrition which went well beyond the "positive" guidance of the Word of Wisdom.

While retaining some of the diversity of the formative years, the predominant perspective on disease during this pioneer period was an essentially naturalistic one, as suggested by Brigham Young's characteristically straightforward description:

> This [is] a healthy country, as healthy as any in which I have lived or traveled; and yet when once a disease gets hold of a person, it is rather apt to terminate one way or the other sooner than in these low countries where a man may always be dying, until some friendly physician shall interpose and quietly put him away according to the most approved and scientific mode practiced by the most learned M.D.'s. The most prevalent diseases here are fevers.[20]

Throughout this period, those in need of medical care continued to be referred to the elders for priesthood blessings, as well as to botanic practitioners or midwives. There was some concern that the afflicted turned a little too quickly to tangible remedies, so a retrenchment on this point was conducted as part of a broader "reformation" in the mid-1850s reaffirming leadership expectations in doctrine and practice. At the same time, the ever-practical Young also advised:

> If we are sick and ask the Lord to heal us, and to do all for us that is necessary to be done, according to my understanding of the Gospel and salvation, I might as well ask the Lord to cause my wheat and corn to grow without my plowing the ground and casting in the seed. It appears consistent to me to apply every remedy that comes within the range of my knowledge, and to ask my Father in Heaven, in the name of Jesus Christ, to sanctify that application to the healing of my body.[21]

Isolated in their western settlements, Mormon pioneers could almost guarantee what sort of medical care was allowed in their communities, as well as what type was not. Young had instructed those brethren who, at his prompting, had volunteered for military service during the Mexican War and had therefore traveled west separated from the main body of Mormon pioneers, "If you are sick, live by faith, and let the surgeon's medicine alone if you want to live, using only such herbs and mild foods as are at your disposal."[22] The assigned military surgeon had other ideas, however, and forced calomel into anyone who fell ill. Not surprisingly, therefore, on establishing themselves in Utah, the Mormons quickly passed a law barring the dispensing of most orthodox medical remedies ("deadly poisons")

> without first explaining fully, definitely, critically, simply, and unequivocally [to the patient and his friends] . . . in plain, simple, English language, the . . . design of said poison . . . and procuring . . . unequivocal approval, approbation and consent.

Offenders were subject to a one-thousand dollar fine or not less than a year at hard labor.[23]

However progressive this early notion of "informed consent," public-health concerns, in the modern sense, remained unappreciated and low on the pioneer agenda. There was some progress. Immigrating converts were advised to avoid specific routes found to be unusually sickly, as well as the dangerous months of summer. Quarantines were enforced on any incoming companies with smallpox. The Mormon reformation of the mid-1850s even included in its lengthy mandatory catechism the question, "Do you wash your bodies once a week," though in answering on behalf of himself Brigham Young announced that he did not, that he had tried it and found it "was not for everybody."[24]

Several decades later, a still imperfectly informed Mormon physician recalled other public-health aspects of these "safe" pioneer years when

> the early settler could pile around him the offal and waste of living—the excreta from the pig-sty and out-house, the contents of the swill barrel could ferment alongside the larder—all these things could be had with little risk, for the "germs" were not [yet] present to . . . do their work of spreading contagion.[25]

Along the same lines, a frustrated Salt Lake City watermaster later wrote in his personal journal of an 1855 confrontation with Brigham Young, who had diverted through his hog pen the city creek that supplied virtually all the city's water. So far as Brother Brigham was concerned, "if he could drink his own filth he did not think others should complain." Although the watermaster eventually prevailed, similar or related problems were endemic in pioneer Utah as late as the 1870s, when a locally assigned military surgeon attributed the allegedly excessive childhood mortality among the Mormons in large part to contamination of the well water used for drinking and culinary purposes by the

> organic matters that settle down from the surface of the streets, yards, gutters, drains, water-closets, & etc., . . . and, as a consequence it becomes a purgative mixture, especially to strangers and the amount of bowel disease, and deaths from its effects, is simply frightful, particularly among the children.[26]

However limited the understanding of the pioneer Mormons of things medical (in fact they differed little from other Americans), and despite popular reports of excessive mortality rates, the sexton's reports again fail to show Salt Lake City to have been much different in rates and distribution of deaths than many other American towns. Death rates were high nearly everywhere, and a large majority of those who died were always children. A notable exception to this generally comparable record is found during the period immediately following the exodus from Nauvoo, during which the Mormon vanguard endured winter quarters on the Missouri River. Those encamped there suffered greatly from malaria, water-borne diseases, and, ultimately, scurvy. Overall death rates were perhaps three to four times higher than before or after, and infant mortality approached a staggering thirty-three percent of all births.[27] Another wave of pioneers shortly thereafter faced the second pandemic of cholera, though this time without the editorial fanfare of the 1832–1833 encounter. The Great Basin, by contrast, was almost without malaria, and dietary deficiencies were not usually a problem. It was also sufficiently isolated to escape, for the most part, epidemics of smallpox and cholera. Thus endemic water-borne diseases (for example, typhoid and dysentery) again dominated the cemetery records.

Like the earliest phase of the Mormon medical experience, the pioneer period was thus marked by a combination of ideology, ignorance, and pragmatism—with the last named, if anything, most prominent. Even the divine promises of the Word of Wisdom, which still could be—and occasionally were—supported by reference to the latest medical thinking, were amenable to commonsense characterization. As one apostle explained, those who were wise enough to adhere to the health code would "walk & not be weary run & not faint," because "they would have wisdom enough to stop before they got weary."[28] Perhaps no one could top the rank-and-file diarist who recorded that when a painful tooth failed to respond to both a herbal remedy and administration of consecrated oil, he suddenly realized that faith without works was dead, and simply reached in and extracted the offending tooth which, "praise be to God," had not hurt him since.

Late Nineteenth Century, 1870–1900

The final decades of the nineteenth century saw several significant changes in the Mormon perspective on health and medical care. The first Mormons sent east to orthodox medical schools, at the behest of Brigham Young, received their training in the early 1870s, just as modern "scientific medicine" was beginning to emerge. These recently trained, medically orthodox Mormon physicians staffed the first small Mormon hospitals. Church-sanctioned schools for midwives and nurses were also begun. In part, this burst of activity was a response to the opening of non-Mormon hospitals staffed by some of the growing body of well-trained non-Mormon physicians who came to Utah following the completion of the transcontinental railroad in 1869. It also reflected leadership concerns that the medical problems of women appropriately remain within the domain of women practitioners. Several of those sent east for training were women, and on their return these early women physicians joined hospital staffs and provided the principal instruction for midwives and mothers.

The influence on the Utah community of these well-trained physicians, and those who followed them, was considerable. Disease and health came increasingly to be viewed in entirely naturalistic terms. Whereas repeated violation of the Word of Wisdom still was believed to predispose one to chronic (and some acute) disorders—a notion receiving welcome support from the new scientific medicine—sanitary reform and the germ theory of disease addressed more directly the most pressing medical problems.

Within two decades "scientific" medical practice had replaced botanical treatment as the order of the day in Mormon Utah, at least among the educated leadership. This transition was not entirely uneventful, for as word got around that "the President of the Church and the chief officers . . . had regularly attended physicians whose services were actually called into use even when the sickness was not serious, it was something of a shock."[29] Almost of necessity, any remaining notion of the primacy of faith healings for most illnesses, which still were overwhelmingly of an infectious nature, was further eroded in this process. The suggestion was even heard—from the new Mormon physicians—that the salutary effect of consecrated oil derived in part from the physical effect of its application or consumption. Also discarded at this time, some four decades after its adoption, was the practice of "rebaptism" for health (or other) purposes.

Mormon Utah also began its first meaningful improvements in the distribution of drinking water during these years. Pipes rather than open ditches appeared in the 1870s, about the time when Young recommended in some of his sermons that drinking water be boiled. By 1887 a new church presidency formally advised its membership:

> Much disease can be avoided by frequent ablutions, simple diet and the destruction or removal of all refuse. Cleanliness is part of godliness. Filth is obnoxious to the spirit of the Gospel. It is the breeding place for epidemics. Our bodies, our houses, our gardens and outhouses should all be kept free from uncleanly accumulations. Individual effort in this direction is a necessity, and this should be supplemented by organized regulations in the various wards [congregations] so that the atmosphere may not become charged with the germs of disease and death.[30]

By the turn of the century, death rates had fallen well below the national average, with reported infant mortality in Salt Lake City about half the national figure.

Finally, a new, but largely polemical, medical issue emerged during this period. For the first time, abortion and family limitation were addressed at length in Mormon discourse, both being roundly condemned as equivalent to infant murder. The message, however, was not directed at the near-maximally fertile Mormon community; rather, it was aimed at critics of Mormonism in an attempt, prompted by a national anti-abortion campaign, to respond in kind to charges of polygamous immorality among the Saints.

The Public Health Years, 1900–1929

Mormons abandoned polygamy about the turn of the century, but a new mark of their distinctiveness soon emerged as compliance with the Word of Wisdom (that is, total abstinence from coffee, tea, tobacco, and alcohol) was made a prerequisite to good standing in the church. This new requirement derived from several developments, including increased medical evidence of the harmful effects of some of the proscribed items, the prohibition movement, and the ascendency within the church of individuals long associated with the view that any divine health code should be considered a "commandment." However, while compliance with the Word of Wisdom was now technically a mandatory prerequisite to participation in important church ordinances or advancement to positions of local leadership, allowances were regularly made for those with long-established habits.

Prominent church leaders joined the Utah public-health association and strongly supported vaccination and other health-reform measures. Also, in 1902, the church opened a modern, well-equipped hospital devoted to the latest in scientific medical care, the first of fifteen modern "LDS" hospitals (eventually totalling some two thousand beds) to be built over the next few decades. An editorial in the church-owned *Deseret News* explained: "Remedies are provided by the Great Physician or by Nature as some prefer to view them and we should not close our eyes to their virtues or ignore the skill and learning of the trained doctor."[31] Priesthood blessings (with anointing now applied only to the crown of the head) assumed a symbolic but unmistakably supplemental status; in the words of a prominent Mormon apostle, "We must do all we can, and then ask the Lord to do the rest, such as we cannot do. Hence we hold the medical and surgical profession in high regard. . . . When we have done all we can then the Divine Power will be directly applicable and operative."[32]

As Mormons turned increasingly for care to those with specialized training, earlier concerns that "female conditions" be treated by women passed into history. This was apparently the result of several factors, including the declining status of midwives and the fact that individual members—men or women—no longer were "called" by church leaders to become doctors. For these and other reasons the relative proportion of women physicians, including those in obstetrics, apparently dwindled.

The still well-entrenched pro-herbal, anti-orthodox medical tradition present in large segments of the Mormon community delayed the implementation of a number of attempted state health reforms. Compulsory vaccination of Utah school children was barred in 1901 by the Mormon-dominated state legislature, over the governor's veto, leaving the state with one of the highest rates of smallpox infection in the nation (albeit relatively low by nineteenth-century standards). Indeed, Utah was (probably incorrectly) believed to be the source of outbreaks of smallpox abroad, via letters or packages sent to Mormon missionaries. While a few other public-health measures also encountered popular opposition, eventually virtually all the tradition-bound obstacles were overcome.

The emergence of a national "birth control" movement in the early twentieth century forced church leaders to consider this subject in earnest for the first time. Responding to the inquiry, is it ever right "intentionally to prevent, by any means whatever, the spirits . . . from obtaining earthly tabernacles," church president Joseph F. Smith responded in 1908 that, "In a general way, and as a rule, the answer . . . is an emphatic negative. I do not hesitate to say that prevention is wrong." In addition to bringing in its wake selfishness and a "host of social evils," it would also "disregard or annul the great commandment of God to man, 'Multiply and replenish the earth.' " Smith added, however, that "I am now speaking of the normally healthy man and woman. But that there are weak and sickly people who in wisdom, discretion and common sense should be counted as exceptions, only strengthens the general rule."[33] Later, amidst a growing national and local enthusiasm over eugenics, he added as a second exception those with "impurities that would be entailed on their posterity." Even in such exceptional cases, the only legitimate preventive was "absolute abstinence."

Mormon fertility, down perhaps twenty-five to thirty percent from mid–nineteenth-century rates, fluctuated somewhat during the first two decades of the century, then plunged during the years of economic depression (which began in Utah in the early 1920s) to levels half those seen just a few years earlier. Although always about eleven to twelve births per thousand population (and roughly one and a half children per family) above national rates, twentieth-century Mormon fertility rates have paralleled closely the variations seen nationally. Nonetheless, as early as the 1920 census, Mormonism was singled out as a rare illustration of the clear impact of religion on family size.[34]

Mormon death rates, including infant mortality, remained well below national figures, prompting Mormon authors for the first time to attempt truly scientific arguments in support of the benefits of their health code. The comparative data then available, failing to make important allowances for varying age structures, led church authors unfamiliar with epidemiology to make claims about low rates of kidney, lung, and nervous system disorders, as well as diabetes and tuberculosis, which have proved to be in error. Similar claims for heart disease and cancer eventually proved correct, and probably accounted for much of the reduced total mortality then noted.

Overall, the philosophical harmony between Mormonism and medicine was probably closer during this phase of Mormon history than it has ever been. Medical support for its Word of Wisdom was greater than at any time since the 1830s; the medical community was generally aligned with church beliefs in the area of birth control; and great strides were made in integrating fully into conventional health-care systems.

Mid-Twentieth Century, 1930–1969

As medical evidence of the deleterious effects of alcohol and tobacco continued to mount, the Word of Wisdom remained a dominant theme in leadership discourse. By 1960 complete abstinence from coffee, tea, tobacco, and alcohol was truly an absolute prerequisite to achieving most of the innumerable leadership "callings" in Mormon congregations, or to attending the sacred rituals performed in Mormon temples. Unofficially the prohibition against coffee and tea was held to derive from the presence of caffeine or related drugs; therefore decaffeinated coffee was not considered in violation of the code. Conversely, caffeinated soft drinks came under a cloud, though they were never officially included on the list of prohibitions.

Ultimately the vast majority of "active" Mormons adhered to the restrictions of their health code. Indeed, those who failed to conform on this point tended to slide into inactivity and be lost to the general fellowship of the church. It has been suggested, though as yet without adequate study to establish the case, that those who follow this unfortunate path are prone to fall into patterns of more serious alcohol abuse.

A clear evolution in leadership thinking on family planning took place during these years, manifested initially by a decade of relative silence during the years of economic depression and low Mormon fertility. By the mid-1940s, strongly pro-family counsel nonetheless condoned, "when the health of the mother demands it, the proper spacing of children . . . by seeking medical counsel, by compliance with the processes of nature, or by continence."[35] The apogee in this progression came almost two decades later with the observation by a member of the church's presiding First Presidency that "the Latter-day Saints believe in large families wherever it is possible to provide for the necessities of life, for the health and education of their children, and when the physical and mental health of the mother permits."[36]

An unprecedented *Sensible Sex Guide for the L.D.S. Bride and Groom*, forthrightly dealing with marital sex and the technical aspects of birth control, was published in 1968 by a leading Mormon physician.[37] Mormon families, meanwhile, remained larger than the national norm, but birth rates dropped during the 1960s even below those prevailing during the depths of the Great Depression. Surveys showed this to be largely through the widespread use of modern contraceptives.

The church was by now irrevocably committed to modern scientific health care, supplemented by priesthood blessings. In the few areas of potential conflict, common sense and modern medicine prevailed. Members were reassured that those whose health might be affected should not participate in the monthly twenty-four–hour fasts held throughout the church. Those entering hospitals were counseled that sacred undergarments, worn day and night by faithful members, need not be worn if they impeded medical care. Finally, the growth of the church nationally and internationally, as well as the emigration of Utahans in search of better economic opportunities, foreclosed for most Latter-day Saints any chance of obtaining medical care from a fellow Mormon; however, when the opportunity presents, most members still seem to seek out an LDS physician.

Only one exception to this near-total embrace of conventional medical care remained: the field of mental health. When administered by non-Mormon therapists, and particularly since the turn of the century, psychiatric care was widely held to be incompatible with traditional Mormon notions of sin and personal accountability. A popular compendium of "Mormon doctrine" published in 1958 (and again in 1966) only partially overstated leadership concerns when it cross referenced "Psychiatry" to "Church of the Devil."[38]

While perhaps more susceptible than the average American to the overtures of "natural" health faddists, Mormons have virtually rejected their herbal heritage. A notable exception was, and continues to be, the small minority of schismatic, excommunicated "Fundamentalists," who also continued to follow most of the other practices and beliefs of the mid–nineteenth-century church, including polygamy. Vaccination was no longer disputed, though a vestige of the old days may have been evident in the continued refusal of Utahans to allow fluoridation of public water supplies.

Recent Developments

The past few years have seen more church interest and activity in the medical arena than at any time in the twentieth century. One way or another these have involved virtually all facets of the Mormon interface with health and medicine.

The now well-demonstrated success of the Mormon lifestyle in dramatically reducing the incidence of cancer, heart disease, and several other disorders has led church leaders to recast the Word of Wisdom into somewhat of a proselyting tool—as a sign of the prophetic insight of Joseph Smith. Beginning in the mid-1970s, leading medical journals have carried an increasing number of studies showing convincingly that Mormons have dramatically lower incidences of many cancers, heart disease, cirrhosis, and birth defects than most Americans. Much of this can be credited to abstinence from tobacco and alcohol—particularly the former—as well as to low levels of promiscuity and early child-bearing. A substantial proportion of the reduction in mortality remains unexplained, although most Mormons believe it relates to the avoidance of coffee and tea, or to the less stressful lifestyle they assume they lead. Curiously, some of the health gains documented among Mormons do not correlate with degree of participation in Mormon congregations, and thus, by implication, with conformity to officially sanctioned life-styles.

In contrast to this record, in recent years anecdotal reports have been used to argue that there is a high incidence of depression among Mormon women. The only quantitative study of the question to date failed to find an increased incidence of depression among married Mormon women in Utah (in comparison to married non-Mormon women). The fact of a significant incidence of emotional problems among the membership, however high or low it might be in comparison to non-Mormon society, led to a reconsideration of the previous attitude toward professional counseling. It was concluded that carefully selected professional therapists should be used throughout the church to assist local ecclesiastical leaders with difficult cases. In addition, regional social-services networks were established, and traveling staff psychologists were made available to church leaders throughout the United States.

In conjunction with these general developments, Mormon psychologists and counselors organized their own professional association, and several began developing a well-publicized "gospel-based" psychotherapy. Hailed by some church leaders, the idea behind this approach was to incorporate revealed gospel insights into a therapeutic model superior to that available in "secular" psychiatry. However, while Mormon counselors continue to counsel Mormon patients in a distinctively Mormon context, this more ambitious project has been abandoned as premature and inadequate to present needs.

A marked drift toward doctrinal fundamentalism among the leadership during recent years has not been accompanied by any modification in the church's position on health care. When the recent national enthusiasm for unorthodox, "natural" remedies struck a responsive chord among some of the faithful, an official message from the church leadership sternly warned those members "with serious illnesses . . . [to] consult competent physicians, licensed under the laws of the land to practice medicine." Members were further reminded that "our belief in the divine power of healing should in no way preclude seeking competent medical assistance."[39]

While priesthood administration remains a common source of hope and reassurance within the church, Mormons are also able to smile at the trace of truth in the definition of "blessing" recently offered by a Mormon humorist: "The ordinance of anointing and laying on hands to heal the sick; most commonly done to those not sick enough to need a doctor or so sick the doctors have given up hope."[40] This notwithstanding, elders are regularly assigned to visit and administer to those in hospitals, and most LDS families often turn in faith and confidence to this source of help.

The church leadership in recent years also has reconsidered its role as a formal provider of health care and divested itself of all its hospitals. While it still pays for the health services of needy members under some circumstances, actual health-care delivery is no longer by church-salaried professionals—except for the clinical psychologists who provide regional support to local congregations. On the other hand, for the first time health professionals—principally public-health specialists—are now sent along with full-time proselyting missionaries to upgrade the health environment of converts in many developing nations.

The tension between church and societal thinking on emerging medical–ethical issues was probably greater in the 1970s than at any time in a century. Confronted with the successful movement to legalize abortion, the church first dealt at length with this issue. However, much like the record on birth control, an initially absolute stand against abortion (unless the mother's life was endangered) subsequently has been qualified to allow exemptions in the case of lesser health risks, rape, incest, and—unofficially—some serious fetal defects. Similarly, artificial insemination with donor semen, initially condemned, has come to be viewed in much less judgmental terms.

On the other hand, homosexuality and sex-change surgery, both subjects of new and strongly condemnatory church guidance in recent years, officially remain grounds for excommunication. Even in these instances, however, there are suggestions of an unannounced softening of the official stance. Aversion therapy for homosexuality came briefly into vogue among some church-supervised psychologists, but has been discontinued.

The new medical technologies of the past decade, such as in vitro fertilization and genetic engineering, have not been publicly addressed by the church leadership. In practice, judgments about the use of such techniques have been left to the individuals directly involved.

Future Direction

In conclusion, a word might be offered on the future direction of church counsel regarding these and similar issues. Several generalizations emerge from the record which may prove predictive, if not prophetic.

First, contrary to its media image, the church (that is, the First Presidency) often chooses *not* to express itself formally on issues with obvious ethical or theological overtones, deferring rather to the "free agency" and personal accountability before the Lord of individual members. This is especially true when the issues are extraordinarily complex or when important scientific questions remain unanswered.

Second, when the church does comment on such issues, the initial guidance is usually only given privately, in response to questions from those most directly involved. Insofar as medical–ethical issues are concerned, there appear to be no twentieth-century exceptions to this general rule.

Third, when formal public statements finally appear, they generally are not until relatively late in the public discussion. By this time, it is not unusual for individual members and local leaders already to have reached independent judgments. While inevitably leading to some confusion, given the Mormon notion of free agency, this basic process is not necessarily viewed as bad. Only on the relatively infrequent occasions when the public statement reverses previously given private guidance (as, for example, was the case with sex-change surgery) does this pose much of a problem; even then it is highly localized.

Fourth, with the passage of time there almost always is an evolution in church guidance on specific medical–ethical issues. The public phase of this evolution invariably has been in the direction of greater conformity to the general medical or social consensus on the subject. One can see this, among other places, on the issues of birth control, sterilization, artificial insemination, abortion, sex-change surgery, and medical practice in general.

Fifth, to some extent this evolution is accompanied by the emergence of what in retrospect might be termed the core of ethical concern that motivated the guidance from the outset. This core is generally expressed in terms unambiguously tied to central tenets of the faith: the centrality of marriage and children, the overriding importance of maintaining family harmony and stability and protecting the health and well-being of mother and child, the preservation of free agency and personal accountability, and the total unacceptability of decisions based on "selfish" rationales.

Sixth, where core beliefs themselves are modified, this generally reflects a reassessment in the light of new knowledge simply unreconcilable with the previous view. This development does not pose as much a challenge to church authority as might be supposed. Accepting as a tenet of Mormon faith that the gospel encompasses all truth, secular and religious, it is implicit that periodically this sort of refinement will take place.

In 1983 a Mormon surgeon replaced the heart of a Mormon patient with an artificial heart, a symbolically fitting last stop for our review. There perhaps can be no more emphatic illustration of the commitment of most Mormons to the very latest in modern medicine. In its brief 155-year history, Mormonism has encountered, responded to, and ultimately been transformed by the medical revolution which has to varying degrees shaped all American religions. The distinctive setting in which it began and its unique pioneer-community heritage have given several chapters of Mormon medical history a slightly different shading, but the basic outlines of the story should be familiar to those of many faiths.

Notes

1. The 1611 Authorized Version of the Bible, or King James Version, is the semi-official Bible within Mormonism, and until recently was the only one quoted by church leaders.
2. *Doctrine and Covenants of the Church of the Latter Day Saints: Carefully Selected from the Revelations of God* (1835, reprinted Independence, MO, 1971), pp. 207–208 [Section 80, dated February 1833, later redesignated Section 89].
3. *Doctrine and Covenants,* p. 123 [Section 13, dated February 1831, later redesignated Section 42].
4. "The Cholera," *Evening and Morning Star,* September 1832.
5. Joseph Smith, *History of the Church of Jesus Christ of Latter-day Saints, Period I,* ed. B.H. Roberts, 6 vols., (Salt Lake City, 1902–1912) 2:80, 114.
6. Smith, *History of the Church* 1:83.
7. Joseph Smith, Junior, *The Book of Mormon* (Palmyra, NY, 1830), p. 582; now usually cited by the chapter and versing introduced later, as Moroni 8:22.
8. Lorenzo Snow, *Desert News,* June 15, 1901, p. 1; on the most important sermon by Joseph Smith on the subject, see Stan Larson, "The King Follett Discourse: A Newly Amalgamated Text," *Brigham Young University Studies* 18 (1978):193–208; and Van Hale, "The Doctrinal Impact of the King Follett Discourse," *Brigham Young University Studies* 18 (1978):209–225.
9. See, for example, Joseph Smith in *Times and Seasons* 1 (1840):132, later adapted as *Doctrine and Covenants,* Section 122; Orson Pratt, "The Pre-existence of Man," *The Seer* 1 (1853):97–98; and, recently, Truman Madsen, *Eternal Man* (Salt Lake City, 1966), expecially chap. 5, "Evil and Suffering."
10. *Doctrine and Covenants,* p. 123 [Section 13]; p. 116–117 [Section 11, dated December 1830, later Section 35].

11. *Doctrine and Covenants,* p. 123 [Section 13].
12. The Mormon hierarchy, as fully developed, was headed by a First Presidency, usually composed of three men, and a Quorum of Twelve Apostles. These men, together with a larger body of assistants called Seventies are termed General Authorities of the church, and are in its full-time employ. All regional and congregational leaders ("stake presidents" and bishops, respectively) are lay ministers. These titles are in distinction to individual ranks of priesthood, which are held by virtually all male members over the age of twelve. Most adult males are "elders," for example, and this term is commonly used to refer to any adult priesthood holder.
13. *Wilford Woodruff's Journal, 1833–1898 Typescript,* 9 vols. (Midvale, UT, 1983–1984), 8:355.
14. Donald Q. Cannon and Lyndon W. Cook, eds., *Far West Record: Minutes of The Church of Jesus Christ of Latter-day Saints, 1830–1844* (Salt Lake City, 1983), p. 96; Smith, *History of the Church* 6:59.
15. Smith, *History of the Church* 5:357.
16. *Latter Day Saints' Messenger and Advocate* 1 (November 1834):22–23.
17. *Wilford Woodruff's Journal* 1:348, 350.
18. See *Boston Medical and Surgical Journal* 63 (1860):438–440; *St. Louis Medical and Surgical Journal* 19 (1861):270–272; *Pacific Medical and Surgical Journal* 4 (1861):343–347.
19. On this see Lester E. Bush, Jr., "Mormon 'Physiology,' 1850–1875," *Bulletin of the History of Medicine* 56 (1982):218–237.
20. *Deseret News,* December 13, 1851.
21. *Journal of Discourses,* 26 vols. (Liverpool, England, 1854–1886), 4:24.
22. Sgt. Daniel Tyler, *A Concise History of the Mormon Battalion in the Mexican War, 1846–1847* (1881, reprinted Glorieta, NM, 1969), p. 146.
23. Offenses Against Public Health; Acts, Resolutions and Memorials Passed at the Several Annual Sessions of the Legislative Assembly of the Territory of Utah [1850–1855], Chap. XXXII, Title IX, Sections 106, 107.
24. Gene A. Sessions, *Mormon Thunder: A Documentary History of Jedediah Morgan Grant* (Urbana, IL, 1982), p. 221.
25. *The Salt Lake Sanitarian* 2 (May 1889):47–48.
26. "Report of Surgeon E.P. Vollum, USA," in John Shaw Billings, *War Department Surgeon General's Office Circular No. 8, "Report on the Hygiene of the United States Army,"* May 1, 1875 (Washington, DC, 1875), pp. 344–345.
27. Maureen Ursenbach Beecher, "Women in Winter Quarters," *Sunstone* 8 (July–August 1983):16.
28. *Wilford Woodruff's Journal* 4:10, quoting Amasa Lyman.
29. *Mormon Democrat: The Religious and Political Memoirs of James Henry Movle,* ed. Gene A. Sessions (Salt Lake City, 1975), p. 11.
30. James R. Clark, ed., *Messages of the First Presidency of the Church of Jesus Christ of Latter-day Saints, 1833–1964,* 6 vols. (Salt Lake City, 1965–1975) 3:123–124.
31. *Deseret News,* January 6, 1905.
32. *Deseret News,* December 17, 1921.
33. *Improvement Era* 11 (1908):959–961; a general history of this subject is Lester E. Bush, Jr., "Birth Control Among the Mormons: Introduction to an Insistent Question," *Dialogue: A Journal of Mormon Thought* 10 (Autumn 1976):12–44.

34. Warren S. Thompson, *The Ratio of Children to Women, 1920* (Washington, DC, 1931), p. 184.

35. Letter of David O. McKay, then of the First Presidency, May 27, 1946, copies of which were later circulated widely.

36. Hugh B. Brown, *You and Your Marriage* (Salt Lake City, 1960), pp. 135–136.

37. Lindsay R. Curtis, *And They Shall Be One Flesh: A Sensible Sex Guide for the Bride and Groom* (Salt Lake City, 1968).

38. Bruce R. McConkie, *Mormon Doctrine* (Salt Lake City, 1966), p. 610.

39. *Church News,* February 19, 1977.

40. Orson Scott Card, *Saintspeak: The Mormon Dictionary* (Salt Lake City, 1981), no pagination.

CHAPTER 15

The Christian

Science Tradition

Rennie B. Schoepflin

Christian Science was born in 1866 when Mary Baker Eddy's spontaneous recovery from a severe injury authenticated her "discovery" that reality is completely spiritual and evil is only an illusion. Her understanding of the mind–body relationship and her healing techniques owed much to the principles of homeopathy and the practice of Phineas Parkhurst Quimby, and her ideas bore many similarities to those of a swarm of religious enthusiasts, mesmerists, spiritualists, and health reformers who, in the words of historian Robert Peel, appealed to "a restless people reaching out blindly for new sources of power, of assurance, of spiritual hygiene."[1] Nevertheless, her consistent emphasis upon the spirituality of the world distinguished her teachings from those of most other mind-healing sects. Struggling to give a distinctive sound to her message, Eddy devoted much of her time after 1866 to teaching, healing, and writing, finally publishing the first edition of *Science and Health,* a textbook of her teachings, in 1875. But her movement grew slowly, and when in 1879 she and her followers organized the Church of Christ, Scientist, in Lynn, Massachusetts, they numbered only twenty-seven. Undeterred, she moved her headquarters to cosmopolitan Boston, where in 1881 she chartered the Massachusetts Metaphysical College to educate practitioners in Christian Science healing.

During the 1880s, mind healers of all kinds spread out from New England to touch new places and new people. Warren Felt Evans, who had been cured by Quimby of a serious nervous disorder in 1863, devoted his life to the refinement, dissemination, and practice of mental healing, exerting through commentaries such as *The Mental Cure* (1869) and *The Primitive Mind Cure* (1885) a formative influence on the development of what came to be known as New Thought. Calling themselves by various names—mind curists, mental curists, and metaphysical healers—these adherents to New Thought diverged widely on the particulars of their views, but they shared in common a confidence in the power of the mind to cure disease and solve human problems and belief in a quasi-religious, often idealist, philosophy that seemed to explain the healing process. Eclectic and independent-minded like Evans, these healers drew upon the mystical writings of the eighteenth-century Swedish philosopher Emanuel Swedenborg, Oriental as well as Judeo-Christian teachings, and the marvels of spiritualism and science to supplement and defend their world views.[2]

Many Americans discovered mind healing in the Christian Science of Eddy's textbook, *Science and Health.* Eager for a cure from their diseases or for the comfort of belief in a benevolent world, these persons often failed to notice any significant difference between Eddy and other mentalists, each with his or her own brand of doctrine. Concerned primarily with the broad picture and unworried by obscure ideological distinctions, large numbers of New Thought adherents and Christian Scientists drifted on a tide of ideas, changing their beliefs or practices to accommodate the latest book they had read or to emphasize a nuance they themselves had discovered.

Busy with her various Boston affairs and confronted by numerous local challenges, Eddy found it increasingly difficult to deal with her far-flung followers. Among other local challenges, religious critics derided her "bogus" Christianity and, comparing her to the purveyor of a popular patent medicine for female complaints, dubbed her the "Lydia Pinkham of the Soul"; former students and eclectic mentalists altered her teachings and questioned her prophetic authority; Julius A. Dresser and his wife Annetta Seabury, former patients and students of Quimby's, accused Eddy of stealing their teacher's ideas. Eddy, convinced that God had revealed the truths contained in *Science and Health,* celebrated her Christian roots, asserted the unreality of matter more adamantly than ever, and moved to unify her followers and define "orthodox" Christian Science by emphasizing her divinely sanctioned authority, clarifying doctrines, and solidifying organizations.

In an effort to provide regular guidance and encouragement to her distant students, Eddy in 1883 established and edited the *Journal of Christian Science* (renamed the *Christian Science Journal* in 1885), a monthly publication intended to shield her students from the "unorthodox" teachings of rival Scientists. She also encouraged the graduates of her Normal Classes at the Metaphysical College to fan out across country, teaching, healing, and establishing institutes of healing and instruction. In the key growth states of Iowa and Illinois alone, Eddy's students established sixteen institutes during the 1880s and 1890s. Occupying an intermediate level of church organization between Eddy and local churches until their closing after the 1890s, these institutes served as successful regional schools for the teaching and spread of Christian Science. To further guard her students from heresy, Eddy encouraged the formation of a National Christian Scientist Association in the spring of 1886. At annual meetings of the Association, she exhorted her own students and those of other teachers to remain committed to her brand of Science.

Many of Eddy's admirers, however, chafed under what they believed to be her excessively authoritarian methods. Some, like A.J. Swarts, acknowledged her unique contributions to mind healing, but insisted that individuals should search for truth outside of *Science and Health* and the Bible and follow it wherever it led without continually seeking her approval. He suggested that mind healers unite Evans's Mental Cure and Eddy's Christian Science into Mental Science. Others, such as Emma Curtis Hopkins, Luther M. Marston, and Ursula N. Gestefeld (all former students of Eddy), objected to Eddy's efforts to establish herself as the only true expositor of Christian Science and to her criticisms of their publications and their schools. Although the teachings of these healers and their students differed in some respects from Eddy's, their shared emphasis on physical healings and their continued use of the name Christian Scientist, even after their separation or expulsion from Eddy's church, justifies labeling them "generic" Christian Scientists.

Many of these generics, having studied with Eddy or one of her students, encouraged an attitude of respect for the woman and her teachings. But they refused to submit to her as the final authority of truth, preferring to trust their own ability to judge truth. At the turn of the century, generics and New Thoughters, fractious as ever, moved again toward organization, forming loose alliances that eventually resulted in the International New Thought Alliance (1914).

New Thought and generic Christian Science find their most numerous descendants in Unity, Religious Science, and Divine Science. Each of these organizations helps people to realize the perfect harmony that exists between God and his creation and thereby to experience that reality through healed bodies and solved financial and emotional problems. Unlike most faithful members of the Church of Christ, Scientist, members of these organizations, most of whom live in the United States, do not eschew modern medicine, choosing rather to supplement mind healing with good health practices and to cooperate with physicians and other health-care professionals when necessary. The Unity School of Christianity exerts the widest influence, employing over five hundred workers and annually circulating over 200,000 copies of the healing journal *Unity* (1891). Together, Religious Science and Divine Science list 277 churches and 613 practitioners in the United States.

Questions among orthodox Christian Scientists over Eddy's authoritarian and arbitrary leadership led in 1888 to a major schism that decimated the church and prompted Eddy to disband all major church organizations and retire to New Hampshire for a period of spiritual reflection. From her retreat near Concord, Eddy embarked on an intensive campaign to stimulate the growth of her movement and place it on a sounder organizational footing. In 1892 she established a central church organization, the Mother Church, in Boston and appointed a board of directors to oversee its affairs and implement her instructions to organize evangelistic lectures and monitor educational standards. Six years later she founded the Christian Science Publishing Society to spearhead worldwide evangelism through the printed word, including *The Christian Science Monitor* (1908). These missionary activities enhanced the growth of Christian Science, spreading it across the oceans from America's urban areas to touch Europe and the Orient by the early twentieth century. During this period of consolidation and outreach, membership exploded from only 8,724 in 1890 to about 55,000 (seventy-two percent of whom were women) by 1906, and the United States Government Census of 1936, counting only members of the Mother Church in the United States, reported 268,915 Christian Scientist adherents. Although no more recent statistics are available because Eddy forbade their publication, local churches now number about three thousand worldwide, with the vast majority of Christian Scientists living in North America (especially the United States) or Western Europe (especially Great Britain and West Germany).[3]

The tenets of orthodox Christian Science, finally settled upon in the early 1890s, have undergone little change. In the eighty-ninth and final edition of the *Manual of the Mother Church* they appeared as follows:

1. As adherents of Truth, we take the inspired Word of the Bible as our sufficient guide to eternal life.

2. We acknowledge and adore one supreme and infinite God. We acknowledge His Son, one Christ; the Holy Ghost or divine Comforter; and man in God's image and likeness.

3. We acknowledge God's forgiveness of sin in the destruction of sin and the spiritual understanding that casts out evil as unreal. But the belief in sin is punished so long as the belief lasts.

4. We acknowledge Jesus' atonement as the evidence of divine, efficacious Love, unfolding man's unity with God through Christ Jesus the Wayshower; and we acknowledge that man is saved through Christ, through Truth, Life, and Love as demonstrated by the Galilean Prophet in healing the sick and overcoming sin and death.

5. We acknowledge that the crucifixion of Jesus and his resurrection served to uplift faith to understand eternal Life, even the allness of Soul, Spirit, and the nothingness of matter.

6. And we solemnly promise to watch, and pray for that Mind to be in us which was also in Christ Jesus; to do unto others as we would have them do unto us; and to be merciful, just, and pure.[4]

Although much of the language used here is traditionally Christian, its meaning often varies from that of historical Christianity and must always be interpreted through a study of *Science and Health* and *Key to the Scriptures,* which Eddy appended to *Science and Health* in 1883.

Today, Christian Scientists participate in eleven-o'clock services on Sunday not unlike those in Protestant denominations, with singing, praying, and reading from the Bible and *Science and Health* constituting the main elements. On Wednesday evenings members attend meetings similar to Baptist prayer meetings to testify to what Christian Science has done for their lives, thereby encouraging others and strengthening their own experience. Having no ordained clergy, each Christian Science branch church elects two Readers from its congregation who preside over services and publicly read from the Bible and *Science and Health.*

Christian Science sprang forth from a New England rich in tradition but also fertile for the political, religious, and medical innovations that animated nineteenth-century America. Jacksonian democrats, religious revivalists, and medical sectarians all damned the authority of "experts" and praised the principles of individualism that characterized the so-called age of the common man. However, despite their occasional criticisms of scientists, churchmen, and physicians, these nineteenth-century Americans displayed a fascination with the wonders of the spiritual and natural worlds. Guided by their commonsense belief that God, the author of both nature and revelation, would never contradict himself, they often reconciled dazzling new scientific discoveries with dusty religious doctrines by revising spiritual truths or devising new spiritual pathways. Questions about human nature and the care of the body and soul especially preoccupied nineteenth-century Americans and led to repeated attempts to reconcile science, medicine, and religion. Each decade seemed to bring some new understanding of human nature that required adaptation to Christianity: phrenology in the 1830s, mesmerism in the 1840s, and spiritualism in the 1850s.[5]

Mesmerism, or animal magnetism as it was popularly called, proved especially effective in leading Americans to relax nervous tensions, relieve spiritual ennui, and restore physical health. First widely publicized across New England by the public lecture tour of Charles Poyen in 1836, mesmerism (similar to the hypnotism of today) fascinated Americans with its bizarre manifestations of clairvoyance, somnambulism, anesthesia, and ecstatic utterance. Professor and peasant alike were attracted to the phrenologists, physicians, spiritualists, and preachers who used mesmerism to awe, cure, or hoodwink.

Phineas Parkhurst Quimby (1802–1866), a thirty-six-year-old clockmaker, listened attentively to Poyen's 1838 lecture in Belfast, Maine, and became intrigued by the medical applications of animal magnetism.

After careful study and experimentation, Quimby concluded that the success of the magnetic healer lay not in his or her control of animal magnetism, but in the patient's confidence in the healer. Believing that a patient's positive mental attitude could effect a cure, Quimby embarked on a career that soon established his reputation as the foremost mentalist of Portland, Maine. He vicariously experienced his patients' symptoms, visited with them to instill a positive mental attitude, and rubbed their head or manipulated their limbs to give them concrete evidence that he was doing something. Although he practiced healing for less than two decades, he exerted an important influence on the birth of both spiritual healing and mind cure in America. During the two years of 1862 and 1863, three major contributors to the early development of American mind healing—Mary Baker Eddy (1821–1910), Warren Felt Evans (1817–1889), and Julius A. Dresser (1838–1893)—received treatment at his hands.[6]

Discovery and Dissent: 1821–1880

Born near Concord in the township of Bow, New Hampshire, on July 16, 1821, and raised in Sanbornton Bridge, only about eighty miles from Portland, Maine, Mary Baker Eddy experienced the religious tensions and medical vagaries of Jacksonian America.[7] As a child and young woman, she suffered from a persistent host of physical and mental illnesses and religious anxieties that severely restricted her activities, dampened her energetic spirit, and hindered her formal education. At one time or another she endured colds, fevers, chronic dyspepsia, lung and liver ailments, backache, nervousness, gastric attacks, and depression. An ambitious child who hoped one day to make her mark as an author, she read and studied when possible, but her ill health and weak constitution prevented her from receiving more than sporadic formal education and occasional tutoring from family members.

When local physicians provided only partial relief of her suffering, Mary turned to self-help remedies and sectarian cures, all of which proved only temporarily effective. During the early 1830s the health reformer Sylvester Graham sought to improve the lives of Americans by promoting a vegetarian regimen that featured the consumption of coarse whole-wheat bread and pure water. Mary first tried Grahamism in 1837 and returned to it occasionally throughout the next twenty-five years, but it never brought her more than transitory relief. In the 1840s she became interested in mesmerism and learned of its power to control or manipulate human thoughts and behavior and to effect surprising cures. During the next decade she discovered homeopathy, a medical theory that encouraged patients to consume minute dilutions of drugs that would, if administered to a healthy person, produce symptoms similar to their own. After some successful experiences with homeopathic treatment, she began to study its principles and to experiment with a variety of medicinal dosages, often treating herself or friends and acquaintances. Observing that her patients recovered even when the solutions they used were so diluted that they contained virtually no medicine, she concluded that their faith in medicine—not the medicine itself—had caused their recovery.

At the same time, a variety of religious problems led Mary to reevaluate traditional Christianity, embracing some of its primitive roots but rejecting other orthodox tenets. Her staunch Congregationalist parents so firmly instilled principles of Christian doctrine and moral behavior into their daughter that at times the intense fervor made the young girl ill. When she was about eight, she heard unknown voices calling her name. On the advice of her mother, who undoubtedly believed that her child represented a fulfillment of the "last days" prophecy of *Acts* 2:17—"your sons and your daughters shall prophesy, and your young men shall see visions"—Mary responded in the words of Samuel: "Speak, Lord; for thy servant heareth" (1 *Sm.* 3:9).[8] Heated theological debates with her father over the doctrine of predestination at times created such mental anxiety that she succumbed to spells of sickness that required a physician's care. While preparing for membership in her parents' church at age seventeen, Mary refused to admit that a good God would damn some souls to eternal hell, but her pastor admitted her anyway.[9] Her later belief in a universe without evil probably derived, at least in part, from her aversion to the contradictions she believed inherent in predestination.

In these early medical and religious experiences we glimpse the origin of important facets of Eddy's personality and teachings and begin to understand how she learned to exert control over herself and others by conjoining religion and health. Her medical odyssey confirmed the impotence of medicine and provided hints for its transformation, while her religious odyssey established her divine calling and revealed how illness could be used to manipulate people and gain power over them.

Disgruntled by the failure of nineteenth-century medicine to cure her permanently, but intrigued by her experiences with mesmerism and homeopathy, Eddy continued to search for solutions to her deteriorating health, turning in 1862 to the now-famous Quimby of Portland. His ministrations effected an immediate but temporary cure; she returned to him in 1863 and remained through the winter, receiving treatments and serving as his faithful disciple. Upon departing in the spring, she took up the occasional practice of Quimbyism, but she could not rid herself of her patients' symptoms, vicariously acquired, and she returned to her mentor for release.

While travelling on icy streets in Lynn, Massachusetts, in February 1866, less than a month after she had learned of Quimby's death, Eddy slipped and fell unconscious. A summoned homeopathic physician did what he could for her severe head, neck, and back pains, but her friends feared for the worst. In pain and depression Eddy turned to her Bible for encouragement, and while reading about the healings of Jesus she discovered the "healing Truth" of Christian Science and experienced a spontaneous recovery. She later recalled that "ever after [I] was in better health than I had before enjoyed."[10] According to Christian Science tradition, it was during this experience that God revealed the truth that distinguishes Christian Science from all other forms of mind healing: "there is but one creation, which is wholly spiritual."[11] Her later recollections to the contrary notwithstanding, after her discovery Eddy continued to struggle against the symptoms of her patients, whom she treated with Quimby-like methods, and to endure occasional relapses of her own assorted maladies. Only two weeks after her fall, she wrote to Julius Dresser, another of Quimby's students, reporting the return of a "terrible spine affection" and "a paralysis of the bowels and digestive functions" and entreating him to take her as a patient.[12] He refused, but sent her words of encouragement and advised her not to place her intelligence in "matter."[13]

Equally unsettling was her need to replace the vital financial and emotional support lost because of her recent marital separation and the death of her teacher and healer. Widowed by the death of her first husband (George Washington Glover) in 1843, and separated from her philandering second husband (Daniel Patterson) after 1866, Eddy for a time moved among various relatives and boarding houses, seeking kind family members and acquaintances to uplift her spirits and provide room and board. Drawing upon her early experiences with homeopathy, mesmerism, and Quimbyism to supplement her spiritual "discovery," she spent much of her time studying the Bible, rehearsing her healing techniques, and sketching the views of reality, sin, and sickness that she believed God had revealed to her. The largess of her hosts proved short-lived, however, forcing her to cast about for some avenue of financial support. Turning to the one thing she knew best, healing, she took out advertisements during the summer of 1868 in the spiritualist journal *Banner of Light,* optimistically claiming for her method "a success far beyond any of the present modes" of healing and an "unparalleled success in the most difficult cases."[14]

In the spring of 1870, she moved to Lynn, Massachusetts, where she used her early pamphlet *The Science of Man, By Which the Sick are Healed* to instruct students in an early form of her teachings, "Moral

Science," and in her healing techniques. Later Eddy called her system Metaphysical Science or simply Metaphysics, before finally settling on Christian Science. She soon formed a partnership with a student, Richard Kennedy, whose income from a successful healing practice supported her teaching and afforded her the free time necessary for the reflections that would bear fruit in the publication of her textbook of Christian Science, *Science and Health* (1875).

At the heart of Eddy's teachings lay her affirmation that there inheres "no Life, Substance, or Intelligence in matter. That all is mind and there is no matter."[15] Her radical idealism denied the existence of anything but God and asserted that humans and the universe are perfect ideas that proceed from God and reflect his harmonious and eternal existence. Only God, his manifestations, and synonyms that express the completeness of his nature—Mind, Spirit, Soul, Principle, Life, Truth, and Love—exist; and all else, especially body, matter, death, error, and evil are merely illusions, the nonexistence of which is proven by humans' reflection of God. With this understanding, rather than with doctrines like predestination that needed to be believed and feared, Eddy thought that she had learned the way to cast out error, heal the sick, raise the dead, and understand the spiritual encounters of her troubled youth. She believed that she had discovered the essence of Christ's life and teachings.[16]

Eddy eventually called her religion Christian Science because her teachings combined her discovery that the power of Christ's words had been in the demonstration of their truth through miracles of healing with her contemporaries' conviction that science could transform nature and ensure human progress. Because most humans did not share her picture of reality, they needed to be taught through a "scientific" process of reasoning and demonstration that emphasized the centrality of healing. She trusted in the inherent logic of her doctrines, convinced that together they formed a unified, coherent, and persuasive picture of reality. For example, if God is all that exists and he is spirit, then matter, sickness, mental illness, and death do not exist. Or, because God is all that exists and he is good, then evil and sin do not exist; they merely reflect the tenacity of false beliefs in their existence and the undue attention paid to the false reports of the senses. Because such claims were difficult to grasp in the abstract, Eddy urged that the truthfulness of her Science be tested in the laboratory of life by healing sickness or overcoming besetting sin. To describe this kind of experimental, and experiential truth, she used the word *demonstrate,* declaring that "the best sermon ever preached is Truth demonstrated on the body, whereby sickness is healed and sin destroyed."[17]

Despite Eddy's continual denial of the existence of matter, it was the practical, concrete evidence of physical healing—eyesight restored, lameness cured, cancer removed—and not just the spiritual healings from sin and a misunderstanding of truth that attracted early followers, provided the best advertisement for Christian Science, and most persuasively demonstrated her metaphysics. In theory, health represented the total "harmony of man," but in reality, improved physical health, increased vitality, and greater longevity proved the real attraction of Eddy's doctrines.[18] These were the results for which patients hoped and the power that practitioners dreamed of possessing. Christian Science did not merely provide Americans with a modified Christian metaphysics that emphasized the healing ministry of Jesus and the salvation of the soul; it also offered them a set of healing techniques that could cure people and earn practitioners a comfortable income. Eddy had experienced healing in her own body and had begun to enjoy the financial independence that followed its practice; thus it is not surprising that she emphasized the advantages of physical healing in her public ministry.

Christian Science, with its philosophical denial of matter and evil, almost openly invited some adherents to embrace human immorality, and such would have been the case more often if Eddy had not retained the strict principles and practical exercises of her father's fierce moralism. Eddy believed that her scientific reform of Christianity comprised a restoration of the full apostolic faith, which had fallen into decay and abuse over the past centuries, but adherents required a spiritual regimen of regular, daily study of the Bible and *Science and Health,* prayer, and the prod of suffering to unlock their Scientific understanding and demonstrate the reality of health. Although suffering does not appease God and ideally speaking does not exist, it inevitably follows sin, sickness, and death; jolts one from one's illusions about reality; and moves one down the path of spiritual understanding. She insisted on strict moral uprightness, even in matters of diet. Echoing Graham, she denounced "depraved appetites for alcoholic drinks, tobacco, tea, coffee, [and] opium."[19] This strong emphasis on personal morality and exclusive commitment to the Bible and *Science and Health* distinguished Eddy and her followers from many generic Christian Scientists and mind healers.

During 1872 Eddy experienced the first real challenges to her fragile authority when a former student, Wallace W. Wright, accused her in a Lynn newspaper of practicing mesmerism, and her associate Kennedy refused her command to reduce the amount of rubbing and manipulating in his practice. Stung by both the partial truth of Wright's charge and the insubordination of Kennedy, Eddy dissolved her partnership with Kennedy, ceased manipulation, and branded as mesmerism all schools of metaphysical healing that differed from her own. Increasingly embattled and suspicious, she gathered her most faithful followers around her to ward off the evil influences of magnetic forces, "malicious animal magnetism," that she felt her enemies were directing against her. During these trying years she gained great courage and support from her future husband, Asa Gilbert Eddy, a converted sewing-machine salesman, whom she married in 1877.

Beginning in 1875 Eddy and her students met sporadically for worship services; in April 1879, she and twenty-six members took the decisive step of establishing a church later designated as the Church of Christ, Scientist, with Eddy as pastor. Lynn remained the hub of Eddy's activities, but not for long. Feeling the tug of cosmopolitan Boston, she and her followers worked to establish their reputations there by starting healing practices, distributing Christian Science literature from door to door, and holding publicly advertised lectures.[20] Her resolve to move from Lynn was further strengthened by the defection of some of her church members, who charged Eddy with "frequent ebullitions of temper, love of money, and the appearance of hypocrisy"—charges that only convinced her shrinking but faithful remnant of the dangers of malicious animal magnetism and led them publicly to proclaim Eddy the "chosen messenger of God" who "had little or no help, except from God, in the introduction to this age of materiality of her book, *Science and Health*."[21]

Completely committed to Boston as the new base for her activities, Eddy moved to build prestige for her movement by chartering the Massachusetts Metaphysical College in 1881 as an institution for health education. The school's 1882 prospectus advertised Eddy as "Professor of Obstetrics, Metaphysics, and Christian Science" and listed the names of cooperating physicians in the Boston area, but the only difference between graduating from the college and completing one of Eddy's courses was the diploma from a state-chartered school.[22] In either case, a graduate received instruction in Christian Science doctrines and in proper healing techniques as well as encouragement to establish a healing practice.

Practicing Christian Science Healing: 1881–1890

In a broad sense, every Christian Scientist was a practitioner who could "demonstrate" over (cure) "false claims" (sickness and sin), but from the start of her movement Eddy encouraged students to earn a living by the practice of healing. Most of these full-time practitioners were women, outnumbering men five to one by the 1890s and eight to one by the early 1970s.[23] For generations, American women had provided primary medical care for their families, but cultural and social pressures had restricted their access to formal medical training and professional standing. During the mid-1800s, owing in part to a large number of broad-based reforms often organized and led by women, women acquired the education and social freedom necessary to establish medical careers—especially as sectarian physicians and for female patients. Christian Science, with its friendly doctrine of a bisexual God and its model of female success in Eddy, provided a similar opportunity.[24]

Many full-time practitioners of Christian Science sensed a strong conviction that signalled their divine calling to the vocation of healing, and although they may not have personally overcome all of their physical and spiritual problems, they had at least "demonstrated" over obvious illness or immorality. Most important, they had settled into the teachings of Christian Science to such an extent that their understanding of the perfection of human nature could not easily be shaken by their patients' reports of moral imperfections or disease symptoms, and they could respond with humility and love during treatments. Theoretically, a believer could train herself to become a practitioner by studying the Bible, *Science and Health,* and Eddy's other writings, but ideally she sought class instruction from Eddy at her Metaphysical College or in public classes. For three hundred dollars a student received a Primary Course of twelve lessons and earned the right to use the title Bachelor of Christian Science (C.S.B.). After three years of practice and the successful completion of a one-hundred-dollar Normal Course, which tested a practitioner's orthodoxy, she could practice as a Doctor of Christian Science (C.S.D.), although numerous generic and some orthodox Christian Scientists advertised as "Doctor" whether they had completed the Normal Course or not.[25]

Often advertising themselves as scientific physicians in the 1870s, but thereafter usually as Christian Scientists, practitioners entered a community as itinerant or resident evangelist–physicians. They advertised in the newspaper, on a signpost, or door-to-door; presented lectures and distributed literature; and performed astounding healings. Charging about the same fees as regular physicians—two dollars for the first visit and one dollar for each subsequent treatment—practitioners treated patients until their symptoms disappeared, which might vary from one to dozens of visits, or until they quit coming. Some earned a consistent income of one hundred dollars per week and in good weeks could reach two hundred dollars, but nineteenth-century practitioners who advertised as specialists—in "dentistry" (especially the use of Christian Science to control pain), "obstetrics" (the use of Christian Science to control the illusions of childbirth, that is, belief in the reality of anatomy, physiology, physical intercourse, and pain), or "absent healing" (the use of Christian Science to treat a patient who was not physically present)—no doubt earned more.[26]

When a patient first visited a Christian Science practitioner he or she expected to be carefully quizzed about symptoms, but the practitioner did not need an exhaustive recital of the patient's "supposed" diseases and symptoms to inform her diagnosis. She needed only to get a general feeling for the patient's problem, whether it be chest pains or infidelity, so that she could "act more understandingly in destroying it."[27] During the late 1870s and the 1880s Christian Scientists differed among themselves regarding the state of mind or expectations that patients must bring to the practitioner before their difficulties could be resolved. Some argued that a patient needed no faith but depended solely on the practitioner's understanding—a characteristic that supposedly distinguished Christian Science from ordinary faith healing—while others claimed that a patient's desire for good was crucial to a positive outcome. Much of the discussion hinged on how much faith and to what purpose. Eddy seemed deftly to straddle both sides of the issue by arguing that one needed at least enough faith to come for help, but that confidence in the procedure was unnecessary. She claimed that dramatic healings occurred for people who only "tried it . . . because their friends wished them to."[28] As the movement entered the twentieth century, Scientists lay less emphasis upon healing as the cure of a particular physical or moral problem effected by the practitioner, and more on healing as a divine process whereby the patient grew in understanding and enlightenment. As a result, Christian Scientists increasingly stressed a patient's responsibility to contribute as much or more to the process as the practitioner.

After the practitioner had diagnosed the patient's problem, she began the treatment, or "argument." Christian Scientists viewed healing essentially as the consequence of a rational conviction that sickness, sin, and death do not exist; the healer, because of her better understanding of that truth, served as midwife or assistant who helped patients recognize their health by arguing that their symptoms and diseases did not exist. The practitioner sought to allay fears by denying their problems and affirming that evil does not exist. For example, she could mentally declare that pain does not exist and continue by arguing: All that exists comes from God; God is Good; therefore, God has not made pain. If the patient appeared receptive, she would perhaps conclude with a brief introduction to the Scientist's metaphysical theory of sickness and pain.[29]

The practitioner was not to use a memorized formula of her own or one of Eddy's that had proven successful in similar cases, nor was she mindlessly to repeat affirmations of truth or denials of errors like an incantation or chant. She was simply to remain open to the leadings of truth for each patient. In an effort to emphasize the scientific nature of their practice and to simplify the writings of Eddy or Evans into handbooks of healing that could be used like cookbooks, many generic

Christian Scientists and undoubtedly some orthodox Scientists as well described step-by-step formulas for healing that were virtually guaranteed to work every time. In her early editions of *Science and Health* and the *Science of Man,* Eddy herself presented her healing instructions in an almost formulaic manner, but later she altered her instructions to become less rigid and denounced those "schismatics" like Luther M. Marston and Ursula N. Gestefeld who persisted in their own efforts to revise her work. Eddy reasoned that she had the clearest view of truth and that those who tried to simplify her work would only confuse truth and detract from the centrality of her discoveries.

When skeptics or patients with little or no knowledge of Christian Science visited practitioners, their cases had to be handled very cautiously in order to avoid further antagonism toward truth. Generally, the practitioner would argue silently in her mind against false understandings and for truth in an effort to correct the ideas of the patient by thought alone, while making sure not to confuse the patient with Christian Science principles that he or she was ill-prepared to understand. Only when the practitioner thought that the patient was ready did she turn to audible arguments.

Christian Scientists believed that the speed of healing depended on the patient's understanding of Christian Science—the clearer the understanding, the faster the healing—and they reserved special prestige for those who could effect speedy and long-lasting results. Other Christian Scientists eagerly sought healing or instruction from such charismatic figures, whose popularity or overweening pride moved Eddy on occasion to restrict their activities and administer reprimands. When they refused Eddy's restraints, they often separated from the discoverer to establish their own heterodox branches of generic Christian Science or to join the eclectic descendants of Evans in the New Thought movement.

When a patient experienced healing, Christian Scientists asserted that the practitioner and patient had "demonstrated" over the malady. "Demonstrate" captures both the fact of sensory demonstration—the patient no longer exhibited symptoms—and the confidence that a metaphysical argument had logically revealed the true nature of reality and had given birth to a spiritual awakening. Treatments did not so much destroy disease as remedy an ignorance of health. Because humans appeared to be what they thought they were, thinking the truth about themselves caused all sickness, sin, suffering, and death to dissolve into the nothingness that they had always been. Sometimes healing was slow and sometimes rapid, but it never failed, except in the sense that one had not yet gained a complete understanding of the true goodness of reality, and never in the sense that reality had proven to be evil.

Because practitioners adamantly denied the existence of sickness and its symptoms, sought to avoid the mental influence of such beliefs, and insisted that their treatments could not fail, they sometimes appeared callous and unsympathetic toward their patients. Although Eddy told her students that "The sick deserve our sympathy and should claim our efforts more even than the sinner," some practitioners feared that a display of sympathy might only strengthen a patient's symptoms or that they themselves might acquire the patient's symptoms.[30] In 1903 a practitioner warned readers of the *Christian Science Journal,* that "The time has passed when the tyro in Christian Science can feel justified in answering tales of suffering and grief with the assertion, 'There is no such thing as pain, and there is nothing in the world to grieve about.'"[31] And to this day Christian Scientists deny the charge of insensitivity, arguing that they exhibit true compassion when they lift a person out of trouble by opening truth to them, not by sharing distress.

Theoretically, Christian Science could overcome all types of sickness, but in the first edition of *Science and Health* Eddy gave a hint of the doctrinal flexibility that usually kept her authority intact, if not untarnished, by allowing her followers to consult surgeons for bonesetting. This concession recognized the difficulty of denying the senses when confronted by a compound fracture, for example, and conformed to Eddy's principle that "in the present infancy of this Truth so new to the world" Christian Scientists should "act consistent with its small foothold on the mind."[32] Christian Scientists claimed that the final result of the healing process and the ultimate demonstration of Science was victory over the error of death itself, but because of the pervasive nature of the belief in death among humans, demonstrations rarely occurred. However, they believed that as time progressed more and more demonstrations over death would occur and that even the incidence of death would decrease.

In the late 1880s Eddy appeared to have weathered the worst of the public criticism and to have established organizational bases for the perpetuation and control of her movement, but her tranquility was shattered in 1888 by the death of a mother and child during a practitioner-attended birth. Although Eddy had advertised herself in 1882 as a "Professor of Obstetrics" and many women had testified to their belief that the principles of Christian Science had reduced or eliminated their pain during childbirth, Eddy had not offered a course on metaphysical obstetrics until 1887. Responding to growing requests by women for such instruction, Eddy began offering classes in the application of Science to the errors of childbirth and preparing her students for potential careers as specialists in painless midwifery.

When Abby H. Corner, a Christian Science practitioner in a suburb of Boston, was indicted for manslaughter in 1888 because of the death of a mother and infant she had attended as metaphysical midwife, Eddy entertained second thoughts about the wisdom of her classes, and rather than publicly defend Corner, she pursued a low-profile path that critics interpreted as merely face-saving. Although the legal case ended in acquittal, Christian Scientists suffered much adverse publicity and the incident raised public questions about the safety and legality of their healing practices. In an effort to defuse the situation, Eddy instructed her followers hereafter to work with physicians in cases of childbirth, echoing her recent accommodation to medicine that had allowed a group of Christian Scientists to pursue medical studies so that they could unite regular obstetrics with the techniques of Christian Science, especially pain control.[33] Such efforts demonstrated again Eddy's adaptive ability and no doubt saved future Christian Scientists much grief, but many of her followers interpreted her failure to defend Corner as evidence of a lack of principle. Disillusioned and disaffected, one-third of her Boston followers left the church, rejecting her authority and decimating the ranks of leadership. In response, Eddy left Boston and withdrew first to Vermont, and then to Concord, New Hampshire, to reassess her mission and the future of her movement. Over a period of two years, she gave up editorship of the *Journal* and divested herself of organizational control of the church—dissolving the Christian Science Association, the Massachusetts Metaphysical College, the Church, and the National Christian Scientist Association. When she emerged again into public life, she launched her movement into the twentieth century with new institutions and a spirit of evangelical outreach.

Consolidation and Outreach: 1890–1910

It may be true that Eddy best displayed her genius through a subtle interplay of prophetic charisma and administrative savvy, for when she again spoke after her months of reflective seclusion, most of her remaining followers held her in even greater esteem and willingly carried out her instructions for the administrative, doctrinal, and missionary reorganization of the movement. In the fall of 1892, she named four devoted followers to serve as members of a Christian Science Board of Directors, delegating to them the responsibility of implementing and enforcing her instructions. Moreover, she deeded to them a parcel of land—with instructions to begin construction in Boston on a new central church headquarters, the Mother Church, to which all truly orthodox Christian Scientists would belong. Building from this administrative base, Eddy worked throughout the 1890s to stabilize her doctrinal authority over members of the Mother Church and to exert discipline through words of advice or threats of excommunication. During these years she intensified her claims to divine insight and literary independence, arguing that "The Bible was my only text-book," and tersely dismissed critics who claimed that she had borrowed her ideas from other mental healers or idealist philosophers.[34]

Eddy especially focused her followers' attention upon the authority and inspiration of *Science and Health,* finally elevating it in 1894 to the level of church pastor. Heretofore, many Christian Science congregations had been led by pastors who preached sermons based upon their understanding of Christian Science. But such sermons, especially when preached by powerful speakers, sometimes developed a following for particular pastors or peculiar doctrines and led parishioners away from Eddy and orthodox Christian Science. Hence, by ordaining her book as an "impersonal pastor" from which assigned passages would simply be read and not commented upon at church services, Eddy eliminated the need to maintain doctrinal purity among human clergy and lessened the possibility that personality cults would develop around talented speakers.

In 1895 she published the first edition of a *Church Manual* that "became the ultimate authority for all action by the church" and codified the numerous bylaws and instructions that emanated from her residence, Pleasant View, outside of Concord.[35] With the ordination of *Science and Health* as church pastor and the codification of church policy in the *Manual,* Eddy needed only to reestablish her control of teaching to complete her mastery over the doctrinal integrity of "true" Christian Science. She accomplished this in 1898 by calling on her students to close down their regional institutes, which she replaced with a centralized Board of Education to direct the instruction of new teachers and to monitor their orthodoxy.

That same year Eddy established a Board of Lectureship to deal with missions. The Board appointed and governed public lecturers, whose primary mission was to present the truths of Christian Science to nonbelievers in public "evangelistic" campaigns. The lecturers' efforts received support from one-man Committees on Publication, who surveyed the public press for any "misinformation" about Christian Science and responded with defenses and explanations. Eventually every state and country that Christian Science entered had a Committee on Publication under the general direction of the Committee on Publication of the Mother Church. Through them, Christian Science sought to direct public opinion and defend the church.

The turn of the century witnessed the establishment and growth of institutions devoted principally to the specific mission of healing. First recommended for churchwide use at the Annual Association Meeting in 1889, Christian Science Missions and Dispensaries offered science publications and free treatments to the worthy poor. Often located in the poor districts of urban centers, dispensaries represented the hope of Christian Scientists that such philanthropy would "raise the vocation of Scientists from being looked on by the world as primarily a means to a livelihood." Within one year the *Journal* reported the establishment of twenty-nine dispensaries across the country.[36] Practitioners treated acute problems on the dispensary premises, but referred patients with chronic problems to practitioners in the community who possessed the necessary expertise. Because dispensaries infringed too much on the income of private practitioners, dispensary managers soon began to charge fees adjusted to the income of individual patients. To avoid further conflict with private practitioners, many dispensaries quit offering treatments near the turn of the century, while continuing to serve as literature distribution centers under the name of their sister organization, the Reading Room. Primarily designed to disseminate literature, Reading Rooms also provided a retreat for traveler, tourist, and businessperson, a place where they could find "not only peace and quiet, but healing as well."[37]

At first glance, the largest and most influential healing institution of Christian Science, the Christian Science Publishing Society, does not even appear to be a health-related institution. But given the importance of right thinking for a Scientist and its close connection with the study of truth-filled literature, one begins to understand the significance of a society that ensures the publication of genuine Christian Science literature. Established in 1898 to publish and distribute healing words to a world searching for health and peace, the Society assumed responsibility for publishing the *Christian Science Journal* and *Christian Science Sentinel* (official organs of the Mother Church), the international *Christian Science Monitor* (1908), and numerous books and pamphlets.

For Christian Science practitioners, the two decades from 1890 to 1910 represented a period of professionalization during which they sought to regulate and strengthen their practices while withstanding the legislative pressures of state governments and regular physicians. These years coincided with a period of political awakening for medical doctors who, increasingly confident in their scientific therapies and eager to reap the social and economic benefits of professionalization, embarked on a campaign to pass public-health ordinances and to license medical practitioners. Although a few states, particularly in New England, granted Christian Scientists immunity from medical practice acts, during the last years of the century Christian Scientists frequently appeared in courts for breaking vaccination laws, failing to report contagious diseases, practicing medicine without a license, or for killing their patients.[38] Between 1887 and 1899, over twenty cases against orthodox Christian Scientists went to trial.[39] Rather than immediately conforming to the new laws, the church fought them by claiming that the state should have no jurisdiction over an individual's liberty to practice healing and no control over a patient's right to choose his or her own healer. In some instances—for example, in the Milwaukee, Wisconsin, case of 1900 against practitioners Crecentia Arries and Emma Nichols—judges agreed with such defenses. Charged with violating the medical practice act of 1897 by practicing medicine without a license, both Milwaukee women won acquittal on appeal by claiming that the law discriminated against Christian Scientists and by emphasizing that they had administered no drugs, performed no surgery, nor even touched their patients. The decision infuriated orthodox physicians, but the legal way had been opened for Christian Scientists to heal in Wisconsin.[40] The easiest solution to such difficulties would have been to deemphasize physical healing slowly, but the church refused, in part because it recognized, in the words of influential lecturer Carol Norton, that "The Cause prospers most through the genuine results obtained in regeneration and physical healing."[41]

Christian Science leaders did, however, make efforts to improve their public image and to tighten controls over their members, and in time they granted some concessions to legislative pressures and persistent physical maladies. During the 1890s the church discouraged specialization by labeling it "quackery," the *Journal* tightened the rules controlling practitioner advertising in its columns, and the Publication Committee restricted the use of the C.S.B. and C.S.D. titles.[42] Although Eddy had urged her followers in the mid-1880s not to use the title "Doctor," she finally included in the *Church Manual* a prohibition against its use, unless they had received it "under the *laws* of the *State*."[43] Therapeutic adaptations followed as well. In 1901 Eddy instructed parents to submit their children to compulsory vaccination, and the same year she rid herself of the last vestiges of the Corner case by declaring that "Obstetrics is not Science, and will not be taught."[44] Such conciliatory efforts, joined occasionally by First Amendment pleas, bore fruit as the cases against Scientists declined to about ten for the years 1900–1915. Persistent maladies also received some concessions as when Eddy, after occasionally using morphine to deaden the pain of kidney stones, sanctioned the use of painkillers for bouts of intense pain in her 1905 revision of *Science and Health* and when the Publishing Society approved the publication of Eddy's books in braille.

Anxious for the future of her church, Eddy spent her final days fine-tuning the organization that she had created and publicly defending her mental stability in the face of scurrilous charges. Finally, weakened by a long life of struggles and triumphs, she "passed on" in December 1910 after a bout of pneumonia, leaving Scientists the task of coming to terms with their prophetic and sectarian past in a modern world that often derided the supernatural and worshipped scientific medicine.

Christian Science in the Modern World: Since 1910

With the passing of Eddy, Christian Scientists lost not only the steady stream of spiritual insight that they had grown almost to worship, but also the one person whose hard-earned authority could settle disputes, regulate doctrinal change, and update practices without jeopardizing belief in the movement's integrity. Thus her passing presented a dilemma. Should they strive to live in absolute obedience to the instructions of the person who had revealed the clearest understanding of truth since the manifestation of the Christ (the true idea of God) in Jesus, or should they emulate her personal example of adaptation and continue to move along a pathway toward deeper truth? If they chose the former, who would interpret her instructions? If they chose the latter, how would they discern the proper path?

In 1916, disputes arose between the Board of Directors of the Mother Church and the Board of Trustees of the Christian Science Publishing Society that precipitated debate over who should define orthodox Christian Science practice and belief. Before her passing, Eddy retained final control over both Directors and Trustees, but which body now had authority to control the doctrinal content of church publications? Reconciliation proved futile as the debate boiled into open conflict during the following five years and spilled over into the courts of Massachusetts, where judgment finally supported the claims of the Board of Directors. Favored by a majority of church members, this 1922 victory for the Directors gave them full control of Eddy's writings. Subsequent developments indicate that they moved to protect her legacy by cautiously encouraging the adaptation of her teachings to the modern world.[45]

If anything, esteem for the Founder or Leader, as Christian Scientists often call Eddy, has grown since her death. Members still revere *Science and Health* as their source of truth, and healing continues to play a central role in their beliefs and practices, representing in its fullest sense, according to the Board of Directors' influential *Century of Christian Science Healing,* "the rescue of men from all that would separate them from the fullness of being."[46] They still insist that the practice of healing cannot be separated from a true understanding of the nature of reality, but hasten to add that such an understanding often dawns agonizingly slowly. Hence, while Scientists continue to avoid physicians, psychiatrists, and psychologists, they wear hearing aids, receive blood transfusions, allow medical doctors to set broken bones and advise "on the anatomy involved" in difficult cases, and employ obstetricians at childbirth.[47] Arthur Nudelman's study of Christian Science university students in the late 1960s concluded that they regularly used eyeglasses, received dental care when necessary, and "utilize[d] medical services more frequently for mechanical problems than for ailments of other types"; however, on the whole they appeared to make little use of medical facilities.[48] In recent years some Christian Scientists have detected the influence of their beliefs and practices in the work of physicians who, in holistic fashion, increasingly emphasize the interrelation of mind, body, and soul.

Death, the most striking evidence of mortality and the reality of evil, continues to challenge many Scientists, poignantly reminding them of their need to advance further into truth. Struggling to affirm their conviction that death is only, in the words of Robert Peel, "one phase, however grievous it may seem, of men's present imperfect sense of life," Christian Scientists who have lost a loved one must struggle not only with their grief and the occasional insensitivity of friends and fellow church members, but often with the added burden of handling the disappointment and doubt resulting from the apparent failure of Christian Science treatment.[49] Confronted by the failed demonstration, they can only fall into the arms of their metaphysical system, affirm the unreality of death, and trust that their understanding will grow. To aid the development of that understanding, most Christian Scientists refuse to speak of "dying," preferring to use the phrase "passing on." In addition, some do not hold funeral services, which would only remind them of death; those who do (probably the majority) participate in a quiet service comprising readings from the Bible and *Science and Health,* either at home or in a funeral parlor. If the body has not been cremated, the casket remains closed.[50] Despite the difficulty of death, Christian Scientists see it as a challenge to be met and not as an escape; therefore, the church reminds those who might be tempted to use euthanasia to overcome pain and hardship that death does not exist.

Conscious that critics often accuse Christian Scientists of being insensitive to suffering because they think members just pretend that evil does not exist, Christian Scientists have gone out of their way to exhibit an attitude of compassion. The Christian Science Benevolent Association, established in 1916, organized and built two sanatoriums, located near Boston and San Francisco, to serve as retreats where sufferers could withdraw from the ordinary routines of life while receiving nursing care and treatment.[51] In these and numerous other certified retreats, nursing, approved by Eddy in 1908, has come into its own during the last thirty years. Clearly subordinate to practitioners, just as medical nurses are to physicians, Christian Science nurses try to keep their thoughts pure and assist practitioners by creating an atmosphere that aids their work. Although practitioners might deny it, there is a sense in which "curing" has increasingly become their domain, while nurses have assumed responsibility for "caring." In a recent journal article that lauded the satisfaction to be found in a nursing career, Marco Frances Farley stated that "The nurse dresses wounds and keeps the body clean, comfortable, and nourished so that it intrudes less on the patient's thought."[52] Within the last few years the church has moved to improve the training of private-duty nurses, sanatorium nurses, and visiting nurses by standardizing nursing education and including classroom instruction and practical training in Christian Science sanatoriums.

For years the Pleasant View Home for the aged in Concord, New Hampshire, provided a concrete response to critics who wondered "Why does not your own church care for its elderly people?"[53] Although it closed in 1975, the Pleasant View home has been replaced by numerous other nursing homes and retirement facilities that provide a setting of compassion and care in which "to prove what Christian Science is doing for humanity in meeting and mastering the needless limitations erroneously associated with advancing years."[54]

Notwithstanding their confidence, as expressed in the book *Century of Christian Science Healing,* that "The healing of physical disease is one of the most concrete proofs that can be offered of the substantiality of Spirit," since the mid-1920s Christian Scientists have more consistently than before emphasized a broad definition of health that does not extol physical healing over emotional and spiritual harmony.[55] This change paralleled the increased confidence of Americans in scientific medicine and undoubtedly reflected Christian Scientists' efforts to highlight those aspects of their doctrines best suited to the current demands of the public. Rather than point to their nineteenth-century roots in sectarian medicine, Christian Scientists now tend to emphasize that they represent a long, mainstream tradition of Christian healing and take pride in the increased influence they believe their radical metaphysics has had in moderating traditional medical practices and expanding religious horizons. Although the varieties of spiritual healing that have recently swept through other American denominations follow different methods and reflect beliefs different from true Christian Science, Christian Scientists see a common spirit of service and a common aim of healing the sick in Christ's name.[56]

Although they do not focus attention on the body, Christian Scientists do pursue a generally healthful lifestyle that includes good food, adequate clothing and housing, and habits of personal hygiene and sanitation. In the words of Alan A. Aylwin, former associate editor of the *Christian Science Journal,* Christian Science "shows the way of escape from all forms of addiction, whether to heroin, tobacco, alcohol, caffeine, masturbation, or just plain overeating."[57] Members of the Church of Christ, Scientist, do not use alcohol or tobacco, not simply because of their impact on the body but because they can quickly become habits that represent a sacrifice of mental freedom.[58] Some evidence from the early 1950s suggested that Christian Scientists lived shorter lives on average than the general population, with death rates due to malignancies and heart disease higher than the national average.[59] Birth control, a matter of contemporary ethical concern, receives scant attention from Christian Scientists, who leave matters of family planning up to the individual couples involved. The church takes no official stand against abortion or "the pill," but because Christian Scientists frown on medical operations and drugs, they probably prefer barrier methods, withdrawal, or abstinence (when both partners agree).

Capitalizing on contemporary themes, practitioners have increasingly applied their essentially unchanged techniques to such problems as homosexuality, drug addiction, obesity, marital troubles, and tensions of the workplace, while emphasizing the overall joys of healthful living that accompany the acceptance of Scientific principles. Practitioners have also broadened their efforts beyond the personal sphere to encompass a wide range of social issues, thus serving as a kind of "world conscience." During the 1920s the *Christian Science Monitor* stood firmly in favor of prohibition and during both world wars the Mother Church distributed food and clothing to the needy in Europe and Asia, and today Christian Scientists work mentally to heal the world of famine, war, unemployment, racial discrimination, and ecological disaster. Often these efforts initially take the form of money, food, and clothing donated by the Mother Church or individual members to alleviate emergency conditions throughout the world, but always these efforts are accompanied by the deeper mental work necessary to heal the world of the misconceptions about reality that constitute the true source of disaster. For example, the *Christian Science Monitor* recently publicized "Hunger in Africa" in a four-part series that fairly and accurately discussed the political, cultural, and climatic dimensions of starvation in East Africa, including in its concluding article entitled "What Can You Do To Help?" the names and addresses of fourteen aid and relief agencies that accept donations.[60] However, in the daily "Religious Article" of the issue that began the series, the anonymous author emphasized that a proper view of reality would provide the best aid and concluded that "we can help those who may be thousands of miles from us, not only through charitable giving but through potent prayer."[61]

Christian Scientists have continued their turn-of-the-century legal efforts to defend their rights to practice healing, but as emphasis on physical healing has declined, they have increasingly shifted their ground of defense to First Amendment guarantees of the freedom of religion. Both individually and institutionally, Christian Scientists have intensified efforts to lobby for concessions in legislative bills that might touch their lives. Their attacks on the World War I-era movement to legislate compulsory health insurance proved decisive in defeating such legislation in California and New York (although they have negotiated with insurance companies to ensure coverage of treatment by Christian Science practitioners), and vigilant Committees on Publication still negotiate exemptions for Christian Scientists on a wide variety of laws, including compulsory vaccination for school children and compulsory physical examinations.[62] Although Christian Scientists have increasingly joined the mainstream of American society, they have continued to stand firmly and unobtrusively for their beliefs.

Notes

1. Robert Peel, *Christian Science: Its Encounter with American Culture* (New York, 1958), p. 11.
2. Charles S. Braden, *Spirits in Rebellion: The Rise and Development of New Thought* (Dallas, 1963), pp. 89–128.
3. Henry King Carroll, *The Religious Forces of the United States Enumerated, Classified, and Described* (New York, 1912); A.J. Lamme III, "Christian Science in the U.S.A., 1900–1910: A Distributional Study," Discussion Paper Series, Department of Geography, Syracuse University, no. 3, April 1975.
4. Mary Baker Eddy, *Church Manual of The First Church of Christ, Scientist, in Boston, Massachusetts,* 89th ed. (Boston, 1925), pp. 15–16.
5. See John D. Davies, *Phrenology—Fad and Science: A 19th-Century American Crusade* (New Haven, 1955); Robert C. Fuller, *Mesmerism and the American Cure of Souls* (Philadelphia, 1982); and R. Laurence Moore, *In Search of White Crows: Spiritualism, Parapsychology, and American Culture* (New York, 1977).
6. Braden, *Spirits in Rebellion,* p. 89.
7. Married three different times, Eddy went by numerous names over her lifetime: Mary Morse Baker, Mary Baker Glover, Mary M. Patterson, Mary Baker Eddy. To avoid confusion, I refer to her as Mary when discussing her childhood and youth and as Eddy for her adult years. The following biographical paragraphs are patterned after Ronald L. Numbers and Rennie B. Schoepflin, "Ministries of Healing: Mary Baker Eddy, Ellen G. White, and the Religion of Health," in *Women and Health in America: Historical Readings,* ed. Judith Walzer Leavitt (Madison, WI, 1984), pp. 376–389.
8. Mary Baker Eddy, *Retrospection and Introspection* (Boston, 1916), pp. 8–9.
9. Eddy, *Retrospection,* p. 13; Robert Peel, *Mary Baker Eddy,* 3 vols. (New York, 1966–1977), 1:23, 50–51.
10. Mary Baker Eddy, *Miscellaneous Writings, 1883–1896* (Boston, 1924), p. 24.

11. Peel, *Christian Science,* p. 90.
12. Letter from Mary M. Patterson to Julius Dresser, February 15, 1866. Archives of The Mother Church, Christian Science Center, Boston.
13. Letter from J.A. Dresser to Mrs. Patterson, March 2, 1866. Archives of The Mother Church, Christian Science Center, Boston.
14. Peel, *Eddy,* 1:221; Julius Silberger, Jr., *Mary Baker Eddy: An Interpretive Biography of the Founder of Christian Science* (Boston, 1980), p. 257, n. 10.
15. Mrs. Mary Baker Glover, *The Science of Man, By Which the Sick are Healed* (Lynn, MA, 1876), p. 5.
16. Ibid., p. 7.
17. Mary Baker Eddy, *Science and Health* (Boston, 1875), p. 147. The third through fifteenth editions (1881–1885) each appeared in two volumes.
18. Eddy, *Science and Health,* 1875, p. 393; 1881, 1:89.
19. Eddy, *Science and Health,* 1881, 1:203–204.
20. Reminiscences of Mary Baker Eddy by Miss Julia S. Bartlett, pp. 14–15. Archives of The Mother Church, Christian Science Center, Boston.
21. Peel, *Eddy,* 2:96, 99.
22. Ibid., pp. 80–82, 111.
23. Stephen Gottschalk, *The Emergence of Christian Science in American Religious Life* (Berkeley, CA, 1973), p. 244; Margery Q. Fox, "Power and Piety: Women in Christian Science," Ph.D. dissertation, New York University, 1973, p. 143.
24. Only in the third edition of *Science and Health* (1881) did Eddy use feminine pronouns to refer to God, but she continued to believe that God exhibited both male and female characteristics.
25. See *Christian Science Journal* 3 (1886):215.
26. In regard to income, see James Neal Reminiscence; Letter from Julia Bartlett to Eddy, [April 9, 1884]; and Letter from Ursula N. Gestefeld to Eddy, July 24, 1884. Archives of The Mother Church, Christian Science Center, Boston. See also George Rosen, *Fees and Fee Bills: Some Economic Aspects of Medical Practice in Nineteenth Century America* (Baltimore, 1946).
27. Mary Baker Eddy, "Fallibility of Human Concepts," *Christian Science Journal* 7 (1889):159–160.
28. Mary Baker Eddy, "Questions and Answers," *Christian Science Journal* 3 (1885):77.
29. See, e.g., Eddy's suggestions in *Science and Health,* 1881, 1:186–205.
30. Ibid., p. 239.
31. Louise Delisle Radzinski, "Sympathy in Christian Science," *Christian Science Journal* 21 (1903):274.
32. Eddy, *Science and Health,* 1875, p. 400.
33. Peel, *Eddy,* 2:236–240.
34. Mary Baker Eddy, "To the Christian World," *Christian Science Weekly* 1 (December 29, 1898):4–5.
35. Peel, *Eddy,* 3:90.
36. "Notice," *Christian Science Journal* 7 (1889):100–101; E.J. Foster Eddy, "Address of Dr. E.J. Foster Eddy Before the N.C.S. Association, June 27, 1890," *Christian Science Journal* 8 (1890):144.
37. Caroline E. Linnell, "The Christian Science Reading Room," *Christian Science Sentinel* 11 (1909):885–886.

38. On medical licensing, see Richard Harrison Shryock, *Medical Licensing in America, 1650–1965* (Baltimore, 1967); and Alexander Wilder, *History of Medicine* (New Sharon, ME, 1899), pp. 776–835.
39. These cases were all reported in the *Journal*.
40. Elizabeth Barnaby Keeney, Susan Eyrich Lederer, and Edmond P. Minihan, "Sectarians and Scientists: Alternatives to Orthodox Medicine," in *Wisconsin Medicine: Historical Perspectives,* eds. Ronald L. Numbers and Judith Walzer Leavitt (Madison, WI, 1981), pp. 60–61.
41. Carol Norton, "Working for the Cause," *Christian Science Journal* 21 (1903):204.
42. A[lfred] F[arlow], "Questions and Answers," *Christian Science Journal* 8 (1891):497; ibid. 10 (1892):413.
43. Mary Baker Eddy, *Church Manual,* 11th ed. (Boston, 1899), pp. 56–57.
44. Eddy, *Church Manual,* 25th ed. (Boston, 1901), p. 70.
45. Charles S. Braden, *Christian Science Today: Power, Policy, Practice* (Dallas, 1958), pp. 61–95.
46. *A Century of Christian Science Healing* (Boston, 1966), p. 239.
47. Peel, *Eddy,* 3:238–242.
48. Arthur Edmund Nudelman, "Christian Science and Secular Medicine," Ph.D. dissertation, University of Wisconsin, 1970, pp. 138–139.
49. Robert Peel, "Christian Science and Death," unpublished manuscript, p. 2. A version of this paper appeared in *Religion and Bereavement,* eds. Austin H. Kutscher and Lillian G. Kutscher (New York, 1972).
50. Ibid.; Lucy Jayne Kamua, "Systems of Belief and Ritual in Christian Science," Ph.D. dissertation, University of Chicago, 1971, pp. 116–118.
51. Lewis Hubner, "The Function of Our Sanatoriums," *Christian Science Journal* 92 (1974):149–150.
52. Marco Frances Farley, "Nursing: A Truly Satisfying Career," *Christian Science Journal* 97 (1979):666.
53. "From the Directors: The Christian Science Pleasant View Home," *Christian Science Journal* 43 (1925):509.
54. Board of Directors, "The Christian Science Pleasant View Home," *Christian Science Journal* 44 (1926):490–491.
55. *Century of Christian Science Healing,* p. 254.
56. See, e.g., Gottschalk, *Emergence of Christian Science;* and *Century of Christian Science Healing.*
57. Alan A. Aylwin, "Help for the Addict," *Christian Science Journal* 89 (1971):539.
58. Nathan A. Talbot, "The Question of Drinking," *Christian Science Sentinel* 84 (1982):1742–1746. See also DeWitt John, *The Christian Science Way of Life* (Boston, 1962).
59. Gale E. Wilson, "Christian Science and Longevity," *Journal of Forensic Sciences* 1 (1956):43–60.
60. *Christian Science Monitor* 77 (November 27–30, 1984).
61. *Christian Science Monitor* 77 (November 27, 1984):14.
62. Ronald L. Numbers, *Almost Persuaded: American Physicians and Compulsory Health Insurance, 1912–1920* (Baltimore, 1978), pp. 81, 90–91.

CHAPTER 16

The Adventist
Tradition

RONALD L. NUMBERS
DAVID R. LARSON

Most Adventists trace their religious ancestry back to the Millerite movement of the early 1840s, when William Miller (1782–1849), a Baptist farmer–preacher from upstate New York, aroused the nation with his prediction that Christ would return to Earth in 1843 or 1844. Following the "great disappointment" of October 22, 1844, the date on which many Millerites had pinned their hopes, the movement splintered into several factions, the largest of which became the Evangelical Adventist and Advent Christian churches. Although these two bodies attracted the majority of prominent Millerites, they did not prosper for long. The former had disappeared entirely by the early twentieth century, and the membership of the latter has remained at about thirty thousand for decades.

A third Millerite faction, initially very small, evolved into the Seventh-day Adventist church. These Millerites were distinguished by their belief that Christ had entered the Most Holy compartment of the heavenly sanctuary on October 22, 1844, by their observance of Saturday as Sabbath, and by their possession of the "spirit of prophecy" in the person of Ellen G. White (1827–1915), who as a seventeen-year-old semi-invalid reported having visions during which she received divine instruction. In 1846 she married James White (1821–1881), an erstwhile schoolteacher and Millerite preacher, whose organizational and promotional skills led, in 1863, to the formation of a General Conference of Seventh-day Adventists, with headquarters in Battle Creek, Michigan. At the time of its incorporation, the infant church supported twenty-two ordained ministers and comprised about 3,500 members, concentrated in the region east of the Missouri River and north of the Confederacy.

Although Ellen White viewed her "testimonies" as a "lesser light" designed to lead people to the "greater light" of the Bible, she at times equated her inspiration with that of the biblical prophets. And although she never assumed formal leadership of the church, she wielded enormous influence in matters of both doctrine and policy—especially after the death of her husband in 1881. By the time of her own death in 1915, many Adventists regarded her writings as authoritative for all areas of thought and action.

In 1874, Seventh-day Adventists dispatched their first foreign missionary, to Switzerland. Other appointments followed in quick succession, first to the largely white, Christian populations of Europe, Australasia, and South Africa, later to the nonwhite peoples of Africa, Asia, and Latin America. By 1900 the church was sponsoring nearly five hundred foreign missionaries, and over fifteen percent of the more than 75,000 Seventh-day Adventists were living outside North America. During the next eighty-five years, membership swelled to over four million, roughly eighty-five percent of whom resided outside of the United States. In order to provide for the growing needs of its missions, as well as to shield its youth from worldly influences, the church developed one of the most extensive systems of denominational education in the world. In 1901 the General Conference headquarters were moved from Battle Creek to the outskirts of Washington, DC, where they remain today.

Over the years the Seventh-day Adventist church gave birth to numerous schismatic movements, most of which repudiated Mrs. White's authority. The most successful of these offshoots was the Church of God (Adventist), which grew out of a controversy in the 1860s. It merged in 1949 with a group of former dissidents from its own ranks, took the name Church of God (Seventh Day), and established a General Conference in Denver, Colorado. By the early 1980s its membership stood at about forty thousand. More prosperous—and less directly related to the Seventh-day Adventists—was the Worldwide Church of God (formerly Radio Church of God), created by Herbert W. Armstrong, an ambitious Church of God (Adventist) minister, who in the 1930s launched an independent ministry that grew into one of the largest Saturday-keeping Christian bodies in the world. Of all the Adventist bodies, however, only the Seventh-day Adventists developed a distinctive philosophy of health.

The Millerites, a heterogeneous group unified by little more than their belief in the imminent return of Christ, collectively espoused no distinctive health principles or practices. Their magazines occasionally reported "cases of bodily cure by the power of faith," but they rarely condemned medicine generally. Millerites aimed their most pointed criticisms of the medical profession at physicians who cared for the insane and who gave credence to the popular notion that the Second Advent message was driving people mad. In fact, during the middle years of the century American asylums admitted scores of patients suffering from symptoms purportedly caused by the Millerite excitement. The great majority of this number were marginally functional persons drawn to the fringes of the movement. Only a handful were Millerites who became mentally ill because of the intense emotional experience or the constant noise, loss of sleep, and abstinence from food sometimes associated with protracted Millerite meetings. Although Millerites vehemently denied that their teachings caused insanity, they did not dispute a connection between religious belief and mental health. The sermons of their opponents, they charged, had driven many a person insane, while the "blessed hope" of Christ's soon return had been known to cure the mentally disturbed.[1]

A number of Millerites embraced the popular temperance and health-reform movements of the day. William Miller himself, who discerned the hand of God in agitation to curtail the consumption of alcohol, warned his followers that those who imbibed would be "wholly unprepared" for the Second Coming of Christ. Other Millerites joined the crusading Sylvester Graham (of cracker fame) in adopting a vegetarian diet and an abstemious lifestyle. Four years after the great disappointment, Larkin B. Coles, a Boston physician and preacher who had worked closely with Miller, published the most comprehensive statement on health to come from the Millerite community: *Philosophy of Health: Natural Principles of Health and Cure* (1848), which followed Graham in promoting the benefits of fresh air and exercise, a meat-free diet, sexual purity, drugless medicine, abstention from stimulants, and sensible dress. Coles taught that it was "as truly a sin against Heaven, to violate a law of life, as to break one of the ten commandments." Unlike postmillennial health reformers, who looked forward to the virtual eradication of disease in a millennium of perfect well-being, Coles viewed obedience to the laws of health primarily as a requirement for entry into heaven and secondarily as a means of living a more enjoyable life on earth. By the time of his death in 1856, 44,000 copies of his book had passed into circulation.[2]

In the years following the disappointment of 1844, a number of former Millerites, like many other Americans, grew increasingly suspicious of orthodox medicine and enamored of so-called natural methods of healing, especially hydropathy or the "water cure." In the early

1860s, Dr. James Caleb Jackson's water-cure establishment in Dansville, New York, became a favorite retreat for ailing Sunday-keeping and Saturday-keeping Adventists, including the prominent editor and evangelist Joshua V. Himes, who occasionally invited Jackson to contribute to the "Health Department" of his magazine *Voice of the Prophets*. James and Ellen White joined the ranks of water-cure enthusiasts early in 1863, after successfully employing hydropathic remedies to treat their sons during a diphtheria epidemic.[3]

Although the majority of ex-Millerites accepted the traditional Christian view of the immortality of the soul, those who coalesced into the Advent Christian and Seventh-day Adventist churches rejected the notions that consciousness continues after death and that the wicked burn forever, believing instead that immortality is conditional upon acceptance of Christ and that the dead are unconscious during the time between death and resurrection. The most influential statement of this belief in conditional immortality appeared in a pamphlet entitled *An Enquiry: Are the Souls of the Wicked Immortal?* (1842), written by the Methodist-turned-Millerite preacher George Storrs. According to Storrs, "Men are really dying, according to the strict and literal meaning of the term, soul as well as body, or the whole man." This rejection of a dichotomy between body and soul eventually became the theological foundation of the Seventh-day Adventist concern for "the whole person." It also served as a dike against spiritualism and eternal torment, views abhorrent to Ellen White, who as a child had suffered extreme mental anguish over the prospect of perpetual punishment and who as an adult feared being identified as a spiritualist.[4]

Ellen White's own history also played a crucial role in the development of Seventh-day Adventist attitudes toward sickness and health. A childhood accident, at about age nine, left her a semi-invalid for years, and throughout her early adult life she suffered from chronic lung, heart, and stomach ailments, frequent "fainting fits," paralytic attacks, and breathing difficulties.[5] Finding that physicians could do little to help her but that prayer sometimes brought relief, in 1849 she instructed her little band of disciples to have nothing to do with physicians: "If any among us are sick, let us not dishonor God by applying to earthly physicians, but apply to the God of Israel. If we follow his directions (*Jas.* 5:14, 15) the sick will be healed. God's promise cannot fail. Have faith in God, and trust wholly in him." During the 1850s, in the wake of criticism following the death of an Adventist sister who had refused medical assistance, White softened her stand against physicians. And in 1860 she condemned as "fanaticism" the notion that it was wrong to seek medical advice, writing that "in some cases the counsel of an earthly physician is very necessary." Nevertheless, for years Adventists continued to avoid the medical profession, especially physicians who prescribed harsh drugs.[6]

Health reform remained a peripheral issue among the sabbatarian Adventists before the 1860s. However, as early as the 1840s White began speaking out against tobacco, tea, and coffee, condemning them not so much because of their injurious effects, but because the money spent on such items was needed by "the cause." (Alcohol was apparently so obviously evil, or so little abused by Adventists, she did not mention it at this time.) In 1854 she criticized the consumption of "rich food" for the same reasons. There seems to have been little practical response to these early admonitions before 1855, when sabbatarian leaders launched a decade-long campaign against tobacco. By the late 1850s, most Saturday-keeping Adventist ministers had forsaken tobacco, and it had become impossible for users to obtain a "card of recommendation" licensing them to preach. Among the laity, however, the habit did not die out until the 1860s.[7] Thus despite the fact that many former Millerites and converts to Adventism had embraced particular aspects of health reform by the early 1860s, it had not yet become a central concern of any of the Adventist sects. And although many Adventists resorted to prayer and avoided regular physicians in times of illness, therapeutic choice remained a private decision.

Visions of Health: 1863–1915

No event in Adventist medical history assumes greater importance than Ellen White's vision on June 5, 1863, which gave the divine seal of approval to health reform and hydropathy and set the medical agenda for her fledgling church. Above all, the 1863 vision elevated healthful living into a moral obligation for Seventh-day Adventists. In language virtually identical to that used earlier by Coles, she declared "It is as truly a sin to violate the laws of our being as it is to break the ten commandments." Henceforth, health reform was to be as "closely connected with the third angel's message [i.e., Adventism] as the hand is with the body." It was not, however, to become "the message," nor even the leading theme of the message.[8]

White's gospel of health, first sketched in a thirty-two–page essay published in 1864 and elaborated over the years, initially stressed the evils of drugs as then used and the benefits of water and other natural remedies. "I was shown," she wrote, "that more deaths have been caused by drug-taking than from all other causes combined. If there was in the land one physician in the place of thousands, a vast amount of premature mortality would be prevented." Instead of dosing themselves with harmful medications, Adventists were to rely on "God's great medicine, water, pure soft water," as well as fresh air, sunshine, simple food, exercise, and cheerful faith.[9]

In the fall of 1864, James and Ellen White spent three weeks observing activities at Dr. Jackson's establishment in upstate New York, and the next year they returned for three months to seek a cure for James, who had suffered a stroke. When her husband failed to improve, and when she discovered that Jackson's theology did not conform to what she had "received from higher and unerring authority," Mrs. White grew disillusioned with the situation at Dansville. Finally, in frustration she removed James from the premises. Shortly thereafter, she learned in a vision that Adventists should open their own water cure so that they would not have to patronize "popular water-cure institutions . . . where there is not sympathy for our faith."[10]

In 1866, in response to this instruction, the Seventh-day Adventists opened the Western Health Reform Institute in Battle Creek, Michigan, the first link in what would become a worldwide chain of Adventist medical institutions. The mission of the new institute, as defined by Ellen White, was "to relieve the afflicted, to disseminate light, to awaken the spirit of inquiry, and to advance reform." To further these goals, Horatio S. Lay, chief physician at the institute and one of the few Adventists with medical experience (though not an M.D.), began publishing a popular magazine, *The Health Reformer*.[11]

After a rocky first decade, the institute began to prosper under the direction of John Harvey Kellogg (1852–1943), a protégé of the Whites who became superintendent in 1876 at age twenty-four. During his sixty-seven–year tenure as head of the renamed Battle Creek Sanitarium, he turned the poorly equipped water cure into a world-famous medical institution. Over the years the talented and ambitious doctor gradually eclipsed the prophetess as Adventism's most visible authority on health. By 1886 he could accurately describe himself in a letter to Mrs. White as "a sort of umpire as to what was true or correct and what was error in matters relating to hygienic reform, a responsibility which has often made me tremble, and which I have felt very keenly." Largely through Kellogg's efforts, the church developed an extensive system of sanitariums, treatment rooms, and vegetarian restaurants. To staff these institutions, he opened a school of hygiene in 1878, a school of nursing in 1883, and a medical school, the American Medical Missionary College, in 1895. By the turn of the century, the Kellogg-controlled International Medical Missionary and Benevolent Association, the medical arm of the church, employed more workers than the General Conference, and physicians enjoyed more power and prestige than their ministerial colleagues, a source of increasing tension. Ellen White believed that the Adventist physician occupied "a position even more responsible than that of the minister of the gospel," but she warned that the "right arm" of the church—that is, the medical work—was not "to become the whole body."[12]

Part of the tension between the medical and ministerial branches of the church resulted from the conflicting motives that prompted the Adventists' medical activities. Initially, the sanitarium in Battle Creek had been established to provide care for ailing Adventists in an atmosphere compatible with their distinctive therapeutic and theological beliefs. Mrs. White, who had long resented having "worldlings sneeringly [assert] that those who believe present truth are weak-minded, deficient in education, without position or influence," had also supported Kellogg's enterprises as a means of improving the church's image. Above all, she had come to see medical institutions as a vehicle for breaking down theological prejudice and paving the way for evangelism. Nothing, she observed in 1899, converted "the people like the medical missionary work." The following year she published a volume of testimonies urging that the health work be used as "an entering wedge, making a way for other truths to reach the heart."[13]

Kellogg, who disliked sectarian labels of any kind, appealed to the healing ministry of Christ in advocating that the medical work be oriented primarily toward relieving suffering rather than winning converts. As early as 1893 he spoke out against the feeling in some Adventist quarters "that work for the needy and suffering unless done with a direct proselytizing motive was of no account and that it was not in the interests of the cause." White, on the contrary, found it difficult to support medical projects unrelated to evangelization. "Our sanitariums," she stressed over and over again, "are to be established for one object,— the advancement of present truth."[14]

On November 10, 1907, Kellogg was disfellowshipped from the Seventh-day Adventist church for being antagonistic "to the gifts now manifest in the church" (that is, White's prophetic gift). The doctor had, in fact, accused some of Mrs. White's associates of manipulating her testimonies and had suggested that the prophetess herself sometimes borrowed from other writers more freely than she acknowledged. However, the excommunication of the czar of the Adventist medical work probably owed less to such indiscretions (or to his alleged pantheistic beliefs) than to his arrogant attempts to control the church, which aroused the ire of such influential ministers as A.G. Daniells, president of the General Conference, and Willie White, Ellen's son. The consequences of this episode for Adventist medical history were immense. The church lost Kellogg and several other prominent physicians as well as the Battle Creek Sanitarium and the American Medical Missionary College. Deprived of the medical school, White and her supporters immediately sought to establish an orthodox educational center in southern California, at Loma Linda, where they had recently purchased a sanitarium. In 1909 they obtained a charter for the College of Medical Evangelists, the forerunner of the present-day Loma Linda University School of Medicine. The Kellogg affair also consolidated White's authority and aggravated the tensions between Adventist physicians and ministers.[15]

In the years immediately following her omnibus 1863 vision on health reform, Ellen White focused considerable attention on sexual issues, particularly masturbation. Her very first book on health, *An Appeal to Mothers* (1864), identified this "solitary vice" as "the great cause of the physical, mental, and moral ruin of many of the children of our time." It also described in graphic detail what she had seen in vision about the dire consequences of self-abuse: "Everywhere I looked I saw imbecility, dwarfed forms, crippled limbs, misshapen heads, and deformity of every description."[16]

A second vision on sex, in 1868, prompted her to begin speaking out on abuses of the marriage relation, particularly the "excessive" sex demanded by some husbands seeking to "gratify the animal propensities." Although she never defined exactly what she meant by "excessive," some Adventists have surmised that she frowned on having intercourse more often than once a month, because such advice, from another author, appeared in an expanded version of *An Appeal to Mothers*. But the vagueness of her advice left Adventists with no fixed rules limiting the frequency of sexual intercourse. Similarly, her silence regarding contraception and abortion meant that these matters, too, were left to individual discretion. After the 1860s, White tended to leave these sensitive subjects to Dr. Kellogg, whose *Plain Facts about Sexual Life* (1877) became a late-century best-seller.[17]

Most Victorian Seventh-day Adventists associated Mrs. White's health message not so much with sexual purity as with dietary reform: a twice-a-day regimen of fruits, grains, nuts, and vegetables. On the basis of her 1863 vision, White had originally proscribed the use of eggs, butter, and meat (as well as alcohol, tobacco, tea, coffee, cheese, spices, and rich foods). She later distinguished between meat, on the one hand, and butter and eggs, on the other, allowing that the latter might help to prevent malnutrition. This distinction encouraged many Adventists to adopt a meatless diet that included eggs and dairy products, the so-called lacto-ovo vegetarian diet. Her advice on meat-eating also underwent substantial revision, particularly with respect to the distinction found in the Levitical law between "clean" and "unclean" flesh. (Clean animals had cloven hooves and chewed their cuds; clean fish had fins and scales.) Before her 1863 vision, White not only ate pork and other unclean meat, but censured those Adventists who attempted to ban the consumption of swine's flesh. After her vision she condemned the eating of all meat, especially pork, but said little until late in the century about the clean–unclean dichotomy. By 1890, however, she was arguing that the Old Testament distinction between "articles of food as clean and unclean" was not "a merely ceremonial and arbitrary regulation, but was based upon sanitary principles." Nevertheless, except for pork, she did not proscribe any particular meats on this basis.[18]

The dietary practices of Seventh-day Adventists seem to have fluctuated greatly during the nineteenth century. In 1870, James White boasted that Adventists "with hardly an exception" had discarded flesh-meats and suppers, but only five years later his wife complained that "our people are constantly retrograding upon health reform." Late in the century Kellogg estimated that all but "two or three" Adventist ministers ate meat, and in 1890 Ellen White herself admitted to straying occasionally from a vegetarian diet. In 1894, however, she vowed to abstain completely from flesh of all kinds and thereafter joined forces with Kellogg in calling for a "revival in health reform." Although she resisted efforts to make the consumption of meat a test of fellowship, by the twentieth century it was clear that the church would not tolerate the eating of unclean foods.[19]

The emphasis of her rationale for abstaining from meat varied considerably over time. During the early years of her health crusade, Ellen White stressed that meat-eating caused disease and stirred up the "animal passions," but in 1905, when she published *The Ministry of Healing,* her last and most mature treatise on health, she dropped sexual arousal from her list of "reasons for discarding flesh foods." She now argued that meat transmits cancer, tuberculosis, and "other fatal diseases" to humans and that meat-eating is cruel to animals.[20] Her comment that "Among those who are waiting for the coming of the Lord, meat eating will eventually be done away" led some of her followers to conclude that only persons who abstained from all meat would be "translated" to heaven without dying.[21]

No aspect of her health-reform campaign proved more frustrating to Ellen White than her attempt to change the style of dress worn by Adventist women. Since her youth, she had associated plain dress with spiritual health, and after 1863 she joined other reformers in calling attention to the anatomical and physiological problems created by fashionable dresses, especially hoop skirts. For over a decade after her vision, she crusaded to put her Adventist sisters into a costume consisting of a "short" skirt over pantaloons (similar to the so-called Bloomer dress), a design she reported having seen in her vision. Her efforts, like those of the women's rights reformers, encountered stiff resistance, and in 1875 she received divine permission to abandon the reform. Henceforth she insisted only that Adventists dress plainly, modestly, and healthfully.[22]

As their medical work expanded under the guidance of White and the administration of Kellogg, Seventh-day Adventists came to rely less on the healing power of prayer and more on the skill of physicians. Adventist ministers continued to anoint and pray for the seriously ill, but they came to have mixed feelings about miraculous healings, which they increasingly regarded, along with other forms of religious enthusiasm, as possible satanic delusions. After the opening of the Western Health Reform Institute, Ellen White advised Adventists not to entertain "the idea that the Institute is the place for them to come to be raised up by the prayer of faith. That is the place to find relief from disease by treatment, and right habits of living." During the last years of her life, she dropped her earlier practice of calling in the church elders to pray for her own recovery, fearing that failure to effect an immediate cure would lead to skepticism and disappointment. And because so many persons she had healed turned out to be unworthy, she expressed reluctance to pray for the healing of others.[23]

In *The Ministry of Healing,* White developed the view that God heals "through the agencies of nature" while Christian physicians "assist nature's work of healing."[24] This approach differed from the exclusive reliance on "faith healing" that characterized the thinking of some of the early Adventists and that later became popular among some conservative Protestants. White's emphasis on cooperating with the laws of nature also distinguished her approach from such "mind-healing" movements as Christian Science. In the tradition of Storrs, who had rejected the dichotomy between the immortal soul and the mortal body, and Coles, who had advocated physiological reform, White stressed the religious and moral importance of the human body in her philosophy of health and healing.

Throughout her ministry, Ellen White condemned all forms of "mind cure," especially hypnotism, and she described "the sciences of phrenology, psychology, and mesmerism" as channels through which Satan could exert his influence. To combat mental illness, she recommended strengthening the willpower and exercising the physical body, the efficacy of which she had learned firsthand while treating her husband during his illness in the mid-1860s. Prayer, she thought, should supplement—not supplant—these natural therapies.[25]

Like many nineteenth-century writers on psychiatry, Ellen White tended to view mental illness as a somatic condition resulting from a diseased brain. She never doubted that demonic possession could also cause insanity—and had done so in biblical times—but in discussing mental illness in her own day, she almost always pointed to natural causes: genetic, chemical, physiological, or psychological. She identified the "main cause" of insanity as intemperate behavior—"improper diet, irregular meals, a lack of physical exercise, and careless inattention in other respects to the laws of health"—either on the part of the sufferers themselves or their ancestors. Writing shortly after her 1863 vision, she traced much of the world's "deformity, disease, and imbecility . . . directly back to the drug-poisons, administered by the hand of a doctor." At various other times she attributed mental illness to masturbation, religious excitement, frustrated ambition, excessive grief, guilt, gossip, novel-reading, and even the wearing of wigs.[26]

White's extensive writings on sin, sickness, and death include a variety of explanations of human suffering and why God allows it. Her dominant theme, especially after 1863, was that disease and suffering result from violations of divinely ordained physiological laws and are not the consequence of direct interventions from God. However, she frequently interpreted her family's mental and physical ailments as afflictions from Satan and his evil angels, who had made her and her husband "the special objects" of their attention. In her best-known statement on the origin of evil, in *The Great Controversy between Christ and Satan* (1888), she wrote that "Nothing is more plainly taught in Scripture than that God was in nowise responsible for the entrance of sin" and its woeful consequences. Nevertheless, she occasionally implied that God allowed—and sometimes even sent—suffering as a blessing in disguise: to perfect character or, by laying some persons prematurely in their graves, to guarantee salvation.[27] Differing opinions about the nature and meaning of suffering have persisted among Adventists down to the present.

Growth and Adjustment Since 1915

Ellen White's death in 1915 left Seventh-day Adventists with the task of finding continuing sources of energy and unity and of discovering ways of adapting their Victorian legacy to the rapidly changing circumstances of the twentieth century. In principle at least, White's testimonies remained authoritative for Adventists around the world. And her guidance continued to flow from the presses as the White Estate, custodians of her literary heritage, drew upon her articles, letters, and other manuscripts to compile new books: *Counsels on Health* (1923), *Medical Ministry* (1932), *Counsels on Diet and Foods* (1938), *Temperance* (1949), and *Mind, Character, and Personality* (1977). Church leaders attached special importance to her ideas that seemed to correspond with modern medical science, arguing that such congruences provided "cogent evidence that compels acceptance by the mind, of the inspiration of the agent of the Spirit of Prophecy, Ellen G. White." When her counsel conflicted with current scientific knowledge, they usually expressed confidence that further research would confirm what she had written.[28]

Although the officers of the White Estate made no attempt to suppress Ellen White's writings on sex (and in fact incorporated some of her early statements in the new books they prepared), they let her first works on the subject go out of print. For decades, Adventists who attempted to fill the need for sexual guidance adopted the content and tone, though not the graphic language, of Mrs. White's works. Not until the appearance in 1974 of Charles Wittschiebe's *God Invented Sex,* an Adventist best-seller that cheerfully encouraged sexual spontaneity and inventiveness within marriage, did an Adventist writer substantially depart from the church's Victorian view of sexual activity.[29]

Because White's authority was at stake, masturbation remained a particularly difficult issue for Adventist authors—even for those who believed that her views on this subject lacked scientific support.[30] Homosexuality, a topic ignored by White, received little attention in Adventist circles before the gay liberation movement of the 1970s brought the issue to the fore.[31] In response to growing concern within the church, the leadership sponsored the Quest Learning Center in Pennsylvania, where, it was hoped, gay Adventists would learn to curtail their sexual activity if not transform their desires. About the same time, an articulate group of lay Adventist homosexuals formed Kinship, International, which sought, without denominational approval, to provide support for gay Adventists and to persuade others that not all homosexual relationships are morally reprehensible.

Lack of evidence makes it impossible to say how closely twentieth-century Seventh-day Adventists have followed the church's teachings on healthful living. Because abstinence from alcohol and tobacco has long been a condition of continuing membership, it seems probable that most Adventists have neither drunk nor smoked. It is also likely that virtually all of them have refrained from eating "unclean" meats and that the majority have avoided caffeinated beverages. A continuing study of Adventist behavior, begun in California in the 1970s, has revealed that about half of those surveyed adhered to a lacto-ovo vegetarian diet, which included the consumption of eggs and dairy products, while a fifth of them ate meat (presumably clean) at least four times a week. Outside of California, and especially beyond the borders of the United States and Australia, vegetarians no doubt constitute a much smaller percentage of Adventists, perhaps no more than ten percent in some places. Not only have Mrs. White's health writings been unavailable in some countries, but standards of living and food supplies have virtually ruled out a meatless diet. Despite the growing popularity of vegetarianism among non-Adventists in recent years, its appeal may be waning among Adventists, whose purchases of church-manufactured meat substitutes declined in the early 1980s.[32]

Undoubtedly because of their healthful life-style, thirty-five-year-old Adventist males living in California enjoy a six-year advantage in life expectancy, and Adventist women of the same age stand to gain four years. Epidemiological studies, also from California, show that Adventists are much less likely than the general population to die from cirrhosis of the liver and cancer of the mouth, esophagus, and lung—diseases associated with drinking and smoking. They are also less likely to die from nontraffic accidents, diabetes, coronary disease, and cancers of the large bowel, breast, and prostate. Adventist men, but not women, are less prone to suicide. However, with the exception of diseases attributed to the use of alcohol and tobacco, "Adventists die of the same causes that everyone else dies from. They simply die later." Whether they acquire fatal diseases at a more advanced age than most Americans or simply succumb to them later remains to be seen.[33]

Since the days of White and Kellogg, Seventh-day Adventists have eagerly promoted their philosophy of health among those of other faiths. In 1885 they began publishing *Life and Health* (now *Vibrant Life*), a magazine that featured articles on prevention, and in 1948 they launched *Listen,* a hard-hitting, colorfully packaged monthly magazine aimed at combatting alcohol, tobacco, and drug abuse. In a short time it became the most widely circulated temperance journal in the world. In 1960, two Adventists collaborated in developing a "Five-Day Plan" to stop smoking, a group-therapy program that subsequently enrolled millions. Adventists have also sponsored stress-management seminars, vegetarian restaurants and cooking schools, weight-reduction clinics, community surveys of public-health needs, screening programs, marathon runs, and an extensive welfare organization, the Adventist Development and Relief Agency.[34]

During the twentieth century, Seventh-day Adventists continued to expand their worldwide network of health-related facilities, which by the mid-1980s employed approximately one-third of the church's 93,000 workers. The roster of such institutions included 167 hospitals and sanitariums; 246 clinics, dispensaries, and medical boats (which began plying the Amazon River in the 1930s); 47 schools of nursing; 26 health-food companies; and the schools of medicine, dentistry, public health, and allied health professions at Loma Linda University.[35] Adventists entered the health-food business in 1877, when John Harvey Kellogg set up a company in Battle Creek to manufacture the whole-grain crackers and cereals he had developed. (At one point Kellogg offered to give the church the rights to his flaked cereal, but, on Mrs. White's advice, the leaders declined his gift—thus opening the door for the doctor's brother W.K. Kellogg to become the cereal king of America.)

Among the most successful church-owned companies in the twentieth century were Loma Linda Foods in the United States, manufacturers of meat substitutes, cereals, gravies, and a profitable soy milk developed by the medical missionary and Adventist folk hero Harry Miller to combat malnutrition in the Orient; and the Sanitarium Health Food Company in Australia and New Zealand, makers of Weet-Bix, a popular breakfast food.[36]

In North America the development of Seventh-day Adventist hospitals occurred along two distinct lines. The increasingly businesslike church-owned hospitals followed the national trend toward consolidation by merging in the early 1980s into the Adventist Health System/ United States, which retained the advertising agency Doyle Dane Bernbach to promote Adventist health care. Its seventy-one hospitals and various other enterprises earned the newly formed entity "the distinction of being the country's largest Protestant, nonprofit, nationally integrated health care delivery system."[37] However, the very size of the system— and the fact that it employed several disaffected Adventist ministers at substantially increased salaries—led some concerned church members to fear that the denomination might be drifting toward another "Battle Creek" showdown between the church's healers and its ministerial leadership. Besides, some of the system's facilities employed so few Seventh-day Adventists they appeared to be Adventist in name only. Despite the denomination's long-standing opposition to church–state entanglements, institutions within the Adventist Health System readily accepted government funds for capital (though not for operating) expenses.

Self-supporting Adventist hospitals have generally been run by members intent on following Mrs. White's "blue print" for such institutions, especially with regard to lifestyle and therapy. Many of these hospitals, especially in the rural Southeast, trace their origin back to the Madison Sanitarium, founded in 1907 on a site near Nashville, Tennessee, selected by Mrs. White herself. Others, in recent years, have derived their inspiration from the Weimar Institute, a medical–educational complex begun in northern California in the 1970s that self-consciously adopted a back-to-White philosophy. Occasionally these self-supporting institutions were affiliated with urban clinics or vegetarian restaurants; more frequently they were located in secluded, rural settings, where patients could learn to live in harmony with nature's laws. A prominent exception to this pattern was the Harding Hospital, a self-supporting psychiatric institution near Columbus, Ohio, founded in 1916. Until the 1960s, when the denominational medical school at Loma Linda first offered a residency in psychiatry, the Harding Hospital almost single-handedly supplied the church with psychiatrists.[38]

As the number of medicinal drugs of proven value increased in the twentieth century, Adventist hospitals and physicians tended to set aside Ellen White's ban on drugs and her advocacy of water and to practice a brand of medicine therapeutically indistinguishable from that of non-Adventists. The White Estate abetted this transition by warning in 1962 that Mrs. White's strictures against nineteenth-century drugs should not be construed to apply to "tested remedial agencies made through scientific research." Twenty years later, church officials formally endorsed all "accepted and scientifically proven methods." By this time few Adventist physicians remembered Mrs. White's admonition that they were not to "follow the world's methods of medical practice, exacting large fees that worldly physicians demand for their services," or her insistence that they follow "the Lord's plan" of treating only those of the same sex. Most of them had also lost sight of their sectarian roots in nineteenth-century hydropathy and had come to view medical sectarianism in its twentieth-century forms (chiropractic and naturopathy, for example) with disdain.[39]

By mid-century, and probably earlier, the distinctiveness of Adventist medicine lay less in its therapies than in its customs, motives, and philosophical justifications. Adventist medical institutions may have abandoned the water cure, but they visibly retained their religious and health-reforming heritage. They all discouraged drinking, smoking, and meat-eating. Though they remained open around the clock, they tried not to schedule elective surgery and other optional treatments during the Sabbath hours, from sundown Friday to sundown Saturday. In addition to the normal chaplaincy services, they offered doctrinal instruction and free Adventist literature. Although they frowned on charismatic faith healing, they gladly permitted ministers to pray for the sick and to anoint them with oil, a ritual devoid of magical expectations. And if patients allowed it, many Adventist doctors and nurses prayed with them at bedtime or before surgery. Such customs cultivated what Ellen White called "a sense of the presence of God."[40]

Various—and often mixed—motivations impelled Seventh-day Adventists toward careers in the healing professions. There was always the desire to alleviate human suffering (historically advocated by Kellogg) or the opportunity to win converts to Adventism (White's emphasis). However, as the century matured, other motives increasingly surfaced. At the individual level, the medical professions offered Adventist youth a chance to pursue careers that not only provided comfortable livings, purposive work, and social standing, but, because the church allowed medical personnel to render essential services on the Sabbath, created little conflict between occupational and religious loyalties. At the denominational level, profits made from clinics and hospitals overseas were used to subsidize evangelistic activities. Thus, to insure the greatest return on their investment, Adventist institutions in Third World countries sometimes catered to persons in the middle and upper classes, as well as to foreign visitors and American expatriates.

The theological justifications for Seventh-day Adventist involvement in medicine can be seen in the work of Jack Provonsha, a physician on the faculty of Loma Linda University and the denomination's first trained ethicist. In his efforts to provide an Adventist theology of healing, he has emphasized that the purpose of Christian medicine is "to make the *whole* man whole," a concept rooted in Seventh-day Adventism's long-standing refusal to separate body from soul. In Provonsha's opinion, the Adventist adherence to conditional immortality has fostered a uniquely positive view of the physical aspects of life and has thus encouraged both clinical medicine and basic research.[41]

Provonsha, the most influential bioethicist in Adventist circles, rose to prominence in the late 1950s partly because of his answers to questions regarding the dangers of hypnosis and other forms of mind control, which Ellen White had denounced as satanic and which the General Conference banned in Seventh-day Adventist institutions. From the Wesleyan strain in Adventism, inherited through White and others, Provonsha seized upon the idea of human freedom as a criterion by which to determine degrees of value and to judge right from wrong. If to be truly human was to be "endowed with a power akin to that of the Creator—individuality, power to think and to do," as White had said, it followed that the primary moral obligation was to act in ways that increase the human capacity for self-determination. Thus, Provonsha reasoned, "whatever enhances the image of God (Freedom, Self-determination) in man is right. Whatever diminishes that image is wrong." Because hypnosis—along with alcohol, mood-altering drugs, intensely emotional sermons, and charismatic "excess"—increases a person's suggestibility and thereby lessens the capacity for self-determination, it is, concluded Provonsha, morally suspect.[42]

The manner in which Provonsha analyzed the morality of hypnosis and other forms of mind control provides a key to understanding the distinctive direction of recent moral thinking within Adventism. His focus on freedom as partial but genuine self-determination, derived from grappling with the problem of hypnosis, clearly influenced his positions on abortion and euthanasia, developed in the 1960s and 1970s. Although all living creatures are intrinsically valuable, some, according to Provonsha, are more valuable than others because of their greater participation in true freedom. A human embryo, because it possesses the potential for self-determination, has more worth than a tumor, but less value than a freely acting adult. Thus, "whenever the developing embryo or fetus places in jeopardy the mother's physical, mental, or emotional health, and that jeopardy is judged to be of sufficiently serious nature, the potential human symbol, the embryo or fetus, may be sacrificed." Using similar logic, he argued that the capacity for self-determination should help to "determine the amount of effort and expense to be put into maintaining [the] survival" of terminally ill patients. In the 1970s and 1980s, Provonsha turned his attention to the area of human reproduction, warning that such procedures as artificial insemination, in vitro fertilization, and embryo transplantation may lessen the capacity for true self-determination by weakening the family unit in which a child's freedom is nurtured—a view greeted with some skepticism at his own university, where medical students were routinely invited to contribute semen to sperm banks.[43]

Except with regard to practices such as hypnotism that Ellen White condemned, the General Conference generally left difficult ethical decisions to individuals and institutions. In 1982 the General Conference recommended that

Each [medical] institution should develop policies consistent with high moral and ethical standards which recognize the value of human life. Such policies should deal with abortions, death and dying, and related issues. No worker should be asked to violate his/her conscience.

But even on these questions church leaders sometimes offered specific advice. In the early 1970s, for example, they circulated a set of "suggested guidelines" that approved of abortion under the following conditions: when a pregnancy threatens a mother's life, when it is likely to eventuate in a severely deformed or retarded child, when conception is the result of rape or incest, when the mother is unwed and below the age of fifteen, and "when for some reason the requirements of functional human life demand the sacrifice of the lesser potential human value." These views, though perhaps more liberal than those of the average member, reflected the Seventh-day Adventist belief that a new person comes into existence gradually as the fetus develops and not instantly at some precise moment, whether at conception, implantation, quickening, viability, or birth.[44]

The Seventh-day Adventist church rarely addressed bioethical issues before the 1960s, when Provonsha began to prompt discussions at the medical school in Loma Linda, and Roy Branson, a Harvard-educated ethicist now associated with the Kennedy Institute at Georgetown University, began offering training in ethics at the Seventh-day Adventist Theological Seminary in Michigan. Branson not only encouraged several young Adventist ministers to become ethicists (one of whom, Gerald Winslow, subsequently wrote a widely acclaimed book on allocating scarce medical resources[45]), but, as editor of *Spectrum*, the quarterly journal of the Association of Adventist Forums, provided a vehicle for exploring a variety of ethical issues facing the church and society without pretending to speak for the denomination as a whole.

In the early 1980s church officials permitted Loma Linda University's Division of Religion to establish a Center for Christian Bioethics, with Provonsha as its first director and two of Branson's former students on its staff.[46] By this time Adventists, long on the social periphery, were growing accustomed to basking in the positive publicity that their life-style and health-care system had generated. But nothing could have prepared them for the attention they received from all parts of the world in 1984 when a Loma Linda surgical team, headed by Dr. Leonard Bailey, transplanted a baboon's heart into a premature infant known simply as Baby Fae—the first time since 1844, noted Branson, "that an Adventist event in America has also been a national event." The baby died after making medical history, but the controversy regarding the procedure continued long after the event. Some observers applauded it as an appropriate therapeutic advance, with Provonsha defending it as the best available therapy for infants born with fatal defects like Baby Fae's. Others criticized the venture in terms of animal rights, better therapeutic possibilities, fairer allocations of medical dollars, more detailed consent procedures, or religious scruples. Although leaders of the denomination maintained a measured and cautious public profile, they remained quietly supportive. Whether or not Adventist medicine, hitherto respected primarily for its clinical excellence, will increasingly play a prominent role in medical research remains to be seen. But there can be no doubt about the great distance Seventh-day Adventists have traversed between Mrs. White's water-cure establishment in Battle Creek, Michigan, and Dr. Bailey's surgical laboratory in Loma Linda, California.[47]

Notes

1. Francis D. Nichol, *The Midnight Cry: A Defense of William Miller and the Millerites* (Washington, 1944), p. 320; Ronald L. Numbers and Janet S. Numbers, "Millerism and Madness: A Study of 'Religious Insanity' in Nineteenth-Century America," *Bulletin of the Menninger Clinic* 49 (1985):289–320.
2. William Miller, *Evidence from Scripture and History of the Second Coming of Christ, about the Year 1843* (Boston, 1842), pp. 146–148; L.B. Coles, *Philosophy of Health: Natural Principles of Health and Cure,* rev. ed. (Boston, 1853), p. 216; Ronald L. Numbers, *Prophetess of Health: A Study of Ellen G. White* (New York, 1976), pp. 38, 59–61, 77–79; Nichol, *Midnight Cry,* pp. 199–203. On the postmillennial health reformers, see James C. Whorton, *Crusaders for Fitness: The History of American Health Reformers* (Princeton, NJ, 1982).
3. Numbers, *Prophetess of Health,* pp. 47, 72–79.

4. Ibid., pp. 9, 134–135; George Storrs, *An Inquiry: Are the Wicked Immortal? In Six Sermons,* 21st ed. (New York, 1852), p. 14; LeRoy Edwin Froom, *The Conditionalist Faith of Our Fathers,* 2 vols. (Washington, DC, 1965–1966), 2:646–667.

5. Ronald L. Numbers and Janet S. Numbers, "The Psychological World of Ellen White," *Spectrum* 14 (August 1983):22–23.

6. Ellen G. White, "To Those Who Are Receiving the Seal of the Living God" (a broadside from Topsham, Maine, dated 31 January 1849); Ellen G. White, *Spiritual Gifts: My Christian Experience, Views and Labors in Connection with the Rise and Progress of the Third Angel's Message* (Battle Creek, MI, 1860), p. 135; Numbers, *Prophetess of Health,* pp. 31–36.

7. Ibid., pp. 37–44.

8. Ellen G. White, *Christian Temperance and Bible Hygiene* (Battle Creek, MI, 1890), p. 53; Mrs. E.G. White, *Testimonies for the Church,* 9 vols. (Mountain View, CA, n.d.), 1:559, 3:62.

9. Ellen G. White, *Spiritual Gifts: Important Facts of Faith, Laws of Health, and Testimonies Nos. 1–10* (Battle Creek, MI, 1864), pp. 120–151, esp. p. 133; Ellen G. White, manuscript relating the vision of 6 [sic] June 1863 (MS-1-1863, Ellen G. White Estate, Washington, DC).

10. Ellen G. White, "Our Late Experience," *Advent Review and Sabbath Herald* 27 (1866):89–91, 97–99; White, *Testimonies,* 1:485–495; Numbers, *Prophetess of Health,* pp. 88–101.

11. Ibid., pp. 102–111; White, *Testimonies,* 3:165.

12. Ibid. 5:439; Numbers, *Prophetess of Health,* pp. 124–128, 169. On Kellogg's life and work, see Richard W. Schwarz, *John Harvey Kellogg, M.D.* (Nashville, 1970).

13. Ellen G. White, *Testimony for the Physicians and Helpers of the Sanitarium* (n.p., n.d.), p. 8; Ellen G. White, Letter 76, 1899 (Ellen G. White Estate); White, *Testimonies,* 6:327.

14. J.H. Kellogg to Ellen G. White, March 21, 1893 (Ellen G. White Estate); White, *Testimonies,* 7:97. See also Jonathan Butler, "Ellen G. White and the Chicago Mission," *Spectrum* 2 (Winter 1970):41–51.

15. Numbers, *Prophetess of Health,* pp. 191–199.

16. Ellen G. White, *An Appeal to Mothers: The Great Cause of the Physical, Mental, and Moral Ruin of Many of the Children of Our Time* (Battle Creek, MI, 1864), p. 17.

17. White, *Testimonies,* 2:472–478; Numbers, *Prophetess of Health,* pp. 157–159.

18. Ibid., pp. 160–177; Ron Graybill, "The Development of Adventist Thinking on Clean and Unclean Meats" (pamphlet dated April 27, 1981, Ellen G. White Estate).

19. Numbers, *Prophetess of Health,* pp. 166–170.

20. Ellen G. White, *The Ministry of Healing* (Washington, DC, 1905), pp. 313–317.

21. White, *Christian Temperance,* p. 119.

22. Numbers, *Prophetess of Health,* pp. 129–147.

23. Ibid., p. 184; White, *Testimonies,* 1:561.

24. White, *Ministry of Healing,* pp. 111–112.

25. Numbers and Numbers, "The Psychological World of Ellen White," pp. 21–31.

26. Ibid.

27. Ellen G. White, *The Great Controversy between Christ and Satan* (Battle Creek, MI, 1888), pp. 492–493; *Early Writings of Ellen G. White* (Washington, DC, 1945), p. 17.

28. Ellen G. White Estate, *Medical Science and the Spirit of Prophecy* (Washington, DC, n.d.), p. 31.

29. Charles Wittschiebe, *God Invented Sex* (Nashville, 1974). Typical of the older genre were the widely read works of Harold Shryock: *Happiness for Husbands and Wives* (Washington, DC, 1949); *On Becoming a Man* (Washington, DC, 1951); *On Becoming a Woman* (Washington, DC, 1951); and *On Being Married Soon* (Washington, DC, 1968). For more recent views, see the essays on Adventism and sexuality by Alberta Mazat, David R. Larson, and Roy G. Gravesen in *Spectrum* 15 (May 1984).

30. See, e.g., Shryock, *On Becoming a Man*, p. 36; John F. Knight, *What a Young Man Should Know about Sex* (Mountain View, CA, 1977), pp. 178–183; Wittschiebe, *God Invented Sex*, p. 165; and Charles Wittschiebe, *Teens and Love and Sex* (Washington, DC, 1982). Evidence of a liberalizing trend can be seen in Nancy L. Van Pelt, *The Complete Parent* (Nashville, 1976), pp. 142–144; and Alberta Mazat, *That Friday in Eden: Sharing and Enhancing Sexuality in Marriage* (Mountain View, CA, 1981), pp. 145–149.

31. It is possible that Ellen White subsumed homosexuality under terms more commonly used to denote masturbation; see Vern L. Bullough and Martha Voght, "Homosexuality and Its Confusion with the 'Secret Sin' in Pre-Freudian America," *Journal of the History of Medicine and Allied Sciences* 28 (1973):143–155.

32. R.L. Phillips and others, "Influence of Selection versus Lifestyle on Risk of Fatal Cancer and Cardiovascular Disease among Seventh-day Adventists," *American Journal of Epidemiology* 112 (1980):296–314; Marcology 21, "Loma Linda Foods: The Shopper's Perspective," unpublished report submitted to the Loma Linda Food Company, August 1983.

33. F.R. Lemon and J.W. Kuzma, "A Biologic Cost of Smoking: Decreased Life Expectancy," *Archives of Environmental Health* 18 (1969):950–955; R.L. Phillips, "Cancer among Seventh-day Adventists," *Journal of Environmental Pathology and Toxicology* 3 (1980):157–169.

34. Jasper Wayne MacFarland and Elman J. Folkenberg, *How to Stop Smoking in Five Days* (Englewood Cliffs, NJ, 1964). On the health-related activities of Adventists in recent years, see R.W. Schwarz, *Light Bearers to the Remnant* (Mountain View, CA, 1979), pp. 598–614.

35. *Seventh-day Adventist Yearbook 1984* (Hagerstown, MD, 1984), p. 4.

36. Schwarz, *Light Bearers to the Remnant*, pp. 609–610; Numbers, *Prophetess of Health*, pp. 188–189. Regarding Miller, see Raymond S. Moore, *China Doctor: The Life Story of Harry Willis Miller* (New York, 1961).

37. Adventist Health System/United States, *1984 Annual Report*, quotation on p. 5.

38. "Madison Institutions," in Don F. Neufeld, ed., *Seventh-day Adventist Encyclopedia* (Washington, DC, 1976), pp. 827–832; Donald Anderson, "Reminiscing—Seventh-day Adventists and Psychiatry," unpublished manuscript available from the Department of Psychiatry, Loma Linda University School of Medicine.

39. Trustees of the Ellen G. White Estate, Preface (dated November 1, 1962) to the second edition of Ellen G. White, *Medical Ministry* (Mountain

View, CA, 1963), p. xiv; *1982 Annual Council of the General Conference Committee: General Actions* (Washington, DC, 1982), p. 36; Numbers, *Prophetess of Health,* pp. 199–200.

40. White, *Medical Ministry,* p. 33.
41. Jack W. Provonsha, "The Philosophic Roots of a Wholistic Understanding of Man," lecture delivered May 20, 1978, at a conference on "Towards a Theology of Healing," the duplicated proceedings of which are available from the Heritage Room, Loma Linda University Library; Provonsha, *Is Death for Real?* (Mountain View, CA, 1981).
42. *1982 Annual Council,* p. 37; Ellen G. White, *Education* (Oakland, CA, 1903), p. 17; Jack W. Provonsha, "Mind Manipulation: A Christian Ethical Analysis," undated, duplicated paper available from the Division of Religion, Loma Linda University.
43. Jack W. Provonsha, "A Christian Appraisal of Therapeutic Abortion," "Love, Life, and Death," and "Some Ethical Considerations Regarding Artificial Insemination," undated, duplicated papers available from the Division of Religion, Loma Linda University.
44. *1982 Annual Council,* p. 37; Medical Secretary of the General Conference of Seventh-day Adventists, "Interruption of Pregnancy: Recommendations to S.D.A. Medical Institutions," published in abridged form in *Ministry* 44 (March 1971):10–11. See also Gerald Winslow, "Adventists and Abortion: A Principled Approach," *Spectrum* 12 (December 1981):6–17.
45. Gerald R. Winslow, *Triage and Justice: The Ethics of Rationing Life-Saving Medical Resources* (Berkeley, CA, 1982).
46. Information about center activities can be found in its quarterly publication, *The Ethics Center Update,* the first issue of which appeared in the fall of 1984.
47. Roy Branson, " 'You Are My Witness,' " *Spectrum* 16 (April 1985):2. See also the special section on Baby Fae in the same issue, pp. 5–26; and "Reflections Regarding Baby Fae," by staff members of the Center for Christian Bioethics, *Ethics Center Update* 1 (Fall 1984):3–6.

CHAPTER 17

The Jehovah's
Witness Tradition

WILLIAM H. CUMBERLAND

Although Jehovah's Witnesses claim Abel as the first Witness, their modern origins stem from 1879, when a wealthy, young Pittsburgh businessman, Charles Taze Russell (1852–1916), began publishing the magazine *Zion's Watch Tower and Herald of Christ's Presence.* Two years later Pastor Russell, as he was called, founded Zion's Watch Tower Bible and Tract Society, incorporated in 1884 with Russell as president. In 1909 he moved to Brooklyn, New York, where the organization's headquarters, Bethel, remain today. At the time of the move, subscribers to *The Watch Tower* numbered 27,000, a figure Russell estimated represented half the size of his following.[1] After Pastor Russell's death in 1916, Joseph F. Rutherford (1869–1942), a flamboyant lawyer who assumed the honorific title Judge, won an internal struggle to assume control of the organization. Shortly thereafter, in the summer of 1918, Rutherford and seven other Watch Tower officials, who had advised their followers to have nothing to do with the war effort against Germany, were sentenced to twenty years in prison for "conspiring to obstruct or impede the war work of the United States." Released from prison in March 1919, Rutherford reclaimed his shattered movement, which he proceeded to reorganize structurally and doctrinally during the next two decades, giving the movement its distinctive character.

Instead of calling his followers Bible Students, as Russell had done, Rutherford in 1931 adopted the name Jehovah's Witnesses (the scriptural basis being *Isaiah* 43:10–12 and 62:2). Over the years, he also abandoned the traditional congregational form of governance for a highly centralized, authoritarian organization that claimed divine sanction for its actions. The key Witness doctrine during the Rutherford years became the "Vindication of Jehovah's Name," which involved warning the world of the impending disaster of Armageddon so that those who accepted "the truth" might find refuge in God's Kingdom.

According to Witness teaching, the Battle of Armageddon prophesied in *Revelation* 16:16 will soon be fought, and Jehovah's forces, led by Christ, will rid the earth of Satan and his demonic hosts. Only Jehovah's Witnesses will survive the worldwide conflict, which will usher in a millennium of righteousness and peace, during which billions of deceased persons will be resurrected and given a chance to prove themselves worthy of eternal life. Throughout this period an "anointed" class of 144,000 will rule with Christ in heaven as spirit beings, while the "other sheep" (the majority of those loyal to Jehovah) will inherit perfectly restored material bodies and reside upon an earth that will gradually regain its original Edenic qualities.

The year 1914 has assumed great importance in the eschatology of Jehovah's Witnesses. From a study of biblical prophecies, Russell identified that year as the time when Armageddon would begin. In 1925 Rutherford suggested that 1914 marked the time when Satan had been cast from the heavens to the vicinity of earth—an event that explained the increasing turmoil and sinfulness of the twentieth century. Later, when 1914 also came to be seen as marking the beginning of the "last days" leading immediately to Armageddon, Jehovah's Witnesses insisted that the generation living in 1914 would see the destruction of the existing system.

Jehovah's Witnesses strongly emphasize traditional family and moral values. They practice baptism by immersion, teach special creation rather than evolution, and reject such doctrines as the immortality of the soul, hellfire, and the Trinity. They refuse to salute the flag, hold public office, vote in elections, or serve in the armed forces. They eschew higher education, though they welcome well-educated converts such as lawyers and physicians. Most Witnesses do not celebrate individual birthdays, Christmas, or national holidays. Their congregations meet in Kingdom Halls, not churches. They regard all baptized members as ordained ministers, although only a fraction of them serve full-time as administrators or pioneers (who devote much of their time to witnessing and distributing literature). They consistently avoid interfaith cooperation.

Since World War II the movement has grown rapidly. The number of publishers (active members contributing part of their time in door-to-door witnessing) has increased from 115,000 in 1942 to 2,680,274 in 1984. Much of this growth is attributable to the leadership of Rutherford's successor, Nathan H. Knorr (1905–1977), who as president enlarged the productive capacity of the Brooklyn publishing facilities, improved techniques used in preaching, and, in 1943, established a six-month training program for missionaries, Gilead College, at East Lansing, New York.

Today Jehovah's Witnesses are active in over two hundred countries, with the majority of members now living outside of North America.

For years the president of the Watch Tower Bible and Tract Society wielded virtually autocratic power, leaving the corporation directors to serve in a largely honorary capacity. In the mid-1970s, however, the Governing Body assumed *de facto* as well as *de jure* powers, forcing the president to surrender some of his authority to a collegium of eighteen members who determine legislative and judicial matters by a two-thirds majority. In 1975, Witnesses experienced the latest in a series of at least six prophetic failures when the year passed without witnessing the predicted end of the present world and the beginning of Armageddon. The disappointment associated with this experience coupled with the rigid demands imposed upon members by the Governing Body no doubt accounted for many of the 768,000 desertions from the movement that occurred during the 1970s.[2] Since Knorr's death in 1977, Frederick W. Franz (b. 1893) has occupied the presidency.

----◄∞►----

The Jehovah's Witnesses provide an interesting example of how one religious body estranged from the world and expecting its imminent end has responded to health-related concerns. In contrast to many Christian denominations, the Witnesses have not created their own health-care institutions. Although they have readily sought medical assistance from non-Witness doctors and hospitals, their rejection of blood transfusions has frequently brought them into conflict with both the medical establishment and the state. This essay focuses on three broad areas of concern: the interaction between the millennial predictions of the Jehovah's Witnesses and their general attitudes toward sickness and health; the specific question of blood, the central medical issue facing the tradition and one that for Witnesses "involves the most fundamental principles on which they as Christians base their lives"; and the ways in which their strict moral code has influenced their social attitudes and lifestyle.[3]

Prophecy and Health

Although Charles Taze Russell recruited many of his early followers from among the Adventists and borrowed many of his interpretations of biblical prophecy from these spiritual heirs of William Miller, who had mistakenly predicted the return of Christ in the 1840s, he shared none of the enthusiasm for health reform displayed by the Seventh-day Adventists, who also lay claim to the Millerite heritage. He did, however, agree with them that disease was a degenerative process that had begun with Adam's fall from grace. Sin, he maintained, had reduced the human life span from more than nine hundred years to less than three score, a decline that would not be reversed until after Armageddon, when bodily perfection would be restored through the combined efforts of human and divine agents. Russell also recognized a psychosomatic element in illness, asserting that "one half the people in the world are sick because they think they are."[4] At times Witnesses have assigned demons a role in the production of disability and disease. As a recent *Watchtower* article stated, "sinister spirit forces or demons are always against mankind's better interest."[5]

Despite Russell's belief that the age of miracles had ended with the apostles, early Witness literature frequently reported instances of miraculous healing, especially in difficult cases. In recent years, however, Witnesses have insisted that in times of illness "they do not look for some miraculous 'faith healing' cure." A few may still harbor suspicions of the medical profession, reasoning that "if Jehovah God wants me to be well, he will keep me so," but the great majority rely for physical healing on the services of trained medical personnel, including M.D.s, osteopaths, and chiropractors.[6]

Psychiatrists and psychologists, however, are a different matter. Fearful that non-Christian therapists might trace the roots of emotional problems to their patients' peculiar faith, leaders of the movement have discouraged Witnesses from seeking professional help for mental disturbances. Articles in the widely circulated *Watchtower* and *Awake!* magazines report that many members have found relief for such problems as depression and anxiety through weekly Bible studies and congregational meetings. If additional help is needed, mentally disturbed Jehovah's Witnesses are urged to seek the counsel of elders in the congregation, who tend to prescribe right thinking and willpower and who sometimes only increase feelings of guilt and anxiety.[7]

The effect of Witness teachings and practices on the mental health of members is difficult to assess. On the one hand, trusting in Jehovah to work out one's problems could diminish personal responsibility and reduce anxiety, even about mundane matters. "Before we received the truth," testified one Witness in the 1930s, "I would lie awake 'till two or three o'clock in the morning trying to figure how to save this property. Now I go to bed, say the Lord's prayer, and in a few moments I am asleep."[8] Also, the nearness of Armageddon offered hope for relief from pain and persecution, and the prospect of entering the New Age without dying greatly blunted the mystery of death. Rutherford captured that vision in 1920 with the slogan (and book title) *Millions Now Living Will Never Die,* and ever since, Witnesses have emphasized that hope in multimillions of books, magazines, and pamphlets printed by the Watchtower presses.

On the other hand, there is some evidence that Jehovah's Witnesses suffer from a higher incidence of mental illness than the population at large. For example, a study of patients in Western Australian psychiatric hospitals revealed an admission rate for Witnesses of 4.17 per 1,000 compared to 2.54 for the general population and an incidence of schizophrenia three times higher than the average.[9] Such studies do not indicate whether the movement has simply attracted mentally unstable converts or has actually caused emotional disturbances. But it seems likely that persistent demands for group conformity, increasing invasion of privacy by the organizational hierarchy, lack of tolerance for dissenting opinions, denial of meaningful social relationships in an economically competitive world, the tension of living on the precipice of Armageddon, and disillusionment resulting from unrealized millennial predictions have at least contributed to the problem.

During the early decades of the movement, Watch-Tower leaders paid little attention to issues related to sickness and health. Both Russell and Rutherford suffered from serious physical ailments—the former from hemorrhoids and heart problems, the latter from lungs damaged during his prison experience and cancer—but neither paraded his disabilities before the public, and few followers learned of either man's struggle with illness. Russell felt that suffering could be redemptive—that instead of making a person rebellious, it should refine one's character. Saints of all ages, he observed, had learned the "blessings of afflictions and sorrows."[10]

From the beginning, Witnesses have placed publishing and preaching above curing social and physical ills. Once the millennium arrived, they taught, all problems, including those related to health, would be solved. "Like the sun," Rutherford wrote in 1921,

> the great Messianic Kingdom, singing forth with healing beams shall dispel the darkness, drive away the sickness, clean up the minds and morals, point the people to proper food, what to eat and how to eat it, what to think and how to conduct themselves; and above all to give them a full knowledge of the loving kindness of our great God and of the Lord Jesus Christ the dearest friend of all.[11]

Although individual Witnesses sometimes supported charitable activities (despite being told that surplus funds should be donated to the organization to spread the message), the Governing Body generally shied away from any official involvement in caring and curing. It was not the function of the Society, claimed the Watchtower hierarchy, to operate hospitals and clinics just as it was not its function to run police and fire departments.[12] Instead of attempting the impossible task of eliminating suffering and injustice from this world, they would invest in saving souls for the New World. Such evils as war and unemployment were "corporately beyond human power to regulate," wrote Russell, who described efforts at social uplift as "unscriptural and erroneous."[13]

On occasion, Russell offered suggestions for preventing and curing illness, even sharing with readers of *The Watch Tower* his own remedies for cancer and influenza.[14] But the Society's publications devoted little space to such topics until the appearance in 1919 of a second major magazine, *The Golden Age* (renamed *Consolation* in 1937 and *Awake!* in 1946). This shift did not result from a change in official policy, but rather stemmed from the personal idiosyncracies of the magazine's editor, Clayton J. Woodworth, who viewed the medical profession as "an institution founded on ignorance, error and superstition." Woodworth warned his readers of the dangers of such things as aspirin, chlorinated water, aluminum cooking utensils, and vaccination for smallpox. "Thinking people," he explained, "would rather have smallpox than vaccination, because the latter sows the seed of syphilis, cancer, eczema, erisipelas, scrofula, consumption, even leprosy and many other loathsome afflictions. Hence the practice of vaccination is a crime, an outrage and a delusion."[15] Even though the Governing Body did not endorse all of Woodworth's opinions, many Witnesses believed that they represented official Society positions. For example, some young Witness men imprisoned during World War II for violating the Selective Service Act refused to be vaccinated until a Watchtower official visited them and explained that the vaccine was merely a serum and thus did not violate the biblical injunction against taking blood.[16]

Blood Transfusions

No medical issue has assumed greater practical and symbolic importance for Jehovah's Witnesses than blood transfusions. The Witness objection to using blood evolved over a period of several decades. Much of this objection derived from peculiar interpretations of Scripture, but its main source seems to have been Woodworth's hostility toward traditional medicine, evidenced by his espousal of idiosyncratic cures and his rejection of the germ theory of disease.[17]

The Witnesses' preoccupation with blood first surfaced in 1927, when an article in *The Watch Tower* and a paragraph in Rutherford's book *Creation* called attention to Old Testament prohibitions against using blood for food. Until this time, Witnesses such as Russell had taught that these prohibitions applied only to Jews and to early Christians who wanted to avoid offending Jewish converts. Because blood transfusions were still relatively uncommon—the earliest blood bank did not appear until 1937—the debate at first centered on such questions as the eating of improperly bled animals or meat that contained blood as an ingredient.[18] However, the widespread use of transfusions during World War II created increasing concern among Witnesses, who in 1945 officially banned the practice. The article in the *Watchtower* announcing the new policy argued that the Old Testament injunction against consuming blood also applied to transfusions because physicians, according to the *Encyclopedia Americana,* "reasoned that as the blood is the principal medium by which the body is nourished, transfusion, therefore, is a quicker and shorter road to feed an ill-nourished body than eating food which turns to blood after several changes." It went on to warn that "it behooves all worshipers of Jehovah who seek eternal life in his new world of righteousness to respect the sanctity of blood and to conform themselves to God's righteous rulings concerning this vital matter."[19]

The Society based its proscription against blood transfusions on three biblical passages: *Genesis* 9:4, which forbade Noah and his family from eating "flesh with the life thereof, which is the blood thereof"; *Leviticus* 17:13–14, which required the Israelites to pour out the blood of slain animals because "it is the life of all flesh"; and *Acts* 15:29, which decreed that Christians were to "abstain from meats offered to idols, and from blood, and from things strangled." The recipient of a transfusion, Witnesses argued, was "feeding upon a God given soul contained in the blood vehicle of man or of fellow man." Thus there was no difference between taking blood orally and taking it intravenously.[20]

Despite the pronouncement in 1945, blood transfusions did not become a major issue until April 1951, when a recently converted Chicago couple, Darrell and Rhoda Labrenz, learned that their seven-day-old baby daughter, Cheryl, suffered from an insufficiency of red blood cells. The infant's doctors at Bethany Hospital insisted that only a transfusion could save her, but the parents refused permission. The anguished mother explained her dilemma to the press:

> Of course I want my baby to live. And I pray that she does. I've always wanted a little girl. But we can't break Jehovah's law. He gave us these commands. He told us if we follow them, we will live. If we do not, he will cast us off. We believe it is more important to carry out his commands than to deliberately break them by giving my baby blood. If my baby dies, I'll feel sorrow. But it would be bearable because of my beliefs. Perhaps God would be using her as a Witness. If she died she would have a chance for the new earth, but if we broke Jehovah's laws we feel we will lose not only our chance, but the baby's for the new earth.[21]

The local health department, in what would become a common practice, secured a court order charging the Labrenzes with technical neglect and making Cheryl a ward of the court. Mr. Labrenz appealed the case, but the Superior Court of Illinois ruled that the parents could not jeopardize their child's life because of their religious beliefs:

> Parents may be free to become martyrs themselves. It does not follow, however, that they are free in identical circumstances to make martyrs of their children before they have reached an age of full and legal discretion, when they can make that choice for themselves. Laws, while they cannot interfere with religious belief and opinion, may be constitutionally appropriate for interfering with religious practices.[22]

Condemned by both the religious and medical establishments, Darrell Labrenz insisted that the real sinners were those who had forced the issue. The Society, while denying the charge of religious fanaticism, bluntly stated that it was "better to die now maintaining integrity and later be resurrected than to compromise now and live for a brief time, only to be dead forever later on."[23] Although most legal action regarding transfusions has involved the rights of children, in a few instances the courts have forced transfusions on adult Witnesses.

Even after the Labrenz case, the Society waited until 1961 before deciding to disfellowship members who violated the prohibition against transfusions. Ever since, the organization has grown increasingly strict in its application of the ban on blood. (One Watchtower official even condemned using fertilizer made of blood.) When some physicians sought to circumvent Witnesses' objections by resorting to autotransfusions, in which the patient's own blood is used, the Governing Body warned that it was unacceptable to use any blood that had been stored for even a brief period of time. The only permissible form of autotransfusion involved keeping the blood in circulation and not separating it or any of its components from the body.[24]

At first the Society expressed ambivalence about the use of serums, such as diphtheria antitoxin and gamma globulin, that contained a small blood component. This led some members to question the appropriateness of using such injections for the purpose of building up resistance to disease. Did this, they asked, fall into the same category as drinking blood or receiving blood transfusions? The Society's answer revealed its vacillation:

> No, it does not seem necessary that we put the two in the same category, although we have done so in times past. . . . The injection of antibodies into the blood in a vehicle of blood serum or the use of blood fractions to create such antibodies is not the same as taking blood, either by mouth or

by transfusion, as a nutrient to build up the body's vital forces. While God did not intend for man to contaminate his blood stream by vaccines, serums or blood fractions, doing so does not seem to be included in God's expressed will forbidding blood as food. It would therefore be a matter of individual judgment whether one accepted such types of medication or not.[25]

In 1974, however, the Society warned Witnesses not to accept "treatment from serum that comes from blood" and specifically forbade the use of gamma globulin, even for Witnesses who had been exposed to viral hepatitis. In at least one area the Society grew more tolerant: After initially condemning the use of blood particles by hemophiliacs, in the late 1970s it finally approved the practice.[26]

Before 1967 the Society permitted organ transplants. The Governing Body then denounced such operations as a "macabre form of cannibalism"—only to reverse itself in 1980 and recognize the procedure as a matter of individual conscience. Because the donor was not killed to supply food and in fact often willed his or her body parts to be used as transplants, the hierarchy decided that concerns about cannibalism did not apply. They also allowed Witnesses to use heart–lung pumps and dialysis machines as long as they were primed with a non-blood fluid.[27]

The Witnesses' refusal to sanction blood transfusions for members of the faith challenged a highly regarded and widely accepted medical practice and posed ethical and legal dilemmas for many physicians. Should they accept patients who rejected the only procedure that might save their lives? Could they be subjected to criminal charges if they failed to use those techniques when available? What should they do when Jehovah's Witness patients arrived in emergency rooms unable to express their wishes concerning transfusions? Should they subordinate their patients' freedom of choice to their own judgment as doctors? Under what circumstances should they appeal to the courts? The medical profession faced the dual challenge of discovering new medical techniques acceptable to Witnesses and of increasing their own sensitivity to the trauma experienced by patients who found themselves confronted by treatments that violated their religious scruples. As one article in a medical journal phrased it, "Who would benefit if the patient's corporal malady is cured but the spiritual life with God, as he sees it, is compromised, which leads to a life that is meaningless and perhaps worse than death itself."[28]

A number of physicians responded to the special needs of Jehovah's Witness patients by searching for acceptable blood substitutes and new surgical procedures. At the Texas Heart Institute in the 1960s, Dr. Denton Cooley performed open-heart surgery on Witness patients using non-blood plasma expanders—after promising them not to give transfusions under any circumstances, even at the risk of death. "We became so impressed with the results on the Jehovah's Witnesses," he later reported, "that we started using the procedure on all our heart patients. We've had surprisingly good success and used it in our [heart] transplants as well."[29] By the 1970s, Witness patients were routinely undergoing cardiac and other major surgery without the use of blood transfusions, and at least one study showed that they experienced no greater mortality and morbidity for having done so.[30] Relatively few physicians, however, were willing to abandon the use of blood in surgery, believing that no substitute or volume expander could match the benefits of blood.

In response to the adverse publicity generated by their position on blood, which came at a time when hostility appeared to be declining, Witnesses during the 1960s began waging a campaign designed to dispel prejudices and explain their stand. Two publications, *Blood, Medicine and the Law of God* (1961) and *Jehovah's Witnesses and the Question of Blood* (1977), were distributed not only to the faithful, but to doctors and hospitals. These booklets cited the scriptural grounds for opposing transfusions and sought to demonstrate that the procedure was medically dangerous. Even some physicians, the Witnesses noted, were beginning to question the indiscriminate use of blood.[31] Witness doctors pointed out that there were alternative medical procedures acceptable to Watchtower members. These included building up a patient's blood before and after surgery with amino acids and oral or intravenous iron compounds, using non-blood fluids, and employing electrocautery hypotensive anesthesia, or hypothermia.[32]

After World War II more and more doctors encountered Witnesses as patients, but few of them knew much about the special needs of these people. To improve communication with the medical profession, the Governing Body arranged meetings between representatives of the Watch Tower Society and the American Medical Association. As a result, many Witnesses began carrying signed cards bearing the message "No Blood Transfusion!" and indicating that non-blood expanders were acceptable. In cooperation with the American Medical Association, Witnesses designed a form to be presented upon entering a hospital. The 1984 version of this document read:

> I direct that no blood transfusions be administered to me, even though others deem such necessary to preserve my life or health. I will accept non-blood expanders. This is in accord with my rights as a patient and my beliefs as one of Jehovah's Witnesses. I hereby release the doctors and hospital of any liability for damages attributed to my refusal. This document is valid even if I am unconscious, and it is binding upon my heirs or legal representatives.[33]

The pressures on Jehovah's Witnesses anticipating surgery were often enormous. They not only had to find a surgeon willing to operate without blood, but to deal with the realization that violating the ban on blood meant turning one's back on God and facing annihilation at Armageddon. "For the doubtful chance that one might be kept alive for a few more years in this system of things, would it make good sense to turn one's back on God by breaking his law?" asked a Society publication. "If we try to save our life, or soul, by breaking God's law, we will lose it everlastingly."[34]

Not all Witnesses could withstand the demands of so stern a faith, and some have submitted to medical pressure in life-threatening situations. For example, the journal *Anaesthesia* told of a twenty-four-year-old woman who refused blood and blood products following a difficult delivery of twins that produced a posterior cervical tear and considerable bleeding, but who finally agreed to a transfusion after a subsequent episode of fainting and seizures.[35] Such cases would normally come before a local congregational committee for "judicial action." If the erring mother remained unrepentant, she would be disfellowshipped. However, depending on the circumstances surrounding the transfusion and the state of her mind at the time, she might get off with probation, counseling, and surveillance, though the seriousness of her sin would not be minimized.

A survey of the members of a small Denver Kingdom Hall, conducted in the early 1980s, revealed a variety of experiences and attitudes regarding the use of blood in surgery. Among the fifty-nine respondents, seventeen had refused a transfusion, and twenty-seven had either undergone bloodless surgery themselves or had a family member who had done so. Seven, evidently unaware that plasma contained blood, indicated that they would accept plasma, and one approved of autotransfusions. Most members of the congregation felt so strongly about the use of blood in surgery they expressed an intention to sue any physician who resorted to forced transfusions.[36]

Morality, Health, and Lifestyle

Charles Taze Russell seldom addressed health-related issues, but he did warn his Bible students to avoid the use of alcohol and tobacco. Early issues of *The Watch Tower* frequently carried testimonies from recent converts telling of how the Lord had helped them overcome these sinful habits. For example, in 1891 one Witness told of his victory over tobacco:

About a year ago, I asked the Lord in all sincerity and prayer to assist me in quitting the use of tobacco, and promised him in all good faith to use the money formerly spent for it in the advancement of his interests, as I now see it through the light that I have received. I had used tobacco for thirty years and often tried to quit it, but could not resist the strong desire for its use; but since I quit this time, with the help of the Lord, I have lost all desire for it, and only twice, shortly after quitting, have I had the least desire for it.[37]

Although Russell himself was apparently a vegetarian, he did not insist that his followers refrain from eating meat. His most complete instructions concerning diet appeared in the sixth volume of his *Studies in the Scriptures,* where he recommended a balanced diet consisting of all necessary food categories and noted that "where necessary for the sake of economy or for any reason a purely vegetable dietary could be arranged at a very small cost that would nourish the family well, in brain, brawn and vigor." In spite of his own preferences, he assured his followers that the Bible allowed complete freedom in matters of diet.[38] Witness President Joseph F. Rutherford took the same position, declaring in 1939 that all food was "religiously clean." Referring to the Old Testament prohibition against eating the flesh of "unclean" animals, such as pigs, he said "I see no reason why anyone should hold that ham and bacon are unclean."[39]

Although most of Russell's strict moral values remained substantially intact during Rutherford's presidency (1916–1942), a growing laxness toward tobacco and alcohol became apparent. Throughout the 1920s, the Judge expressed grave doubts concerning the efficacy of national prohibition, which he denounced as a "scheme of the Devil," perpetrated by those modern Pharisees, the clergy, who "loudly demand the rigid enforcement of the Prohibition Law against the poor workingman, and yet many of them have their cellars well stocked with the forbidden liquid." Ironically, he himself had apparently developed a drinking problem. One insider complained in the late 1930s that Rutherford had turned the headquarters at Bethel into a Babylon of immorality, notable for its excessive use of liquor and profanity. A sociologist who investigated the movement about that time reported a split between urban and rural Witnesses: Those living in cities tended to consume moderate amount of alcohol, while those in the country demanded total abstinence.[40]

The same scholar also noted an increase in the tolerance of tobacco among Witnesses. Oldtimers who had joined the movement under Russell had begun complaining to Rutherford about the growing use of tobacco by younger members. In response to these protests, the Judge mildly rebuked Witnesses for straying from their original principles. However, he refused to make smoking and chewing tobacco grounds for being disfellowshipped, and he condemned its use not on religious grounds, but because Witnesses "should have something better to do with their time and money."[41]

Upon Rutherford's death in 1942, Nathan Knorr assumed the presidency of the Watchtower Society and sought, as the patriarch of God's family on earth, to impose a standard of morality worthy of those awaiting the millennium. Under his leadership, the emphasis on character building evident during the Russell and Rutherford eras gave way to increased control over even the most intimate details of Witnesses' lives. Values such as personal enjoyment and family life were subordinated to the dictates of the organization as Knorr and his associates built up "a great body of theocratic law." One student of the movement compiled a list of regulations that appeared in *The Watchtower* during the decade 1953–1963. Witnesses, he reported, were forbidden to

> practice gambling, hunt or fish for sport, tell lies among themselves, laugh at dirty jokes, wear mourning clothes for long after the death of a relative, justify themselves, be sterilized, masturbate, become an officer in a union or picket, go out on a date without a chaperone, throw rice at weddings, display affection in public except for momentarily at greetings and partings, become a member of or frequent a nudist colony, participate in prayer led by one not dedicated to Jehovah, give free rein to unbridled passion while having allowed sexual intercourse, use profanity, or do the twist.

Violators faced censure by local judicial committees and, increasingly, the prospect of being disfellowshipped, cut off from all Witness friends and family. During a single year in the 1950s the organization disfellowshipped over 6,500 members.[42]

Because of the nearness of Armageddon and the desire for total commitment to the cause, Watchtower leaders for years discouraged members from marrying. But in 1951 the Governing Body changed its positon and began, with some ambivalence, to approve of marriages among Witnesses. Although Witness writings commonly assigned women a position subordinate to their husbands, Witness women were, according to Barbara Grizzuti Harrison, encouraged "to exercise a degree of autonomy over their own bodies" by such means as giving birth at home, breast-feeding their babies, and using contraceptives. The hierarchy did, however, prohibit artificial insemination by anonymous donors (a form of adultery) and the use of intrauterine devices (which might induce abortions).[43] For years the Society also opposed sterilization, arguing that it violated the natural procreative powers provided by Jehovah and threatened to create marital discord if one of the marriage partners later desired to have a family. In the 1980s, in response to the possibility of successful reversals of sterilization procedures, Witnesses softened their opposition and began treating the issue as a private and personal matter.[44] Abortion—"murder in God's eyes"—was not permitted even when the mother's life was in danger or birth defects seemed likely. Because Witnesses believed that life began at conception, the age of the embryo was never a factor in determining the morality of abortion.[45]

From their earliest days, Witnesses took a rather dim view of human sexuality. "Sexual appetites," warned Pastor Russell, "war against the spirit of the New Creation."[46] Under Knorr the Society stepped up its attack on "unnatural" and "improper" expressions of sex, even condemning too much passion within the marriage relationship and such "perversions" as oral and anal sex. Masturbation, too, was deemed sinful—but forgivable if done during a "state of semi-conscious sleep." Homosexuality, a crime punishable by death in ancient Israel and by disfellowshipping in the Watchtower Society, constituted grounds for permanent exclusion from God's Kingdom.[47]

The Society also devoted increasing attention to drug addiction and the evils of tobacco. After years of discouraging but tolerating the use of tobacco, the Governing Body in 1973 instructed Witnesses to stop smoking within six months or face being disfellowshipped. Tobacco, they argued, defiled both "flesh and spirit," causing disease and damaging morals.[48] Perhaps because of the personal habits of the organization's twentieth-century leaders, the consumption of alcohol escaped such blanket condemnation. The Society spoke out strongly against drunkenness and warned that alcohol should never be used as a "means to escape from the reality of life for boredom," but Watchtower literature insisted that drink was a gift from God to be used in moderation. Those who abused it were encouraged to seek counsel from the elders; if they persisted in their course and showed no signs of repentance, they were disfellowshipped.[49]

Death and Life Eternal

While Witnesses have historically claimed that death entered the world as a consequence of sin, they have also believed that death was not the end that Jehovah envisioned for obedient humans. He designed his universal plan to show that some persons could maintain their integrity and thereby vindicate his name and sovereignty. For Jehovah's Witnesses, death has meant only the termination of conscious existence, not eternal torment. Those who die prior to Armageddon will experience death as a deep sleep, lasting until Jehovah's call to arise from the tomb. A second testing will follow the millennium. At that time Satan and his disciples will be cast into the lake of fire, and death and evil will be vanquished. The righteous will be given eternal life. Thus Witnesses have not viewed death as an event to be feared, but as a door to the New World paradise of Jehovah God.[50]

Witnesses view human life as a precious gift, and they believe that suffering, patiently borne, strengthens character. Thus no matter how difficult a life crisis may be, they reject suicide and active euthanasia, because both violate God's law regarding the sanctity of life, which "may not be taken or surrendered simply because of suffering." They do not, however, object to mercifully letting "the dying process take its due course" or to counseling physicians not to employ "extraordinary and costly measures to keep the patient alive."[51]

The intense faith of Jehovah's Witnesses has called for constant activism, a strict moral code, social ostracism, group conformity, and, in times of illness, the rejection of some lifesaving therapies. Yet this authoritarian, theocratic tradition with its conspiratorial world view and its belief in the imminent climax of history has also provided millions with a sense of security and well-being. The proximity of Armageddon (during which Witnesses will be given refuge) and the prospect of a restored world have enabled many a believer to face illness, pain, and death with serenity. And, as one former Witness has observed, "not even Marxists believe that history is on their side to the extent that the Witnesses of Jehovah do."[52]

Notes

1. Timothy White, *A People for His Name: A History of Jehovah's Witnesses and an Evaluation* (New York, 1968), pp. 41–44.
2. Raymond Franz, *Crisis of Conscience* (Atlanta, 1983), p. 31. See also Joseph F. Zygmunt, "Jehovah's Witnesses: A Study of Symbolic and Structural Elements in the Development and Institutionalization of a Sectarian Movement," Ph.D. dissertation, University of Chicago, 1967, 3 vols., 1:8; and Jerry Bergman, *Jehovah's Witnesses and Kindred Groups: A Historical Compendium and Bibliography* (New York, 1984).
3. Watchtower Bible and Tract Society, *Jehovah's Witnesses and the Question of Blood* (Brooklyn, NY, 1977), p. 19.
4. Charles Taze Russell, *Studies in the Scriptures*, vol. 1: *The Plan of the Ages* (Brooklyn, NY, 1924), p. 206; Russell, *Our Most Holy Faith* (East Rutherford, NJ, 1950), p. 521.
5. "Faith Healing: Does It Really Work?" *Watchtower* 102 (September 1, 1981):3–4. See also M. James Penton, *Apocalypse Delayed: The Story of Jehovah's Witnesses* (Toronto, 1985), pp. 289–290.
6. *Jehovah's Witnesses and the Question of Blood*, p. 27; Herbert Hewitt Stroup, *The Jehovah's Witnesses* (New York, 1945), pp. 106–107.
7. "Aid to the Mentally Ill," *Watchtower* 87 (August 1, 1966):479; Barbara Grizzuti Harrison, *Visions of Glory: A History and a Memory of Jehovah's*

Witnesses (New York, 1978), p. 248; Penton, *Apocalypse Delayed*, pp. 289–290.

8. Quoted in Stroup, p. 110.

9. John Spencer, "The Mental Health of Jehovah's Witnesses," *British Journal of Psychiatry* 126 (1975):556–559. Penton has questioned the validity of such studies; see *Apocalypse Delayed*, pp. 289–292. See also M.J. Pescor, "A Study of Selective Service Law Violators," *American Journal of Psychiatry* 105 (1949):648; Havor Montague, "The Pessimistic Sect's Influence on the Mental Health of Its Members: The Case of Jehovah's Witnesses," *Social Compass* 24 (1977):135–146.

10. Russell, *Our Most Holy Faith*, p. 509. See Alan Rogerson, *Millions Now Living Will Never Die* (London, 1969), pp. 63–66; William J. Whalen, *Armageddon Around the Corner* (New York, 1962), p. 55; "A Faithful Witness," *Consolation* 23 (No. 584):17.

11. Joseph F. Rutherford, *The Harp of God* (Brooklyn, NY, 1921), pp. 349–350.

12. "How Jehovah Prospers His Work," *Watchtower* 82 (May 1, 1961): 278; "Keep the Poor in Mind," ibid. 97 (April 1, 1976):200–202; *1983 Yearbook of Jehovah's Witnesses* (Brooklyn, NY, 1982). pp. 8, 31.

13. Quoted in Stroup, p. 121; see also ibid., p. 105.

14. *Watch Tower* 34 (July 1, 1913):5268; ibid. 36 (May 15, 1915):5689; William H. Cumberland, "A History of Jehovah's Witnesses," Ph.D. dissertation, University of Iowa, 1958, p. 63; Edmond C. Gruss, *Apostles of Denial: An Examination and Expose of the History, Doctrines and Claims of the Jehovah's Witnesses* (Nutley, NJ, 1970), pp. 45–46; Penton, *Apocalyspse Delayed*, pp. 153–154.

15. Quoted in White, *A People for His Name*, p. 391.

16. A.H. Macmillan, *Faith on the March* (New York, 1957), pp. 187–189; William and Joan Cetnar, "An Inside View of the Watchtower Society," in *We Left Jehovah's Witnesses: Personal Testimonies*, ed. Edmond C. Gruss (Grand Rapids, MI, 1975), pp. 64–66.

17. See, e.g., "Pasteur the Fake," *The Golden Age*, Sept. 25, 1936, p. 814. See also White, *A People for His Name*, p. 173; M. James Penton, *Jehovah's Witnesses in Canada* (Toronto, 1976), p. 230; Jerry Bergman, "Jehovah's Witnesses and Blood Transfusions," *Journal of Pastoral Practice* 4 (1980):83–85.

18. Joseph F. Rutherford, *Creation* (Brooklyn, NY, 1927), pp. 112, 164; *1975 Yearbook of Jehovah's Witnesses* (Brooklyn, NY, 1974), p. 222; "Immovable for the Right Worship," *Watchtower* 66 (July 1, 1945):195–204; Bergman, "Jehovah's Witnesses and Blood Transfusions," p. 80. The title of *The Watch Tower* was changed to *The Watchtower* in 1939.

19. "Immovable for the Right Worship," pp. 195–204; White, *A People for His Name*, p. 392.

20. Watchtower Bible and Tract Society, *Blood, Medicine and the Law of God* (1961), pp. 3–15; *Jehovah's Witnesses and the Question of Blood*, pp. 3–24.

21. "Children: Do They Belong to Parents or to the State?" *Awake!* 32 (May 22, 1951):5. See also Bergman, "Jehovah's Witnesses and Blood Transfusions," pp. 82–83.

22. George I. Thomas and others, "Some Issues Involved with Major Surgery on Jehovah's Witnesses," *American Surgeon* 34 (1968):542. See also Mostaga I. Bonakdar and others, "Major Gynecologic and Obstetric

Surgery in Jehovah's Witnesses," *Obstetrics and Gynecology* 60 (1982):590; "Children," p. 5.

23. "Children," pp. 3–8.

24. J. Lowell Dixon and M. Gene Smalley, "Jehovah's Witnesses: The Surgical/Ethical Challenge," *Journal of the American Medical Association* 246 (1981):2471; "Questions from Readers," *Watchtower* 99 (June 15, 1978):29; White, *A People for His Name,* pp. 395–396.

25. "Questions from Readers," *Watchtower* 79 (September 15, 1958):575; "Questions from Readers," ibid. 82 (January 15, 1961):63–64; *Jehovah's Witnesses and the Question of Blood,* pp. 18–22.

26. "Questions from Readers," *Watchtower* 95 (June 1, 1974):351; Penton, *Apocalypse Delayed,* pp. 202–206.

27. "Questions from Readers," *Watchtower* 88 (November 15, 1967):702–704; "Questions from Readers," ibid. 99 (June 15, 1978); "Questions from Readers," ibid. 101 (March 15, 1980):31; Penton, *Apocalypse Delayed,* pp. 112–114.

28. Morris Weinberger and others, "The Development of Physician Norms in the United States: The Treatment of Jehovah's Witness Patients," *Social Science and Medicine* 16 (1982):1719–1723; Bernard Gardner and others, "Major Surgery in Jehovah's Witnesses," *New York State Journal of Medicine* 76 (1976):765–766; Dixon and Smalley, "Jehovah's Witnesses," p. 2472, who quote from Gardner and others.

29. Quoted in *Jehovah's Witnesses and the Question of Blood,* p. 56.

30. Bonakdar and others, "Major Gynecologic and Obstetric Surgery on Jehovah's Witnesses," p. 587.

31. *Jehovah's Witnesses and the Question of Blood,* 1977, pp. 49–54; Penton, *Jehovah's Witnesses in Canada,* p. 235; Bergman, "Jehovah's Witnesses and Blood Transfusions," p. 83.

32. Dixon and Smalley, "Jehovah's Witnesses," p. 2471.

33. "Your Life, Your Integrity and the Card," *Watchtower* 105 (December 1, 1984):25–26. See also *Jehovah's Witnesses and the Question of Blood,* pp. 29–30; Weinberger and others, "Development of Physician Norms," p. 1723; "Medical Alert for Witnesses," *Journal of the American Medical Association* 245 (1982):19; and George I. Thomas and others, "Some Issues Involved with Major Surgery on Jehovah's Witnesses," *American Surgeon* 34 (1968):543.

34. Watchtower Bible and Tract Society, *The Truth that Leads to Eternal Life* (New York, 1968), pp. 168–169.

35. Michael Hetreed, "Large Volume Blood Loss Replaced with Plasma Expanders," *Anaesthesia* 35 (1980):76–77.

36. Larry J. Findley and Paul M. Redstone, "Blood Transfusion in Adult Jehovah's Witnesses: A Case Study of One Congregation," *Archives of Internal Medicine* 142 (1982):606–607.

37. Quoted in Stroup, *Jehovah's Witnesses,* p. 106.

38. James A. Beckford, *The Trumpet of Prophecy* (New York, 1975), p. 17; Charles Taze Russell, *Studies in the Scriptures,* vol. 6: *The New Creation* (Brooklyn, NY, 1924), p. 561.

39. Stroup, *Jehovah's Witnesses,* p. 108.

40. Joseph F. Rutherford, *Deliverance* (Brooklyn, NY, 1926), p. 139; Rutherford, *Light* (Brooklyn, NY, 1930), pp. 26, 75–76. On Rutherford's drinking, see, e.g., Gruss, *Apostles of Denial,* pp. 290–299; and Penton, *Apocalypse Delayed,* p. 225.

41. Stroup, *Jehovah's Witnesses,* p. 106. See also "Tobacco Shortens Life," *Consolation* 22 (June 11, 1941):25–27.
42. White, *A People for His Name,* pp. 385–386.
43. Stroup, *Jehovah's Witnesses,* pp. 113–114; Harrison, *Visions of Glory,* pp. 73–78, quotation on p. 86; Penton, *Apocalypse Delayed,* pp. 261–270. Regarding IUDs, see "Questions from Readers," *Watchtower* 100 (May 15, 1979):30–31.
44. "Questions from Readers," *Watchtower* 80 (1 July 1959):415–416; "Questions from Readers," ibid. 106 (1 May 1985):31. See also Penton, *Apocalypse Delayed,* pp. 202–203.
45. Watchtower Bible and Tract Society, *True Peace and Security* (New York, 1973), pp. 56–57; Watchtower Bible and Tract Society, *You Can Live in Paradise on Earth* (New York, 1982), p. 132; "Is Abortion the Answer?" *Awake!* 56 (August 22, 1975):3–6.
46. Quoted in Harrison, *Visions of Glory,* p. 73.
47. "Where Does Your Church Stand on Homosexuality?" *Watchtower* 94 (June 15, 1973):355–356; "Try to Be Like Him," ibid. 97 (January 1, 1976):13; "Maintaining God's View of Sex," ibid. 104 (June 1, 1983):24–25; Harrison, *Visions of Glory,* pp. 78–79; White, *A People for His Name,* pp. 385–386; Penton, *Apocalypse Delayed,* pp. 111–112.
48. Penton, *Jehovah's Witnesses in Canada,* p. 28; "Keeping God's Congregation Clean," *Watchtower* 94 (June 1, 1973):336–343.
49. Watchtower Bible and Tract Society, *Your Youth* (New York, 1976), pp. 103–104; "Drinking: Do You Share the Bible's View," *Watchtower* 104 (April 15, 1983):25–27; "Drinking Problems: What Can the Elders Do?" ibid. 104 (May 1, 1983):25–27.
50. "How Long Would You Like to Live?" *Awake!* 38 (April 8, 1957):5–8.
51. "Euthanasia and God's Law," *Watchtower* 82 (February 15, 1961):116–118; "Hope Safeguards the Mind," ibid. 82 (May 1, 1961):259–260; "Taking Delight in Suffering," ibid. 93 (March 15, 1972):174–179.
52. Penton, *Jehovah's Witnesses in Canada,* p. 17.

CHAPTER 18

The Evangelical-

Fundamentalist

Tradition

GARY B. FERNGREN

Evangelicalism in its broadest sense represents that movement within Protestantism that has traditionally emphasized the necessity of personal conversion for salvation. The movement had its origins in the Evangelical Revival in England and America in the eighteenth century, which was in turn influenced by continental pietism and its emphasis on personal holiness and good works in the Christian life. It was through his contact with the pietistic Moravians that John Wesley (1703–1791) experienced an evangelical conversion. The preaching of Wesley and George White-field (1714–1770) led to the Evangelical Revival, which was carried to North America by the preaching of Whitefield. A series of revivals in the American colonies between about 1725 and 1760 (the First Great Awakening) was responsible for a widespread evangelical spirit. In England, evangelicalism spread rapidly through the growth of Methodism and the rise of an evangelical party in the Church of England that was later centered in the Clapham Sect. In 1846, evangelicals representing a wide variety of denominations organized the Evangelical Alliance, which was long active in promoting evangelical principles. Later revivals in America produced the Second Great Awakening (from about 1787 to 1825), which led to a resurgence of evangelicalism. The spread of the revivals to the frontier resulted in the rapid growth of evangelical churches. By mid-century, evangelicalism was dominant in most major Protestant denominations. The influence of revivalism remained strong in evangelicalism, notably in the preaching of such prominent figures as Charles G. Finney (1792–1875), Dwight L. Moody (1837–1899), and William ("Billy") Sunday (1862–1935).

In the last third of the nineteenth century, evangelical orthodoxy was challenged by new intellectual currents from Europe, particularly by the theory of evolution, biblical criticism, and theological liberalism. As the new ideas took root in colleges and seminaries, conservative evangelicals resisted them by sporadic counterattacks that included heresy trials and attempts to remove liberals from positions of denominational leadership. By World War I, however, the new thinking had become dominant in many influential colleges and seminaries. Strong opposition to modernism (as theological liberalism came to be called) culminated in the fundamentalist–modernist controversy of the 1920s. The term *fundamentalism* (coined in 1920) was widely used to describe the beliefs of those who subscribed to the basic tenets of evangelical orthodoxy as they were defined in *The Fundamentals,* a series of twelve volumes published between 1910 and 1915. Fundamentalists were largely unsuccessful in stopping the advance of modernism in the large denominations, most of which became theologically inclusive. While many evangelicals remained within the older denominations, others withdrew into smaller, separatist, denominations and independent churches and founded their own seminaries and Bible colleges, as well as journals and mission agencies.

As a result of the theological struggles of the 1920s, some fundamentalists adopted a militant, schismatic, and anti-intellectual stance that was not generally a part of the older evangelicalism. The fundamentalist movement as a whole was widely regarded as reactionary, particularly after the adverse national publicity given to it during the Scopes trial in 1925. The victory of the liberals and the withdrawal of evangelicals from the mainstream of American religious life greatly lessened the visibility and influence of the latter group. But while fundamentalism seemed to have retreated in the 1920s into a theological and cultural backwater and enjoyed little respectability, the number of its adherents, both within and outside the major Protestant denominations, was large.

Evangelicalism turned in a new direction in the 1950s as a number of articulate spokesmen, who styled themselves "neo-evangelicals" (for example, Harold Ockenga and Carl F.H. Henry), sought to reverse the negativism and intellectual and cultural parochialism that they believed characterized much of fundamentalism. The evangelistic crusades of Billy Graham (b. 1918) attracted national attention, and with the founding of the journal *Christianity Today* in 1956, evangelicals acquired an influential voice. In the 1970s, evangelicalism displayed an aggresive, self-confident spirit and began to make itself felt as a national force socially and politically. As evangelicals rapidly accommodated themselves to modern American culture, the movement once more sought to enter the mainstream of religious life.

While evangelicalism is less monolithic in the 1980s than at any time since the 1920s, basic evangelical beliefs have not changed in a century or more. The basis of evangelical theology is a belief in the full inspiration and complete infallibility of the Bible. Most evangelicals would include belief in the following as essentials of an evangelical faith: the deity of Jesus Christ (his virgin birth, sinless perfection, resurrection, and second coming); the total depravity of the human race and each individual's need of a Savior; Jesus' death on the cross as a substitutionary atonement for sin; the necessity of salvation by grace through faith alone; eternal life in heaven for the saved and in hell for the unsaved.

Although most evangelicals share a common core of theological beliefs, the movement is a heterogeneous one that reflects differences of style and emphasis. Its major branches are fundamentalism and mainstream evangelicalism.[1] Fundamentalism, which represents the right wing of evangelicalism, has been greatly influenced in its theology by dispensationalism, a system of literal interpretation of the Bible that places much emphasis on Christ's imminent return and is generally pessimistic about reforming society apart from personal conversion.[2] Fundamentalism advocates separation, both ecclesiastically (from any form of modernism) and personally (from "worldly" practices). It tends to be militant and anti-pentecostal (in its opposition to speaking in tongues and excessive emphasis on healing). Jerry Falwell, while not reflecting all its traditional distinctives, is a leading representative of this movement. The center of the evangelical movement may be called mainstream evangelicalism.[3] It has been deeply influenced by the neo-evangelicals of the 1950s, who sought a position more in line with the older evangelicalism. They encouraged a revival of evangelical scholarship, displayed an openness to modern culture, and sought to revive an evangelical social consciousness. They tended to be more irenic and self-critical and to encourage a greater degree of evangelical cooperation than fundamentalists generally. These emphases have been absorbed into mainstream evangelicalism and have helped to shape its present identity.

Although the evangelical–fundamentalist tradition is often regarded as a unified phenomenon, it is today a diversified movement with many disparate elements. In this essay the tradition (particularly in the twentieth century) is described in a narrow and specific rather than a broad and inclusive sense, as referring to those who form a consciously evangelical movement that is noncharismatic and largely interdenominational in its outlook.[4] Although evangelical churches and individuals are found in most major and minor American denominations, the energies of the movement have been channelled into an extensive network of nondenominational institutions and organizations that have historically provided (as they provide today) its greatest influence. These include colleges (such as Wheaton, Gordon, and Biola); Bible schools (such as Moody); seminaries (such as Dallas, Fuller, Trinity, and Gordon-Conwell); periodicals (such as *Christianity Today, Moody Monthly,* and *Eternity*); parachurch organizations (such as Inter-Varsity Christian Fellowship, Campus Crusade, Young Life, Youth for Christ, and Navigators); mission agencies (such as Wycliffe Bible Translators); and publishing houses (such as Baker, Zondervan, and Eerdmans). According to a recent study, the greatest percentage of those who consider themselves evangelicals live in the South, but evangelicals are distributed in other sections of the country, with the exception of New England, relatively equally. They tend to be heavily represented in rural areas and small towns.[5]

The evangelical tradition has tended until quite recently to view personal well-being almost exclusively in spiritual terms. In reply to the query "What constitutes well-being?" most evangelicals would instinctively have agreed that the well-being of humans in every aspect of their personalities is dependent on their enjoying communion and fellowship with God. The historic stress of evangelicalism on the total depravity of human beings and their need of a Savior has led perhaps inevitably to this perspective. The essence of evangelical religion has traditionally been its emphasis on the necessity of a radical conversion that marks a sharp break from a previous life of sin and a reordering of one's post-conversion life in conformity with biblical standards. Evangelicals have regarded conversion and sanctification as the twin pillars upon which the Christian life is built, as even a cursory perusal of the devotional literature produced by evangelical writers of the past will reveal. Typical is G.W.E. Russell, who wrote of his Victorian upbringing:

> My home was intensely Evangelical and I lived from my earliest days in an atmosphere where the salvation of the individual soul was the supreme and constant concern of life. . . . May my lot be with those evangelical saints from whom I first learned that, in the supreme work of salvation, no human being and no created thing can interfere between the soul and the Creator. Happy is the man whose religious life has been built on the impregnable rock of that belief.[6]

Health and Healing

It is safe to say that concerns of health and healing have not been central to the evangelical–fundamentalist tradition, although they have on occasion been prominent issues in theology or practice. One looks in vain, for example, in *The Fundamentals* for any mention of the subject. In their concern for the defense of Protestant orthodoxy, fundamentalists were too busy fighting other battles to devote much attention to health-related matters. The larger evangelical tradition historically has either reflected the emphases of Protestantism in general or else accommodated itself to the prevailing views of contemporary culture. One cannot, moreover, easily delineate fundamentalist from mainstream evangelical attitudes to health and healing. Both share a common set of core beliefs, but exhibit considerable variation regarding those matters (like healing) not regarded as essential. Evangelicalism and fundamentalism have always been democratic movements. As a result, their theology has usually been popular rather than academic. (*The Fundamentals* and the widely used *Scofield Reference Bible* are good examples.) The Protestant doctrine of the priesthood of the believer has produced much diversity of belief in secondary and tertiary matters. The encouragement of individual Bible study, the predominance of congregational polity, and the lack of concern for (or distrust of) ecclesiastical authority and tradition have contributed to this diversity. Perhaps the public prominence that the leaders of evangelicalism and fundamentalism have enjoyed both within and outside these movements has tended to obscure the pluralism that has always existed in them. One can speak of common themes and underlying assumptions, but it is difficult to make neat distinctions between the two groups.

Traditionally, evangelical attitudes toward health have been ambivalent. At the root of these attitudes is the evangelical emphasis on sanctification, the process by which the Christian life is inwardly transformed in the direction of holiness and godly living. On the one hand, evangelical piety has emphasized that the body is the temple of the Holy Spirit and therefore is to be kept from those habits and vices that would prevent it from glorifying God. On the other hand, evangelicals have usually considered the body of secondary importance in the Christian life, and they have shown little desire (perhaps out of a Protestant aversion to monastic practices) to mortify the body for the sake of the soul, encouraging rather an asceticism of the mind and will.[7] Evangelicals have not ordinarily practiced fasting as a spiritual discipline and vegetarianism has never been a feature of evangelicalism.[8] Warnings against gluttony were (and still are) notable chiefly for their absence.

Two historical influences, however, have shaped evangelical attitudes toward health and its maintenance. The first is the idea of separation from the world, introduced into evangelicalism from pietism through Methodism. Evangelicals sought to promote sanctification by proscribing the use of such addictive substances as tobacco and alcohol. Because such proscription was a feature of Wesleyan practice and later of the Finney revivals and their successors, it became an integral part of the evangelical ethic. Evangelicals gave widespread support to the temperance movement in the nineteenth century, though they were divided on the question of whether temperance called for total abstinence from alcoholic beverages.[9] The influence of the temperance movement declined dramatically in this century after the repeal of the Eighteenth Amendment in 1932, but the evangelical ethic that gave rise to it remains. There has never existed a uniform belief among evangelicals that the use of either tobacco or alcoholic beverages is wrong. Rather, disapproval of them has generally varied according to regional, ethnic, and denominational lines. Nevertheless, their use is still regarded with disfavor among large segments of the evangelical community, particularly among those of Wesleyan or Baptist heritage (but less among those of Presbyterian or Reformed backgrounds). For the former, temperance has become virtually synonymous with total abstinence, which they defended partly on the ground that the Christian's body is the temple of the Holy Spirit, and partly because certain practices were deemed "worldly" owing to their frequent association with the evils that were thought to accompany them. The same arguments have been applied even more strongly to the use of addictive drugs by evangelicals, who have argued that the only acceptable Christian attitude toward them is one not merely of total avoidance, but of the strongest possible condemnation.[10] While most fundamentalists remain strong in their requirement of total abstinence from alcohol, in the 1970s some mainstream evangelicals quietly dropped their insistence that total abstinence is the only consistent evangelical stance. This softening attitude is probably to be explained in part by the accommodation of many evangelicals to modern American culture and the ensuing loss of some traditional distinctives, and in part by the perceived lack of direct biblical support for total abstinence.[11]

A second historical influence that has shaped evangelical thinking about health is the attitude toward faith healing that grew out of the debate over the subject in evangelical circles in the late nineteenth century. No issue related to illness and health has occasioned more discussion in evangelical churches than the matter of faith healing. There was in American Protestantism generally a dramatic surge of interest in religious healing in the nineteenth century. Among those who sought to reclaim for the church the ministry of healing that they believed played a significant role in apostolic times were several evangelicals, the most notable of whom were A.B. Simpson (1844–1919), founder of the Christian and Missionary Alliance, and A.J. Gordon (1836–1895), a nationally prominent Baptist minister in Boston.[12] Both men came to believe in faith healing after they themselves experienced personal healing. Simpson came under the influence of Dr. Charles Cullis, a former Boston physician who maintained an influential ministry of religious healing, and Simpson's belief in faith healing was partly responsible for his decision to leave the Presbyterian ministry for an independent one.[13]

Both Simpson and Gordon came from a Calvinistic tradition that looked with suspicion on any apparent manifestations of modern miraculous healing. The question of the cessation of miracles was much debated by evangelical theologians in the nineteenth century. The traditional Protestant position, since the time of the Reformation, was that miracles had ceased at the end of the apostolic age, and this long remained the view of most Protestants.[14] As late as 1948 the evangelical theologian E.J. Carnell wrote that "the doctrine that miracles no longer occur is one of those fundamental canons which separate Protestantism from Roman Catholicism."[15] The well-known evangelical scholar J. Gresham Machen reflected the same view in distinguishing between miracles, which have ceased, and healing in answer to prayer, which he described as "a very wonderful work of God, but it is not a miracle."[16] In *The Ministry of Healing* (1882) Gordon, appealing to Christ's commands to his disciples to heal (for example, in such passages as *Mark* 16:15–18) and to Christian belief in the unchanging nature of God and His world, argued that miraculous healing was a privilege of Christians of all ages and therefore ought to enjoy a permanent place in the ministry of the church. Gordon's book balanced an emphasis on God's willingness to heal (he cited many examples from the history of the church) with a recognition that God is sovereign in matters of healing. He warned against making healing an end in itself and deprecated fanaticism in the matter.[17]

In *The Gospel of Healing* (1877), Simpson went much farther than Gordon. He argued that sickness, like sin, was caused by Satan and therefore contrary to God's will; Christ came into the world to save human beings both from sin and from the consequences of sin, which included sickness and pain. In his atonement Christ bore both sin and sickness. Hence the Christian could claim divine healing apart from physicians and medicine because it was always God's will to heal.[18] Later in his ministry, Simpson gave less prominence to faith healing and refused to support the healing campaigns that were held in America by the Australian faith healer John Alexander Dowie, thus earning the enmity of the latter.[19]

While faith healing continued to have some evangelical adherents after the turn of the century, it declined appreciably in reaction to the prominence that it came to have in Pentecostal churches. Evangelicals objected to the insistence of Pentecostals that speaking in tongues was normative Christian experience and they were embarrassed by what they regarded as their fanaticism. Pentecostalism came under increasing attack by evangelicals, including Simpson, whom Pentecostals had initially regarded as an ally. A colleague of Simpson's, asked to investigate the new movement, reported: "I am not able to approve the movement, though I am willing to concede that there is probably something of God in it somewhere."[20] By the 1920s, fundamentalists had largely repudiated Pentecostalism.[21]

Faith healing, as championed by Gordon and Simpson, received much criticism from traditional evangelicals. One of the best of the polemical works written against it was *Counterfeit Miracles,* by the redoubtable Princeton theologian Benjamin B. Warfield (1851–1921). Published in 1918, after the heyday of evangelical faith healing, it did more than any other work to influence subsequent evangelical thinking regarding the theology and practice of faith healing. It represented a powerful restatement of the traditional Protestant view that the age of miracles had passed. Warfield's title indicated the position that he took with regard to contemporary claims of miraculous healing. He argued that the function of miracles was to accompany and validate divine revelation and to authenticate a messenger of God.

> Miracles do not appear on the pages of Scripture vagrantly, here, there and elsewhere indifferently, without assignable reason. They belong to revelation periods, and appear only when God is speaking to His people through accredited messengers declaring His gracious purposes. Their abundant display in the Apostolic Church is the mark of the richness of the Apostolic age in revelation; and when this revelation period closed, the period of miracle-working had passed by also, as a mere matter of course.[22]

God's special revelation of himself was complete and contained in the biblical record; it remained only to be spread throughout the world. Of course, every age witnessed apparent manifestations of miraculous phenomena, but they could not be accepted as genuine because they did not authenticate new revelation. Warfield examined in successive chapters the "apostolic gifts" associated with Edward Irving (1792–1834), Christian Science, and Protestant faith healing. He suggested that faith healings of all types were susceptible to natural rather than supernatural explanations (for example, hysteria, credulity, superstition, or exaggeration) and they cured only functional disorders and not organic diseases. He distinguished, however, between divine healing, which he accepted as a continuing phenomenon, and miraculous healing, which ceased after the apostolic age.

> First of all, as regards the *status quaestionis,* let it be remembered that the question is not: (1) whether God is an answerer of prayer; nor (2) whether in answer to prayer, He heals the sick; nor (3) whether His action in healing the sick is a supernatural act; nor (4) whether the supernaturalness of the act may be so apparent as to demonstrate God's activity in it to all right-thinking minds conversant with the facts. All this we believe. The question

at issue is distinctly whether God has pledged Himself to heal the sick miraculously, on the call of His children—that is to say without means— any means—and apart from means, and above means; and this so ordinarily that Christian people may be encouraged, if not required, to discard all means as either unnecessary or even a mark of lack of faith and sinful distrust, and to depend on God alone for the healing of all their sicknesses. This is the issue, even conservatively stated.[23]

Warfield's work was reprinted several times and was widely used in the fundamentalist polemic against Pentecostalism. Nevertheless, many evangelicals were hesitant to accept his premise that miracles had ceased absolutely. While conceding a special role for miracles in authenticating biblical revelation, they wished to leave open the possibility that God still intervened miraculously, particularly in view of the increasingly anti-supernatural emphasis of theological liberalism. Many had heard missionaries describe cases of miraculous healing, and some had observed what they regarded as miraculous healing in their own lives or in the lives of acquaintances. Yet at the same time they vigorously rejected both the claims of Pentecostal faith healers and the theology that lay behind it. Henry W. Frost, in his book *Miraculous Healing* (1931), took a position not far from Warfield's in his criticism of the theology and claims of faith healers, but he was more positive in his conviction of God's continuing willingness on occasion to heal miraculously.[24] In general, evangelical writers from Warfield to the present have stressed God's sovereignty in choosing to heal. They have believed that divine healing is possible, but the exception rather than the rule.

Evangelicals have sometimes cited *James* 5:13–15, which advises calling the elders of the church to pray for and anoint the sick, as a basis for divine healing. The difficulty has been to understand precisely what the passage teaches. Evangelicals have generally accepted one of three interpretations: that the passage speaks of an apostolic rite that ceased with the passing of the age of miracles;[25] that it speaks of spiritual (not physical) healing;[26] that it offers a supernatural means of recovery to those within the church who are anointed with oil and prayed over.[27] Many evangelical churches have embraced the third view and practiced the rite of anointing the sick. However, evangelical scholars have not agreed on whether the oil was meant to be symbolic of the anointing of the Holy Spirit or representative of a medicinal agent. Gordon believed that it was symbolic of the spiritual unction of the Holy Spirit.[28] Warfield agreed that oil might be symbolic of the power of the Holy Spirit, but favored the view that it referred to a medicinal agent, and that the rite involved asking God effectively to use available medicinal means to restore health.[29] The question was thus whether James advised seeking healing apart from the use of means or through means employed with God's blessing. Because evangelicals have not for the most part rejected the use of medicine, the rite has often been used as a last resort after medicine has failed. But the emphasis has usually been on the effectiveness of corporate prayer rather than on the unction, because evangelicals have rejected any idea of sacramental efficacy.

As the ministry of healing advocated by Gordon and Simpson was taken over and increased by Pentecostals, it declined in evangelical churches. Fundamentalism came to be deeply influenced by dispensationalist theology, which held that speaking in tongues and other miraculous gifts had ceased with the age of the apostles. Fundamentalist ministers often refused to have fellowship with Pentecostals because the latter held views that they regarded as unscriptural and unbalanced. Evangelicals were extremely distrustful of faith healers and usually condemned their ministries. An exception was Kathryn Kuhlman, a charismatic evangelist whose ministry of healing attracted favorable comment from some evangelicals.[30]

One finds little denigration of physicians in evangelical literature; in fact, physicians have generally enjoyed high esteem in evangelical churches.[31] Nor is there evidence that evangelicals or fundamentalists have been more prone than the general population to rely on unorthodox or "fringe" cures (for example, Laetrile to treat cancer). There is little indication of tension between evangelical theology and orthodox medicine. Most evangelicals (including fundamentalists) gratefully accept medicine today, as they have in the past, as God's normal provision for healing. But they believe that he sometimes heals apart from means (when they are lacking or fail) by divine intervention, particularly in direct answer to prayer. One often finds the word *miraculous* used in the writings of twentieth-century evangelicals and fundamentalists (especially in popular works) to describe what nineteenth-century writers would have called "special providences." But whether they call the healing a "miracle" or a "special providence" is perhaps a merely semantic distinction.

In the 1970s there was a resurgence of attempts in some mainstream evangelical circles to restore a healing ministry.[32] The movement reflected charismatic or Pentecostal influences, although somewhat modified to suit evangelical theology. Thus far its influence has been very limited, and it is likely to remain so given the traditional evangelical opposition to an emphasis on faith healing.

Suffering, Mental Health, and Humanitarianism

Closely related to the place of divine healing in the church was the
theological understanding of the meaning of sickness and suffering in
the world, for the Christian in particular. In opposition to the theology
of faith healing, which stressed both the connection between sickness
and individual sin and God's desire always to heal sickness, most
evangelical theologians continued to maintain the traditional view of
orthodox Protestantism that there was a place for sickness and suffering
in the life of the Christian.[33] Their arguments were maintained in a
considerable body of literature directed in the late nineteenth and early
twentieth centuries against the views of men like Simpson and Gordon
and in the twentieth century against Pentecostal faith healers.[34] According to this position, sickness resulted directly from the entrance of
sin into the world and thus originated in the Fall. Death (both physical
and spiritual) and disease were imposed by God on all human beings
as a penalty for Adam's sin. As a result of God's curse on a sinful
world, all persons could expect to experience illness, suffering, sorrow,
guilt, and death. Certain diseases and physical disabilities (for example,
venereal disease and cirrhosis of the liver) were linked directly to sin
or moral failing, but they were attributed to the sufferer's failure to
recognize that disobedience to God's moral law sometimes had physical
consequences.

Against the view that it was not God's will that his children suffer
from pain or disease and that the power manifested in Christ's miracles
was available for healing today, traditional evangelicals argued that in
his miracles of healing, exorcism, and raising from the dead, Jesus
provided merely a foretaste of a fully redeemed world that still awaited
fulfillment. Sin was not yet abolished, nor were disease and death yet
banished. Although redeemed, God's people would never experience
perfection either in the spiritual or physical realm in this world. They
lived in two spheres, experiencing all the manifestations of a fallen
world, yet at the same time undergoing the redemption that was being
accomplished in their own lives and in God's world. They groaned
while awaiting the redemption of the body and the destruction of that
final enemy, death. Hence, they argued, Christians should not expect,
while living in a sinful world, to be free from the curse of sickness
and pain.

In contrast to Simpson and later Pentecostals, who believed that
sickness was always caused by Satan and never came from God, their
evangelical opponents maintained that although Satan was the author
of sin, God had ordained sickness, disease, and death as penalties for
sin. They pointed out that God was pictured in the Old Testament as
smiting individuals and nations with disease. They acknowledged that

Scripture also spoke of Satan's being responsible for both sickness and sin as he waged continual warfare against God's kingdom, but they believed that God permitted Satan to engage in activity only within certain limits, which included the spread of sickness and pain. However, God worked to bring good out of the suffering produced by Satan so that his will (not Satan's) was accomplished. Thus behind Satan's activity was a sovereign God effecting his purposes in the world.

In particular, the traditional theologians emphasized that there was no necessary correlation between godliness and health and that sickness and pain had beneficial spiritual effects in God's economy. The proponents of the theology of faith healing believed not only that sickness resulted from the sinful nature of all human beings, but that it was a consequence of a lack of faith or a particular sin in the life of an individual. Traditional evangelicals replied that both Scripture and experience contradicted such a view; simple observation showed that many godly individuals suffered severe affliction and pain, while the wicked all too frequently enjoyed good health and prosperity. These evangelicals argued that individual suffering was not a matter of merit in which God dispensed punishment as retribution for sin. The English Baptist Charles Spurgeon (1834–1892) asserted that it was well that God did not proportion suffering according to righteousness and wickedness, for he would then encourage an insufferable self-righteousness instead of humble dependence on him.[35] "We deny utterly," wrote the Princeton theologian A.A. Hodge (1823–1886), "that in the case of Christians, whose sins are pardoned for Christ's sake, sickness is any part of the punishment of sin."[36] Christ bore the punishment of sin on the cross; thus evangelicals seldom viewed suffering as a sign of God's anger or displeasure.

What, then, was the purpose of illness and suffering in the life of an evangelical Christian? Evangelical theologians replied that suffering was the fatherly chastisement of God, a mark of his love and concern for one's spiritual well-being, not of his anger. They rejected the idea that illness was an unmixed evil, that it was always or even usually caused by a particular sin, that it indicated God's displeasure or was contrary to his will, and that he willed in every case that sickness be healed. They pointed out that the New Testament promised suffering and tribulation for Christians as a mark of discipleship and that it indicated that God's chastisement was a sign of his favor.

Many of the older writers spoke of the benefits of sickness. "I see in it," wrote the evangelical Anglican bishop J.C. Ryle (1816–1900),

> a useful provision to check the ravages of sin and the devil among men's souls. If man had never sinned I should have been at a loss to discern the benefit of sickness. But since sin is in the world, I can see that sickness is

a good. It is a blessing quite as much as a curse. It is a rough schoolmaster, I grant. But it is a real friend to man's soul.[37]

Among its benefits Ryle mentioned the following: A sickness helped to remind human beings of death; it made them think seriously of God; it softened their hearts; it leveled and humbled them; it tried the nature of their religion.[38] Other writers did not hesitate to affirm that God might will sickness in the life of a Christian in order to draw that person to himself or to bring about patience or an attitude of sympathy with the suffering.[39] And finally, evangelical writers argued that suffering prepared Christians for heaven by purifying them and fitting them to meet their Savior, who suffered for their sins. Evangelicals admitted that much suffering could not be explained by the need for chastisement, but they believed that it was sometimes necessary to admit that God is sovereign, to place one's confidence in him, and to seek grace to live with one's questions unanswered. This was not, of course, a strictly evangelical view; one finds it in many of the older Protestant spiritual writers.[40] Although there have been variations in the traditional evangelical view of suffering, it has remained remarkably unchanged in the evangelical and fundamentalist polemic against faith healing since its classic formulation in the nineteenth century.[41]

Until a century ago, pastors routinely dealt with many problems that are now referred to psychiatrists or psychologists.[42] Evangelical views of mental health and disease reflected the older Protestant explanations, which recognized melancholy as a serious disorder that greatly affected the spiritual life, and older treatments of spiritual experience discussed melancholy at length.[43] The older evangelical literature attributed mental illness essentially to three causes: sin, organic disorder, and demonic possession. Evangelicals believed that much mental and emotional suffering was due to sin or moral failings and that therapy should consist primarily of confession and forgiveness. Before the twentieth century, evangelicals, reflecting contemporary medical views, also attributed some forms of melancholy and insanity to lesions of the brain, chemical imbalance, or temperament.[44] They explained at least some mental illness as being the result of demonic possession. Missionaries added credence to the belief that demon-possession was not limited to biblical times by their reports of demonic activity. A work that had great influence in this regard was John L. Nevius' *Demon Possession and Allied Themes* (1892), which described Nevius' experience as a missionary doctor in China.[45] While in much of Protestantism natural and psychological explanations have replaced belief in demonic etiology of mental illness, fundamentalism has produced in this century an enormous literature that testifies to the continuing belief in demonic activity. For example, many evangelicals and fundamentalists ascribed to satanic activity the revival of interest in the occult in the 1970s.[46] Many evangelical theologians and professionally trained psychologists have accepted possession as an authentic phenomenon.[47] They believed that its symptoms differed from those of mental illness and required specifically spiritual therapy, such as prayer or exorcism.

Evangelicals greeted with distrust or hostility the new disciplines of psychiatry and psychology, which gained influence early in the twentieth century. They believed that psychologists were attempting to provide scientific answers to spiritual problems and that psychological theories of religious behavior were invariably reductionist. Doubtless, too, many evangelicals saw in the new psychology speculation that ran counter both to common sense and to their Baconian preference for facts over theories. Evangelicals used similar criticism against Darwinism and higher criticism of the Bible, which they regarded as unscientific and based on unsupported hypotheses.[48] Sigmund Freud, the founder of modern psychoanalysis, came under special attack because of his perceived obsession with sexuality and hostility to religion.[49] While evangelicals and fundamentalists have generally looked with favor on the medical profession and have not insisted on securing medical care from members of their own religious community, treatment of mental and emotional illness has proven to be an exception to this rule. Evangelicals have tended to avoid psychiatric treatment except by evangelical therapists. They feared that the treatment arising out of the perceived anti-Christian presuppositions of modern psychology would be inimical to an evangelical faith.

In the 1950s a few evangelicals, like Henry Brandt and Clyde Narramore, began to adopt in a guarded way psychological perspectives on emotional and mental problems. A trickle of books by evangelical psychologists turned into a stream in the 1960s and a flood in the 1970s, indicating a radical change in evangelical attitudes to psychology.[50] This new emphasis in evangelicalism, which employed psychological techniques without accepting their secular theoretical basis, avoided a confrontation with traditional doctrines. By wedding psychological techniques to conservative theology, evangelical psychologists seemed to make established doctrines more relevant to everyday life, and this might explain why evangelicals responded so readily to their methods. In adopting a problem-centered view of the Christian life (as many did), evangelicals probably reflected the spirit of their age more than they realized. Great numbers of popular books, aimed at an evangelical–fundmentalist audience, have appeared on the market in recent years, dealing with marriage, sexuality, self-fulfillment, depression, loneliness, worry, and peace of mind. Most in some way have combined biblical teaching with insights taken from modern psychology. Films, radio programs, seminars, and conferences on these subjects have become enormously popular. Over fifteen million people have viewed a film series *(Focus on the Family)* by an evangelical child psychologist, James Dobson, who deals with the problems that face the modern Christian family. In many churches, films and panel discussions on problem-oriented themes have replaced preaching in Sunday evening services. Laymen expect evangelical pastors to spend an increasing amount of their time in personal counseling, and the 1970s have witnessed the rapid growth of Christian counseling centers staffed by evangelical psychologists. Seminaries have developed programs and degrees in Christian counseling. At least two evangelical institutions offer Ph.D.s in psychology: Rosemead Graduate School of Psychology, now affiliated with Biola University; and Fuller Theological Seminary's Graduate School of Psychology. Both programs are approved by the American Psychological Association. Their curricula differ from secular ones in their attempt to integrate biblical and theological components into psychological theory and training.

In spite of the marked change in evangelical attitudes toward psychology, there remains a great diversity of approaches. Some evangelical counselors have attempted to integrate the work of secular psychologists with evangelical theology.[51] Others, like Jay Adams, whose self-styled "nouthetic" approach to counseling is popular with many evangelical pastors, have rejected deterministic psychology and the disease model of mental and emotional illness for a moral and biblical one.[52] Still others have attacked modern psychology as dangerous and unbiblical.[53] While evangelicals and fundamentalists have increasingly sought professional help from pastors and Christian counselors for personal problems, many remain reluctant to consult secular psychiatrists and psychologists. Moreover, evangelicals, who are anxious to stress moral responsibility for individual behavior, have resisted modern attempts to define deviant behavior patterns in secular, nonjudgmental ways. Hence they tend to regard alcoholism, for example, as the result of sin rather than as an illness.

Until the modern "psychological revolution" began to influence evangelicalism in the 1950s, evangelicals typically placed little importance on "healthy-mindedness," as psychologists defined the term. "Fundamentally and finally," wrote Vernon Grounds, a well-known Baptist theologian, representing a traditional evangelical view, "Christianity is not concerned about the individual's emotional welfare any more than it is concerned about his physical condition. Fundamentally and finally, Christianity is concerned about the individual's relationship to God."[54] Evangelicals have traditionally emphasized the need for communion with God over a well-adjusted personality and they have placed a higher priority on spiritual than on psychological well-being.

"It is infinitely better," wrote Grounds, "to be a neurotic saint than a healthyminded sinner."[55]

Evangelicals regarded mental (like physical) illness as a possible means of bringing the sufferer into closer communion with God and therefore as being sometimes spiritually beneficial. They did not consider health—whether mental or physical—as a sign of God's pleasure, or as a goal of the Christian life. Was it then to be valued and nurtured? Yes, like all God's gifts it was to be accepted with thanksgiving. It was not an ultimate good, or an end in itself, but rather a means to an end, to serve and glorify God and to enjoy fellowship with him. Many evangelicals today would agree at least in theory with the traditional view, but so great has been the emphasis in recent years on the ability of the gospel to solve all personal and interpersonal problems and to bring about personal satisfaction that for many evangelicals the traditional view has probably lost much of its force.[56] The importance given by the television evangelist Robert Schuller and others to self-esteem and the Christian's need of a positive self-image have provoked vigorous debate in evangelical circles over whether the new emphasis represents a necessary corrective to the theology of the Protestant Reformation or a serious departure from it.[57] While evangelical opinion has been divided, it appears that many evangelicals (and virtually all fundamentalists) have been uneasy with this novel concern, which suggests that traditional views still retain a strong hold on much of the evangelical constituency.[58]

Another contemporary movement to which evangelicals have only begun to respond is holistic (or wholistic or whole-person) medicine. The attempt to humanize health-care by restoring an ecological and pastoral approach has attracted some attention among evangelical professionals.[59] It has been featured most prominently in the emphasis given to the theme by a few well-known evangelicals such as Ruth Carter Stapleton.[60] While the subject has enjoyed a vogue in the 1980s, some evangelicals have expressed concern over the influence that eastern mysticism and occultic, humanistic, and syncretistic elements have had within the holistic healing movement, and Stapleton herself (who died in 1983) remains controversial among evangelicals.[61]

Evangelicalism has historically had a strong philanthropic and humanitarian component, though it is one that has produced some tension within the movement. Many of the well-known humanitarian efforts of the nineteenth century stemmed from evangelical influences in both Britain and America, and they created a tradition of voluntary charitable activity that is still active today.[62] Evangelicals undertook philanthropic work in part out of obedience to Christ's command to clothe the naked, feed the hungry, and visit the ill and imprisoned, and in part as a preliminary step to evangelism. Perhaps the chief motive for human-

itarian work was evangelistic; but a concern for human souls often led
to a desire to relieve the suffering and poverty of those to whom
evangelicals ministered. This compassion resulted in work on behalf of
prisoners, prostitutes, deprived children, and the poor generally. It also
provided a stimulus to active campaigning for humanitarian legislation,
particularly in England, where evangelicals like William Wilberforce
(1759–1833) and the Earl of Shaftesbury (1801–1885) led movements
for factory and prison reform and the abolition of the slave trade.[63]
But they preferred where possible to deal with social problems by
voluntary charity, believing that aid by the state could never duplicate
the compassion and concern for individuals and their souls that motivated philanthropy.

Medical missions did not begin to play an important role in evangelical missionary activity until the second half of the nineteenth century.[64] One estimate put the number of European medical missionaries
in 1852 at a mere thirteen. Most missionary societies initially feared
that medical work might interfere with the primary goal of missions,
the salvation of souls. This attitude gradually underwent reevaluation
and evangelical societies came to recognize medicine as a desirable and
even necessary part of missionary activity. At first, evangelicals thought
its use to be mainly strategic, a means of gaining a hearing for Christianity in areas where missionary work did not find ready acceptance.
Evangelicals were much concerned, however, that medicine be auxiliary
to evangelism, which they still regarded as paramount. This attitude
gave way by the end of the century to the view that the alleviation
of human suffering was a Christian duty, which reflected the compassion
that Christ demonstrated when he healed the sick. Evangelicals came
to view medical missionary endeavors as a practical manifestation of
the gospel, undertaken in obedience to Christ's commands, and not
merely a means of aiding in the conversion of souls. As a result, by
1900 the number of medical missionaries had risen to 650, many of
whom represented evangelical missionary societies.

Evangelicals and fundamentalists have founded few hospitals or
healing institutions in the twentieth century. There are several reasons
for this. The social concern of nineteenth-century evangelicalism was
a casualty of the fundamentalist–modernist controversy. Evangelicals
abandoned it at least in part because of fundamentalist opposition to
the Social Gospel, advocated by many theological liberals, which evangelicals regarded as emphasizing social action at the expense of proclaiming salvation. Moreover, fundamentalist institutions tended to be
decentralized, with the local congregation serving as the focus of the
movement, a factor that discouraged the establishment of hospitals.
Many evangelicals adopted the "faith missions" approach that relied
on God to supply funds, a method pioneered by George Müller

(1805–1898) in his orphanage in Bristol, England, that was not, however, very practicable in the maintenance of hospitals. The belief among fundamentalists in the imminency of Christ's return perhaps also militated against the founding of permanent philanthropic institutions. The fundamentalists' concern with personal salvation led them rather to involvement in such enterprises as slum missions, where philanthropy was closely tied to evangelism.[65]

Passages and Biomedical Issues

Evangelicals have always thought themselves to be, like John Wesley, *homines unius libri* ("people of one book"). They have held that the Bible is fully inspired and authoritative in all its parts. They have considered it alone sufficient to provide the basis of theology and ethics, and they have deemed no position acceptable that does not have the support of Scripture.[66] Thus their procedure in determining matters of faith and practice has been to assemble the relevant data of Scripture in order to reach a conclusion that reflected the truth of God's Word.[67] They fully recognized that allowances had to be made for temporal or cultural differences, but believed that the biblical record, properly interpreted in the plain sense intended by its writers, could provide not merely guidance, but normative teaching on specific questions.[68] Not only evangelicals but orthodox Christians of most Protestant communions held this view until about a century ago.

We may consider the subject of human sexuality as typical of this approach to ethical questions. Evangelical views on the subject were not markedly different from those of Protestantism generally.[69] Evangelicals assumed that there existed a unity in the biblical ethic in spite of differences of time or culture.[70] As part of the creation ordinances (mandates given by God at creation), God had established marriage as the normal sexual relationship between man and woman. He intended that the relationship be monogamous, and within it that sex provide both companionship and the means of procreation. The Fall affected every aspect of human nature, including the sexual function. But, according to evangelical thought, the entry of sin into the world and the frequent perversion of sex did not abrogate the original intention of God. Sexual practices that fell below God's intended standard (for example, divorce, concubinage, polygamy) he sometimes tolerated, while those that were directly contrary to it (for example, adultery, fornication, homosexuality, lesbianism, bestiality) he explicitly condemned in all periods.[71] Among Protestants generally, the traditional consensus that this pattern represented the teaching of Scripture and therefore the normative pattern of human sexuality has broken down since the 1960s.

Evangelicals, however, have vigorously opposed situational ethics.[72] Moreover, a recent survey found that evangelicals ranked highest among the religious groups surveyed in their opposition to homosexuality, pre- and extra-marital relations, divorce, and abortion.[73] There have been recently a few challenges to the nearly unanimous moral consensus that has characterized evangelicals and fundamentalists.[74] But as long as they view Scripture as normative, it is unlikely that most evangelicals will abandon traditional views.

There have always been a number of issues in ethics (for example, abortion, contraception, euthanasia), however, that did not admit of easy solutions because Scripture did not clearly address them. In cases such as these, evangelicals drew inferences from general principles or passing biblical references. While traditional attitudes usually prevailed, there was not (nor is there now) unanimity of opinion. Evangelicals, like Protestants generally, in the nineteenth century accepted the traditional view that artificial birth-control was immoral. As contraceptive information came to be propagated, evangelicals, thinking that it would encourage vice and immorality, joined in organizing leagues for the suppression of contraceptives. Traditional attitudes, based on the assumption that birth control was contrary to Scripture (*Gn.* 38:8–10 was often cited), persisted well into the twentieth century.[75] Yet as evangelicals examined Scripture closely, the presumed objections to contraception no longer seemed compelling.[76] Undoubtedly the Protestant view, dating from the Reformation, that intercourse exists for conjugal pleasure as well as for procreation made it easier for evangelicals than for Catholics to accept birth control.[77]

The question of abortion presented another morally complex issue. Evangelicals, like most other Protestants, accepted the pre-Reformation view that abortion was homicide. They supported their position by citing passages in Scripture (for example, *Jer.* 1:5, *Ps.* 139:15–16, *Lk.* 1:41) that seemed to teach that the fetus was a personal being endued with an immortal soul. Some evangelicals were willing to permit an abortion when the life of the mother was endangered, on the ground that an actual life is of greater value than a potential one. Once this view was accepted, it was possible to argue that there were other (though perhaps rare) cases in which abortion was justified. Thus evangelicals (and Protestants generally) could take a slightly more lenient position than Roman Catholics, though, in fact, many and perhaps most agreed essentially with the traditional view.[78]

As the demand for more liberal abortion laws grew in the 1960s, evangelicals had to define their view more precisely than before. The modern debate over abortion has tended to harden positions, and many evangelicals and fundamentalists have come to consider all abortions wrong. They have been, in fact, in the forefront of opposition to the liberalization of abortion laws, and on few social issues is there so much unanimity among them. A recent poll showed that 95.3 percent of evangelicals opposed abortion (except when the mother's life was in danger), a higher proportion than even Catholics (of whom 90.5 percent were opposed).[79] A film series, *Whatever Happened to the Human Race?*, which featured two well-known evangelicals, Dr. C. Everett Koop (who later became Surgeon General of the United States) and theologian Francis Schaeffer, speaking against abortion and euthanasia enjoyed much success among evangelical audiences.[80] Behind evangelical opposition to abortion has been the belief that the fetus is a potential human being created in the image of God, not merely expendable tissue.

An examination of evangelical views on contraception and abortion reveals an important point: There has been no single evangelical position regarding a number of ethical issues. One has seldom been able to look to official pronouncements of evangelical bodies for guidance. Evangelical and fundamentalist denominations have been reluctant to issue social pronouncements or to speak for their churches. John Eighmy's observation regarding the Southern Baptists that "their conservative theology, religious individualism, and congregational government continue to restrict progressive expression" could be applied to virtually every evangelical denomination.[81] Evangelicals, moreover, have generally refused to be bound by ecclesiastical tradition or reason. On any issue under discussion they have been accustomed to ask, "What does the Bible teach?" On some issues the rejoinder has been either that Scripture did not speak directly to the matter or that its teaching was not clear. Hence on a number of ethical issues a variety of interpretations has been possible.

Evangelicals (like those of other religious traditions) have only recently begun to think seriously about a number of issues in medical ethics (for example, artificial insemination, genetic engineering, in vitro fertilization).[82] But as a group they have tended not to be particularly concerned with issues raised by modern medical technology. They have been more concerned about matters of personal morality (for example, abortion and homosexuality) and these issues have occupied their attention largely to the exclusion of broader issues that they have regarded as peripheral to traditional evangelical concerns. Moreover, the theological conservatism and biblicism of evangelicals and fundamentalists have given them a reluctance to abandon traditional interpretations of Scripture or conservative positions generally, in spite of their formal refusal to recognize the authority of ecclesiastical tradition.

In the eighteenth and nineteenth centuries, frequent reflection on death was characteristic of evangelical religion. Evangelicals viewed life on earth as a vale of tears through which the Christian passed as a preparation for eternal life. Evangelicals regarded the destiny of the soul as being of supreme importance. In evangelical homes, parents taught their children from a young age to think of eternity and they regularly warned them that there was a hell to be shunned and heaven to be gained.[83] Victorian evangelicals brought their children to the deathbeds of family members in order to impress upon them the frailty of life and the necessity of being prepared to meet death.[84] Among many evangelicals, particularly in America, this concern with death gave way to an expectation that the imminent return of Christ might usher Christians into his presence without death. The change in attitude resulted from the widespread growth of premillennialism in evangelical circles in the last third of the nineteenth century. A large proportion of evangelicals (and later fundamentalists) came to believe that they were living in the last days and that signs pointed to the imminent return of Christ to establish his millennial kingdom. This view, called premillennialism, became one of the most significant doctrines of the fundamentalist movement, and many fundamentalists firmly believed (as many continue to believe) that they would see Christ's return in their lifetime.[85] Since about 1960, premillennialism has declined somewhat in its influence within mainstream evangelicalism, although it still retains a strong influence in fundamentalist circles. Evangelical literature today places less stress on "the Blessed Hope" (Christ's Second Coming) than it did a generation ago. The attention given to the joys of heaven and the terrors of hell has declined as well, probably reflecting a greater interest among evangelicals in this world. Instead, contemporary evangelical magazines regularly feature articles, differing little from those produced within other branches of Christianity, on understanding the process of grief or aiding in the emotional adjustment of both the dying and the bereaved.[86]

In caring for the dying pastorally, evangelicals have above all been concerned that those facing death settle the matter of the state of their souls. John Wesley made it a routine part of his busy ministry to visit prisoners condemned to the gallows in order to give spiritual counsel, and evangelical clergy have frequently undertaken a similar ministry to those facing death in institutions. Evangelicals have taken seriously the biblical dictum that "it is appointed unto men once to die, but after this the judgment"—hence their urgency in pressing the question of salvation on those facing death. Since the spread of theological liberalism in the twentieth century, there has been a marked difference between the pastoral concerns of evangelicals, whose theology centers on the question "Is your soul right with God?"; and the concerns of Christians who espouse a theology of universalism, which holds that all persons will be saved. To those of evangelical conviction, all lesser matters have faded in importance when a soul hung in the balance.

Among evangelicals and fundamentalists, assurance of personal salvation has brought to the dying both comfort for the present and hope for the future. Their belief in God's sovereignty has given them confidence that he controls every aspect of life and death and that nothing happens by chance. In this spirit, the well-known evangelical author Joseph Bayly wrote:

> Shortly after our five-year-old died of leukemia, someone asked me how I'd feel if a cure for leukemia were then discovered. My answer was that I'd be thankful, but it would be irrelevant to the death of my son. God determined to take him to His home at the age of five; the means was incidental.[87]

A firm belief in the existence of heaven and hell rather than a vague idea of a future life has strengthened this confidence. Evangelical piety, reflected in popular gospel songs of the late nineteenth and early twentieth centuries (for example, "Face to Face," "When We All Get to Heaven," "When the Roll Is Called Up Yonder"), has centered on the theme of the glorious future that awaits believers with their Savior in heaven.[88] The promise of the resurrection of the body has encouraged those whose bodies were wracked with pain, while those experiencing grief looked forward to a future in which there would be no sorrow. And the greatest of all hopes has been in a future life in which the last enemy, death, will be vanquished. In the face of death, generations of evangelical Christians have found consolation in these beliefs. Because they have held that God alone ought to control human destiny, they have opposed both suicide and active (but not necessarily passive) euthanasia.[89]

In its approach to death, as in its approach to health, sickness, and healing, evangelicalism in its various manifestations has traditionally shown its primary concern to be with salvation and the Christian life in a personal, individualistic manner. Basic to this outlook has been a vital religious experience, a simple but profound faith that Jesus Christ gives meaning to every aspect of life. This attitude is succinctly expressed in the words of the Heidelberg Catechism of 1563, with which evangelicals and fundamentalists, in spite of many differences of style and emphasis, would probably have given warm assent:

> What is thy only comfort in life and death? That I with a body and soul, both in life and death, am not my own, but belong unto my faithful Saviour Jesus Christ; who, with his precious blood, hath fully satisfied for all my sins, and delivered me from all the power of the devil; and so preserves me that without the will of my heavenly Father, not a hair can fall from my head; yea, that all things must be subservient to my salvation, and

therefore, by his Holy Spirit, he also assures me of eternal life, and makes me sincerely willing and ready, henceforth, to live unto him.[90]

Notes

1. For a discussion of these movements, their characteristics, representatives, institutions, and churches, see Donald G. Bloesch, *The Future of Evangelical Christianity: A Call for Unity Amid Diversity* (Garden City, NY, 1983), pp. 24–35. I have substituted the phrase *mainstream evangelicalism* for Bloesch's *neo-evangelicalism*. Because they lie outside the scope of this chapter, I ignore what Bloesch calls confessionalist evangelicalism, charismatic religion, neo-orthodoxy, and catholic evangelicalism.
2. For an excellent discussion of the formation of fundamentalism, see George M. Marsden, *Fundamentalism and American Culture: The Shaping of Twentieth-Century Evangelicalism, 1870–1925* (New York, 1980). For a criticism of Marsden's definition of evangelicalism, see the review by Timothy L. Smith, "Historical Fundamentalism," *Fides et Historia* 14 (1981):68–72.
3. See George M. Marsden, "From Fundamentalism to Evangelicalism," in *The Evangelicals*, eds. David F. Wells and John D. Woodbridge (Nashville, 1975), pp. 122–142.
4. On the problem of defining evangelicalism, see George Marsden, "The Evangelical Denomination," in *Evangelicalism and Modern America*, ed. George Marsden (Grand Rapids, MI, 1984), pp. vii–xvi. Marsden distinguishes between three different definitions of evangelicalism.
5. See James Davison Hunter, *American Evangelicalism: Conservative Religion and the Quandary of Modernity* (New Brunswick, NJ, 1983), esp. pp. 49–69. Hunter's definition of evangelicalism is broader than that used here.
6. Quoted in Ian C. Bradley, *The Call to Seriousness: The Evangelical Impact on the Victorians* (New York, 1976), p. 193.
7. For an evangelical view of asceticism, see Bernard L. Ramm, *The Right, the Good, and the Happy* (Waco, TX, 1971), pp. 57–59. A similar view is expressed by J.A. Ziesler, *Christian Asceticism* (Grand Rapids, MI, 1973), pp. 99–118.
8. For modern evangelical attempts to introduce fasting as a spiritual discipline, see David R. Smith, *Fasting: A Neglected Discipline* (Fort Washington, PA, 1969); and Richard J. Foster, *Celebration of Discipline: The Path to Spiritual Growth* (San Francisco, 1978), pp. 41–53.
9. On the evangelical influence on the temperance movement in the nineteenth century, see Frank Thistlethwaite, "The Anglo-American World of Humanitarian Endeavor," in *Ante-Bellum Reform*, ed. David Brion Davis (New York, 1967), pp. 75–77. On revivalism and temperance, see Whitney R. Cross, *The Burned-Over District: The Social and Intellectual History of Enthusiastic Religion in Western New York, 1800–1850* (New York, 1965), pp. 211–217.
10. See, e.g., Ramm, *The Right*, pp. 103–109.
11. For evangelical concern about this new attitude, see Jerry G. Dunn (with Bernard Palmer), *What Will You Have to Drink? The New Christian Password* (Beaverlodge, Alberta, 1980).

12. See Donald Dayton, "The Rise of the Evangelical Healing Movement in Nineteenth Century America," *Pneuma* 4 (1982):1–18. On A.J. Gordon, see also Ernest B. Gordon, *Adoniram Judson Gordon: A Biography* (London, n.d.), pp. 333–335, 144–148.
13. See A.W. Tozer, *Wingspread* (Harrisburg, PA, 1943), pp. 75–88.
14. For the early Protestant view, see Keith Thomas, *Religion and the Decline of Magic* (New York, 1971), pp. 124–125. For the nineteenth century, see the comments of A.J. Gordon, *The Ministry of Healing* (Harrisburg, PA, n.d.), p. 1.
15. Quoted in Colin Brown, *Miracles and the Critical Mind* (Grand Rapids, MI, 1984), p. 203.
16. J. Gresham Machen, *The Christian View of Man* (1937, reprinted London, 1965), pp. 111–112.
17. See Gordon, *The Ministry of Healing,* pp. 209–223.
18. A.B. Simpson, *The Gospel of Healing,* rev. ed. (Harrisburg, PA, n.d.), esp. pp. 65–68.
19. See Tozer, *Wingspread,* pp. 134–135.
20. Ibid., pp. 132–133.
21. Marsden, *Fundamentalism,* pp. 93–94.
22. B.B. Warfield, *Counterfeit Miracles* (1918, reprinted London, 1972), pp. 25–26.
23. Ibid., pp. 192–193.
24. Henry W. Frost, *Miraculous Healing* (1931, reprinted Grand Rapids, MI, 1979), esp. pp. 113–125.
25. See R.V.G. Tasker, *The General Epistle of James,* Tyndale New Testament Commentaries (Grand Rapids, MI, 1977), pp. 130–132.
26. This is not a widely held view; but see C.E. Putnam, *Modern Religio-Healing: Man's Theories or God's Word?* (Chicago, 1924), pp. 139–149.
27. See, e.g., Gordon, *Healing,* pp. 31–38; and J. Sidlow Baxter, *The Divine Healing of the Body* (Grand Rapids, MI, 1979), pp. 160–171.
28. Gordon, *Healing,* pp. 31–32.
29. Warfield, *Counterfeit Miracles,* pp. 171–173.
30. See, e.g., Baxter, *The Divine Healing of the Body,* pp. 272–277. The well-known British minister and physician, D. Martyn Lloyd-Jones, is more cautious in his assessment of Kuhlman; see *The Supernatural in Medicine* (London, 1971), pp. 3–4, 21.
31. See, e.g., Frost, *Miraculous Healing,* pp. 75–76, in defense of physicians against their denigration by certain faith healers.
32. See Charles E. Hummel, *Fire in the Fireplace* (Downers Grove, IL, 1978), pp. 207–223; and Hummel, *Healing* (Downers Grove, IL, 1982). For an account of a rediscovery of healing associated with a course offered by Fuller Seminary, see the composite work *Signs & Wonders Today* (Wheaton, IL, 1983).
33. For an example of a theology of faith healing, see, e.g., Simpson, *The Gospel of Healing,* pp. 76–86.
34. Against the evangelical healing movement in the nineteenth century, see, e.g., "Prayer and the Prayer-Cure," in A.A. Hodge, *Popular Lectures on Theological Themes* (Philadelphia, 1887), pp. 94–116, esp. pp. 107ff. Against Pentecostal faith healers, see, e.g., Putnam, *Modern Religio-Healing,* pp. 74–154.
35. "Accidents, not Punishments" (a sermon delivered on September 8, 1861), in C.H. Spurgeon, *Metropolitan Tabernacle Pulpit,* 63 vols. (Lon-

don, 1855–1917), 7:484. On Spurgeon's attitude to healing, see Russell H. Conwell, *Life of Charles Haddon Spurgeon: The World's Great Preacher* (Philadelphia [?], 1892), pp. 172–186.

36. Hodge, "Prayer and the Prayer-Cure," p. 109.
37. "Sickness," in J.C. Ryle, *Practical Religion* (1879, reprinted Cambridge, England, 1969), p. 238.
38. Ibid., pp. 238–241.
39. See, e.g., Edward M. Merrins, "Gifts of Healing," *Bibliotheca Sacra* 66 (1909):408–410.
40. See, e.g., "Advantages of Sickness," in Jeremy Taylor, *The Rule and Exercises of Holy Dying* (1651, reprinted Philadelphia, 1846), pp. 79–92.
41. A popular contemporary restatement of the traditional evangelical view of suffering is found in Joni Eareckson and Steve Estes, *A Step Further* (Grand Rapids, MI 1978), esp. pp. 115–185, which discusses the theology of suffering in the context of Eareckson's experience as a quadriplegic.
42. See Michael MacDonald, "Religion, Social Change, and Psychological Healing in England, 1600–1800," in *The Church and Healing*, ed. W.J. Sheils (Oxford, 1982), pp. 101–125.
43. See, e.g., Archibald Alexander, *Thoughts on Religious Experience* (1844, reprinted Edinburgh, 1967), pp. 32–50. For a modern evangelical discussion, see John White, *The Masks of Melancholy: A Christian Physician Looks at Depression & Suicide* (Downers Grove, IL, 1982). A popular evangelical treatment of the subject, written from a pastoral and biblical perspective, is D. Martyn Lloyd-Jones, *Spiritual Depression: Its Causes and Cure* (Grand Rapids, MI, 1965).
44. On physiological and moral causes of insanity, see Alexander, *Thoughts on Religious Experience*, pp. 48–49.
45. See Frederick S. Leahy, *Satan Cast Out* (Edinburgh, 1975), pp. 124–127. A popular modern work that describes purported demonic activity in Borneo is Robert Peterson, *Roaring Lion* (London, 1968).
46. Leahy, *Satan Cast Out*, pp. 152–159. See also Kurt Koch, *Christian Counseling and the Occult* (Grand Rapids, MI, 1965); and John Warwick Montgomery, *Principalities and Powers* (Minneapolis, 1973).
47. See, e.g., White, *The Masks of Melancholy*, pp. 21–39.
48. On evangelicalism's appeal to common sense and Baconian science, see Marsden, *Fundamentalism and American Culture*, pp. 55–62, 212–221.
49. Typical is Philip E. Hughes, *Christian Ethics in Secular Society* (Grand Rapids, MI, 1983), pp. 81–89, 91.
50. See Hunter, *American Evangelicalism*, pp. 91–99.
51. See, e.g., Gary R. Collins, *The Rebuilding of Psychology: An Integration of Psychology and Christianity* (Wheaton, IL, 1977); and H. Newton Malony, ed., *Wholeness and Holiness: Readings in the Psychology/ Theology of Mental Health* (Grand Rapids, MI, 1983).
52. See Jay E. Adams, *Competent to Counsel* (Phillipsburg, NJ, 1970).
53. See, e.g., Paul C. Vitz, *Psychology as Religion: The Cult of Self-Worship* (Grand Rapids, MI, 1977); and William Kirk Kilpatrick, *Psychological Seduction: The Failure of Modern Psychology* (Nashville, 1983).
54. Vernon Grounds, *Emotional Problems and the Gospel* (Grand Rapids, MI, 1976), pp. 109–110.
55. Ibid., p. 110. Contrast William James' description of "The Religion of Healthy-Mindedness" in *The Varieties of Religious Experience* (1902, reprinted New York, 1929), pp. 77–124.

56. See Hunter, *American Evangelicalism,* pp. 98–99.
57. See Robert H. Schuller, *Self-Esteem: The New Reformation* (Waco, TX, 1982). For an evaluation of Schuller, see "Hard Questions for Robert Schuller about Sin and Self-esteem," *Christianity Today* 28 (August 10, 1984):14–20; and Kenneth Kantzer with Paul W. Fromer, "A Theologian Looks at Schuller," ibid., pp. 22–24.
58. See, e.g., Paul Brownback, *The Danger of Self-Love* (Chicago, 1982); and the strong attack on Schuller's theology by John MacArthur, "Questions for Robert Schuller," *Moody Monthly* 83 (May 1983):6–10.
59. See David E. Allen, Lewis P. Bird, and Robert Herrmann, eds., *Whole-Person Medicine: An International Symposium* (Downers Grove, IL, 1980).
60. See Ruth Carter Stapleton, *The Gift of Inner Healing* (Waco, TX, 1976).
61. See, e.g., the special issue of the *SCP* [Spiritual Counterfeits Project] *Journal* 2 (August 1978) devoted to a critical examination of the holistic health movement. On Ruth Carter Stapleton, see Brooks Alexander, "Holistic Health from the Inside," ibid., pp. 14–15.
62. See Bradley, *The Call to Seriousness,* pp. 119–134.
63. On evangelical social reform, see Earle E. Cairns, *Saints and Society* (Chicago, 1960); Timothy L. Smith, *Revivalism and Social Reform* (New York, 1957); Donald W. Dayton, *Discovering an Evangelical Heritage* (New York, 1976); W. David Lewis, "The Reformer as Conservative: Protestant Counter-Subversion in the Early Republic," in *The Development of an American Culture,* eds. Stanley Coben and Lorman Ratner (Englewood Cliffs, NJ, 1970), pp. 64–91.
64. See C. Peter Williams, "Healing and Evangelism: The Place of Medicine in Later Victorian Protestant Missionary Thinking," in *The Church and Healing,* pp. 271–285; and A.F. Walls, " 'The Heavy Artillery of the Missionary Army': The Domestic Importance of the Nineteenth-Century Medical Missionary," ibid., pp. 287–297.
65. See Timothy P. Weber, *Living in the Shadow of the Second Coming* (New York, 1979), pp. 82–104.
66. See Timothy P. Weber, "The Two-Edged Sword: The Fundamentalist Use of the Bible," in *The Bible in America: Essays in Cultural History,* eds. Nathan O. Hatch and Mark A. Noll (New York, 1982), pp. 101–120.
67. For a typical example of this approach to a particular issue, see John Murray, *Divorce* (Philadelphia, 1961).
68. See George M. Marsden, "Everyone One's Own Interpreter? The Bible, Science, and Authority in Mid-Nineteenth-Century America," in Hatch and Noll, *The Bible in America,* pp. 80–81.
69. See, e.g., Otto A. Piper, *The Biblical View of Sex and Marriage,* rev. ed. (New York, 1960).
70. A good example of this approach is John Murray, *Principles of Conduct: Aspects of Biblical Ethics* (London, 1957), esp. pp. 7–9.
71. Ibid., pp. 45–81. See also Hughes, *Christian Ethics,* pp. 149–181. For an older statement of the traditional evangelical view, see Charles Hodge, *Systematic Theology,* 3 vols. (1872–73, reprinted Grand Rapids, MI, 1977), 3:368–421.
72. See, e.g., Norman L. Geisler, *Ethics: Alternatives and Issues* (Grand Rapids, MI, 1971), pp. 60–77; and Hughes, *Christian Ethics,* pp. 70–79.
73. See Hunter, *American Evangelicalism,* pp. 85–86.

74. See Letha Scanzoni and Virginia Ramey Mollenkott, *Is the Homosexual My Neighbor? Another Christian View* (San Francisco, 1978), which argues for an evangelical acceptance of homosexual behavior. For a restatement of the traditional view, see Richard F. Lovelace, *Homosexuality and the Church* (Old Tappan, NJ, 1978).

75. See Lloyd A. Kalland, "Views and Positions of the Christian Church— An Historical Review," in *Birth Control and the Christian,* eds. Walter O. Spitzer and Carlyle L. Saylor (Wheaton, IL, 1969), pp. 448–454.

76. For a list of European and American churches that have taken a positive stance toward birth control, see ibid., p. 459. A good discussion of the arguments on both sides of the issue is found in Geisler, *Ethics,* pp. 211–218.

77. On the Protestant, and particularly Puritan, emphasis on companionability in marriage, see Roland H. Bainton, *Sex, Love and Marriage: A Christian Survey* (Glasgow, 1958), pp. 99–111; and Lawrence Stone, *The Family, Sex, and Marriage in England, 1500–1800* (New York, 1977), pp. 135–142. Evangelical (and most Protestant) discussions of birth control emphasize the importance of sex as a contributing factor to marital companionship; see, e.g., M.O. Vincent, "Moral Considerations in Contraception," in Spitzer and Saylor, *Birth Control and the Christian,* pp. 247–255; and Geisler, *Ethics,* p. 201. There has recently been a spate of books writen by evangelical and fundamentalist authors on the "recreational" aspect of sex within marriage; see, e.g., Tim and Beverly LaHaye, *The Act of Marriage: The Beauty of Sexual Love* (Grand Rapids, MI, 1976).

78. Most discussions of abortion from an evangelical point of view consider abortion to be justifiable on some grounds; see, e.g., Geisler, *Ethics,* pp. 218–223; Hughes, *Christian Ethics,* p. 179; and "A Protestant Affirmation on the Control of Human Reproduction," in Spitzer and Saylor, *Birth Control and the Christian,* p. xxv.

79. See Hunter, *American Evangelicalism,* p. 85.

80. See Francis A. Schaeffer and C. Everett Koop, *Whatever Happened to the Human Race?* (Old Tappan, NJ, 1979).

81. See John Lee Eighmy, *Churches in Cultural Captivity: A History of the Social Attitudes of Southern Baptists* (Knoxville, TN, 1972), p. 199.

82. On genetic engineering, see Hughes, *Christian Ethics,* pp. 133–147. On artificial insemination, see ibid., pp. 228–230. Sterilization, genetic engineering, and artificial insemination are also discussed in several essays in Spitzer and Saylor, *Birth Control and the Christian.* A number of bioethical issues (e.g., organ transplants, sterilization, artificial insemination) are treated in individual articles in Carl F.H. Henry, ed., *Baker's Dictionary of Christian Ethics* (Grand Rapids, MI, 1973).

83. See Stone, *The Family, Sex and Marriage,* pp. 251–253.

84. See Bradley, *The Call to Seriousness,* pp. 187–188.

85. See Timothy P. Weber, *Living in the Shadow,* pp. 43–64.

86. See, e.g., Joseph Bayly, *The Last Thing We Talk About,* rev. ed. (Grand Rapids, MI, 1973); Bayly, "The Suffering of Children," *Christian Medical Society Journal* 12, 1 (1981):2–7; Haddon W. Robinson, *Grief* (Grand Rapids, MI, 1976); Donald Howard, *Christians Grieve Too* (Edinburgh, 1979).

87. Bayly, *The Last Thing We Talk About,* p. 24.

88. See Bradley, *The Call to Seriousness,* p. 192.

89. On suicide, see Geisler, *Ethics,* pp. 236–240; and Henri Blocher, *Suicide,* trans. Roger Van Dyk (Downers Grove, IL, 1972). On euthanasia, see Geisler, *Ethics,* pp. 231–236; and Hughes, *Christian Ethics,* pp. 125–133.
90. *The Psalter: With Doctrinal Standards, Liturgy, Church Order, and Added Chorale Section,* rev. ed. (Grand Rapids, MI, 1947), p. 1 at the rear of the volume.

CHAPTER 19

The Pentecostal

Tradition

GRANT WACKER

Pentecostalism was born in the United States less than a hundred years ago, but in that brief period it has become one of the most conspicuous religious stirrings of the twentieth century. Although no one knows how large the movement really is, scholars estimate that there are several million adherents in the United States and possibly 100 million worldwide. Over the years more than three hundred Pentecostal denominations have sprung up in this country alone. Most are quite small, yet the two largest, the Assemblies of God and the Church of God in Christ, each claim more than two million domestic followers and additional millions in other parts of the world.

Although historians debate the exact origins of the movement, most agree that it grew from the confluence of distinct traditions within evangelical Protestantism in the late nineteenth century. The result of this confluence was a widespread conviction that the conversion experience ought to be followed by another landmark experience known as baptism of the Holy Spirit. The latter was regarded as the necessary foundation for personal holiness and, more significantly, a prerequisite for the impartation of the gifts of the Holy Spirit described in 1 *Corinthians* 12 and 14. Near the turn of the century, this notion combined with numerous reports of miraculous healing experiences to fuel a powerful expectation that the Lord's return was at hand.

In this context of mounting religious fervor, many believers began to look for an indisputable sign, or proof, that they had received the baptism of the Holy Spirit. In 1901 Charles Fox Parham, an itinerant faith healer living in Topeka, Kansas, came to the conclusion that speaking in "unknown tongues" (technically called glossolalia) was the coveted evidence they were seeking. Five years later a black holiness preacher named William J. Seymour carried Parham's message to Los Angeles, where he ignited the Azusa Street revival and, as it turned out, the modern Pentecostal movement.

All of the major Pentecostal denominations emerged in the next two decades. Between 1907 and 1911 several already-thriving Wesleyan sects in the Southeast joined the movement through the influence of persons who had visited the Azusa Mission. These groups included the predominantly black Church of God in Christ, centered in Mississippi and western Tennessee; the Church of God, based in the southern Appalachians; and the Pentecostal Holiness Church, concentrated in the Carolinas and Georgia. After a slow start the Pentecostal message also caught fire among non-Wesleyan evangelicals in the lower Midwest and California. The Assemblies of God, organized in 1914, grew most luxuriantly in Missouri, Oklahoma, and Texas. A doctrinal dispute in the Assemblies of God over the nature of the Trinity prompted the formation of numerous unitarian or "Oneness" groups throughout the Midwest. The largest of these now call themselves the United Pentecostal Church, International, and the Pentecostal Assemblies of the World. In the 1920s Aimee Semple McPherson also broke from the Assemblies of God to establish her own denomination in Los Angeles, the International Church of the Foursquare Gospel.

In the early days Pentecostal churches often named themselves Full Gospel Tabernacles, which meant that they preached the "full" gospel of personal conversion, baptism of the Holy Spirit with the evidence of unknown tongues, divine healing, and the promise of the Lord's imminent return. Contemporary Pentecostals still share these beliefs, but in other ways they have become extremely diverse. Run-down urban missions and Appalachian revival tabernacles contrast with opulent suburban churches and billion-dollar television ministries dominated by Pentecostal celebrities. Moreover, since the 1950s, speaking in tongues has penetrated the Roman Catholic Church and other Protestant denominations, forming a Pentecostal subtradition widely known as the charismatic renewal. Even so, the movement as a whole continues to be bonded by a common conviction that the gospel is still true—not the old-fashioned gospel of the nineteenth century, but the miraculous, wonder-working gospel of the first century.

One could argue that over the years the doctrine and practice of divine healing, along with the doctrine and practice of speaking in tongues, has been the enduring backbone of the Pentecostal tradition. Only a small minority of Pentecostals have ever claimed a miraculous healing themselves, but virtually all would have insisted that God readily breaks into history to heal any believer whose faith is sufficient. Therefore, a historical survey of the Pentecostal view of healing is not so much a description of one aspect of a larger tradition as a portrayal of the social and cultural history of Pentecostalism itself.[1]

Nineteenth-Century Background

Among the legacies of eighteenth-century German pietism was a conviction that New Testament miracles did not cease at the end of the apostolic age but continued to be available for the comfort and edification of the church in all ages. Thus in 1852 a pietist pastor named Johann Christoph Blumhardt established a retreat near Württemberg where the sick were given medical treatment and, more significantly, anointed and prayed for in accord with *James* 5:14: "Is any sick among you? Let . . . the elders of the church . . . pray for him, anointing him with oil." Blumhardt believed that original and personal sin was the principal cause of illness; hence repentance for sin was the basis upon which a believer might claim healing for the body as well as the soul. But sin was not the whole story. Because demons sometimes tormented the bodies of the faithful, exorcism ought to be a regular feature of the healing ministry of the church. Although Blumhardt was careful to say that God might, in his sovereign will, withhold healing, Otto Stockmayer, a Reformed pastor in Switzerland, soon pushed Blumhardt's teaching to its logical conclusion. Drawing upon *Isaiah* 53:5 ("He was wounded for our transgressions . . . and with his stripes we are healed"), and Jesus's repetition of Isaiah's words in *Matthew* 8:16–17, Stockmayer argued that the promise of healing was an integral part of the atonement. Because the ransom Jesus paid with his body secured the healing of our bodies as well as the salvation of our souls, Christians were obliged to seek and expect physical healing just as they were obliged to seek and expect spiritual salvation.[2]

In a closely related development in England, a Plymouth Brethren preacher named George Müller established an orphanage in Bristol in 1835 on the "faith work" principle. The assumption underlying Müller's enterprise was that all necessary material needs would be met if they were committed to God with a "prayer of faith." Although Müller was not a prominent advocate of divine healing, his insistence that Christians should *expect* God to respond favorably to a prayer of faith strongly influenced the healing (and later, healing and prosperity) movements in the United States.[3]

This cluster of beliefs about the relationship among sin, atonement, healing, and the automatic efficacy of the prayer of faith swept across a large part of evangelical Protestantism in the 1870s and 1880s. Not surprisingly, it first took root among holiness Methodists. Because these men and women already believed that conversion ought to be followed by a definable experience of "entire sanctification" that cleansed the heart of "inbred sin," it was easy to conclude that entire sanctification could also cleanse the body of disease. Probably a majority of the holiness leaders resisted the new teaching, but a significant minority, such as Ethan O. Allen, a venerable Methodist pastor in Hartford, and W.B. Godbey, a prolific author and evangelist in the southern wing of the church, found it congenial. "With the coming of the doctrine of entire sanctification," wrote one pioneer, "came also the doctrine of divine healing. A veritable tidal wave of bodily healing swept through the land. . . . There would be healing services at almost every camp-meeting. . . . Many persons were miraculously healed of all sorts of diseases."[4]

The idea that healing was mediated through Christ's atoning and sanctifying work was also popularized by non-Methodist evangelicals with holiness sympathies. Leaders included Carrie Judd Montgomery, an Episcopal laywoman in Buffalo, New York, and William E. Boardman, a well-known Presbyterian evangelist who soon became an organizer of the divine-healing movement in England. By far the most prominent of the popularizers, though, was Charles C. Cullis, an Episcopal layman and homeopathic physician in Boston. In the early 1870s Cullis came to believe that the prayer of faith not only secured entire sanctification for the heart, but also healing for the body. He determined to pray as well as care for the sick, and over the years described the fruits of his ministry in *Faith Cures* (1879), *More Faith Cures* (1881), and *Other Faith Cures* (1885).[5]

Many evangelicals, especially in Baptist and Presbyterian circles, were sympathetic to the atonement-healing theology, but unlike Cullis, they were not willing to link healing with a definable sanctification experience. Moreover, they were, as a rule, strongly influenced by the Plymouth Brethren emphasis upon the nearness of Christ's Second Coming. Thus they characteristically insisted that the healing ministries of the church, described in *James* 5, and the charismatic gifts of healing, described in 1 *Corinthians* 12:8–9 ("For to one is given . . . the gifts of healing by the same Spirit"), had been restored to the church to help spread the gospel and to serve as one of the "signs and wonders" heralding the Lord's return.[6]

A leading advocate of this view was Adoniram J. Gordon (1836–1895), a Baptist pastor in Boston and founder of what is now Gordon College and Gordon-Conwell Theological Seminary. In 1882 Gordon published a biblical and historical defense of *The Ministry of Healing,* which soon became, in the words of one historian, the "standard apologia for the movement." Unlike most advocates of the atonement-healing theology, Gordon did not believe that God had limited his sovereignty in order to make healing an automatic benefit of the prayer of faith. But he did think that the church had fallen prey to the "caged-eagle theory of man's existence." As a result, it had forgotten that the body, being the Lord's creation, was not to be despised, but preserved in good health until fully restored on the resurrection day.[7]

Albert B. Simpson (1843–1919), the founder of the Christian and Missionary Alliance, was less thoughtful than Gordon, but ultimately more influential, at least among Pentecostals. Following a miraculous healing experience, Simpson resigned the pastorate of the Thirteenth Street Presbyterian Church in New York in 1881 in order to devote himself more fully to *The Gospel of Healing,* as his partly autobiographical exposition of the divine healing theology was called. To some extent Simpson's influence grew from his widely publicized Friday-afternoon healing services in the New York Gospel Tabernacle, which he founded in 1889. But the greater part stemmed from his uncompromising insistence that healing, like salvation, must be secured solely by faith in Christ's atoning blood. The ramifications of this claim were far-reaching. For one thing, it meant that the use of medicine or physicians signified deliberate rebellion against God's promises. It also meant that failure to be healed was evidence of inadequate trust in God's Word. "Disease is sin's mortgage," he warned; since Christ has paid the debt at Calvary, "the mortgage is discharged, and my house is free." Undoubtedly Simpson only hoped to underscore the richness of God's grace, but his teaching actually promoted an interpretation of disease in which the victim was doubly blamed—blamed for the sin and faithlessness that caused the sickness in the first place, and blamed again for failing to have sufficient faith for healing. For better or worse, the blame-the-victim theory of illness soon became a hallmark of the Pentecostal understanding of the human condition.[8]

Despite differences about the need for a definable sanctification experience and about the automatic efficacy of the prayer of faith, the general framework of the atonement-healing theology was firmly in place by the end of the century. Faith homes such as Cullis's Faith Cure House in Boston (1882), Simpson's Berachah House in New York (1884), and Montgomery's Faith Rest Cottage in Buffalo (1882) and House of Peace in Beulah Heights, California, (1894) institutionalized it; periodicals such as *Guide to Holiness, Times of Refreshing,* and *Triumphs of Faith* proclaimed it; schools such as The Bible Missionary Training Institute in Rochester, New York, and Simpson's New York Missionary Training Institute (now Nyack College) taught it; annual summer camps such as the Old Orchard Beach Conference in Maine, and conventions such as the 1885 International Conference on Divine Healing and True Holiness in London popularized it.[9]

Near the turn of the century a number of itinerant healers became prominent in evangelical circles and captured considerable attention in the secular press as well. Most worked within the theological traditions and institutional networks described earlier, but some put particular emphasis upon their own ability to effect healings through the empowerment of the Holy Spirit. Especially notable in this respect was Maria B. Woodworth-Etter (1844–1924), a Winebrennerian Churches of God evangelist who joined the Pentecostals about 1912. Convinced that she possessed the apostolic gifts of healing, Etter started to hold mass healing rallies in Indiana and Illinois in the mid-1880s. One feature of her ministry was a tendency for individuals to fall prostrate when she touched them. This event, commonly known as being "slain in the Spirit," or "resting in Jesus," has persisted in some Pentecostal circles to the present. A second feature of Etter's ministry was pandemonium. One reporter judged that her services sounded like the "female ward of an insane asylum." Another said that "one can not imagine the . . . confusion":

> Dozens lying around pale and unconscious, rigid and lifeless as though in death. Strong men shouting till they were hoarse, then falling down in a swoon. Women falling over benches and trampled under foot. . . . Aged women gesticulating and hysterically sobbing. . . . Men shouting with a devilish, unearthly laugh.

Rumors of unrestrained behavior were so persistent that some communities passed ordinances prohibiting minor children from attending her meetings. But for countless men and women none of this mattered; her ability to heal was beyond dispute.[10]

Among Pentecostals, Etter's star still shines brightly, but for a short time her reputation was eclipsed by John Alexander Dowie (1847–1907), an Australian emigrant who established Zion City, Illinois, in 1900 as a communitarian theocracy devoted to holy living and divine healing. Dowie himself never became a Pentecostal, and after 1905 he fell from grace because of alleged financial and sexual irregularities. But at one point or another dozens of men and women who later became Pentecostal leaders associated with and apparently came under the influence of this strangely gifted man.[11]

In the course of his lifetime Dowie wrote literally thousands of pages on the theology of divine healing. None of it was particularly original or systematic. His influence grew, rather, from his extreme hostility to medicine and physicians. Year after year Dowie waged a

"Holy War against Doctors, Drugs, and Devils," insisting that the most dreaded disease of all was *"bacillis lunaticus medicus."*

> What! You doctors think that you can control the whole population from the cradle to grave? We cannot be born without you, we cannot live without you, and we cannot die without you? . . . "Medical science"! Medical bosh! (Laughter) Where is your science? The Homeopath says . . . like cures like. The Allopath says . . . the contrary cures the contrary. The Osteopath says, "You are both fools." The Psychopath says, "You are all three fools." . . . And I agree with them on that proposition. (Laughter and applause.)[12]

Dowie might have been written off as a harmless eccentric if he had not persuaded seven thousand people to move to Zion City where physicians, nurses, veterinarians, morticians, hospitals, and man-made medicines were banned. Most of his followers believed that the Lord had used Dowie to heal them of every imaginable disease. One reporter deadpanned that the prophet's followers routinely claimed to have been cured of everything except "decapitation and *rigor mortis*." Nor was he far wrong. Year after year tourists, journalists, and scholars traveled to Zion City to see the array of crutches, trusses, casts, braces, corrective shoes, pill bottles, wheelchairs, and "instruments of surgical torture" that lined the walls of the tabernacle—"trophies," Dowie boasted, "captured from the enemy."[13]

A few notable evangelicals, such as Arthur T. Pierson, editor of the *Missionary Review of the World,* endorsed the basic principles of the atonement-healing theology but disassociated themselves from the extremism that Simpson, Etter, and Dowie represented. Some, such as the evangelist Dwight L. Moody, privately disavowed all aspects of the divine healing movement, while others, such as Benjamin B. Warfield, the dragon of Princeton Theological Seminary, vigorously attacked it. Most evangelical leaders seem to have ignored the whole business. But among ordinary believers, countless thousands threw away their medicines and vowed to commit their lives and their children's lives to the Lord's care, come what may. This was the context in which Pentecostalism and the Pentecostal message of divine healing for the body was born.[14]

Primitive Pentecostalism (1900–1930)

Modern Pentecostals commonly distinguish themselves from other Protestants by the doctrine and practice of speaking in tongues. This represents a certain loss of historical memory, for an overview of the early literature leaves little doubt that in the beginning divine healing was, if not equally distinctive, at least equally important. Many of the original leaders, including Charles Fox Parham and William J. Seymour, had earned their livings as itinerant healing evangelists. The premier issue of the *Apostolic Faith,* published by the Azusa Mission in Los Angeles in 1906, overflowed with healing testimonials. The cover of the initial issue of the *Latter Rain Evangel,* published in Chicago in 1908, declared that its aim was to proclaim the message of "Jesus the Redeemer, Jesus the Healer." The lead article of the *Pentecost,* launched in Indianapolis in 1908, bore the headline: "Broken Arm Healed." In the mountains of eastern Tennessee the first issue of the *Evening Light and Church of God Evangel* evinced a somewhat broader range of concerns, yet its testimonial columns were similarly filled with stories describing the Lord's assault upon sickness, "the stronghold of the Devil."[15]

The "signs and wonders" of primitive Pentecostalism should not be equated with the ecstatic eruptions that punctuated the revivals of the nineteenth century. Although Pentecostalism certainly had its share of trances, dancing, prostration, screaming, laughing, weeping, and violent jerking, behavior of this sort was never the central focus. The uniqueness of Pentecostalism grew instead from its preoccupation with events that seemed starkly supernatural. "The common heartbeat of every service," David Edwin Harrell has said of a somewhat later period, "was the miracle—the hypnotic moment when the Spirit moved to heal the sick and raise the dead." Every conceivable form of healing—including replacement of missing organs and resurrection from the dead—was reported endlessly, page after page, normally in the jargon of the camp meeting, yet often in the straightforward prose of a daily newspaper. One reminiscence from 1903, drawn virtually at random, intimates the throbbing energy of a Pentecostal meeting:

> People singing, shouting, praying, and many speaking languages that I couldn't understand; while all about the tent were empty cots and wheel-chairs, and numerous discarded canes and crutches were hung round about the tent, while those who had been delivered from using same leaped and shouted and rejoiced.

Visiting journalists often said more about the purported healings than anything else. And for good reason: The claims were so astounding, and recurred with such frequency, in so many contexts, one could hardly fail to take notice.[16]

The formal healing theology of early Pentecostalism resembled the atonement-healing theology articulated by Gordon, Simpson, and some other evangelical writers of the late nineteenth century. Although both stressed the biblical passages that suggested that healing is grounded in the atonement, there were differences of tone and emphasis. The evangelical writers ordinarily emphasized the healing ministry of the church, described in *James* 5, as well as the covenantal promise of *Exodus* 15:26 ("If thou wilt diligently hearken to the voice of the Lord . . . I will put none of these diseases upon thee . . . for I am the Lord that healeth thee"). Pentecostal writers, on the other hand, gave more attention to the special gifts of healing, described in 1 *Corinthians* 12, and the "Great Commission" in *Mark* 16:17–18 ("And these signs shall follow them that believe . . . they shall lay hands on the sick, and they shall recover"). They also were more likely to insist that the record of contemporary experience—the "tidal wave" of miraculous cures sweeping Pentecostal missions in all parts of the world—irrefutably proved that God had truly restored the ministry of healing in these, the final days of history.[17]

The distinctiveness of the new movement became most apparent in the practical and devotional application of this theological brief. To begin with, Pentecostals transformed the healing covenant into a healing contract. "Getting things from God is like playing checkers," said F.F. Bosworth, the most respected healing evangelist of the 1920s. "He always moves when it is His turn. . . . Our move is to expect what he promises . . . before we *see* the healing." E.W. Kenyon, a prolific writer whose works continue to be read by contemporary Pentecostals, explained that genuine faith does not even acknowledge the existence of a disease. To do so is to "sign for the package" Satan has left. Indeed, said Kenyon, "it is not good taste to ask [God] to heal us, for he has already done it. He declared that we are healed; therefore we are."[18]

Given the premise that God always responds to a genuine prayer of faith, the persistence of illness could be explained only two ways: Either one's life was impure or one's faith was shallow. The propensity to blame the victim was, as we have seen, implicit in the work of Simpson and other nineteenth-century writers, but early Pentecostals made it painfully explicit: "Whose fault is it if you stay sick?" demanded Lillian Yeomans, a former physician and prominent convert. "Not the fault of the Lord. If we are not healed we must look for the cause of it in ourselves."[19]

Pentecostal writers were understandably reluctant to dwell upon the real-life effects of this notion, but they left numerous hints that believers who were unable to leave their crutches at the altar either drifted from the movement, or entered a permanent underclass of spiritually second-rate citizens as they struggled to overcome or ignore their symptoms.[20] Thus in a popular tract of 1920 Etter declared: "We must cling to the promises of Jesus instead of looking at our feelings . . . for our senses are false witnesses. . . . In reality we are healed when we believe."

The testimonial literature confirms the depth and pervasiveness of Etter's view. One woman typically explained that she had prayed for healing from diphtheria, but "a raging fever" and continued suffering had tempted her to doubt it. Then the Lord spoke:

> "These are not symptoms of diphtheria, for I healed you of that last night. . . . These are only imitation symptoms kept up by the devil. I healed you when you prayed. . . . I want you to act just as you would if you felt perfectly well, *because* you *are* well." . . . [Then] I saw that God's Word was true and the symptoms were the devil's lie. . . . This is what it means to . . . have faith in God's Word and not in feelings.[21]

From here it was only a short step to the idea that *truly* converted and Spirit-filled believers were protected from illness in the first place. "So long as I keep my soul in contact with the living God," judged John G. Lake, pastor of a large church in Spokane, "no germ will ever attach itself to me," for when you are filled with the Holy Spirit, "it oozes out of the pores of your flesh and kills the germs." This was the preventive part of the Spirit's work. The therapeutic part was divine happiness and health. Because God had promised to preserve Christians "in perfect soundness," one writer asserted, they are "never to be sorrowful for a moment, but to be ALWAYS REJOICING." Pentecostals carefully explained that the "Resurrection Life" did not prevent the normal processes of aging, but it did forestall "brain weariness" and unnatural afflictions of the body prior to the appointed hour of death. Yeomans summed up the Pentecostal position without flinching: "Therefore, not healing only, but absolute immunity from disease is ours in Christ Jesus."[22]

The role of demons in human affairs was another major concern in the practical healing theology of early Pentecostalism. As already noted, in the nineteenth century many evangelical Protestants assumed that demons could oppress or even inhabit the human body. In time this view lost cogency, especially in the older denominations, but Pentecostals continued to view demons as a constant threat, the direct and immediate source of many afflictions. Pentecostals constructed elaborate typologies of the different kinds of demons and the various ways they entered and tormented the body. Ordinary folk, especially, seem to have believed that spirits were prone to penetrate the body at particular places, such as the groin or mouth. Consequently, they often construed divine healing as exorcism of the oppressing demon. One editor proudly explained that "instead of trying to fight disease by means of doctors, drugs and human resources . . . our people rebuke and cast out demons." In many parts of the world, he went on to warn, "belief in Satan and evil spirits" is rapidly disappearing, but among Pentecostals, "demons are seen and recognized as the powers which are afflicting and oppressing human beings."[23]

These, then, were the principal formal and practical concerns of the theology of divine healing in primitive Pentecostalism. Within this general context, however, Pentecostal leaders disagreed about the proper attitude toward medicine and physicians. A large minority acknowledged that medical care was an inferior yet morally permissible alternative for Christians of weak faith, but the majority urged total avoidance of professional help, and many displayed overt hostility toward the medical and especially pharmaceutical professions.[24] Their reasons were complex. Resentment against the higher social status of physicians and druggists undoubtedly played a part, but theological assumptions also entered in. Pentecostals perceived physicians as intruders upon a sacred realm, and regarded patent medicines as evil precisely because the alcoholic and narcotic ingredients in them seemed not natural but demonic in origin.[25]

We know that many ordinary Pentecostals followed their leaders' advice to avoid medical treatment. Editors never liked to advertise the movement's failures, but the evidence repeatedly hints that hundreds of members died or allowed their children to die rather than resort to worldly means.[26] Indeed, one of the constant problems for responsible denominational officials was "extremism," which they defined as refusal to cooperate with nature by washing a wound, wearing eyeglasses, or seeing a dentist. Stomping on demons and choking believers in order to expel demons from their bodies also became a problem from time to time.[27] Nonetheless, it is clear that many—perhaps most—Pentecostals did consult physicians. More often than not the testimonials began by stating that worldly doctors had tried but failed to cure the illness or injury in question—and frequently added that doctors were baffled or even angered when patients returned to show off their healing.[28]

Finally, it is worth noting that the disinclination to seek medical care was part of a larger pattern of renunciative behavior. Pentecostals, like most evangelical Protestants, routinely banned dancing, cosmetics, and the use of tobacco and alcoholic drinks. Unlike most other Protestants, however, they often forbade seemingly harmless pastimes such as chewing gum, eating ice cream, wearing neckties, watching parades, reading novels, attending fairs, and engaging in "sugar coated swearing" (such as saying "my goodness" or "gee whiz"). They also warned against "excess in the conjugal relation" and occasionally urged complete sexual abstinence within marriage.[29]

Altogether, then, primitive Pentecostalism presents a paradoxical picture of a very other-worldly supernaturalism on one hand and a very this-worldly pragmatism on the other. The supernatural was always present and palpably real. At the same time, however, through Herculean feats of faith, Pentecostals struggled to gain mastery over the forces of disease and disability that impinged upon their lives. As the movement moved into the middle decades of the century, it changed in many ways. But, as we shall see, among many ordinary folk this paradoxical determination to manipulate as well as worship the divine persisted without apology.

Mid-century Patterns (1930–1960)

The Pentecostal movement as a whole enjoyed modest numerical growth during the mid-century decades. Yet this is only half the story, for after World War II the social standing of the typical church member dramatically improved. Moreover, after the war most of the established denominations entered a period of sustained centralization and institutional development, characterized by the opening of Bible schools, orphanages, and retirement homes. These modernizing trends seem to have fostered a gradual abatement of healing miracles in Pentecostal worship services, and, at the same time, a corresponding relaxation of the prohibitions against medicines and physicians. By 1950, however, two powerful counter-modernizing pressures had emerged, and both impinged upon the nature and care of the human body.[30]

The first was the New Order of the Latter Rain, a little-known but influential movement that erupted in 1947 in an independent (that is, not denominationally supported) Bible school in North Battleford, Saskatchewan. It quickly spread to the United States and touched Pentecostal missions worldwide. Like early Pentecostalism, the New Order, as it was commonly called, emphasized demons as the source of illness, equated healing with exorcism, and construed these and other charismatic gifts as tokens of the Lord's immediate return. Unlike early Pentecostalism, however, the New Order also emphasized the biblical justification for prolonged (preferably forty-day) fasts, and the restoration of the gifts of healing to specially chosen apostles and prophets rather than to the church as a whole. Prominent figures included Myrtle D. Beall of the Bethesda Missionary Temple in Detroit and Thomas Wyatt of the Wings of Healing Temple in Portland, Oregon. By 1960, New Order teachers generally had been discredited as mavericks and extremists in the more established Pentecostal churches, but they remain visible in the nondenominational charismatic movement today, especially in segments that advocate an authoritarian and patriarchal organizational structure.[31]

The second and more important of the counter-modernizing trends was the rise of independent "deliverance" evangelism in the 1950s and

1960s. This was not a wholly new development. From the beginning, Pentecostals had drawn a distinction between the corporate gifts of healing, resident in the church as a whole, and the personal gifts of healing that individuals such as Etter and Dowie seemed to possess.[32] Early Pentecostals tended to emphasize the value of the former and to minimize the latter. By the end of the 1920s, however, a small number of demonstrably capable healers, such as Aimee McPherson, Fred F. Bosworth, Smith Wigglesworth, and Charles S. Price, had become minor celebrities in Pentecostal (and sometimes non-Pentecostal) circles. A few, such as Sister Aimee, served as denominational officials; most were unaffiliated with, yet well respected by, the established Pentecostal denominations.

At this point the story becomes murky. For reasons far from clear, in the late 1940s and early 1950s a new group of shaman-like healers skyrocketed into national prominence and acquired a broad following among rank-and-file Pentecostals. Initially the most prominent was William Branham, a semiliterate Oneness preacher widely credited with spectacular healings and an eerie ability to diagnose the ailments and personal histories of persons in his audiences. Other notables included A.A. Allen, Jack Coe, T.L. Osborn and, of course, Oral Roberts. Sooner or later most were forced out of their denominations, but the effort to ostracize them predictably backfired. Unfettered by institutional restraints, many of the deliverance evangelists built private empires of seemingly boundless influence and financial support.[33]

Although few denominational officials ever admitted it, the beliefs and practices of the deliverance evangelists in the 1950s and 1960s closely resembled the beliefs and practices of early Pentecostals. But there were differences of style and subtlety. The role of the prayer of faith is a case in point. First-generation leaders unquestionably believed that the prayer of faith was automatically efficacious, but the deliverance evangelists stripped away whatever theological cushioning the notion once may have had and offered it as a foolproof device for healing to the desperate and impoverished folk who crowded their tents. Thus W.V. Grant urged the sick to "look up and say . . . 'Lord . . . give it here' "; if you are God's child "you can have whatever you say." Allen similarly directed his followers to forget about "weakness or pain": "ACT YOUR FAITH. . . . Leave your wheel chair. Throw away your crutches. Walk and run! Leap for joy! . . . Quit 'trying to believe.' Simply believe, and ACT." The mid-century healers frequently implied that their own ability to heal was virtually automatic. In a volume appropriately titled *Everlasting Spiritual and Physical Health*, O.L. Jaggers explained that "fasting and prayer" was the quickest way to acquire the gifts of healing. With these powers, he added, "the Spirit filled minister . . . will do VERY LITTLE PRAYING FOR THE SICK. . . .

HE WILL GIVE COMMANDS THAT THE SICKNESS LEAVE." Indeed, with these gifts modern "spiritual giants" will be able to "unlock the doors to God's dynamite vaults!"[34]

As we have seen, early Pentecostals were never reluctant to claim incredible healings, including resurrections from the dead, but the mid-century evangelists routinely claimed healings that seemed not so much miraculous as simply preposterous. Decayed teeth were filled, halos photographed, screaming demons tape-recorded, and bloody cancers coughed up and put on display. Allen told of one woman whose stomach had been surgically removed:

> Before an audience of thousands in Baltimore, God touched her instantly. She arose from her stretcher, and danced in the Spirit back and forth across the front of the tent. Then, she ate a hamburger and drank a Pepsi-Cola.[35]

Franklin Hall represented the most extreme wing of the movement. His (still-flourishing) ministry was heralded in books that bore titles such as *FORMULA FOR RAISING THE DEAD* and *SUBDUING THE EARTH* (or how to "control the weather . . . stop whirlwinds, etc."). Hall's specialty was the ministry of "Bodyfelt Salvation," which led to healing "so intense that it becomes fire or heat upon the body . . . leaving us covered with the warm or hot tangible miracle SUBSTANCE from Jesus' body." Claiming that Bodyfelt Salvation was "700% greater than ordinary healing power," Hall insisted that it not only prevented aches, tiredness, and grumpiness, but also replaced natural body odors with the "Hallelujah Cologne Fragrance," making believers "insect proof, or a Holy Ghost exterminator."[36]

Independent deliverance evangelism reached the peak of its influence in the early 1960s. By the end of the decade most of the big tents were gone and most of the stars were dead or disgraced by persistent rumors of financial or sexual irregularity. A few, such as Oral Roberts and Rex Humbard, survived by modernizing their methods and diversifying their interests. It is tempting to believe that the rise and fall of the celebrity healers was a final outburst that marked the exhaustion of the old values and the beginning of a new style of life and worship in the established Pentecostal denominations. But the extraordinary appeal in the 1970s and 1980s of prosperity and television evangelism suggests that the changes may have been more apparent than real.

Pentecostals in a Modern World (1960–1985)

It is important to remember that thousands of Pentecostals are not affiliated with any of the established Pentecostal denominations and thus rarely show up in official tabulations and scholarly studies of the movement. Little is known about them, but scattered evidence suggests that they gather in homes, cinderblock missions, and ramshackle buildings on the outskirts of small towns. Their ministers are typically traveling evangelists or television preachers who stress health and wealth through fasting, exorcism, and such techniques as rubbing anointed handkerchiefs, books, cassette tapes, and fluorescent statues.[37]

Another important (and often-overlooked) stream within the Pentecostal movement consists of persons who belong to one of the established Pentecostal denominations, yet strongly identify with a variety of independent (and usually denominationally opposed) ministries. These folk are the main supporters of prosperity evangelism, or the "Faith Confession" movement as it is often called. Although virtually all of the independent deliverance evangelists and many television celebrities, including Roberts and Humbard, endorse Faith Confessionalism to some degree, the principal leaders are Fred Price in Los Angeles, Kenneth Copeland in Fort Worth, and T.L. Osborn and Kenneth Hagin in Tulsa. Hagin's Rhema Bible Training Center, which enrolls five thousand students, is considered the movement's primary institutional center.[38]

The major premise of Faith Confessionism is that there are foundational spiritual laws in the world which, like the laws of physics, are universal and immutable. One of these laws is that financial contributions to the Lord's work that go beyond tithing and a prudent calculation of one's ability to give invariably bring a manifold return on the initial "investment." Roberts call this the *Miracle of Seed-Faith,* as one of his books, which has sold more than two million copies, is titled. The minor premise of the Faith Confession is that God expects his children to prosper financially as well as spiritually. The main prooftext is 3 *John* 2–4 ("Beloved, I wish above all things that thou mayest prosper and be in health"). But there are many others. Copeland points out, for example, that the prodigal-son parable in *Luke* 15 shows that the son who stayed home went unrewarded "because of the littleness of his thinking." The prosperity evangelists constantly regale their readers and listeners with stories of new cars and lavish homes they can have if their lives are upright and faith in God's promises is unwavering. In a booklet aptly called *God's Pact for Life's Best: Go for More in '84,* Osborn explains that "God's WINNING message includes His BEST for people! And His BEST is for happiness, health, success and prosperity. . . . When people find out that God is never mad at them . . . real happiness and success and health can begin."[39]

The extreme claims of the Faith Confession message have prompted some thoughtful Pentecostals to attack the theological and financial integrity of the prosperity evangelists. But the criticism has had little impact; in the mid-1980s the movement appears more robust than ever.

And to be fair, most of the prosperity preachers seem sincerely to believe that sick, impoverished, or unhappy Christians have failed God as much as themselves. The plain truth, says Copeland, is that God commands his children to put him to the test: "The world's shortages . . . should have no effect on us here who have made Jesus the Lord of our lives."[40]

The established Pentecostal churches of the 1980s also tend to couple stark supernaturalism with shrewd pragmatism. Outsiders are often astonished at the extent to which an archaic world-view still covers all aspects of life, even in wealthy suburban congregations, and this is especially evident in matters of health and healing. Denominational officials carefully insist, for example, that divine healing is *essentially* different from any natural form of healing, and they warn believers not to be fooled by the modern supposition that demonic disturbances are "simply a result of mental illness [or] split personalities."[41] One of the consequences of the persistence of the older beliefs is that many of the ethical and moral questions that trouble mainline Christians simply do not trouble Pentecostals, who still prohibit, for example, the use of alcohol, tobacco, and marijuana without a second thought. An addiction to one of these substances is regarded not as a tolerable weakness, much less as a disease, but as the predictable result of deliberately sinful choices.[42] Denominational publications reflect virtually no interest in bioethical questions such as euthanasia or artificial fertilization. Although family planning is encouraged (without openly endorsing contraception), nonmarital sexuality, including masturbation, is treated with utmost severity.[43] Life-cycle discussions are limited to childrearing and aging. Writings about the former ordinarily stress the importance of Godly discipline, while comments on the latter tend to emphasize God's command to honor fathers and mothers.[44] Death is redefined as a transition to a higher and better stage of life (for the saved). Early Pentecostals sometimes said that a person had been "transferred" from earth to heaven; modern Pentecostals commonly say that those who have "died in Christ" have been "coronated" or have "gone to be with the Lord."[45] Although problems of mental health are no longer routinely attributed to demonic influences, non-Pentecostal psychologists and psychiatrists are distrusted. Indeed, when church publications discuss mental health they often display a bouncy, pep-talk attitude, which suggests above all else that Pentecostals still do not take the subject entirely seriously.[46]

The distance between the modern and the Pentecostal world-views is particularly evident in matters closely related to the orders of creation. The Church of God, for example, states that it remains "unalterably opposed" to abortion (except when the mother's life is imperiled), adding that: "We abhor the usual circumstances that cause abortion." In an official position paper on homosexuality, the Assemblies of God similarly insists that homosexuality is not a "psychological problem" nor an "alternate life-style." Rather it "is sin because it is contrary to the principles . . . God established in the beginning. . . . When people choose to be homosexuals, they reject God's principles." Warning against "the sentimental credulity which results in tolerance of this behavior," the denomination urges Christians to distinguish between homosexuals "who honestly want God's salvation and those who may be recruiting sympathizers."[47]

Just as the Pentecostal world-view continues to reflect the heightened supernaturalism of the early years, Pentecostal behavior continues to reflect the same determination to master life's perils by harnessing and disciplining one's faith. Denominational publications still feature testimonials of miraculous healings (as well as deliverances from peculiarly modern problems such as overeating and addiction to television watching), and ordinary believers still routinely seek the healing ministrations of their pastor (or a call-in television evangelist) in times of need.[48]

It would be unfair, however, not to acknowledge the changes that have taken place in both the cognitive and behavioral realms. Although the basic structure of the old atonement-healing theology is still very much intact, occasionally one can discern subtle bulges in the direction of modernity. In recent years several Pentecostal writers have intimated, for example, that healing is rooted not so much in the atonement as in God's essentially compassionate nature.[49] A few have acknowledged that efficacious faith is a gift bestowed—or not bestowed—by God in his sovereign judgment.[50] Some have allowed that God may withhold healing for reasons beyond human ken.[51] Others have admitted that God is not honored by a believer's determination to deny pain or the symptoms of illness.[52]

If the theology of modern Pentecostals is inching toward modernity, it may be because their behavior has already raced far ahead. Perhaps the most striking change is their willingness, especially since World War II, to seek the best of modern medical care. Prescription drugs are routinely accepted and physicians highly esteemed.[53] Indeed, the handful of Pentecostals who still refuse professional treatment, such as the snake-handlers in the southern Appalachians, are an acute embarrassment to their brethren. New attitudes toward health and healing are also evident in the institutional developments of the 1970s and 1980s. As noted before, after World War II most of the major Pentecostal denominations made significant commitments to orphanages, adoption agencies, nursing homes, and retirement centers. In recent years, however, Pentecostals have measurably broadened the scope their concerns, as demonstrated by the establishment of a wide variety of denominationally sanctioned health-related ministries. A notable example is

Heritage Village, a 1,600-acre family recreation park in Fort Mill, South Carolina, owned by the PTL Club Television Network. The park includes camping and (luxurious) hotel facilities, a retirement community, an adoption agency, a residence for unmarried mothers, and a year-round tabernacle where divine healing is prominently featured. Another example is Teen Challenge International, which maintains drug treatment centers in 136 cities. Each is run by nonprofessional Christian staffworkers who emphasize rehabilitation through conversion and rigorous moral and physical discipline. In contrast, at Emerge Ministries and Counseling Center in Akron, Ohio, professionally trained Christian staffworkers use clinical techniques as well as prayer to treat emotional problems.[54]

By far the most spectacular venture by Pentecostals into institutional health care is Oral Roberts's 150-million-dollar City of Faith Medical and Research Center started in Tulsa in 1978. Roberts predicts that by 1988 the center will be generally regarded as the "Mayo Clinic of the Southwest." And with good reason. The complex includes accredited (and flourishing) graduate schools of medicine, dentistry, and nursing; a sixty-story clinic; a thirty-story hospital; and a twenty-story laboratory specializing in aging, cancer, and heart disease. Believing that both prayer and scalpels are God's instruments for healing, Roberts's staff assigns a physician, a nurse, and prayer partner to each entering patient. This holistic view of health care is reflected in the motto of Oral Roberts University: "To educate the whole man in spirit, mind and body." It is also reflected in the school's requirement that all students and faculty must meet exacting weight and physical fitness tests or be dismissed. One university official may have revealed more about modern Pentecostalism than he intended when he remarked, "You can't be much of a witness [for Christ] if you are a loser."[55]

Conclusion

Standing beside the City of Faith, Roberts recently explained that in his right hand he is able "to pick up the presence of Satanic power tormenting people." The scenario is a paradigm of modern Pentecostalism. It reveals a very other-worldly supernaturalism and very this-worldly pragmatism still locked in a curiously compatible marriage that has lasted longer than anyone can quite remember. Admittedly, over the years both partners have changed. The supernaturalism has become less stark, and the pragmatism has grown more resourceful, now embracing state-of-the-art technology along with the prayer of faith. But the essential structure of the relationship, the essential paradox, remains intact. Another way of putting it is to say that under the canopy of a

first-century cosmology, divine healing rituals and high-tech hospitals
have proved to be equally functional devices for getting along in the
real world.[56]

Even so, there is more to Pentecostalism than supernaturalism or
pragmatism, and questions about the role of health and healing cannot
be adequately answered unless one also considers the enduring satis-
factions the movement has afforded. The choruses of the songs Pentecostals have loved to sing tell a major part of the story:

> It is joy unspeakable and full of glory
> Full of glory, full of glory;
> Oh, the half has never yet been told.
>
> * * * * *
>
> This is like heaven to me
> I've crossed over Jordan to Canaan's fair land
> And this is like heaven to me.

Or as one Amanda Smith phrased it in a letter to an editor in 1910,
"This blessed way never gets old; always new and juicy, never dry.
Hallelujah!"[57]

And finally there is the religious question. The centrality of divine
healing in the Pentecostal tradition underscores the timeless bond between physical infirmity and religious anxiety on one hand, and between
physical health and religious assurance on the other. This means that
for Pentecostals, divine healing and other miracle experiences have
effectively functioned as sacraments, palpable symbols of those rare but
unforgettable moments of grace in the life of the believer. This is
especially true of the first generation, the men and women who chose
to endure pain rather than resort to wordly means. Even those who
were not healed, and thus suffered the opprobrium of "shallow faith,"
could still interpret their ability to persevere as confirmation of the
genuineness of their salvation. Simply stated, an adequate interpretation
of brokenness and healing in the Pentecostal tradition must take account
of the human longing for redemption. For the secret of movements of
this sort is not the social and cultural conditions that make them possible,
but the religious impulses that make them inevitable.

Notes

I wish to thank the Reverend Wayne E. Warner, Archivist, International Head-
quarters of the Assemblies of God, Professor Russell P. Spittler of Fuller
Theological Seminary, and Professor Ruel W. Tyson, Jr., of the University of
North Carolina for critical and bibliographical suggestions.

1. Walter J. Hollenweger, *The Pentecostals: The Charismatic Movement in the Churches,* trans. R.A. Wilson (Minneapolis, 1972), chap. 25; E. Mansell Pattison, et al., "Faith Healing: A Study of Personality and Function," *Journal of Nervous and Mental Disease* 157 (1973):398; William M. Clements, "Faith Healing Narratives from Northeast Arkansas," *Indiana Folklore* 8 (1975–76):21, and "Ritual Expectation in Pentecostal Healing Experience," *Western Folklore* 40 (1981):139–148.

2. R. Kelso Carter, *Pastor Blumhardt* (Boston, n.d. [ca. 1885]), pp. 22–82. Stockmayer's influence is described in A.J. Gordon, *The Ministry of Healing: Miracles of Cure in All Ages* (Brooklyn, NY, 1882), pp. 163–165. Surveys of the nineteenth-century background I have drawn upon include Gordon, *Ministry of Healing,* chap. 8; Arthur T. Pierson, *Forward Movements of the Last Half Century* (1900, reprinted New York, 1912), chap. 30; Raymond J. Cunningham, "From Holiness to Healing: The Faith Cure in America, 1872–1892," *Church History* 43 (1974):499–513; Edith L. Waldvogel, "The 'Overcoming Life': A Study in the Reformed Evangelical Origins of Pentecostalism," Ph.D. diss., Harvard University, 1977, chap. 4; Donald W. Dayton, "Theological Roots of Pentecostalism," Ph.D. diss., University of Chicago, 1983, chap. 5. I am especially indebted to Dayton's work.

3. Dayton, "Roots of Pentecostalism," pp. 150–152.

4. Ibid., pp. 169–173; C.B. Jernigan, *Pioneer Days of the Holiness Movement in the Southwest* (Kansas City,1919), p. 155.

5. Cunningham, "Holiness to Healing," pp. 501–505.

6. George M. Marsden, *Fundamentalism and American Culture: The Shaping of Twentieth-Century Evangelicalism: 1870–1925* (New York, 1980), pp. 94, 256.

7. Gordon, *Ministry of Healing,* p. 194; Cunningham, "Holiness to Healing," p. 504.

8. A.B. Simpson, *The Gospel of Healing* (1888, reprinted Harrisburg, PA, 1915), pp. 157–175, and *The Lord for the Body* (1903, reprinted Harrisburg, PA, 1959), p. 115. The phrase *blame-the-victim* is taken from Margaret Poloma, *The Charismatic Movement: Is There a New Pentecost?* (Boston, 1982), p. 98.

9. There is no book-length study of these developments, but the best brief survey in print is Donald W. Dayton, "The Rise of the Evangelical Healing Movement in Nineteenth Century America," *Pneuma: Journal of the Society for Pentecostal Studies* 4 (1982):1–18.

10. The reporter's comments are in the San Francisco *Examiner,* January 11, 1890, and Muncie *Daily News,* September 21, 1885, both quoted in Wayne E. Warner, *The Woman Evangelist: The Life and Times of Charismatic Evangelist Maria B. Woodworth-Etter* (Metuchen, NJ, in press). Biographical data are taken from Warner and Maria Woodworth-Etter, *A Diary of Signs and Wonders* (1916, reprinted Tulsa, n.d.).

11. Dowie's influence upon Pentecostalism is assessed in Edith L. Blumhofer, "The Christian Catholic Church and the Apostolic Faith: A Study in the 1906 Pentecostal Revival," in *Studies of Pentecostal-Charismatic Experiences in History,* ed. M. Cecil Robeck (Peabody, MA, 1986). For brief surveys of Dowie's career, see Alden R. Heath, "Apostle in Zion," *Journal of the Illinois State Historical Society* 70 (1977):98–113; and Grant Wacker, "Marching to Zion: Religion in a Modern Utopian Community," *Church History* 54(1985):496–511.

12. For Dowie's remarks, see, respectively, *Leaves of Healing*, October 21, 1899, quoted in Gordon Lindsay, *John Alexander Dowie: A Life Story of Trials, Tragedies and Triumphs* (1951, reprinted Dallas, 1980), pp. 161–162; *Leaves of Healing*, June 14, 1895, p. 563; *Zion Banner*, June 5, 1901, p. 54.

13. Dowie, *Leaves of Healing*, March 22, 1895, pp. 416, 407. The reporter was James L. Dwyer, "Elijah the Third," *American Mercury* 11 (1927):294.

14. Pierson, *Forward Movements*, pp. 394–400, and *The Holy Care of the Body* (New York, n.d.), pp. 5–6, 16. Moody's resistance is described in Waldvogel, " 'Overcoming Life,' " p. 123. For Benjamin B. Warfield, see his *Counterfeit Miracles: The Thomas Smyth Lectures* (New York, 1918). For other critiques by evangelical leaders, see Waldvogel, " 'Overcoming Life,' " pp. 129–133, 141–146; Cunningham, "Holiness to Healing," pp. 509–512.

15. [Sarah E. Parham], *The Life of Charles F. Parham: Founder of the Apostolic Faith Movement* (Baxter Springs, KS, 1930), pp. 32, 39, 68–69; Douglas J. Nelson, "For a Time Such as This: The Story of Bishop William J. Seymour and the Azusa Street Revival," Ph.D. diss., University of Birmingham, England, 1981, pp. 163, 166–167; *Apostolic Faith*, September 1906. *Latter Rain Evangel*, October, 1908, p. 1; *Pentecost*, August 1908, p. 1; *Evening Light and Church of God Evangel*, March 1, 1910, p. 8.

16. David Edwin Harrell, Jr., *All Things Are Possible: The Healing and Charismatic Revivals in Modern America* (Bloomington, IN, 1975), p. 6. The reminiscence is from A.W. Webber, "Revival of 1903 in Galena, Kansas," *Apostolic Faith* [Baxter Springs, KS], May 1944, p. 11. For autobiographical accounts, most of which describe healing and related phenomena, see Wayne E. Warner, ed., *Touched by the Fire: Eyewitness Accounts of the Early Twentieth-Century Pentecostal Revival* (Plainfield, NJ, 1978). See also Robert Mapes Anderson, *Vision of the Disinherited: The Making of American Pentecostalism* (New York, 1979), pp. 42, 48–49, 58–59, 93–96, 103–105, 150.

17. This is a brief summary of what was, in fact, a nuanced theological position. See, for example, William Hamner Piper, "The Covenant at Marah: Divine Healing in the Atonement," *Latter Rain Evangel*, March 1909, pp. 18–22; B. Freeman Lawrence, "Healing for the Body," *Pentecost*, April 1910, p. 5; Ralph Riggs, "The Great Physician," *Trust*, January 1915, pp. 12–17; F.F. Bosworth, "Is Healing for All?" *Exploits of Faith*, April 1929, pp. 1–6.

18. F.F. Bosworth, *Christ the Healer: Sermons on Divine Healing* (n.p., 1924), pp. 98–99; E.W. Kenyon, *Jesus the Healer*, p. 20, quoted in Charles Farah, Jr., "A Critical Analysis: The 'Roots and Fruits' of Faith-Formula Theology," *Pneuma: Journal of the Society for Pentecostal Studies* 13 (1981):6.

19. Lillian B. Yeomans, M.D., *Health and Healing* (1938, reprinted Springfield, MO, 1973), pp. 33–34, 56.

20. For the anxiety insiders felt, see, for example, *Evening Light and Church of God Evangel*, July 1, 1910, p. 8; Charles S. Price, *The Real Faith* (1940, reprinted Plainfield, NJ, 1972), pp. 7–8. For examples of outsiders' attacks on this score, see Rowland V. Bingham, *The Bible and the Body or Healing in the Scriptures* (Toronto, 1921), preface; and C.E. Putnam, *Modern Religio-Healing* (Chicago, 1924), pp. 157–159.

21. Maria B. Woodworth-Etter, *Divine Healing: Health for Body, Soul and Spirit* (Indianapolis, n.d. [ca. 1920]), pp. 1–4; Edith Shaw, "How God Taught Me the Principles of Faith," *Trust,* July 1915, pp. 16–17.

22. Gordon Lindsay, ed., *The John G. Lake Sermons on Dominion over Demons, Disease and Death* (Dallas, 1982 [sermon ca. 1910]), p. 108; Henry Proctor, "Christ Our Full Redemption," *Trust,* May-June, 1930, p. 14, for "resurrection Life" and "always rejoicing"; Carrie Judd Montgomery, *The Prayer of Faith* (Beulah Heights, CA, 1917), p. x, for "brain weariness"; Lillian Yeomans, M.D., *Healing from Heaven* (Springfield, MO, 1926), p. 46. For a tortured attempt to distinguish between natural deterioration and unnatural disease, see F.M. Britton, *Pentecostal Truth* (Royston, GA, 1919), pp. 91–93.

23. G.B. Studd, "Christ or Satan," *Upper Room,* November 1910, p. 3. For exorcism and folk beliefs, see W.H. Cossum, "Some Valuable Points," ibid., July 1910, p. 3; *John G. Lake Sermons,* p. 11; Frederick G. Henke, "The Gift of Tongues and Related Phenomena at the Present Day," *American Journal of Theology* 13 (1909):204. For demon typologies, see [William H. Piper?], "The Masterpiece of Satan," *Latter Rain Evangel,* March 1909, p. 13; "Anonymous," "A Helpful Discussion on Demon Obsession," ibid., December 1908, pp. 9–10.

24. For examples of the former, see Montgomery, *Prayer of Faith,* pp. 88–91; E.N. Bell, *Questions and Answers* (Springfield, MO, 1923), pp. 54–55; P.C. Nelson, *Does Christ Heal Today? Messages of Faith, Hope and Cheer for the Afflicted* (Enid, OK, 1941), appendix, p. "R." For examples of the latter, see Yeomans, *Healing from Heaven,* pp. 14, 69–72; Britton, *Pentecostal Truth,* p. 89; A.S. Worrell and John J. Scruby, *What Is Divine Healing?* (Dayton, OH, n.d.), p. 19.

25. Yeomans, *Healing from Heaven,* pp. 14, 19; *Evening Light and Church of God Evangel,* May 15, 1910, pp. 5–6; ibid., July 11, 1914, p. 1. Some of the nontheological reasons for hostility to medicine and physicians are suggested in Heath, " 'Apostle,' " pp. 103–105.

26. Lindsay, *Dowie,* pp. 214–218; Farah, "Critical Analysis," p. 4, and *From the Pinnacle of the Temple: Faith vs. Presumtion?* (Plainfield, NJ, n.d.), pp. 53–54, 121–122; Weston LaBarre, *They Shall Take up Serpents: Psychology of the Southern Snake-Handling Cult* (1962, reprinted New York, 1969), pp. 23–26, 46–50.

27. Bell, *Questions and Answers,* pp. 56–57, 82; Britton, *Pentecostal Truth,* pp. 92–93; Nelson, *Does Christ Heal,* appendix, p. V.

28. See, for example, "Broken Arm Healed," *Pentecost,* August 1908, p. 1, in which it is claimed that an enraged physician deliberately rebroke an arm that had been healed by prayer. However, it is risky to assume that references to physicians were necessarily factual. Clements notes that Pentecostal testimonials, like healing narratives in the New Testament, usually followed a pattern in which the first unit was the alleged helplessness of worldly physicians. "Faith Healing Narratives," pp. 15–39. See also Rudolf Bultmann, *Form Criticism: Two Essays on New Testament Research,* trans. Frederick C. Grant (1934, reprinted New York, 1962), pp. 37–39.

29. For proscriptions against chewing gum, etc., see *Book of Minutes . . . of the Church of God* (Cleveland, TN, n.d. [1922]),p. 278; *Pentecostal Holiness Advocate,* December 13, 1917, p. 7; *Church of God Evangel,* October 13, 1917, p. 2; ibid., November 10, 1917, p. 3; Vinson Synan,

The Holiness-Pentecostal Movement in the United States (Grand Rapids, MI, 1971), pp. 67, 180. Regarding "excess in the conjugal relation," see Gordon Lindsay, ed., *The Sermons of John Alexander Dowie: Champion of the Faith* (Dallas, 1979 [orig. sermon ca. 1900]), p. 101; "The Marriage Question," *Upper Room*, August 1909, p. 3; Nelson, "William J. Seymour," p. 78.

30. Harrell, *All Things Are Possible*, pp. 14–20.

31. L. Thomas Holdcroft, "The New Order of the Latter Rain," *Pneuma: Journal of the Society for Pentecostal Studies* 2 (1980):46–60; and Richard Riss, "The Latter Rain Movement of 1948," ibid., 4 (1982):32–45.

32. Bell, *Questions and Answers* (1923), p. 54; [Parham] *Parham* (1930), p. 33; Robert A. Brown, *Divine Healing* (New York, n.d. [ca. 1945]), p. 6.

33. Harrell, *All Things Are Possible*, chaps. 3–5; Hollenweger, *Pentecostals*, pp. 354–367.

34. W.V. Grant, "You can Have Whatever You Say," *Herald of Deliverance*, March 4, 1951, p. 7; [A.A. Allen ?], *Preministerial . . . Correspondence Courses* (Miracle Valley, AZ, n.d.), Course #1, p. 10; O.L. Jaggers, *Everlasting Physical and Spiritual Health* (Dexter, MO, 1949), pp. 108, 100, 110.

35. *Hall Deliverance Foundation 1980 Newsletter*, p. 5, regarding teeth; Harrell, *All Things Are Possible*, p. 87, 116, regarding cancers and halos; A.A. Allen, *Miracle Revival Recordings* #111, cited in Hollenweger, *Pentecostals*, p. 383, regarding demons; A.A. Allen, "Pastor's Wife Eats Anything," *Miracle Magazine*, June 1959, p. 8, regarding Pepsi.

36. Franklin Hall, "Deeper Experiences," *Divine Healing Newspaper*, July 1982, p. 8; "How I May Be a Believer" [tract]; "Catalogue of Writings." These (and much more) are available upon request from Hall Deliverance Foundation, Box 11157, Phoenix, AZ 85017. See also Harrell, *All Things Are Possible*, pp. 212–214.

37. Harrell, *All Things Are Possible*, chap. 8. Howard Elinson, "The Implications of Pentecostal Religion for Intellectualism, Politics, and Race Relations," *American Journal of Sociology* 70 (1965):403–415; Leslie K. Tarr, "Canadian Better Business Bureaus Warn against Humbard . . . ," *Christianity Today*, September 21, 1984, pp. 70–71.

38. There is no adequate study of prosperity evangelism. In addition to primary sources, I have drawn upon Harrell, *All Things Are Possible*, passim; Farah, "Critical Analysis" and *From the Pinnacle*; Vinson Synan, "Faith Formula Fuels Charismatic Controversy," *Christianity Today*, December 12, 1980, pp. 65–66.

39. Oral Roberts, *Miracle of Seed-Faith* (Tulsa, 1970), esp. p. 39; Kenneth Copeland, *The Laws of Prosperity* (Fort Worth, 1974), pp. 94–95, 13, 47; T.L. and Dr. Daisy Washburn Osborn, "Run with Winners," *Miracle Faith Digest*, July 1984, pp. 12–14. See also Kenneth E. Hagin, *"You Can Have What You Say"* (Tulsa, 1979), and "How God Taught Me about Prosperity," *Word of Faith*, September 1984, pp. 2–4, 10.

40. Copeland, *Laws of Prosperity*, pp. 10–11. For critiques of prosperity evangelism by Pentecostals, see Farah, *From the Pinnacle*; and Gordon D. Fee, "The 'Gospel' of Prosperity—an Alien Gospel," *Pentecostal Evangel*, June 24, 1979, pp. 5–8.

41. Gwen Jones, ed., *Conference on the Holy Spirit Digest*, 2 vols. (Springfield, MO, 1983), I:236, 250.

42. Lulu Carpenter, "Alcoholism a Disease?" *Pentecostal Evangel,* June 24, 1983, p. 31; Jimmy Swaggert, "Four Conditions for Being Included in the Rapture," ibid., September 12, 1982, pp. 19, 21; Charles T. Crabtree, *This I Believe* (Springfield, MO, 1982), p. 144.

43. Raymond T. Brock, *The Christ-Centered Family* (Springfield, MO, 1977), pp. 73–77; Betty Jane Grams, *Families Can Be Happy* (Springfield, MO, 1981), pp. 11–12, 49.

44. Richard D. Dobbins, "When Children Rule the Home," *Pentecostal Evangel,* March 21, 1982, p. 19. One writer found it necessary to remind Pentecostal parents not to kick, club, or "strike a child in the face." Grams, *Families,* p. 68.

45. For early and recent illustrations of death redefinition, see *Evening Light and Church of God Evangel,* March 1, 1910, p. 8; and Faith Campbell, *Stanley Frodsham: Prophet with a Pen* (Springfield, MO, 1974), pp. 138–141.

46. See, for example, C.M. Ward, "How to Avoid a Nervous Collapse," *Pentecostal Evangel,* April 25, 1976, pp. 4–5; Betty Swinford, "How I Avoided a Breakdown," ibid., July 21, 1974, pp. 8–9. See also Hollenweger's remarks on the role of psychiatrists (*Pentecostals,* pp. 380, 384), which my research confirms.

47. "Resolution on Abortion," *Church of God Evangel,* April 23, 1984, p. 23; *Assemblies of God General Presbytery Report on Homosexuality,* August 14, 1979, pp. 4–5, 9–10.

48. Pattison, "Faith Healing," pp. 398, 404; Clements, "Faith Healing Narratives," p. 38, and "Ritual Expectation," pp. 139–148; Poloma, *Charismatic Movement,* pp. 87–92.

49. Bill Popejoy, *The Case for Divine Healing* (Springfield, MO, 1976), pp. 33, 58–59; Pierre Hegy, "The Healing of Brokenness: A New Spirituality," *Journal for the Scientific Study of Religion* 17 (1978):181–184.

50. Charles S. Price, *The Real Faith* (1940, reprinted Plainfield, NJ, 1972), pp. 11–13; L. Thomas Holdcroft, *Divine Healing: A Comparative Study* (Springfield, MO, 1967), pp. 49–51; Kathryn Kuhlman, "Healing in the Spirit," *Christianity Today,* July 20, 1973, pp. 4–10.

51. Farah, *From the Pinnacle,* pp. 139–142; Richard G. Champion, "Our Greatest Obligation," *Pentecostal Evangel,* September 30, 1984, p. 3; G.M. Burge, "Problems in Healing Ministries within the Charismatic Context," paper presented to the Society for Pentecostal Studies, Cleveland, TN, November 1983.

52. Jones, ed., *Holy Spirit,* II: 292; Gordon Wright, "While We Wait for Healing," *Pentecostal Evangel,* September 30, 1984, pp. 4–5.

53. One indication of this change is that physicians are coveted as speakers in Pentecostal churches and meetings. See, for example, the address by K. Dewayne Piker, M.D., in Jones, ed., *Holy Spirit,* II:290–293.

54. Some of these developments are summarized in Poloma, *Charismatic Movement,* pp. 104–107; [Richard G. Champion], "Healing the Brokenhearted," *Pentecostal Evangel,* March 17, 1985, pp. 10–12; Philip Yancey, "The Ironies and Impact of PTL," *Christianity Today,* September 21, 1979, pp. 29–33; Mary McLendon, *Jim Bakker and Friends* (Charlotte, NC, 1981), pp. 60–67. See also the standard denominational histories, for which the handiest guide is Charles Edwin Jones, *Guide to the Study of the Pentecostal Movement,* 2 vols. (Metuchen, NJ, 1983).

55. Holly G. Miller, "Science and Prayer: Keys to the City of Faith," *Saturday Evening Post,* July-August 1979, pp. 22–26; "Obesity and Bias," *New York Times,* April 13, 1980; Peggy Wehmeyer, "Oral Roberts Opens His Tulsa Hospital," *Christianity Today,* December 11, 1981, pp. 41–42; Landrum R. Bolling, "Oral Roberts' 'Impossible Dream,'" *Saturday Evening Post,* September 1983, pp. 42–45, 110–111.
56. Lloyd Billingsley, "Oral Roberts . . . Asks for Money," *Christianity Today,* February 18, 1983, p. 29.
57. Amanda Smith, *Pentecost,* March 1910, p. 3.

CHAPTER 20

The

Afro-American

Traditions

ALBERT J. RABOTEAU

There are today approximately 28 million Afro-Americans in the United States, the vast majority of whom descend from 400,000 Africans enslaved in North America between 1619 and 1808, the year Congress ended the slave trade. Brutally separated from their homelands, Africans could not re-create their cultures in America. Nevertheless, they did transmit to their descendants fundamental perspectives about health, medicine, and religion, as well as a great deal of concrete lore and custom. African religious and medical traditions survived in a variety of folk traditions and even converged with some aspects of the Christian faith that black Americans adopted.

During the colonial period, Christianity made little headway among the slaves. Slaveowners were hostile or indifferent to instructing their slaves, and the efforts of missionaries were weak. The religious revivals that periodically swept parts of the nation in the last half of the eighteenth century first brought slaves to conversion in large numbers. The emotional preaching and plain doctrine of the Methodist and Baptist revivalists proved successful among black Americans during the era of the Revolution, when the Methodist denomination and some individual Baptists went on record against slavery.

These revivalistic denominations also attracted black members because they permitted black men to preach. As early as the 1770s, black preachers organized congregations of black Baptists. By the end of the century, black Methodists had followed suit, and in 1816 they formed themselves into an independent denomination, the African Methodist Episcopal Church. In the antebellum period, independent black churches grew in number and size throughout northern black communities. Most black Americans lived as slaves in the South, however, where they attended church, if at all, with whites. Some were allowed their own services, under white supervision. Occasionally, slaves met in secret to worship God free of white control.

Following Emancipation, the freedmen swarmed out of white-controlled churches to form their own. By the end of the century, the Baptists had taken the lead numerically, with the Methodists a distant second. But both had lost membership, after 1880, to a new religious movement called Holiness, which promoted the doctrine of complete sanctification and revived the emotional style of worship from which Methodists and Baptists had allegedly strayed. At the turn of the century, black Holiness church members took the lead in spreading a related movement known as Pentecostalism, which emphasized the experience of glossolalia (speaking in tongues) as evidence of the true faith.

By 1900, there were 2.7 million church members in a black population of 8.3 million. Of this number, the overwhelming majority was Protestant and rural. Until 1910, ninety percent of black America lived in the South. Starting in that decade and gaining momentum during World War I, rural blacks migrated to northern and western cities in steadily increasing numbers. Urbanization introduced black migrants to new religious movements, which took root in the hundreds of storefront and house churches that dotted the burgeoning black ghettos of the large cities. Spiritualism, heterodox versions of Judaism and Islam, and a host of leader-centered cults appealed to thousands of urban black folk disaffected from traditional Protestant Christianity. And, by mid-century, migrants from the Caribbean had introduced Cuban santeria and Haitian voodoo into the major cities of the country.

Despite the new religious options of urban America, the largest religious denominations among Afro-Americans remain those that they first adopted in the late eighteenth century, the Baptists and the Methodists, with the latter being challenged numerically by the rapidly growing Holiness-Pentecostal churches. Today, black Baptists number over nine million and black Methodists roughly four million. The churches constituting the black Holiness-Pentecostal family probably account for another four million members. Afro-Americans in white churches should be added to these figures, though most denominations do not report membership by race.

Because Afro-Americans belong to a variety of religious communities, their views on medicine and health have been shaped by many of the faith traditions treated in this volume. But alongside these faiths other religious traditions have endured—partly derived from Africa, partly developed in America—which have helped to form the attitudes of Afro-Americans toward health, sickness, and curing. These traditions, commonly called "folk beliefs" or more pejoratively, "superstitions," do not constitute a single creed—indeed, they are by nature eclectic— but they do convey several consistent and coherent perspectives about health and medicine. It is the goal of this essay to trace the African origins of these perspectives, their persistence in Afro-American culture, and their interaction with Christianity and other faith traditions adopted by black Americans from the period of slavery to the present.

The African Heritage

In the West and Central African societies from which the ancestors of black Americans came, religion, medicine, and magic constituted inter-related parts of coherent cultures, articulated in age-old myths and rituals in which Africans explained why the world was as it was and what to do if things went awry. Traditional African religions portrayed life as basically good. Ideally, in the natural order of things people should achieve health, fertility, prosperity, and status—in a word, ful-fillment. Actually, their world was filled with evil forces that might disturb the harmony of life and frustrate each individual's destiny by causing illness, barrenness, poverty, disgrace, or untimely death. The essence of religion (inclusive of medicine and magic), then, was to "prevent misfortune and maximize good fortune."[1]

Africans sought security in the world in two basic ways: by acquiring the protection of the gods and ancestors and by making use of protective charms and sacred medicines. God, the Supreme Creator, was believed to be benevolent but uninvolved in human affairs. It was his children, the gods, and the deceased ancestors who interceded in people's daily lives for good or ill. The gods resembled humans to the extent that they had personalities, likes, and dislikes. Unlike humans, they could control the forces of nature, with which they were frequently identified, and they held sway over the fate of individuals and communities. The ancestors too stood watch over the behavior of the society and the kinship groups that they had founded. Gods and ancestors had the power to reward those who pleased them and to punish those who angered them—not in some future world, but in the here and now. Placating them established and maintained harmony in the personal, natural, and social spheres of life.

In African cultures the person, nature, and society were seen as intimately connected. Africans conceived of the individual self, for example, as constituted by a web of kinship relations. Each person existed only in relation to a community. In this holistic view of the person, strained or broken social relations were the major cause of disease. Africans believed that anger, jealousy, and hatred, in a word, antisocial behavior, literally led to illness. An ordered and harmonious relationship with one's community, both present and past (as represented by the ancestors) was essential for health and well-being. Similarly, an ordered relationship with the forces of nature, personalized in the figures of the gods, was also essential for preserving the health of the community and the individual. In this traditional world view, aspects of life and nature that moderns view as impersonal were seen as personal and relational. Although Africans knew very well that illness had natural causes, they believed that, fundamentally, sickness resulted from discordant relations between the person and the natural or social worlds in which he or she lived. Long before western medicine recognized the fact, African traditional healers stressed that interpersonal relations affected people's health.

To maintain or restore harmony between the person, nature, and community, Africans turned to priests, diviners, mediums, and healers who were skilled in various methods of mediating divine power. Divine power became accessible to humans in three ways: possession, divination, and sacrifice. During religious festivals, the priests and mediums of the gods went into trance states, which they perceived as states of divine possession. The personality of the god temporarily displaced the personality of the medium, who then spoke to the community on behalf of the god. Trained in the lore of the god, the initiated medium danced out in religious festivals the movements and the character of her patron deity, literally "incarnating" the divinity and his or her power. The gods, through their mediums, diagnosed problems including illness, prescribed cures, and warned against future physical ailments or misfortunes. Typically, the deity's prescription for curing and preventing sickness included the offering of a ritual sacrifice.

Frequently, the divine message addressed the emotional as well as the physical problems of the medium's community. In describing the psychological impact of possession upon the medium herself, Benjamin Ray, a scholar of African religion, has suggested that the gods acted as "magnified symbols" of the people they possessed. Possession trances served, according to Ray, as occasions for "the devotee to express certain unconscious aspects of the self and to integrate his or her total personality."[2] A striking example of the psychological import of ceremonial spirit possession was recorded by Pierre Verger, an authority on the religion of the Yoruba in Nigeria and its cognates in Brazil. A woman who had lost all of her babies in childbirth became possessed by the god Ogun, who spoke through her the following message to the people of her town:

> See the new *iyaworisha* [medium]; it is *Ogun* that chose her. . . . It is because I have seen the death on her that I took her. Now she is not going to die; no more danger for her; she is going to have a lot of children, boys and girls. I am going to tell her father and her husband what they must do now. Because she is not the same any more; the husband must not beat her any more; he must leave her in peace. If the husband has anything to say, he must tell it to me. It is *Ogun* now who is the father. Everybody must hear, men and women.[3]

Although this incident occurred in the mid-twentieth century, the tradition it represents is centuries old. Possession served a therapeutic function in traditional African societies by placing people in contact with the power of the gods represented by the priests and mediums in possession trance. The gods in rituals of possession healed people of physical illness by revealing the causes of the disease and prescribing the appropriate sacrifices to cure it. Likewise, the gods cured social "sickness" in the community by empowering individuals to voice emotional problems and sometimes solutions.

Ritual sacrifice exemplified African belief in reciprocity between gods and people. Just as humans depended upon gods for protection and well-being, so gods depended on humans for food and praise. By offering sacrifice, people placated the gods and strengthened their power to help. Because the gods governed the forces of nature and the forces of life, people neglected them at considerable risk. In other words, humans had to pay careful attention to how they related to those forces in the world that lay ultimately beyond their control—such as wind, storm, lightning, drought, chance, accident, and disease. In addition to the gods, the ancestors required sacrifice and praise. As the founders of society and the inventors of its rules, the ancestors were especially concerned with the behavior of individuals in community. Whenever anyone acted selfishly or anti-socially, the ancestors' anger was roused. People, in other words, forgot the rules of social behavior at their own peril.

Thus, offering sacrifices to gods and ancestors symbolized the Africans' belief that people must attend carefully to their relationships with nature and society, because their happiness, their health, indeed their lives, depended on it. If things went awry, systems of divination— some complex, some simple—would reveal what the problem was and prescribe methods to set things right. Diviners were consulted by the sick or by those concerned to ward off illness. First the diviner discovered the cause of the disease and then instructed his client on the appropriate cure which usually required the patient to offer a sacrifice and to take herbal medicines. Frequently, diviners were skilled in the use of natural medicines and treated the client's malady themselves. The best protection, however, was prevention, for which there were charms to ward off all kinds of misfortune and disease.

Angry gods and disapproving ancestors might deflect any person's destiny from its proper course. So, too, might the ill will of others (including family and friends). To protect themselves from the evil unleashed, consciously or unconsciously, by human anger and jealousy, Africans turned primarily to sacred medicines, material charms that embodied spiritual power. These charms were assembled by experts who knew not only which material objects to use, but which rituals to enact in order to activate the spiritual power latent within the physical. Once activated, the spirit within the charm protected its owner against illness and misfortune unless overcome by the power of a stronger charm. Hence, the spirit within the charm needed to be strengthened by moistening it periodically with food and drink. These sacred medicines had a judicial, as well as protective, function. Once the litigants in a legal dispute, for example, agreed upon a settlement, they sealed their agreement by driving pieces of metal into the body of a charm. If either party later reneged, the spirit of the charm would hunt him down no matter how far he fled. When people cheated, lied, stole, or otherwise aggrandized themselves at the expense of others, they faced severe retribution from the spirits housed in communal charms. Sacred medicines, according to African belief, were given by God not only to protect individual well-being, but also to insure societal well-being. They were meant to heal the body social as well as the body personal.[4] Charms served as outer manifestations of the inner tensions within all societies, tensions exacerbated within small, intimate communities. The very family and friends who supported and inspired trust also threatened and created mistrust.

Africans knew that disease had physical causes, and they developed herbal medicines to treat them. African healers called upon a vast store of knowledge about medicinal roots, herbs, and leaves, which contemporary medical doctors in some areas of Africa have found well worth consulting. For the African traditional healer, however, medicine was not enough to effect a cure without the presence of ritual that made medicine effective. Ritual was necessary because illness and cure involved the spiritual, not just the material. Africans did not think that material causes were sufficient explanations for the source of illness, which they located in the anger of gods, the displeasure of ancestors, or the hatred of other people. In this world view, forces that the modern mind thinks of as impersonal—for example, nature, accident, probability, social tensions—were symbolized as personal. Because the experiences of the African ancestors of black Americans were so radically social and interpersonal, it is not surprising that they thought of health and medicine in personal, rather than impersonal, terms.[5]

Even though African religions were transformed by contact with Native American and European religions, slaves in the New World interpreted their experiences and dealt with their problems in many of the old, familiar ways. In Haitian voodoo and Cuban santeria, for example, the prevalence of African gods, spirit possession, ritual sacrifice, divination, and sacred medicines clearly demonstrate that African traits simply overpowered whatever features these Afro-Caribbean religions inherited from Christianity. As a result of religious and demographic factors that need not detain us here, African theology and ritual did not persist as fully in the United States as they did in the Caribbean and parts of Latin America. But the personal cosmology of African traditional thought with its emphasis on spirit possession and sacred medicines lived on in the worship of black "shouting" churches and in the practice of conjure.

Shouting Churches

It was no accident that slaves began converting to Christianity in large numbers during periods of revival. The revivals made Christianity attractive to more black Americans than ever before, because revivals encouraged ecstatic behavior, that is, the outward physical expression of religious experience, so reminiscent of African worship. Overcome by the emotional fervor of the revival meetings, converted sinners, white and black alike, wept, shouted, sang, jerked, danced, and fainted in response to the powerful pleas of the revival preachers. Slaves readily approved of these "physical exercises," as they were called, and quickly incorporated them into their regular religious services. In this ecstatic behavior, fostered by Protestant revivalism, the slaves discovered a Christian analogue to African spirit possession. To be sure, there were differences. The slaves believed that they were filled by the Holy Spirit, not possessed by Ogun or some other god. But the rhythmic drumming, repetitive singing, and constant dancing, characteristic of possession ceremonies in Africa, were replicated on the plantations of the antebellum South. Slaves used hands and feet to approximate the rhythms of the drum, they substituted spirituals for the hymns to the gods, and they danced in a counterclockwise circular ring, called the shout, the steps of which bore a striking resemblance to possession dances in Africa and the Caribbean.[6] When educated ministers tried to stamp out the practice after Emancipation, former slaves argued that the shout was "the essence of religion" and asserted that "without a ring, the Spirit will not come."[7]

Just as spirit possession was central to many African religions, the experience of conversion was essential to the revivalistic Protestantism that the slaves made their own. Hints in the historical record suggest that some slaves in Virginia in the 1830s thought of Christian conversion and baptism as similar to the initiation rituals of spirit possession. Henry Brown, a former slave from Virginia, remarked that when his sister "became anxious to have her soul converted" she "shaved the hair from her head, as many of the slaves thought they could not be converted without doing this."[8] Shaving the head of the initiate, according to African custom, prepared the individual for possession by his or her patron god.

Besides the ritual similarities between African spirit possession and Afro-American shouting traditions, there were important therapeutic similarities as well. As anthropologist I.M. Lewis has demonstrated in his book *Ecstatic Religion,* religious ecstasy offers individuals of low status—the poor, the oppressed, the alienated—an opportunity to experience power and to gain prestige as mediums of the divine in societies that block them from other channels to status. In the antebellum South, for example, black preachers converting white sinners, or at least moving them to tears with the force of their eloquence, represented important, if temporary, reversals of racial status.[9] Similarly, the prevalence of women as mediums in possession cults and as shouters in Protestant revival churches may be explained, at least partially, by the status attached to this role. The experience of the Spirit enhanced the self-esteem of the slave, surrounded by a world that constantly asserted his or her inferiority. The conversion narratives of former slaves attest to the deep emotional and psychological impact that the experience of conversion had upon them. Many who did not know the date of their actual birth recalled with pride the moment of their "rebirth."

Although conversion was an individual experience, the general pattern of the conversion accounts is consistent enough to justify a general outline. The individual feels weighted down with cares, worries, or sinfulness. She may be ill or severely depressed (common symptoms, too, for individuals chosen by the gods to become their mediums in African possession belief). Her condition worsens and she falls into a trance in which she perceives another self. This other or inner self faces death or damnation, frequently visualized as a deep, dark pit. Suddenly, a messenger, in the form of an angel, a "little man," or Jesus, saves her from annihilation and ushers her into the presence of God, who lovingly informs her that she is saved and chosen as one of his children. Awakening from the vision, the convert is filled with joy and feels totally renewed. In the words of Ogun cited earlier, "she is not the same anymore." Or, as the former slaves expressed it, "my hands and feet were new," and "I loved everything and everybody."

From sadness to joy, from darkness to light, the imagery of the conversion experience illustrated an experience of transformation in the inner life, the psyche of the converted slave. In this experience, slaves and their descendants internalized a sense of their own self-worth despite the degradation of slavery and discrimination. Conversion, in the words of anthropologist Paul Radin, represented "a new individuation, an inward reintegration," which served to preserve emotional wellness among countless Afro-Americans during slavery and after.[10] Conversion and the ecstatic experience of shouting frequently had a physical as well as emotional impact upon the convert. "Being made new" described the sense of well-being that came with conversion. "Sin-sickness," that is, states of nervousness, depression and lethargy, frequently associated with loss of sleep, appetite, and weight were replaced by feelings of vitality, energy, and health attached to a new sense of identity, purpose, and confidence.

Although conversion was fundamentally individual, shouting churches also had a significant impact on the emotional health of the community gathered for worship. A glimpse of this communal dimension was provided by a former slave, asked to describe what worship was like in the old days:

> The old meeting house caught on fire. The spirit was there. Every heart was beating in unison as we turned our minds to God to tell him of our sorrows here below. God saw our need and came to us. I used to wonder what made people shout, but now I don't. There is a joy on the inside, and it wells up so strong that we can't keep still. It is fire in the bones. Any time that fire touches a man, he will jump.[11]

In this context of worship, individuals transcended their troubles in the common ecstasy of worship. Some critics have condemned this type of religion as "compensatory" and "other-worldly," a distraction from political action. Whatever the merits or deficiencies of this criticism, who can gainsay the value of the shouting churches for relieving the pent-up frustration, the rage, the depression, and the anxiety of an enslaved and oppressed people? By giving them a sense of control over their own lives, independent of whites, the shouting churches served as an agency of emotional health for slaves and free blacks, helping to counter the destructive effects of racism upon human personality, effects that had physical as well as psychological consequences. Over the years following Emancipation, black shouting congregations were criticized as old-fashioned and ignorant. They were called "countrified" or "holy rollers." But even as educational levels rose and as rural blacks became urban, the hold of ecstatic religion remained firm. When one congregation became too sedate, there was always another in which the "old time" religion endured. For many black Americans the experience of the power of the spirit remained "the essence of religion" as well as a major source of emotional healing. And in some shouting churches, as we shall see, members believed that the spirit that had cured people in biblical times was miraculously healing their physical ills too.

Conjure

If the ring-shout represented the transformation of African spirit possession into Christian revivalism, conjure symbolized the translation of African sacred charms into Afro-American magical medicine. Conjure, also known as hoodoo or root-work, was widespread in the nineteenth-century South and still exists today wherever southern blacks have migrated. Conjure was grounded in the belief that illness was caused by the enmity of others. In this system of explanation, conjurers or root-workers were believed to have the power to make charms, for a fee, that could harm and even kill the intended victim.[12]

Charms consisted of various materials, but all were activated by spirits or forces that gave them power to harm or to cure. Some materials, such as graveyard dirt, which derived its power from being the spirit of the dead, were believed to make powerful charms. Similarly, any object that had been worn or used by the victim or pieces from his body, such as fingernail or hair clippings, were potent charms because they conveyed access to his or her spirit. Charms buried along a roadside or under a porch had the capacity to attack only the intended victim while leaving other passersby untouched. As in Africa, charms embodied spiritual power in the world of Afro-American conjure.[13]

It was axiomatic that a conjured person could only be cured by a conjurer. Other medicines and doctors were useless. If an illness proved resistant to treatment, or if a series of inexplicable mishaps struck, it was probable that the victim had been conjured by someone who hated him or her. Various techniques indicated whether conjure was involved or not, but the only remedy was to hire a conjurer to "lift the fix." In a rough kind of retributive justice, the conjurer could, upon request, turn the charm back upon its original sender.

Mysterious and feared figures in the black community, conjurers held the power to hurt or cure. Their gift came from a spiritual source: either God or the Devil. Usually distinguished by unusual features, such as red eyes or blue gums, conjurers or hoodoo doctors, as they were called, cultivated an aura of mystery which lent credibility to their craft. Unusual attire, crooked canes, and the conjure bag were the accoutrements of the trade of the old-time, rural conjurer. People believed that the conjurer could harm with a glance and that his knowledge was supernatural.

The first part of the conjurer's treatment was to determine whether a client was hexed or not. The conjurer might ask the client to hold a piece of silver in his or her hand for several minutes. If the metal turned black, it was a certain sign that the person had been conjured. Once it was established that the illness was due to conjure, the conjure doctor had to locate the charm. Chickens with frizzly feathers were particularly adept at digging up charms buried in front yards, but the conjurer could turn to many other methods for discovering the location of the charm victimizing his patient. After finding the charm, the conjurer analyzed its components and prepared a more powerful charm to counteract its effects. If the charmed object had somehow been introduced into the victim's body, the conjurer would remove it or give the patient an antidote to ingest. One of the more gruesome—and frequently described—symptoms that conjurers alleviated for their clients was the feeling that snakes, spiders, or lizards were roaming around inside their bodies. In case after case, witnesses claimed to have observed conjurers expelling live reptiles from people.

Besides curing victims of conjure, the hoodoo doctors made charms to ward off danger of disease and ill fortune. They also read the signs, that is, interpreted what meaning natural events, such as an owl's screeching, had for people's lives. The multifaceted skills of the conjurer were described by Rosanha Frazier, a former slave from Mississippi, who blamed the loss of her eyesight upon conjure:

> Dey powder up de rattle offen de snake and tie it up in de little old bag and dey do divilment with it. Dey git old scorpion and make bad medicine. Dey git dirt out de graveyard and dat dirt, after dey speak on it, would make you go crazy.
>
> When dey wants conjure you, dey sneak round and git de hair combin' or de finger or tonail, or anything natural 'bout you body and woks de hoodo on it.
>
> Dey make de straw man or de clay man and dey puts de pin in he leg and you leg gwineter git hurt or sore jus' where dey puts de pin. Iffen dey puts de pin through de heart you gwineter die . . .
>
> Dey make de charm to wear round de neck or de ankle and dey make de love powder too out de vine, what grow in de wood. Dey bites de leaves and powders 'em. Dey sho' works, I done try 'em.[14]

Faith in conjure survived incidents of failure. If one conjurer's charms didn't work, the client chose another. Then, too, a clever conjurer could always excuse failure by blaming the client for misunderstanding instructions. Even the skeptical could be driven by necessity to suspend disbelief. Moreover, conjure did work. Many conjurers were skilled herbalists. They put their knowledge of medicinal (and poisonous) plants and roots to use. Conjurers were also adept observers of human nature and resolved many of their clients' problems, especially those of the heart, by sound advice if not by magic potion. Finally, whether one appeals to automatic suggestion or para-psychological phenomena as an explanation, the conjurer's charms worked because people believed they would work.[15]

In part, conjure appealed to people because of its explanatory power. Why does someone fall ill? Why do accidents happen? To these questions conjure supplied an answer: because of the hostility of others. This answer became all the more convincing when medicine failed, or when the victim showed unusual symptoms, such as mental disorder, that seemed to have no physical cause. Conjure also appealed to people who distrusted or could not afford medical doctors. The emotional relief that came from receiving a diagnosis and the reassuring confidence of the conjurer must have gone a long way toward helping a patient wondering whether he or she had been "fixed." Some conjurers even offered their patients control over the future by "reading the signs" for coming events.

Furthermore, conjure presented a forum for people to vent their feelings about others—the petty jealousies, grudges, and sheer ill-will to which all communities fall prey. Feelings that could never be expressed openly could be stated secretly (and effectively) by means of conjure. Although slaves, for example, disagreed about the possibility of conjuring whites, some tried. They did so in order to avoid punishment, to gain better treatment, and to get revenge. For a largely powerless people, conjure functioned as a symbolic assertion of power. In story after story, black folklore celebrated the ability of conjurers to manipulate whites as well as blacks. The fictional triumph of the conjurer in these stories was a source of vicarious enjoyment and power for people who experienced little of either in real life. The counter-cultural strain in conjure was revealed by the universal description of conjurers as "African" and the assertion that Africa was a place of powerful magic. The contention that the white doctor's medicine was useless against the charms of the black conjurer represented a subtle but effective rejection of white supremacy in matters medical and magical. And the sight of white clients patiently waiting upon the skills of black conjurers proved the same point.[16]

Like conjure, Christianity offered the slaves and their descendents an explanation for disease and misfortune couched in a personal idiom. Illness was due to the will of God, the malevolence of Satan, the commission of sin, or all of these. The relationship of conjure to

Christianity was ambiguous. Some people dichotomized the two, making conjure the realm of the Devil and Christianity the realm of the Lord. Others spoke of conjure in either naturalistic terms, as an ability due to accident of birth (being born with a caul, the seventh son of a seventh son, after twins), or in supernatural terms, as a gift from God. On the practical level, conjure and Christianity were complementary. Christianity offered a language rich in the vocabulary of morality, a language well suited for describing the ultimate cause of things and the ultimate end of history, a language in which personal salvation and ritual commerce with the Supreme Being were well articulated. For all that, Christianity as a language suffered from an impoverished vocabulary for describing how one could make one's way securely in this world. Day-to-day concerns, such as fertility, health, sustenance, good fortune, and personal relationships were the primary issues for conjure. While these concerns were not absent from the ethical norms of Christianity, personal morality and personal salvation took primacy of place. Protestantism had underdeveloped ritual technology for dealing with such everyday realities as security and danger.

It was precisely those functions—explanation of misfortune, effective cure of illness, prediction and control of future events, and symbolic expression of social conflict—that conjure fulfilled and that the Protestant vocabulary failed to address (until the development of Holiness-Pentecostal Protestantism in the late nineteenth century, as we shall see). To effect cures, Protestantism offered prayer; to know the future, dreams or randomly selected scripture verses. For relief of social tension, proscriptions against scratching the very itch that needed scratching, that is, no "backbiting," no coveting, no fighting. Christianity as a language was dominated by a syntactical structure of right and wrong. Yet there were experiences in life that fell outside the categories of morality, experiences of danger and safety or the threat of power and the use of power in a "dog eat dog" world, for example. These formed the syntactic structure, as it were, of conjure. Slaves (and their descendents), practical realists that they were, spoke both languages, Christianity and conjure, depending upon which proved more appropriate to the particular concern at hand.

A World of Spirits

Conjurers claimed the ability to cure illness by manipulating the power or spirit enveloped in material charms. The whole system of conjure rested upon the fundamental belief that the world is suffused with spiritual forces, including things that moderns view as inanimate. Conjurers instructed their clientele to moisten their charms with liquor in order to "feed" them and so keep up their strength. Charms embodied some of the spirit of the sender, augmented by the powers wrapped within the charm. From this perspective, it made perfect sense for a conjure woman named Mymee to refer to her protective charm as "Li'l Mymee." This sense that the world is populated with spirits has undergirded Afro-American folk beliefs about witches, ghosts, and graves from the nineteenth century down to the present.[17]

Witchcraft, Afro-Americans believed, caused illnesses, especially those associated with symptoms of exhaustion, loss of weight, and lethargic behavior—all of which were attributed to witches who left their bodies at night, turned their victims into animals, and rode them wherever they willed. Constant tiredness was a sure symptom of "being rid by haunts." Weight loss indicated an even more serious malady—one's soul was being consumed by a witch. Antidotes to witchcraft varied. Two of the most popular took advantage of the witch's obsession with counting. A sieve placed at the door before retiring or newsprint pasted on the wall would prevent a witch from attacking, because she could never count all the holes in the sieve or all the letters in the newspaper before sunrise robbed her of her power. If the skin of a sleeping witch could be found and rubbed with cayenne pepper or salt while she roamed at night, the skin would shrink and the soul of the witch would not be able to fit back into her body when she returned. Those suspected of witchcraft usually turned out to be elderly women, persons living apart from the community, or individuals perceived as different.[18]

Besides witches, the nocturnal world was populated by the souls of the dead and by the souls of the living, both of which could roam the world, thus causing people to dream. For this reason, it was dangerous to sweep dirt out of the house after dark, lest one disturb a wandering spirit. Bottles were sometimes hung on tree branches to catch and entrap ghosts until sunrise could destroy them. Even today, bottle trees can still be seen in sections of the South.[19]

Much of the witchcraft and ghost lore of black Americans closely paralleled that of white Americans, but several distinctive funeral customs indicate that they thought differently about the dead. Grave decorations for black Americans have differed significantly from those of whites. In addition to the standard headstone and cross, the graves of American black communities have been marked with shells, mirrors, lamps, and the possessions of the deceased. These objects, as art historian Robert Farris Thompson persuasively argues, reflect funeral customs derived from Central Africa. Their presence suggests that Afro-American beliefs about the dead have been heavily influenced by the cosmology of the Kongo region, the source of perhaps one-third of North American slaves.[20] In Kongo thought, the world of the dead, characterized by wisdom, mirrors the world of the living, characterized by energy. The worlds are joined by spirits of the dead who reenter the world through reincarnation in children. The living can contact the world of the spirits through the door to their world, the grave.

In both Kongo and Afro-American practice, the grave was customarily marked out by an enclosure, formed by a border of bottles, shells, or other materials such as wood or concrete. The enclosure was intended to protect the deceased from intrusion by outsiders and to guard the living from the awesome power of the dead. Mirrors and glass embedded in Afro-American gravestones reflected the Kongo concept that the boundary between this world and the other is water, which is both transparent and reflects light. The flash of light playing on the glass illustrated the belief that the underworld was the world of sight, of understanding, represented by the color white. Lamps placed on black American graves lit the way of the dead to the underworld, especially those who died at night. Pipes or culverts, stuck in the grave, acted as channels for communication to pass between the other world and this. Representations of white chickens symbolized the ancestors and the mediation of sacrifice by which the power of the spirits was invoked. Trees planted on the graves reminded the living that the spirits were immortal. Shells, covering the graves, "stand for the sea," according to Bessie Jones, a descendent of slaves from the Sea Islands of Georgia. "The sea," she explained, "brought us; the sea shall take us back. So the shells upon our graves stand for water, the means of glory and the land of demise." Placing the last object used by the deceased upon the grave, "lays the spirit," that is, prevents the person from returning to get them. The grave, then, has been viewed as a crucial space in black folk-culture, the place of passage between this world and the next, a passage, however, that leads two ways. The spirits of the dead, in this tradition, are not gone and buried; they are buried and accessible.[21]

Another tradition that encouraged black Americans to commune with the spirits of the dead developed out of mid-nineteenth-century Americans' interest in mesmerism, spirit rapping, and clairvoyance. Spiritualism, like Kongo religion, taught that the world of matter and the world of spirit interpenetrate. Indeed, matter was simply the lowest form of spirit and spirit the highest form of matter. Those gifted with clairvoyance could see beyond the realm of matter to the world of spirit, and the spirits of the dead could communicate with the living by means of trance mediums, speaking on their behalf. Through mediums, the spirits gave advice, diagnosed illnesses, and prescribed therapies for those still entrapped in the less refined material world.

The spiritualist movement by its very nature tended to be unstructured, based in independent congregations, and centered on individual mediums. As a result, it is impossible to date the beginnings of organized spiritualism among black Americans. However on July 29, 1865, the following spiritualist advertisement appeared in the *Christian Recorder,* the official organ of the African Methodist Episcopal Church.

> The services of Madame Julian, a remarkable (and only public colored) Clairvoyant and Trance Medium, have been secured, who will give diagnosis and prescriptions for diseases in the abnormal condition.

Self-promotion may have led Madame Julian to claim to be the only black spiritualist professional. During the late nineteenth century, spiritualist ideas spread in black America, and during the first decade of the twentieth century black spiritualist churches began to appear in Chicago, New Orleans, and other cities. These churches added elements of belief and ritual from the Baptist, Holiness, Pentecostal, and Roman Catholic traditions to spiritualism. The world of the spirits was nothing if not eclectic.[22]

The Faith That Heals

While mainline Christian churches in the last decades of the nineteenth century were criticizing clairvoyant seers and entranced mediums as heretics and humbugs, a new movement in American Christianity, Holiness, was reemphasizing the role of the Holy Spirit in the experience of Christians. Typical of the conflict between these two spirit-oriented religions is the following account of a conversion from one to the other:

> A brother who had been a spiritualist medium and who was so possessed with demons that he had no rest, and was on the point of committing suicide, was instantly delivered of demon power. He then sought God for the pardon of his sins and sanctification, and is now filled with a different spirit.[23]

The Holiness movement and the Pentecostal tradition that developed from it in the early twentieth century stressed that Christians in the modern world, no less than those of the apostolic period, should receive the Holy Spirit and the gifts that accompanied his presence. These gifts, as outlined in 1 *Corinthians* 12:4–11, consisted of speaking in unknown tongues, prophesying, interpreting, performing miracles, and healing. Black Christians actively participated in the Holiness movements and led the 1906 Azusa Street revival in Los Angeles from which Pentecostalism spread.

The centrality of healing in Holiness-Pentecostal piety is illustrated by the following reports published on the first page of the first issue of *The Apostolic Faith,* the newspaper of the Azusa Street revival:

Many have laid aside their glasses and had their eye sight perfectly restored. The deaf have had the hearing restored. . . . A man was healed of asthma of twenty years standing. Many have been healed of heart trouble. . . . A little girl who walked with crutches and had tuberculosis of the bones, as the doctors declared, was healed and dropped her crutches and began to skip about the yard.[24]

Sickness, *The Apostolic Faith* declared, resulted from original sin, and because Christ had atoned for sin, he had freed Christians from illness which is "of the devil."[25] The power to cast out demons, given by Jesus to his disciples, past and present, included the power to cast out the diseases that demons caused. Preachers and evangelists transmitted the healing power of the Spirit by the laying on of hands. Healing in the Holiness-Pentecostal tradition came also by anointing with oil, by using blessed water, and by applying prayer cloths to the sick body.

One had only to listen to broadcasts of Holiness or Pentecostal church services on black radio stations to learn how important physical and emotional healing is to this faith tradition. Given the poverty of many black Americans and the high cost of medical care, given the cultural distance between black communities and predominantly white medical facilities, given the lack of rapport between black patients and white medical professionals, it is not surprising that alternate forms of healing became important for Afro-Americans, especially in the days when black doctors were rare.

The sanctified church, as those in the Holiness-Pentecostal tradition were called, offered health directly through faith healing and indirectly through moral codes and styles of worship. Sanctification required that church members refrain from tobacco, alcohol, narcotics, gambling, and "worldly" amusements. Thus alcoholism, drug addiction, and tobacco-related diseases were combatted by the ethical rules of the sanctified community. Honesty, thrift, hard work, and discipline were encouraged. This pattern of behavior gave order, structure, and meaning to people's everyday lives. In other words, sanctification, as preached in Holiness-Pentecostal churches, gave to black Americans, many of them poor and oppressed, a coherent set of values by which they could order their lives. These values promoted upward mobility (within the limits of discrimination) and enhanced the communal identity of "the saints," thus helping them to stave off the anomie and hopelessness that ghetto life produced.

Proscribing secular entertainment, the sanctified churches became little social worlds that replaced the recreational excitement denied members in the outside world. The music and the ecstasy of their churches offered tired and downtrodden people a catharsis that was truly "recreative." These black "saints" believed the Gospel adage "Your faith has made you whole" and applied it to the body as well as the soul. In the ecstasy of worship they reaffirmed their belief experientially. The healing effects of faith proved to them that their faith was real. Although the Holiness and Pentecostal revivalists taught that there was only "one faith and one spirit" by which people were to be saved, black Americans in the twentieth century confronted a bewildering array of faiths, each promising health in its own way.

Therapeutic Pluralism

Among the many new religions black people encountered in an increasingly pluralistic America, two represented the outright rejection of Christianity as a religion for whites only. Black Jews and Black Muslims, despite their considerable differences, were united in preaching a new religio-racial identity for American blacks. Black people were not Negroes, Afro-Americans, or Colored; their true identity, stolen from them by slavery, was, alternately, Muslim or Jewish. Black people were really "Moors," according to the Moorish Science Temple; "the lost tribe of Shabazz," according to the Nation of Islam; or the "descendents of the lost tribes," according to various groups of black Jews. These mythic histories symbolized a strong rejection by blacks of the dominant racist stereotypes depicting them as descendents of "primitive" Africans. The new identity, in each case, was buttressed by new rituals and new laws. Consumption of liquor, tobacco, and pork was forbidden, as was dancing and other displays of so-called "black culture," especially emotional worship. Cleanliness, sobriety, honesty, and industry were stressed. Like the sanctified congregations, Black Muslims and Black Jews created an effective ethic of social control with great potential for transforming the lives of individuals. *The Autobiography of Malcolm X* is only one of many testimonials to the ability of the Muslims to rehabilitate convicts, addicts, and alcoholics. Health and diet were major concerns of Elijah Muhammad (1897–1975), long-time leader of the Nation of Islam, who attacked "unclean" foods and habits forced upon black people by slavery and exhorted his disciples to adopt the healthful diets and life-style of the Muslims. In a weekly newspaper column, he offered detailed advice on "How to Eat to Live." A diet of one meal a day, eaten at the same hour, consisting mainly of "vegetables, fruits, pure fresh milk, and pure whole wheat bread," would, according to Elijah Muhammad, prolong life and cure many diseases. Meat, fatty foods, and foods prepared in grease or oil were to be avoided entirely or eaten sparingly. This natural diet which Allah had intended for mankind had been corrupted by the unrighteous. As a result, the human life-span had grown shorter and people suffered all kinds of illnesses brought on by excessive eating and unhealthy foods. Disease, Messenger Muhammad explained, could be alleviated by diet because "we get all our energy and our health through eating and drinking." Even "poison germs" picked up from the atmosphere "can be removed from our bodies most of the time—by eating the proper foods at the proper time." Birth control was condemned by the Black Muslims as racial suicide because whites outnumbered blacks in America by a ratio of nine to one. Although critical of some physicians for commercialization, Elijah Muhammad and the Nation of Islam favored medical science and advertised for "highly learned doctors" to set up a department of medicine in their projected Islamic University. They also planned to establish a hospital under the auspices of the Nation.[26]

Some Afro-Americans sought salvation not in these new and heterodox versions of Islam and Judaism, but in a number of religious communities gathered around new messiahs. The best known nationally was Father Divine (1877–1965), who was credited by his followers with having the power to heal regardless of the distance. Numerous testimonials from converts claimed that the mere mention of his name or meditating upon his benevolence had cured them of tuberculosis, heart trouble, paralysis, and other ailments. Divine, influenced by the positive thinking philosophy of the New Thought movement, taught his disciples that illness and death resulted from failures in faith. If the faithful simply thought of Father during times of trouble, their problems would vanish. The more faithfully they lived his teachings, the closer they came to divinity and immortality. The followers of Divine avoided alcohol, tobacco, gambling, racial prejudice (including even the mention of race), and sexual intercourse. As the testimony of one convert reveals, bodily healing and moral reformation coincided in the person of Father Divine:

> I want to tell the people . . . what my Father did for me. I had a sinful body and a wicked soul. I had weak lungs, bad kidneys, and a nervous breakdown. For three years I had been getting worser and worser. When he came into my life I realized he was God and was made whole. Now, I have no heart trouble, no lung trouble, and no nerve trouble. I was a great adulteress, never without a boy friend or a husband. I don't need these now as Father Divine gives me everything I want.[27]

Father Divine offered salvation in this world. His interracial communities or "heavens," as they were called, became famous for their sumptuous banquets, which were served even during the worst years of the Depression as visible proof of Father's beneficence. Flamboyant as Father Divine seemed, his mission, as he expressed it to a hostile black critic, appealed to thousands and inspired a movement that survived his death: "Because your god would not feed the people, I came and I am feeding them. Because your god kept such as you segregated and discriminated, I came and I am unifying all nations together. That is why I came, because I did not believe in your god."[28] Divine's emphasis on this-worldly salvation from disease, from hunger, from poverty, and from discrimination addressed the discontent of those tired of deferring happiness to some other world.

The desire to control one's own destiny, including health and prosperity, prompted some blacks to turn to the occult, the mysterious lore of the supernatural known only to the initiated. *Occult* as a term covers a great variety of beliefs and practices, from mail-order magic to tarot cards, from High-John the Conqueror root to palmistry, from blessed candles to astrology.[29] They all, however, have one thing in common: a technology of the supernatural. Devotees feel that with the right expertise, they can use secret knowledge to solve problems and avoid misfortune. In every sizable black community, occult professionals and occult shops promise their clientele diagnosis, treatment, and prognosis for every conceivable illness. "Spiritual Advisors" columns in the black popular press advertise the services and the wares of contemporary conjurers, healers, and seers. Ironically, the very success of modern scientific technology has seemingly influenced some people to search for security in occult systems of knowledge that science long ago displaced or discredited.

African Gods in America

In a world that seems to grow increasingly impersonal and bureaucratically controlled, is it any wonder that people adhere to personal cosmology and personal control offered by traditional religions? The traditional religions of Africa, brought to mid-twentieth-century America by immigrants from Cuba, Puerto Rico, and Haiti, have spread to cities across the country. In American santeria and voodoo centers, the gods of Africa are worshipped today as they have been for centuries.

Santeria and voodoo are syntheses of African religions and Roman Catholicism created by slaves and their descendants in Cuba and Haiti. The term *santeria* refers to an essential aspect of these religions, namely, the veneration of African gods identified with Catholic saints. Similarly, *voodoo* derives from the word *vodun,* which means divinity among the Fon people of Dahomey. The gods or saints rule the lives and destinies of humans and need to be propitiated by praise and sacrifice so that they will guard their devotees from illness and misfortune.

Initiation places the individual in close and continuing contact with his or her patron god and makes the god's power accessible. In santeria, a seriously ill person may undergo initiation in order to be cured and strengthened by his or her saint.

Possession, sacrifice, and divination occur in New York, as well as in Haiti, Cuba, and Nigeria and with similar therapeutic effects. Possessed santeros (santeria initiates) may heal the members of their community by channeling to them the power of the gods. Diviners can diagnose illness and prescribe cures by manipulating sea shells or pieces of coconut rind. Cures usually involve prayer and sacrifices to one or more of the gods depending upon the nature of the illness. Chickens and other animals make the best sacrifices because blood is believed to be the most powerful source of energy, but even smoking a cigar or lighting a candle releases energy (smoke, light, heat) which may be offered to invoke the aid of the saints. Food offered to the gods may be shared among the faithful who view it as an especially powerful medicine for restoring or preserving health.

Voodoo priests and initiated santeros possess a great deal of knowledge about medicinal herbs and frequently prescribe potions, teas, ointments, and other treatments for sick patients. A recent book on santeria describes santeros using herbal medicines to treat a wide range of diseases and disorders, including cancer, epilepsy, headache, earache, syphilis, dysentery, sunstroke, cuts, and fractured bones.[30] Knowledge and power to heal, however, derives ultimately from the gods. So the santeros and voodooists take care to maintain altars for the gods and to honor their presence represented by statues, holy pictures, and other emblems. They arrange elaborate celebrations to observe the annual feast days of the gods confident that in return the gods bless them with good health and happiness.

How well the gods will continue to serve their people in the modern world is an open question. But African religions have shown an amazing resiliency because of their ability to absorb and transform traditions from other sources. A graphic example of their resilience is the *botanica* or religious-goods store that can be found in black and Hispanic sections of most major cities. Within the *botanicas,* statues of the saints, herbal medicines, emblems of African gods, spiritualist books, blessed candles, and tarot cards all crowd the shelves. The *botanica* symbolizes the plurality of religious traditions that have informed Afro-American attitudes about health and suggests that some have valued therapeutic pluralism, whatever their denominational identity.

Conclusion: Modern Medicine and Traditional Thought

For much of their history, therapeutic pluralism in the form of alternative forms of medicine was a necessity for black Americans because they had limited access to modern medical treatment. During slavery, the master decided whether an ill slave's condition warranted a doctor's care. After Emancipation, freedmen were left to seek out medical assistance on their own in a world where scientific medicine was overwhelmingly the preserve of whites. This situation began to change slowly as black medical schools were founded and began producing an increasing number of black physicians in the last three decades of the century. Between 1869 and 1907, twelve black medical colleges were founded. However, only two of these, Howard and Meharry, survived, and most of the rest lasted only a few years. Founded by freedmen's aid societies or the missionary organizations of northern white churches, the black medical schools could not be sustained by an impoverished black community and depended heavily upon the philanthropy of northern whites. When these funds proved inadequate or simply dried up, the schools closed. Between 1890 and 1910, the number of black doctors in the United States increased from 909 to 3,077, due mainly to the black medical schools. The demise of many of these schools undoubtedly decreased the opportunity for medical education among black Americans. Between 1910 and 1950, the number of black physicians rose from 3,077 to 3,660, an increase of a mere 583 doctors over a period of forty years! Today there are over 13,000 black physicians in the United States. Black doctors have played a crucial role in the delivery of scientific medical care to the black community. They have also served as important symbols of the rise of an oppressed people to a new level of education, professionalism, and power.[31]

Although most contemporary black Americans share the assumptions of modern medical theory and practice, the old religious magical medical ways live on. They live on because they continue to offer effective physical and psychological healing to thousands of patients dissatisfied with or deprived of scientific diagnosis and treatment. Certainly, the majority of churchgoing black Americans identify themselves as Protestant and would, if asked, condemn conjure and other forms of folk belief as supersitition or worse. Yet herbalism, conjure, spiritualism, and other alternate forms of healing still thrive in black communities, urban as well as rural, because for many people they meet needs that Christianity does not. Nor does belief in Christianity necessarily conflict with these alternate traditions in their minds. One and the same person may turn to God, a medical doctor, and a root worker or conjurer for relief from illness, with no sense of inconsistency. And those who do perceive some conflict may prefer pluralistic therapy to intellectual consistency. Traditional beliefs persist in the modern world because they reflect a view of life that many people find more adequate to their experience than science. Because they experience life as primarily personal, or at least think that it should be so, they regard their relationships with other persons, divine and human, as the ultimate cause of health and sickness. For them, explanations that identify viruses as the causes of illness might seem valid but incomplete.

Ultimately, the question "Why does anyone become ill?" is, like the problem of evil, a religious issue, beyond the scope of medicine. Yet, scientific and traditional medicine can agree upon one important belief: Health and healing depend profoundly on one's relations to the other persons with whom life is shared.

Notes

1. Willy Decraemer, Jan Vansina, and Rene Fox, "Religious Movements in Central Africa," *Comparative Studies of Society and History* 18 (1976):460–461, 467–468.
2. Benjamin C. Ray, *African Religions: Symbol, Ritual, and Community* (Englewood Cliffs, NJ, 1976), p. 70.
3. Cited in Ray, *African Religions,* pp. 68–69.
4. Robert Farris Thompson and Joseph Cornet, *The Four Moments of the Sun: Kongo Art in Two Worlds* (Washington, DC, 1981), pp. 37–41.
5. Robin Horton, "African Traditional Thought and Western Science," *Africa* 37 (1967):50–71, 155–187.
6. Albert J. Raboteau, *Slave Religion: The "Invisible Institution" in the Antebellum South* (New York, 1978), pp. 59–72.
7. Cited in Raboteau, *Slave Religion,* p. 69.
8. Charles Stearn, *Narrative of Henry Box Brown* (Boston, 1849), pp. 17–18.
9. I.M. Lewis, *Ecstatic Religion: An Anthropological Study of Spirit Possession and Shamanism* (Baltimore, 1971); Raboteau, *Slave Religion,* pp. 314–317.
10. Clifton H. Johnson, ed., *God Struck Me Dead: Religious Conversion Experiences and Autobiographies of Ex-slaves* (Philadelphia, 1969), p. vii.
11. Johnson, ed. *God Struck Me Dead,* p. 74.
12. Loudell F. Snow, "Folk Medical Beliefs and Their Implications for Care of Patients," *Annals of Internal Medicine* 81 (1974):82–96; Hans A. Baer, "Toward a Systematic Typology of Black Folk Healers," *Phylon* 43 (1982):327–343.
13. Raboteau, *Slave Religion,* pp. 275–278.
14. Cited in Raboteau, *Slave Religion,* pp. 277–278.
15. Leonora Herron and Alice M. Bacon, "Conjuring and Conjure-Doctors," *Southern Workman* 24 (1895):117–118, 193–194, 209–211; Raboteau, *Slave Religion,* pp. 281–282.
16. Eliott J. Gorn, "Folk Beliefs of the Slave Community," unpublished manuscript; Newbell Niles Puckett, *Magic and Folk Beliefs of the South-*

ern Negro (New York, n.d.), p. 275; Eugene D. Genovese, *Roll, Jordan, Roll: The World the Slaves Made* (New York, 1974), pp. 217–218.

17. Puckett, *Magic and Folk Beliefs*, pp. 232–234; Ruth Bass, "Mojo," in *Mother Wit from the Laughing Barrel: Readings in the Interpretation of Afro-American Folklore*, ed. Alan Dundes (Englewood Cliffs, NJ, 1973), pp. 380–387.

18. Savannah Unit, Georgia Writers' Project, Works Progress Administration, *Drums and Shadows: Survival Studies Among the Georgia Coastal Negroes* (Athens, GA, 1940); "Hags and Their Ways," *Southern Workman* 23 (1894):27.

19. Thompson, *Four Moments*, pp. 178–181.

20. Ibid., pp. 181–203; Robert Farris Thompson, *Flash of the Spirit: African and Afro-American Art and Philosophy* (New York, 1983), pp. 132–142.

21. *Drums and Shadows*, p. 128; Frances Butler Leigh, *Ten Years on a Georgia Plantation Since the War* (London, 1883), p. 77; Thompson, *Four Moments*, p. 200.

22. Hans A. Baer, *The Black Spiritual Movement: A Religious Response to Racism* (Knoxville, TN, 1984), pp. 17–30.

23. *The Apostolic Faith* 1 (September 1906):1.

24. Ibid.

25. Ibid. 1 (September 1907):2.

26. *Muhammad Speaks*, April 21, 1967, p. 11.

27. Cited in Robert Weisbrot, *Father Divine and the Struggle for Racial Equality* (Urbana, IL, 1984), p. 82.

28. Arthur Huff Fauset, *Black Gods of the Metropolis: Negro Cults in the Urban North* (Philadelphia, 1944), pp. 52–67; Weisbrot, *Father Divine*, pp. 8, 62–64.

29. Loudell F. Snow, "Mail Order Magic: The Commercial Exploitation of Folk Belief," *Journal of the Folklore Institute* 16 (1979):44–74.

30. Migene Gonzalez-Wippler, *Santeria: African Magic in Latin America* (New York, 1973), pp. 70–75.

31. Todd L. Savitt, "The Education of Black Physicians at Shaw University, 1882–1918," in *Black Americans in North Carolina and the South*, eds. Jeffrey J. Crow and Flora J. Hatley (Chapel Hill, NC, 1984), pp. 160–188; Savitt, "Lincoln University Medical Department—A Forgotten 19th Century Black Medical School," *The Journal of the History of Medicine and Allied Sciences* 40 (1985):42–65; Herbert M. Morais, *The History of the Afro-American in Medicine* (Washington, DC, 1976), pp. 40–48.

A Guide to

Further Reading

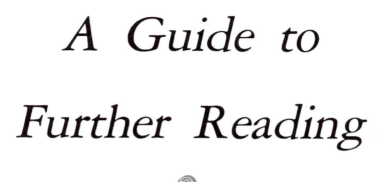

Despite a wealth of publications on medicine and religion, historical surveys of the subject are rare. In 1973 Morton T. Kelsey brought out *Healing and Christianity: In Ancient Thought and Modern Times* (New York), described on the jacket as "the first comprehensive history of sacramental healing in the Christian church from biblical times to the present." Although it provides a useful introduction to the subject, the author's theological agenda—"to offer a rationale for practicing healing in the church today"—mars its value as history. His selection of sources relating to the early centuries of Christianity, for example, distorts the attitudes of the Church Fathers toward suffering, sickness, and healing. A more critical, though less comprehensive, look at the subject can be found in W.J. Sheils, ed., *The Church and Healing,* volume 19 of *Studies in Church History* (Oxford, 1982), a collection of twenty-two essays originally presented to the Ecclesiastical History Society. *Health/Medicine and the Faith Traditions* (Philadelphia, 1982), a volume edited by Martin E. Marty and Kenneth L. Vaux, includes a 110-page survey of medicine and religion from pre-Christian antiquity to the present. On the Quaker tradition, which unfortunately is not covered in the present volume, see Robert A. Clark and J. Russell Elkinton, *The Quaker Heritage in Medicine* (Pacific Grove, CA, 1978).

The Jewish Tradition

Readers interested in a brief overview of the history and ideology of Judaism would probably do best by consulting general encyclopedia articles on the subject. A more thorough, but highly readable, intro-duction can be found in Robert M. Seltzer, *Jewish People, Jewish Thought: The Jewish Experience in History* (New York, 1980).

While many of the medieval and modern primary sources on Jewish medical ethics (especially the responsa) are available only in Hebrew, some of the central texts of the Jewish tradition have now appeared in English. They include the Hebrew Bible (available in many trans-lations); the *Mishnah* translated and annotated by Philip Blackman, 6 vols. (London, 1951–1956); the *Talmud*, 18 vols. (London, 1935); and Maimonides' *Mishneh Torah*, translated as *The Code of Maimonides*, 21 vols. (New Haven and London, 1949–1979).

The first, and still the most comprehensive, treatment of Jewish bioethics is *Jewish Medical Ethics* by Immanuel Jakobovits (New York, 1959). That is a good source for many of the primary materials, but one must be aware that it is written from an Orthodox point of view. A good presentation of the varying views of contemporary Jews on medical issues can be found in Alex J. Goldman, *Judaism Confronts Contemporary Issues* (New York, 1978).

There is a paucity of material on the history of the development of Jewish medical thought and practice. Two works that treat the history of medicine in Judaism during biblical and talmudic times are more collections of sources than histories: Fred Rosner, *Medicine in the Bible and Talmud* (New York, 1977), and Julius Preuss, *Biblical and Talmudic Medicine,* trans. Fred Rosner (New York, 1978). A much more historically aware treatment of these issues, for the Middle Ages, is *Jewish Magic and Superstition* by Joshua Trachtenberg (New York, 1939, reprinted 1961). A collection of interesting and, at times, resourceful articles on specific aspects of Jewish medical history can be found in Harry Frie-denwald, *The Jews and Medicine,* 2 vols. (Baltimore, 1944). A history of Jewish medical practice in the modern, scientific era has not yet been written.

The Early Christian Tradition

Histories of the early church abound. F.F. Bruce, *New Testament History* (Garden City, NY, 1972) provides a reliable survey of the New Testament church. The most recent comprehensive treatment of the early centuries of Christianity is by W.H.C. Frend, *The Rise of Christianity* (Philadel-phia, 1984). This volume has thorough narrative bibliographies at the end of each chapter, which greatly enhance its value. More specialized studies that help to provide one with an understanding of the spiritual, theological, and social context of issues of health and healing in the early church are J.N.D. Kelly, *Early Christian Doctrines,* 5th ed. (New

York, 1976); Bernard Cooke, *Ministry to Word and Sacraments: History and Theology* (Philadelphia, 1976); Igino Giordani, *The Social Message of the Early Church Fathers,* trans. Alba I. Zizzamia (Boston, 1977); and E.R. Dodds, *Pagan and Christian in an Age of Anxiety* (New York, 1970).

On healing and faith in early Christianity, the following works are useful: Klaus Seybold and Ulrich B. Mueller, *Sickness and Healing,* trans. Douglas W. Stott (Nashville, 1978), is a critical discussion of the understanding of sickness and healing in the Old and New Testaments. Victor G. Dawe, *The Attitude of the Ancient Church Toward Sickness and Healing* (unpublished Th.D. dissertation, Boston University School of Theology, 1955) deals with both the New Testament and the early church (first four centuries). Evelyn Frost, *Christian Healing: A Consideration of the Place of Spiritual Healing in the Church of Today in the Light of the Doctrine and Practice of the Ante-Nicene Church,* 2nd ed. (London, 1954) is especially valuable as a collection of pertinent statements of primary sources.

The Medieval Catholic Tradition

The Catholic Church was such an integral part of all facets of life in the Middle Ages that a general introduction to the medieval ethos is extremely helpful for the nonspecialist. Francis Oakley, *The Medieval Experience: Foundations of Western Cultural Singularity* (New York, 1974), provides a short but exceedingly insightful orientation. R.W. Southern, *Western Society and the Church in the Middle Ages* (Baltimore, 1970), is a very reliable guide to the history of medieval Catholicism.

On healing and faith, the following works are useful: Peter Brown, *The Cult of the Saints: Its Rise and Function in Latin Christianity* (Chicago, 1981), is a creative and sensitive analysis of the development of the cult of saints and relics from the late fourth through the sixth centuries. Broader in scope, both chronologically and thematically, is Jonathan Sumption, *Pilgrimage: An Image of Medieval Religion* (Totowa, NJ, 1975). Ronald C. Finucane, *Miracles and Pilgrims: Popular Beliefs in Medieval England* (Totowa, NJ, 1977), examines the miracle registers of seven English and two French shrines between 1066 and 1300. The perspicacious introductory and concluding sections of Benedicta Ward, *Miracles and the Medieval Mind: Theory, Record and Event, 1000–1215* (Philadelphia, 1982), make this work a temporally broader guide to the place of the miraculous in medieval society than the title indicates.

Insight into medieval attitudes toward health and sickness can be enhanced by an examination of the history of a disease that had a special religious significance during the Middle Ages, as provided by S.N. Brody, *The Disease of the Soul: Leprosy in Medieval Literature* (Ithaca, NY, 1974).

There is no single, reliable survey of medieval medical history. Numerous regional or national studies are available, the majority of which are not in English. The following three quite different volumes, although they focus on England, make some comparisons and contrasts with continental practices: Wilfrid Bonser, *The Medical Background of Anglo-Saxon England: A Study in History, Psychology and Folklore* (London, 1963); C.H. Talbot, *Medicine in Medieval England* (London, 1967); and Edward J. Kealey, *Medieval Medicus: A Social History of Anglo-Norman Medicine* (Baltimore, 1981).

The Roman Catholic Tradition Since 1545

The most recent general history of the Roman Catholic Church since Trent can be found in the last three volumes of Roger Aubert et al., eds., *Nouvelle histoire de l'église*, 5 vols. (Paris, 1963–1975); so far only the fifth volume has appeared in English (London, 1978). This broad treatment can best be supported by special studies, of which John Bossy, *The English Catholic Community, 1570–1850* (New York, 1976) and James Hennesey, *American Catholics: A History of the Roman Catholic Community in the United States* (New York, 1981) stand as excellent examples.

There is no satisfactory treatment in English of casuistry and moral theology during the tridentine period; the best source remains the manuals themselves, notably the good summary in Alphonsus Liguori, *Compendium theologiae moralis* (Rome, 1849). An excellent monograph on the relationship between parish priest and people is Timothy Tackett, *Priest and Parish in Eighteenth-Century France* (Princeton, NJ, 1977).

A good introduction to the development of modern sexual mores at a formative stage is C.B. Paris, *Marriage in Seventeenth-Century Catholicism* (Montreal, 1975). On the final rite of passage, the overarching study by Philippe Aries, *The Hour of Our Death*, trans. Helen Weaver (New York, 1981), provides, from a variety of sources, insight into tridentine patterns of thought and action.

Health care was and continues to be a strong concern of tridentine Catholics. Useful treatments of the early period include William A. Christian, Jr., *Local Religion in Sixteenth-Century Spain* (Princeton, NJ, 1981) and Carlo M. Cipolla, *Faith, Reason, and the Plague in Seventeenth-Century Tuscany* (Ithaca, NY, 1979). On miraculous healings, see Thomas A. Kselman, *Miracles and Prophecies in Nineteenth-Century France* (New Brunswick, NJ, 1983) and R.T. Trotter and J.A. Chaviera,

Curanderesmo (Athens, GA, 1981), which looks at faith healing in a contemporary setting. On the development of medical ethics, see David F. Kelly, *The Emergence of Roman Catholic Medical Ethics in North America* (New York, 1979).

The Eastern Orthodox Tradition

For a general introductory overview of the life, teaching, history, faith, practice, and worship of the Orthodox Church, two books are especially valuable: Timothy Ware, *The Orthodox Church,* rev. ed. (New York, 1980) and Fotios K. Litsas, ed., *A Companion to the Greek Orthodox Church* (New York, 1984).

A ground-breaking book that revised the impression that Eastern Orthodoxy lacked a history of social involvement is Demetrios J. Constantelos, *Byzantine Philanthropy and Social Welfare* (New Brunswick, NJ, 1968), which provides a wealth of information regarding Byzantine philanthropy, especially as it addressed illness.

On Byzantine medicine, see John Scarborough, ed., *Byzantine Medicine,* vol. 38 of the *Dumbarton Oaks Papers* (Washington, DC, 1984), and Timothy S. Miller, *The Birth of the Hospital in the Byzantine Empire* (Baltimore, 1985). Also useful is Harry J. Magoulias, "The Lives of the Saints as Sources of Data for the History of Byzantine Medicine in the Sixth and Seventh Centuries," *Byzantinische Zeitschrift* 57 (1964):127–150.

Little has been written in the area of bioethics from the perspective of Eastern Orthodox Christianity, but see Stanley S. Harakas' survey in *The Encyclopedia of Bioethics* (New York, 1978), 1:347–355, which has been republished in booklet form under the title *For the Health of Body and Soul* (Brookline, MA, 1980). See also his *Contemporary Moral Issues Facing the Orthodox Christian,* rev. ed. (Minneapolis, 1982) and *Let Mercy Abound: Social Concern in the Greek Orthodox Church* (Brookline, MA, 1983), which address a number of bioethical issues.

The Lutheran Tradition

Luther's extensive writings are readily available in modern English translation in *Luther's Works,* 55 vols. (Philadelphia, 1955–), edited by Helmut Lehmann and Jaroslav Pelikan. The first twenty-nine volumes are composed of Luther's biblical lectures and commentaries. The latter part of the set includes his tracts, sermons, and letters. The Lutheran Confessions are also available in English translation, by Theodore G. Tappert, *The Book of Concord* (Philadelphia, 1959). Of special interest is the collection of Luther's reflections and advice on all areas of wellness and illness: Theodore G. Tappert, ed., *Luther: Letters of Spiritual Counsel* (Philadelphia, 1955).

Among the overwhelming amount of secondary literature on Luther, the Lutheran Confessions, and the history of Lutheranism, two volumes are particularly helpful: Vilmos Vajta, ed., *The Lutheran Church Past and Present* (Minneapolis, 1977); and Eric W. Gritsch and Robert W. Jenson, *Lutheranism: The Theological Movement and Its Confessional Writings* (Philadelphia, 1976). The Vajta volume contains eighteen essays by leading Lutheran scholars on the faith, life, and history of the Lutheran churches. Its usefulness is further enhanced by the inclusion of a bibliography, statistics of the Lutheran churches worldwide as of 1976, and a list of addresses of important Lutheran agencies and organizations. The Gritsch and Jenson volume is an excellent, succinct introduction to what the authors, both Lutheran seminary professors, term the "Lutheran option in ecumenical Christianity." A valuable reference work containing sketches of Lutheran history, institutions, persons, and beliefs is Julius Bodensieck, ed., *The Encyclopedia of the Lutheran Church,* 3 vols. (Philadelphia, 1965). A recent effort to assess Lutheran convictions and attitudes on the basis of information from a scientifically selected sample of laity and clergy has been edited by Roger A. Johnson, *Views from the Pews: Christian Beliefs and Attitudes* (Philadelphia, 1983). The contributors are leading Lutheran sociologists and theologians.

The only comprehensive volume on Lutheran health concerns, attitudes, and practices is Martin E. Marty, *Health and Medicine in the Lutheran Tradition* (New York, 1983). Specific aspects of Luther's contributions to health issues are explored by two European scholars. Aarne Siirala, a Finnish Luther-scholar teaching in Canada, relates psychotherapeutic healing and salvation, medicine and theology, from the standpoint of his experience in medical and pastoral work in *The Voice of Illness: A Study in Therapy and Prophecy* (Philadelphia, 1964). The famous Hamburg theologian and preacher Helmut Thielicke discusses life and death from his own experiences and biblical reflections arising out of World War II in *Living with Death,* trans. Geoffrey W. Bromily (Grand Rapids, MI, 1983). This is a revision of Thielicke's earlier volume *Death and Life* and includes an excursus, "Human Death in Luther."

The Reformed Tradition

For background on the Reformed tradition, the late John T. McNeill's *The History and Character of Calvinism* (New York, 1954) is a valuable introduction, as is McNeill's *A History of the Cure of Souls* (New York,

1951), which places the approach of this particular tradition to matters of faith and caring in the larger Christian tradition. Richard Baxter in "Directions for the Sick," *The Practical Works of Richard Baxter,* 4 vols. (London, 1954), 1:522–547, gives a detailed analysis of the seventeenth-century Puritan approach to health and healing. Cotton Mather in *The Angel of Bethesda,* ed. Gordon W. Jones (Barre, MA, 1972), a younger contemporary of Baxter, wrote the earliest and longest treatise on medicine in the American colonies, although the volume was not published until the twentieth century. Seward Hiltner, a twentieth-century American and a pivotal figure in the field of health, healing, and pastoral counseling, published *Religion and Health* (New York, 1943) and *Preface to Pastoral Theology* (Nashville, 1958). James Gustafson in *The Contribution of Theology to Medical Ethics* (Milwaukee, 1975), Kenneth Vaux in *Health and Medicine in the Reformed Tradition* (New York, 1984), and William F. May in *The Physician's Covenant: Images of the Healer in Medical Ethics* (Philadelphia, 1985) continue to explore dimensions of this subject from the perspective of the Reformed tradition.

American Presbyterian denominations have taken some leadership in exploring the relationship between faith and problems of modern medicine, as in the case of the Presbyterian Church in the United States (now the Presbyterian Church [U.S.A.]) *The Nature and Value of Life* (Atlanta, 1981) and the United Presbyterian Church in the United States of America (now Presbyterian Church [U.S.A.]) *The Relation of Christian Faith to Health* (New York, 1960).

The Anglican Tradition

For a history of the Church of England from the sixteenth century to the present, along with some explanation of the Anglican Communion, see Stephen Neil, *Anglicanism* (Harmondsworth, 1958). There is no adequate history of the Episcopal church, but James Thayer Addison's *The Episcopal Church in the United States, 1789–1930* (New York, 1951) is helpful.

Fundamental to an understanding of basic attitudes toward health and medicine in the Anglican tradition are the Books of Common Prayer. See especially *The Book of Common Prayer 1559: The Elizabethan Prayer Book,* ed. John E. Booty (Charlottesville, VA, 1976), which has explanatory notes as well as text; *The Book of Common Prayer* [1979] (New York, published since 1976), the current order of worship of the Episcopal Church; and *Prayer Book Studies* (New York, 1950–), an ongoing series of publications of the Standing Liturgical Commission of the Episcopal church.

Of great importance for the history of health and medicine are the reports of the Lambeth Conference of Bishops from 1867 to 1978. Collections of documents from these conferences will be found in *The Six Lambeth Conferences, 1867–1920* (London, 1920), compiled by Lord Davidson of Lambeth, and *The Reports of the 1920, 1930, and 1948 Conferences, with Selected Resolutions from the Conferences of 1867, 1888, 1897, and 1908* (London, 1948). For the Episcopal church, see *General Convention: Journals of the Protestant Episcopal Church in the United States of America,* published since 1789. More specifically concerned with health and medicine is *Church and Society: Social Policy of the Episcopal Church,* Executive Council and General Convention, December 1967–April 1979 (New York, n.d.).

There is a valuable collection of essays in *The Church and Healing,* ed. W.J. Sheils, *Studies in Church History,* vol. 19 (Oxford, 1982). Charles W. Gusmer has presented a detailed study concentrating on healing and the prayer book in *The Ministry of Healing in the Church of England: An Ecumenical-Liturgical Study,* Alcuin Club Collections, No. 56 (Great Wakering, 1974). Lawrence Stone's *The Family, Sex, and Marriage in England, 1500–1800* (New York, 1977) is a massive study of importance for any consideration of health and the Anglican tradition. Narrower in scope, but still of value, is Michael MacDonald's *Mystical Bedlam: Madness, Anxiety, and Healing in Seventeenth-Century England* (Cambridge, 1981).

The Anabaptist Tradition

For the general history of Anabaptism, one can do no better than to consult George H. Williams, *The Radical Reformation* (Philadelphia, 1963), still the most comprehensive history of the whole movement, even though more recent research has dated some of its conclusions. [C. Henry] *Smith's Story of the Mennonites* (Newton, KS, 1981), edited by C. Krahn, provides the most detailed information on Mennonites, Hutterites, and Amish from the seventeenth century to the present.

The four-volume *Mennonite Encyclopedia* (Scottdale, PA, 1955–1959), edited by H.S. Bender and C. Krahn, includes articles on medicine, hospitals, and deaconesses—virtually the only published histories of these subjects. A second reference work, *Mennonite Bibliography 1631–1961,* edited by N. Springer and A.J. Klassen, 2 vols. (Scottdale, PA, 1977), lists all Mennonite, Hutterite, and Amish literature according to geographical region. Extensive author and subject indexes make this a major research tool.

Anabaptism in Outline: Selected Primary Sources, introduced and edited by W. Klaassen (Kitchener, Ont. and Scottdale, PA, 1981), the

third volume of the series *Classics of the Radical Reformation,* comprises the most comprehensive collection of Anabaptist source materials available at present and contains a selected bibliography of secondary literature. D.F. Durnbaugh's *The Believers' Church: The History and Character of Radical Protestantism* (London, 1968), a historical and theological work, deals with major aspects of the Anabaptist tradition in both descriptive and analytical fashion.

In an innovative and interesting study, *Anabaptists Four Centuries Later* (Scottdale, PA, 1975), J.H. Kauffman and L. Harder demonstrate both continuity and discontinuity between modern Mennonites and their sixteenth-century predecessors. The most important modern studies of the Hutterites and Amish are two historical and sociological volumes by John A. Hostetler: *Amish Society* (Baltimore, 1963) and *Hutterite Society* (Baltimore, 1974).

The January 1982, issue of the *Mennonite Quarterly Review* (vol. 56) is devoted entirely to articles on the history and theory of Mennonite mental-health activities, written by persons closely associated with that work. A comprehensive history of Anabaptist involvement in medical matters remains to be written.

The Baptist Tradition

The best general history of the Baptists is Robert G. Torbet, *A History of the Baptists,* 3rd ed. (Valley Forge, PA, 1980). It is comprehensive in scope, covering current issues in Baptist historiography as well as providing a good overview of Baptist origins and development. An excellent collection of primary sources in Baptist history is William H. Brackney, ed., *Baptist Life and Thought: 1600–1980* (Valley Forge, PA, 1983). To sort out some of the differences between Baptists in America, one should consult Samuel S. Hill, Jr. and Robert G. Torbet, *Baptists North and South* (Valley Forge, PA, 1964).

No book exists on Baptist health and medical practices per se, though some work has been done on the role of medicine in Baptist missions. Franklin T. Fowler, "The History of Southern Baptist Medical Missions," *Baptist History and Heritage* 10 (1975):194–203, relates the southern Baptist experience; and John Spencer Carman, *Rats, Plague, and Religion: Stories of Medical Mission Work in India* (Philadelphia, 1936), describes some of the unique problems facing western Christian doctors in an eastern religious and cultural setting.

Rufus Spain, *At Ease in Zion: A Social History of Southern Baptists, 1865–1900* (Nashville, 1961), and George Kelsey, *Social Ethics Among Southern Baptists, 1917–1969* (Metuchen, NJ, 1973), document how Baptists in the American South translated some of their health concerns, especially those relating to alcohol and tobacco, into overt political action. Unfortunately, nothing of a similar nature has been done on northern Baptists.

On the subject of the spiritual dimensions of physical suffering, the classic work (1652) is Roger Williams, *Experiments of Spiritual Life and Health*, ed. Winthrop Hudson (Philadelphia, 1951), written to his wife after a severe illness nearly took her life. Also helpful is Edwin Scott Gaustad, ed., *Baptist Piety: The Last Will and Testament of Obadiah Holmes* (Grand Rapids, MI, 1978), which shows how a persecuted Baptist pioneer handled suffering. In Billy Graham, *Till Armageddon: Perspectives on Suffering* (Waco, TX, 1981), there is a more recent view by the twentieth century's most famous Baptist clergyman. For a controversial and atypical Baptist approach to faith healing, there is A.J. Gordon, *The Ministry of Healing* (Houston, 1882).

The Wesleyan-Methodist Tradition

Essential primary sources on the origins and character of Methodism include *The Works of John Wesley* (the critical edition of which is edited by Frank Baker and published by Oxford University Press, then Abingdon Press), and the doctrinal and organizational regulations of the church from 1743 to the present, several of which are found in *The Book of Discipline of the United Methodist Church, 1972* (Nashville, 1972). John Wesley's handbook of medical remedies, *Primitive Physick,* is a key document for understanding his views about medicine and health and is available in an uncritical edition entitled *Primitive Remedies* (Beverly Hills, CA, 1973).

The best biography of Wesley is that by V.H.H. Green, *John Wesley* (London, 1964), and Richard P. Heitzenrater has recently provided a thoughtful, documentary review of past and present attempts to understand Wesley, as well as called for major new studies of his life and thought in *The Elusive Mr. Wesley*, 2 vols. (Nashville, 1984).

Modern histories of Methodism tend to focus on developments in England and America. Especially valuable are several of the essays in the integrated collection edited by Rupert Davies and Gordon Rupp, *A History of the Methodist Church in Great Britain*, 3 vols. (London, 1965–1983). Also helpful, but less consistent in quality and coherence, is Emory Stevens Bucke, ed., *The History of American Methodism*, 3 vols. (New York, 1964). Social and intellectual developments within Methodist history are also explored in the three volumes published under the title *Methodism and Society:* Richard M. Cameron, *Methodism and Society in Historical Perspective* (New York, 1961), Walter G. Muelder, *Methodism and Society in the Twentieth Century* (New York,

1961), and S. Paul Schilling, *Methodism and Society in Theological Perspective* (New York, 1960).

Given the important place of medicine and health in the Methodist tradition, it is remarkable that so little research has focused on these aspects of Methodist history. Except for John Wesley's career and the temperance and prohibition campaigns, topics regarding both healing and health have been essentially unresearched in the Methodist heritage.

The Unitarian and Universalist Traditions

Russell Miller's two-volume encyclopedic history of Universalism, *The Larger Hope* (Boston, 1979, 1985), which surveys the entire North American history of the movement; and Ernest Cassara, *Universalism in America: A Documentary History of a Liberal Faith* (Boston, 1971) provide the best sources for the reader wishing to explore the Universalist tradition.

Unitarianism lacks a comprehensive history; however, C. Conrad Wright, *The Beginnings of Unitarianism in America* (Boston, 1953), stands as a classic, unsurpassed in its critical analysis of the decline of Puritanism, the rise of Arminian theology, and the eventual development of Unitarianism. Octavius Brooks Frothingham's *Boston Unitarianism: 1820–1850* (New York, 1890) focuses on the ministry of Frothingham's father, a representative example of the conservative faction of Boston ministers. Daniel Walker Howe, *The Unitarian Conscience: Harvard Moral Philosophy, 1805–1861* (Cambridge, MA., 1970), surveys the major leaders on the conservative side of the denomination during its first half-century and provides superb notes on original sources.

There is no systematic examination of health and medicine for either tradition or the merged denomination. Gerald N. Grob's recent biography, *Edward Jarvis and the Medical World of the Nineteenth Century* (Knoxville, TN, 1978), details the life of a Concord-born Unitarian physician, close associate of major nineteenth-century ministers, and a leader in a variety of causes (public health, mental illness, temperance) in which large numbers of Unitarians and Universalists participated. *The Collected Works of William Ellery Channing* (Boston, 1885) includes numerous sermons and lectures reflecting Channing's progressive attitude toward such issues as health, work, temperance, ministries to the poor, and freedom of thought.

Two recently reprinted works by women reformers within the movement offer additional progressive perspectives on issues relating to sexuality and women's development. Antoinette Brown Blackwell's *The Sexes Throughout Nature* (1875, reprinted Westport, CT, 1976) challenges the sexist assumptions of other well-meaning writers of the period. Elizabeth Blackwell, *Essays in Medical Sociology*, 2 vols. (1902, reprinted New York, 1972) discusses in frank detail "The Human Element in Sex" and "Conscience in Medicine," among other issues. Thomas Wentworth Higginson's *Outdoor Papers* (Boston, 1863) reflects the earlier views of Theodore Parker and Charles Follen regarding the importance of exercise, care of the body, and the relation of religion to good health. Harriet Martineau, an English Unitarian and noted author, who visited American Unitarians in the 1830s, later wrote *Life in the Sick-Room* (Boston, 1844) reflecting upon her own extended illness.

The Disciples of Christ-Church of Christ Tradition

The best general history of the Disciples of Christ is William E. Tucker and Lester G. McAllister, *Journal in Faith* (St. Louis, 1975). David Edwin Harrell, Jr. is the author of a two-volume social history of the Disciples: *Quest for a Christian America* (Nashville, 1966) and *The Social Sources of Division in the Disciples of Christ 1865–1900* (Athens, GA, 1973). A sketchy study of the social views of Disciples, useful mostly for the twentieth century, is James A. Crain, *The Development of Social Ideas Among the Disciples of Christ* (St. Louis, 1963). A doctoral dissertation that documents the paucity of material on health themes in early Disciples literature is William C. Creasy, "A Study of the Development of the Popular Motives of Health, Wealth, Power and Success in Practical Theology of the Early Disciples of Christ," Doctor of Divinity thesis, Vanderbilt University, 1971.

The best broad sampling of Alexander Campbell's thought may be found in Alexander Campbell, *Popular Lectures and Addresses* (Philadelphia, 1863). The official record of the Christian Church (Disciples of Christ) is the *Yearbook and Directory of the Christian Church (Disciples of Christ)* (publication information varies), which has been published since 1885.

In the absence of a strong central organization through much of the movement's history, Disciples thought must be traced largely through the numerous religious periodicals its preachers have published. In the first generation, the most important were Alexander Campbell's two magazines, *The Christian Baptist* (1823–1830) and *The Millennial Harbinger* (1830–1870); and Barton Stone's *Christian Messenger* (1826–1845). Two of the most important later journals have been indexed: *The Christian–Evangelist Index, 1863–1958*, 3 vols. (St. Louis, 1962) and *Christian Standard Index, 1866–1966*, 6 vols. (Nashville, 1972). The most popular conservative journal of the twentieth century is the *Gospel Advocate* (1855–present).

The Mormon Tradition

The best general histories of The Church of Jesus Christ of Latter-day Saints are Leonard J. Arrington and Davis Bitton, *The Mormon Experience: A History of the Latter-day Saints* (New York, 1979), a thematic history written for a non-Mormon audience; and James B. Allen and Glenn M. Leonard, *The Story of the Latter-day Saints* (Salt Lake City, 1976), a detailed chronological history aimed at a Mormon audience.

Recent scholarly studies on sub-themes broadly related to health and medicine are Lawrence Foster, *Religion and Sexuality: Three American Communal Experiments of the Nineteenth Century* (New York, 1981), which compares Mormons, Shakers, and Oneida Perfectionists; and Klaus J. Hansen, *Mormonism and the American Experience* (Chicago, 1981), especially chapters 3 and 5 on death and sexuality.

The best works specifically on Mormon health and medicine are the two issues of *Dialogue: A Journal of Mormon Thought* devoted to the subject. The first, Volume XII, Number 3 (Autumn 1979), includes essays on the herbal medicine tradition among the Mormons, Brigham Young's views on physicians, the non-Mormon view of nineteenth-century Mormon health, the initial Mormon encounter with cholera, and Mormon medical–ethical guidelines. The second, *Dialogue,* Volume XIV, Number 3 (Fall 1981), has essays on the initial context and later history of Mormonism's health code, the Word of Wisdom.

The recent appearance of *The Journal of Collegium Aesculapium,* a semiannual publication of the newly formed Brigham Young University Academy of Medicine, also has provided a regular forum for those interested in issues of health and medicine within the Mormon context. Initial issues (December 1983, July 1984) have included, among others, thoughtful essays on quackery among the Mormons, the church and international health, Mormon health, and moral issues for LDS physicians.

Additional secondary works of value include Ralph T. Richards, *Of Medicine, Hospitals, and Doctors* (Salt Lake City, 1953), which was the first book-length survey of health and medicine in Utah; and Robert T. Divett, *Medicine and the Mormons: An Introduction to the History of Latter-day Saint Health Care* (Bountiful, UT, 1981), which is the most recent. The latter, an uneven work both in coverage and analysis, is useful because it incorporates into a single work the substance of several important secondary sources. It also includes an excellent bibliography.

An important primary source is *The Doctrine and Covenants of the Church of Jesus Christ of Latter-day Saints* (Salt Lake City, 1981), originally published as *Doctrine and Covenants of the Church of the Latter Day Saints: Carefully Selected from the Revelations of God* (Kirtland, OH, 1835) and recently reprinted (Independence, MO, 1971). The Word of Wisdom appears in this as Section 89 (1981 edition); passing health-related references are found in several other places, including Section 42 on faith healing and the use of herbs; Sections 24, 35, 46, 66, and 84 on faith healing; and Section 49 on the use of meat. Some minor variations in wording appeared over the years, and the numbers assigned to the sections have varied.

The Christian Science Tradition

Although there is no standard history of Christian Science, Norman Beasley's *The Cross and the Crown: The History of Christian Science,* (New York, 1952), written from the perspective of a nonmember, provides a fairly reliable introduction to the years during Mary Baker Eddy's lifetime, and his *The Continuing Spirit: The Story of Christian Science Since 1910* (New York, 1956) carries the story to the mid-twentieth century. Charles S. Braden's *Christian Science Today: Power, Policy, Practice* (Dallas, 1958) draws upon more hostile sources to cover the recent period. Two books by Christian Scientists—Stephen Gottschalk's *The Emergence of Christian Science in American Religious Life* (Berkeley, CA, 1973) and Robert Peel's *Christian Science: Its Encounter with American Culture* (New York, 1958)—place the tradition within the context of American religious and cultural history.

The best source of information on Eddy and Christian Science during her lifetime is Robert Peel's scholarly three-volume biography, *Mary Baker Eddy* (New York, 1966–1977). Eddy's own often revealing but highly selective autobiography, *Retrospection and Introspection* (Boston, 1891), can inform, but the numerous editions of her *Science and Health* (Boston, 1875–1882) and *Science and Health with Key to the Scriptures* (Boston, 1883–1910) provide a more reliable guide to her thinking.

There is no systematic historical analysis of Christian Science healing, but *A Century of Christian Science Healing* (Boston, 1966) uses testimonies of healing to explore a wide variety of healing experiences and to convey a sense of their centrality to a Scientist's life.

Charles S. Braden's indispensible introduction to America's numerous mind-healing sects, *Spirits in Rebellion: The Rise and Development of New Thought* (Dallas, 1963), brings order to chaos by placing the sects within the context of Christian Science and New Thought. Donald Meyer's influential *The Positive Thinkers: A Study of the American*

Quest for Health, Wealth and Personal Power from Mary Baker Eddy to Norman Vincent Peale (New York, 1965, and reissued under a slightly altered title in 1980) interprets Christian Science and mind cure as pop psychology.

The Adventist Tradition

There is no standard history of Seventh-day Adventists, but Richard W. Schwarz, *Light Bearers to the Remnant* (Mountain View, CA, 1979), designed as a college text, serves as a reliable introduction. A valuable reference work, containing numerous historical sketches of individuals, institutions, and beliefs, is Don F. Neufeld, ed., *Seventh-day Adventist Encyclopedia*, rev. ed. (Washington, DC, 1976).

Like the church as a whole, Ellen White has failed to receive the scholarly attention she deserves. One exception is Ronald L. Numbers' critical analysis of her health-related activities, *Prophetess of Health: A Study of Ellen G. White* (New York, 1976); another is Ronald D. Graybill's Ph.D. dissertation, "The Power of Prophecy: Ellen G. White and the Women Religious Founders of the Nineteenth Century" (Johns Hopkins University, 1983), which explores White's domestic life and her role as a denominational leader. Although apologetic in tone and uncritical in method, the six-volume official biography, *Ellen G. White* (Washington, DC, 1981–1986), by Arthur L. White, a grandson of the prophetess, offers a detailed account of White's life and work. The best entrée to White's own voluminous writings is the splendid three-volume *Comprehensive Index to the Writings of Ellen G. White* (Mountain View, CA, 1962–1963). A laser-disk concordance is available in most Seventh-day Adventist college libraries.

Three books trace the rise and progress of Seventh-day Adventist health concerns from a triumphalist point of view: Dores Eugene Robinson, *The Story of Our Health Message* (Nashville, 1943), by a grandson-in-law and former secretary of White's; George W. Reid, *A Sound of Trumpets: Americans, Adventists, and Health Reform* (Washington, 1982), by an Adventist minister and editor; and Warren L. Johns and Richard H. Utt, eds., *The Vision Bold: An Illustrated History of the Seventh-day Adventist Philosophy of Health* (Washington, DC, 1977), an attractive volume that includes contributions by several Adventist historians.

The Jehovah's Witness Tradition

The Watch Tower Society's literature is an excellent source for those interested in the history and doctrines of the Jehovah's Witnesses. The basic, though somewhat biased, historical account is *Jehovah's Witnesses in the Divine Purpose* (New York, 1959). The *1975 Yearbook of Jehovah's Witnesses* updates the movement's history and explains how the opposition to blood transfusions developed. *The Watchtower* (spelled *The Watch Tower* until 1939), published since 1879, provides the authoritative doctrinal message, while *Awake!* (formerly the *Golden Age*, 1919–1937, and *Consolation*, 1937–1946) offers a newsy look at the movement. Charles Taze Russell's six-volume *Studies in the Scriptures* (Allegheny, PA, 1886–1904) and the more than twenty books authored by Joseph F. Rutherford are out of print, but can be found in some major libraries.

Non-Witness scholars have written few objective accounts of the movement. One of the earliest is Herbert Hewitt Stroup's *The Jehovah's Witnesses* (New York, 1945), a sociological analysis. The best is M. Alan Rogerson's *Millions Now Living Will Never Die* (London, 1969), which treats beliefs and attitudes with considerable insight. Over forty dissertations and theses have been written on the Jehovah's Witnesses, including William H. Cumberland's "A History of the Jehovah's Witnesses" (University of Iowa, 1958) and Joseph F. Zygmunt's three-volume "Jehovah's Witnesses: A Study of Symbolic and Structural Elements in the Development and Institutionalization of a Sectarian Movement" (University of Chicago, 1967).

Some of the most revealing accounts have been written by former Witnesses. Among the best are M. James Penton, *The Jehovah's Witnesses in Canada* (Toronto, 1976); Barbara Grizzuti Harrison, *Visions of Glory: A History and a Memory of Jehovah's Witnesses* (New York, 1978); and Timothy White, *A People for His Name* (New York, 1967), published pseudonymously by a Stanford-trained Ph.D. who was a Witness at the time. Penton, a professional historian, has also published a superb analysis of the entire movement: *Apocalypse Delayed: The Story of Jehovah's Witnesses* (Toronto, 1985). Raymond Franz, *Crisis of Conscience* (Atlanta, 1983), by a former member of the Governing Body, provides a fascinating inside view.

Jerry Bergman's *Jehovah's Witnesses and Kindred Groups: A Historical Compendium and Bibliography* (New York, 1984) lists over five thousand references, including over a hundred articles, mostly from medical journals, on the blood issue. The only book-length study of the Jehovah's Witnesses and the blood-transfusion issue is Alfred Derek Farr's *God, Blood and Society* (Aberdeen, Scotland, 1972).

The Evangelical–Fundamentalist Tradition

An excellent history of the formation of fundamentalism is George M. Marsden, *Fundamentalism and American Culture: The Shaping of Twen-*

tieth-Century Evangelicalism, 1870–1925 (New York, 1980). For a useful series of essays on evangelical beliefs, history, and attitudes, see David F. Wells and John D. Woodbridge, eds., *The Evangelicals: What They Believe, Who They Are, Where They Are Changing* (Nashville, 1975). A penetrating study of the changing attitudes of contemporary evangelicals, based on a Gallup survey conducted for *Christianity Today* in 1978–1979, is James Davison Hunter, *American Evangelicalism: Conservative Religion and the Quandary of Modernity* (New Brunswick, NJ, 1983).

There is no historical treatment of evangelical views of health and healing, but for a discussion of evangelical attitudes of the past to faith healing, see J. Sidlow Baxter, *Divine Healing of the Body* (Grand Rapids, MI, 1979). Two older works that continue to influence evangelical views of faith healing are Henry W. Frost, *Miraculous Healing* (reprinted Grand Rapids, MI, 1979), and B.B. Warfield, *Counterfeit Miracles* (reprinted London, 1972).

A number of issues related to sexual and biomedical ethics are discussed at length in Norman L. Geisler, *Ethics: Alternatives and Issues* (Grand Rapids, MI, 1971); and in short but informative articles in Carl F.H. Henry, ed., *Baker's Dictionary of Christian Ethics* (Grand Rapids, MI, 1973). Extensive discussions of birth control, abortion, and biomedical ethics are found in Walter O. Spitzer and Carlyle L. Saylor, *Birth Control and the Christian: A Protestant Symposium on the Control of Human Reproduction* (Wheaton, IL, 1969). A valuable treatment of all aspects of abortion is found in R.F.R. Gardner, *Abortion: The Personal Dilemma* (Grand Rapids, MI, 1972).

The Pentecostal Tradition

The handiest survey of worldwide Pentecostalism is Walter J. Hollenweger, *The Pentecostals: The Charismatic Movement in the Churches*, trans. R.A. Wilson (Minneapolis, 1972). Chapter 25 is devoted to the history of divine healing in the United States and other parts of the world. The best—albeit highly critical—study of the emergence of Pentecostalism in the United States, per se, is Robert Mapes Anderson, *Vision of the Disinherited: The Making of American Pentecostalism* (New York, 1979). Anderson places divine healing and related practices in the social and cultural context of the period. A more sympathetic survey, which emphasizes the Wesleyan origins and complexion of the movement as a whole, is Vinson Synan, *The Holiness Pentecostal Movement in the United States* (Grand Rapids, MI, 1971).

Although there is no comprehensive study of the Pentecostal view of health, healing, and the body, the theological roots of the movement's outlook are sketched in Donald W. Dayton, "The Rise of the Evangelical Healing Movement in Nineteenth Century America," *Pneuma: Journal of the Society for Pentecostal Studies* 4 (1982):1–18. *John Alexander Dowie: A Life Story of Trials, Tragedies and Triumphs* (Dallas, 1980), by Gordon Lindsay, is an uncritical yet informative biography of the father of modern healing evangelism. The proliferation of independent deliverance ministries in the mid–twentieth century is traced in David Edwin Harrell, Jr., *All Things Are Possible: The Healing and Charismatic Revivals in Modern America* (Bloomington, IN, 1975). One of the virtues of this exceptionally interesting book is its extensive bibliographic essay on hard-to-find primary materials. See also David Edwin Harrell, Jr., *Oral Roberts: An American Life* (Bloomington, IN, 1985).

Many of the original sources are, however, readily available. For a judicious formulation of the theological premises that undergirded the Pentecostal outlook, one should see Adoniram J. Gordon, *The Ministry of Healing: Miracles of Cure in All Ages* (Brooklyn, NY 1882). More uncompromising statements, which reflect a preoccupation with demonology and extreme hostility to the medical profession, include Lillian B. Yeomans, M.D., *Healing from Heaven* (Springfield, MO, 1926); and Gordon Lindsay, ed., *John G. Lake Sermons on Dominion over Demons, Disease and Death* (1928, reprinted Dallas, 1982). The gospel of prosperity is propounded in Oral Roberts's best-seller, *Miracle of Seed-Faith* (Tulsa, 1970). A thoughtful recent defense of the Pentecostal view of health and healing is L. Thomas Holdcroft, *Divine Healing: A Comparative Study* (Springfield, MO, 1967).

The Afro-American Traditions

The best summary of black church history is still Carter G. Woodson's classic but outdated *History of the Negro Church* (Washington, DC, 1921), which has been reprinted several times. For the African religious background and its continuing influence on Afro-American views of the world, Robert Farris Thompson has written the most comprehensive and persuasive analysis in his marvelously illustrated study, *Flash of the Spirit: African and Afro-American Art and Philosophy* (New York, 1983). The transformation of African religion and the development of Christianity among the slaves of the United States are sketched in Albert J. Raboteau, *Slave Religion: The "Invisible Institution" in the Antebellum South* (New York, 1978). A comprehensive survey of black folk thought during slavery and after has been written by Lawrence W. Levine, *Black Culture and Black Consciousness: Afro-American Folk Thought from Slavery to Freedom* (New York, 1977). An important study of medicine among slaves is Todd L. Savitt, *Medicine and Slavery:*

The Diseases and Health Care of Blacks in Antebellum Virginia (Urbana, IL, 1978).

A valuable collection of essays on black folklore, including folk magic and medicine, has been edited by Alan Dundes, *Mother Wit from the Laughing Barrell: Readings in the Interpretation of Afro-American Folklore* (Englewood Cliffs, NJ, 1973). A veritable treasure trove of black magical and herbal medicine may be found in two large collections: George P. Rawick, ed., *The American Slave: A Composite Autobiography,* 19 vols. (Westport, CT, 1972), and Harry M. Hyatt, ed., *Hoodoo, Conjuration, Witchcraft, Rootwork,* 5 vols. (Washington, DC, 1970).

The new religious options that confronted black migrants to the cities of the North in the early twentieth century have been treated from the perspective of a social scientist by Arthur Huff Fauset in *Black Gods of the Metropolis: Negro Cults in the Urban North* (Philadelphia, 1944). The only full-length study of the spiritualist churches among black Americans is a recent book by Hans A. Baer, *The Black Spiritual Movement: A Religious Response to Racism* (Knoxville, TN, 1984). Migene Gonzalez-Wippler articulates the appeal of santeria from the perspective of a member of the religion in her popularly written book, *The Santeria Experience* (Englewood Cliffs, NJ, 1982). Jacquelyne Johnson Jackson critically surveys the literature on medical care among "Urban Black Americans" in *Ethnicity and Medical Care,* ed. Alan Hardwood (Cambridge, MA, 1981).

Index